SECOND EDITION

Consumer Health and Integrative Medicine

Holistic View of Complementary and Alternative Medicine Practices

Linda Baily Synovitz, RN, PhD
Professor Emeritus of Health Education, Southeastern Louisiana University

Karl L. Larson, PhD, MCHES
Associate Professor of Health Education, Gustavus Adolphus College

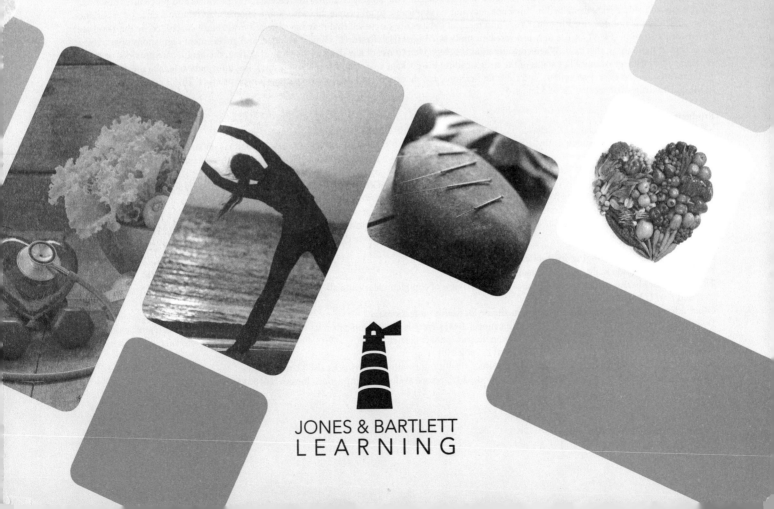

JONES & BARTLETT
LEARNING

MW01077023

World Headquarters
Jones & Bartlett Learning
5 Wall Street
Burlington, MA 01803
978-443-5000
info@jblearning.com
www.jblearning.com

Jones & Bartlett Learning books and products are available through most bookstores and online booksellers. To contact Jones & Bartlett I
directly, call 800-832-0034, fax 978-443-8000, or visit our website, www.jblearning.com.

Substantial discounts on bulk quantities of Jones & Bartlett Learning publications are available to corporations, professional associations,
other qualified organizations. For details and specific discount information, contact the special sales department at Jones & Bartlett Learni
via the above contact information or send an email to specialsales@jblearning.com.

Production Credits

VP, Product Management: David D. Cella
Director of Product Management: Cathy L. Esperti
Product Assistant: Allyson Larcom
Director of Production: Jenny L. Corriveau
Vendor Manager: Molly Hogue
Director of Marketing: Andrea DeFronzo
VP, Manufacturing and Inventory Control: Therese Connell
Composition and Project Management: Exela Technologies
Cover Design: Kristin E. Parker

Text Design: Kristin E. Parker
Director of Rights & Media: Joanna Gallant
Rights & Media Specialist: Merideth Tumasz
Media Development Editor: Troy Liston
Cover Image (Title Page, Part Opener): © ifong/Shutterstock;
    © lsarat/Shutterstock; © Yellowj/Shutterstock;
    © Africa Studio/Shutterstock
Printing and Binding: Bang Printing
Cover Printing: Bang Printing

Library of Congress Cataloging-in-Publication Data

Names: Synovitz, Linda Baily, author. | Larson, Karl L., author.
Title: Consumer health and integrative medicine : holistic view of complementary and alternative medicine practices / Linda Baily Synovitz
    and Karl L. Larson.
Other titles: Complementary and alternative medicine for health professionals
Description: Burlington, MA : Jones & Bartlett Learning, [2018] | Preceded by: Complementary and alternative medicine for health professionals/
    Linda Baily Synovitz, Karl L. Larson. Burlington, Mass. : Jones & Bartlett Learning, c2013. | Includes bibliographical references and index.
Identifiers: LCCN 2018013477 | ISBN 9781284144123 (pbk. : alk. paper)
Subjects: MESH: Complementary Therapies | Consumer Health Information | Holistic Health | United States
Classification: LCC R733 | NLM WB 890 | DDC 610–dc23 LC record available at https://lccn.loc.gov/2018013477

6048

Printed in the United States of America
23 22 21 20 19   10 9 8 7 6 5 4 3 2

I dedicate this text to my late husband, Robert J. Synovitz, who started me on the path to becoming a health educator and who supported me throughout my doctorate program and ensuing career.

–Linda Baily Synovitz

I dedicate this book to my wife Kathy and our three wonderful kids, Danielle, Evan, and Brenden.

–Karl L. Larson

Contents

PART 3 Complementary and Alternative Medicine and Health Care   63

Chapter 6 CAM, Integrative Medicine and Health, and Early Pioneers... 64

Chapter 7 Complementary and Alternative Health Care: Historical Foundations of Holistic Healing 81

Chapter 8 Alternative Medical Systems: Ayurveda and Its Practices....... 91

Chapter 9 Alternative Medical Systems: Traditional Chinese Medicine 112

Preface

We are delighted to offer the second edition of *Complementary and Alternative Medicine for Health Professionals: A Holistic Approach to Consumer Health* that has been retitled *Consumer Health and Integrative Medicine: Holistic View of Complementary and Alternative Medicine Practices*. We retitled the second edition to better target teachers of both consumer health and alternative medicine. Integrative medicine is increasingly becoming a standard of care across this country, and because we devoted much information about integrative medicine in the first edition, we believed that the term needed to be added to the title. We also saw the need to update information already presented in our first edition and to add more recent research studies, facts, and references.

Throughout our many combined years of teaching consumer health courses, we began to learn much about nontraditional healing methods, namely, those medicinal practices considered complementary and alternative medicine (CAM). Because of that, we began to introduce these practices into our consumer health classes, and our students expressed an increasing interest in the exploration of more topics related to CAM. We realized the need for a textbook that would meet our view for this course. Unfortunately, we came to find that there were no consumer health texts available that explored in detail the topic of alternative health practices and methods of healing in addition to coverage of the core consumer health topics. There were a few that contained a chapter or so, but it became evident that a new approach was needed, and from that need the first edition of this text was conceived. We hoped to aid our students and readers in learning more about CAM practices, so they might become more savvy health consumers. The text was well received by many teachers across the country and they expressed a wish for a second edition.

Today, being a health consumer not only encompasses more than being knowledgeable about traditional medicine and health practices, but also includes the necessity to be knowledgeable about the expanding field of CAM here in the United States.

We realize that health professionals cannot learn much about alternative modalities within one or two chapters, as is the norm in other consumer health texts. Therefore, our outline for both the first and second editions of this text includes chapters about the major alternative medicine systems and healing modalities, including Ayurvedic medicine, traditional Chinese medicine, naturopathy, homeopathic medicine, chiropractic medicine, massage, reflexology, and herbals or botanicals.

Our vision for the consumer health portion of the text was to make the information fun to learn and applicable to students' lives. We have gone to great lengths to provide accurate and meaningful information on a vast array of practices, as well as information on how to evaluate treatments and quackery, and leave the consumer to explore more and make their own conclusions. The mission was to increase the reader's knowledge base, not to make up their mind for them. We all make better choices related to our own personal health care practices when we are informed consumers.

▶ Organization of This Text

We opened the text with an introduction to **"Consumer Health, Conventional Medicine, and Complementary and Integrative Health,"** a chapter that introduces the purpose of learning about health consumerism and the costs involved. Often, we strive for good health by purchasing agents or services that we believe will make us healthier. This includes the traditional or orthodox practices (seeing a medical doctor, joining a fitness facility, purchasing exercise equipment) or the alternative medicine practices (seeing a chiropractor, getting a massage, or buying some herbal preparations). If we purchase health-related resources, we need to become knowledgeable health consumers. We also need to engage in positive health practices for the right reasons, not necessarily to avoid becoming ill but to enhance our lives.

We included **Chapter 2, "Scientific Method,"** so that readers could learn more about the characteristics of research design, types of research, and where to find valid health information. We should decide if a health product or practice meets certain scientific criteria, and if it does not, we need to consider the reasons why not. We, then, can make an intelligent health purchase. We can also use this knowledge when we read or listen to advertising blogs. **Chapter 3, "Advertising Health Products,"** helps us to consider the methods used to influence consumers of health products and information.

The cost of healthcare in the United States is spiraling even higher. **Chapter 4, "Cost of Health Care in the United States,"** outlines the reasons for rising healthcare costs, the expenditures, and ways to control costs. Healthcare programs in the United States and the healthcare delivery system are complex. **Chapter 5, "Conventional Medical and Health Care,"** reviews how care is provided in the United States. First, we discuss self-care and the options and choices available to consumers over the counter, and then provide an explanation of the professionals, services, and facilities that provide care.

Integrative medicine is found in the central unit of the book, **Part 3, "Complementary and Alternative Medicine and Health Care."** The reason for placing this in the middle third of the text is based on the authors' experiences in structuring the course, primarily that teaching the course was more fun by starting with traditional consumer health information, then a component related to alternative medicine practice, followed by more traditional consumer health information.

Chapter 6, "CAM, Integrative Medicine and Health, and Early Pioneers," introduces the reader to the meaning of integrative medicine and integrative medicine clinics. Early pioneers who have promoted integrative medicine and alternative healing modalities, and the reasons people seek alternative forms of medical care are highlighted. **Chapter 7, "Complementary and Alternative Health Care: Historical Foundations of Holistic Healing,"** gives the historical foundations of holistic healing and the reasons that people seek alternative forms of medical care. Key historical healing modalities and events that have impacted present-day healing methods, from shamanism to current-day spiritual approaches, are discussed.

Each of the chapters on the **Alternative Medical Systems (Chapters 8 through 13)** describe the historical foundations, what it is, the main principles or beliefs, the diagnostic techniques, the therapies, and related scientific studies. **Chapter 14, "Mind-Body Intervention,"** includes six forms of meditation, the meditation positions, and techniques. The chapter includes a history of yoga, how it works, and offers results of clinical studies. Also included in the chapter is information about therapeutic hypnosis and how it is used; the Alexander technique and benefits; the origins of biofeedback, how it works, and its effectiveness; and prayer and faith healing. **Chapter 15, "Energy Therapies,"** contains historical information and how each is used as a healing modality. Topics are tai chi ch'uan, qi gong, Reiki, Therapeutic Touch and bioelectromagnetic therapies.

Following the alternative medicine chapters is **Chapter 16, "Frauds and Quackery."** We need to realize that quacks operate out of both conventional and alternative medicine healing fields. This chapter provides a brief history of fraudulent products and some of the most notorious purveyors of those products.

Chapter 17, "Protection and Rights of American Consumers," is devoted to showing students their rights as U.S. consumers. Many agencies are available to help us when we feel we have been a victim of fraud, and this chapter identifies several. The last chapter, "Health Insurance in the United States," gives an in-depth look at health insurance in the United States, including an overview of the impact of the Affordable Care Act. Available health insurance options are described and other forms of insurance related to personal health are differentiated.

Finally, an **Appendix** explains how to find trusted conventional health resources and websites to access and evaluate CAM practices.

▶ Features of This Book

Case Studies: Chapters contain one or more case studies so that reader can apply chapter concepts in a more personal way. Case studies are presented as scenarios intended to evoke analytical thinking skills. Application of concepts presented is made easier because of the ways in which scenarios are presented.

In the News: This feature is intended to engage the reader in an active learning process because these relate to the chapter topics. We offer questions concerning the news feature that encourages analytical thinking and which makes the situation or problem personally relevant.

Suggestions for Class Activities: As in any college course, we believe that students learn better when they are actively engaged in the classroom. Therefore, suggestions for classroom activities are included at the end of each chapter. This gives students an opportunity to present in the classroom, work in a group, or engage in an activity. A classroom activity may also involve bringing in a practitioner who explains his or her practice and who then engages the class in a particular activity.

Review Questions: Several review questions can be found at the end of each chapter. These are intended to help the reader conceptualize and reflect on the main points discussed in the chapter.

▶ What's New to the Second Edition?

- ■ **NEW!** The title of the book has been changed to place a greater light on the consumer health and integrative medicine aspects of the text.
- ■ **UPDATED!** Changes in terminology to comply with updated NIH terminology.
- ■ **REVISED!** Chapter 5, "Conventional Medicine and Health Care," has brand new information on

health insurance coverage and cost of personal health in lieu of the Affordable Care Act (ACA). All new considerations on how the ACA has impacted American health care.

- ■ **REVISED!** A brand new section in Chapter 14 addressing "Mindfulness" and its role in "Mind–Body Intervention."
- ■ **REVISED!** A brand new section in Chapter 15 regarding the human biofield, as well as a whole new section of classroom activities.
- ■ **REVISED!** Chapter 16 now addresses the Ephedra controversy of the early 2000s, and also addresses more specific types of quackery by topic area (such as HIV, cancer treatment, and sexual function).
- ■ **REVISED!** Chapter 17 of the previous edition has been shortened and incorporated as part of Chapter 5 for a more streamlined, organized informational layout.
- ■ **UPDATED!** New research and statistics have been incorporated throughout the book regarding the various complementary and alternative methodologies. We have strengthened our information on evidence-based research into CAM and incorporated more information as to how these fit into the current Western medicine environment.

Acknowledgments

We could not have completed this project without the help and support of many others. First, I would like to thank my co-author, Dr. Larson, for working with me as we moved through this book-writing journey. He was most cooperative and a diligent writer. I would like to thank my family and friends for their support during the writing of this second edition.

–Dr. Synovitz

I would like to thank Dr. Synovitz for her work in leading the completion of the second edition. She is a true professional and a valued colleague. I thank my administrative and teaching colleagues at Gustavus Adolphus College for their support along the way. And finally, my wife Kathy, for her support and love throughout the process of completing the text.

–Dr. Larson

We also thank the team at Jones & Bartlett Learning for their hard work on behalf of this book: Cathy Esperti, Allyson Larcom, Molly Hogue, Roxanne Klaas, Merideth Tumasz, Troy Liston, Andrea DeFronzo, and Therese Connell. We also thank the production staff who brought this book to fruition. We especially give a huge thank you to Indraneil Dey, Project Manager, who managed our book's production. He examined and gave feedback on every detail throughout all chapters of this book.

There were several individuals and organizations that helped greatly when writing the first edition and we remember their help, for without it, this second edition might not have occurred.

- Kanani Kauka from the Kaiser Family Foundation.
- American Hospital Association Resource Center.
- Early pioneers: Dr. Andrew Weil and Dr. Bernie Siegel for their personal correspondence and permission to use their photos.
- Bravewell Collaborative, Duke Integrative Medicine Center, and University of Wisconsin Health.
- Random House, Inc. (contact Carol Christiansen) for use of Deepak Chopra's *Dosha Quiz*.
- Terra Rafael for subdosha descriptions published in her book, *Ayurveda for the Childbearing Years* (2009).

- Lawrence Michail for use of the *Five Elements Chart*.
- Associated Bodywork & Massage Professionals for excerpts about tuina touch.
- Ken Chow, Dipl. OM, DNM, CBP, an acupuncturist from Baton Rouge, Louisiana, for photos of him conducting acupuncture and cupping.
- Subhuti Dharmananda, PhD, founder and director of the Institute for Traditional Medicine in Portland, Oregon, for his review of Chapter 9 and for his *Fifteen Most Commonly Used Chinese Herbals* information.
- The Bach Centre in Oxon, England. Stefan Ball was invaluable for providing and sharing information about Bach® Original Flower Remedies. Stefan reviewed the chapter section on *Bach® Original Flower Remedies* and made several suggestions for revision.
- Don McLeod from the Centers for Medicare and Medicaid Services and Karen Migdail of the Agency for Health Resources and Services Administration at the U.S. Department of Health and Human Services for e-mail correspondence, telephone calls, and input regarding permission to use government data.
- William C. Andress, DrPH (Department of Health and Exercise Science, La Sierra University), Martha Dallmeyer, PhD (Department of Family and Consumer Sciences, Bradley University), Ari Fisher, MA (Department of Kinesiology, Louisiana State University), Debra C. Harris, PhD, MST (Department of Human Kinetics and Health, University of Wisconsin: Oshkosh), Joseph Hudak, PhD (Department of Health Science, Ohio University Eastern), Dr. Garry Ladd (Department of Health and Exercise Science, Southwestern Illinois College), Dr. Kirsten Lupinski (assistant professor, Health and Physical Education, Albany State University), Linda Pina, PhD, RN (Department of Nursing, California University of Pennsylvania), and Barbara Wright, MS (Department of Health and Physical Education, Virginia Western Community College) for their valuable guidance in reviewing the first edition.

▶ Reviewers

In addition, many professionals from across the country reviewed chapters, and we thank the following reviewers for their valuable feedback:

Wanda Hawkins Burrell, MS
Tennessee State University

Laura Durbin, MSN, RN, CNE
West Kentucky Community and Technical College

Ethel Elkins, DHSc, MHA, MA
University of Southern Indiana

Jalynn Garcia, PhD
California State University, Fullerton

Gary Garrison, MSE, MS
Maranatha Baptist University

Diane L. Habash, PhD, MS, RDN, LD
Ohio State University College of Medicine

Charlene G. Harkins, EdD, RD, LD, FADA
University of Minnesota, Duluth

Wendelyn Inman, PhD
Tennessee State University

Audrey McCrary-Quarles, PhD
South Carolina State University

Dawn Pisarski, MS
South Florida State College

Amy L. Versnik Nowak, PhD
University of Minnesota, Duluth

About the Authors

Linda Baily Synovitz, RN, PhD
Professor Emeritus, Health Education
Department of Kinesiology and Health Studies
Southeastern Louisiana University

Dr. Synovitz obtained a degree in nursing in 1964 and a PhD in Curriculum & Instruction/Health Education from Kent State University in 1993. She nursed for 12 years in Peoria and Macomb, Illinois. Dr. Synovitz then went back to school at Western Illinois University (WIU) obtaining a degree in School Health Education in 1981 and Masters in Community Health Education in 1985. During that time, she raised two sons (Blake and Jared Baily), taught Medical Assisting at Robert Morris College in Carthage, Illinois, became director of nursing at a shelter care home in Macomb, Illinois, taught at WIU in the health sciences department, and remarried in 1985 to Dr. Robert Synovitz. She and her husband moved to Kent, Ohio, where in 1993 she obtained a Doctorate in Curriculum & Instruction/Health Education at Kent State University. Her dissertation about Sexual Victimization of College Females was honored as the Dissertation of the Year. Dr. Synovitz then taught for 4 years at Northern Illinois University until moving to Hammond, Louisiana, in 1996, where she began teaching at Southeastern Louisiana University (Southeastern) in the Department of Kinesiology and Health Studies, moving from assistant to tenured associate professor and then full professor. Dr. Synovitz is a widow and still resides in Hammond, Louisiana.

Dr. Synovitz received many honors during her undergrad and master's years. As a professional, she was the recipient of the national Honor Award as the representative of the Southern District Alliance for Health, Physical Education, Recreation and Dance; the Distinguished Service Award for American School Health Association, the recipient of American Association for Health Education (AAHE); National Health Education Professional of the Year, College/University category; Louisiana Association for Health, Physical Education, Recreation and Dance (LAHPERD) Scholar Award; recipient of College of Nursing and Health Sciences President's Award for Excellence in Research; and many more.

Dr. Synovitz is a Fellow of the American School Health Association. She served on the Editorial Board of the Journal of School Health, was a member of Rutgers University Medical Advisory Board, and acted as a contributing editor of the *LAHPERD Journal*. Dr. Synovitz retired in May 2014.

Karl L. Larson, PhD, MCHES
Associate Professor, Health Education
Department of Health and Exercise Science
Gustavus Adolphus College

Dr. Karl L. Larson is an Associate Professor of Health Education, Department Chair, and Public Health Program Director at Gustavus Adolphus College in St. Peter, Minnesota. Dr. Larson earned his PhD in Community Health Education from Southern Illinois University-Carbondale, and is a Master Certified Health Education Specialist (MCHES). After several years in the public and corporate sectors, and four years teaching at the University of Southern Indiana, Dr. Larson began his work at Gustavus in 2005. He is currently the President of the Minnesota Chapter of the Society for Public Health Education (SOPHE). He is the author of three books and the creator of the National Case Study Competition in health education. In 2018, he was awarded the Karen Denard Goldman Mentor Award from SOPHE.

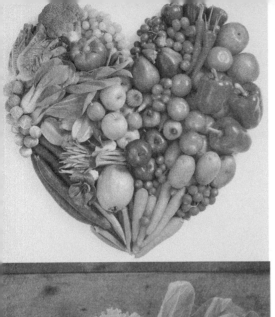

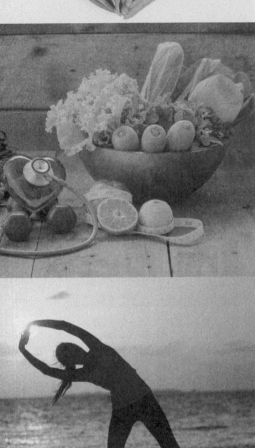

PART 1

Understanding the Basics

Consumer Health, Conventional Medicine, and Complementary and Integrative Health

Note: Throughout this text, our use of the word "healthcare" will refer to a system that offers, provides, or delivers health care to individuals. Also, our use of the phrase "health care" will refer to care given to a patient by medical or health professionals.

▶ Why Learn About Health Consumerism and CAM

This chapter is intended to get you motivated to become a better health consumer and to learn initial information regarding complementary and alternative medicine (CAM). All of us "consume" health by buying products and services to treat illnesses or to prevent disease or disorders. Traditional therapies might include obtaining physician examinations, blood laboratory tests, physical therapy taking prescription drugs, vitamins, minerals, and other over-the-counter (OTC) drugs. Complementary and alternative medicine therapies might encompass taking herbal supplements; and getting massages, reflexology, **acupuncture**, and **acupressure**.

As health **consumers**, not only do we buy those previously mentioned products and services, we join fitness centers or clubs where we "work out," swim, or play tennis. We use walking, running, or bicycle trails. We join golf clubs. So that youth can have a safe place to skateboard, many cities are building skateboard tracks within their city parks or other sites. To participate in many of these activities, we need to buy proper clothing: tennis or running shoes and outfits, swimsuits, and so forth. We attempt to eat more nutritiously and thus, we pay more. For example, we are eating more fruits and vegetables and buying organic foods grown without the use of chemicals such as fertilizers and pesticides. We buy meats grown without antibiotics being placed in their food chain. We buy eggs grown from chickens allowed to be free to roam. As a result of our fitness-seeking lifestyle we spend a lot of money, and we need to learn to spend wisely. We can only do that if we are knowledgeable about the products and services we are purchasing.

Why do we buy health products or engage in fitness activities? Why do we believe it's important to make better food choices when we go to the grocery store? Why do many people look for, and select, organic foods? It seems that we are chasing after good health.

▶ How Costly Is Chasing After Good Health?

People want to be healthy because they perceive that healthy people feel and look better, appear more youthful, and they want to live longer with higher quality of life. Because of this, individuals of every race and culture seek ways to become healthier and, in so doing, they collectively spend billions of dollars. It is wonderful that people want to become healthier, but improving health of a nation requires financing. Part of the funding for health comes from private- and government-funded programs. For undeveloped countries (low or middle income), publicly financed **development assistance for health (DAH)**[1] is available in the form of financial resources and improved effectiveness of resources. Dieleman and colleagues[1] examined data from 1990 to 2014 to identify health areas that received funds and the amount of money that was provided. Findings revealed that during this period of time, $458 billion was provided, and of that, the United States (U.S.) government gave $143.1 billion—$12.4 billion in 2014 alone. Private philanthropy provided $48.2 billion or 10.5% of DAH.[1] The Bill & Melinda Gates Foundation has contributed much since 1999—$21.6 billion. Disbursement of money flows through channels such as the United Nations agencies (i.e., World Health Organization [WHO] and United

Nations International Children's Emergency Fund [UNICEF]), The Global Fund, and the Bill & Melinda Gates Foundation. Money from those entities then goes to specific targets or institutions that implement use of the funds (i.e., HIV/AIDS, maternal health, newborn and child health, tuberculosis, ebola and other infectious diseases, Noncommunicable disease, and more).

The Centers for Disease Control and Prevention (CDC) reports that the five leading causes of death (heart disease, cancer, chronic lower respiratory disease, stroke, and unintentional injuries) have a huge economic impact.[2] People with these chronic diseases put a strain on the healthcare system and they miss work which decreases productivity. The CDC estimates that 69 million workers per year report missing days at work, which decreases economic output by $260 billion.[2] More information regarding the cost of health care in the United States is in Chapter 4.

As can be seen, we value our health and we spend great amounts of money to increase health status. We also contribute to the cost of health care due to the diseases we acquire. It is important, therefore, to gain an understanding of the meaning of health and disease/illness conditions.

▶ What Is the Meaning of Disease/Illness and Health?

Disease and Illness

Mental or physical conditions can cause disease or disorders. An example of a mental disease is depression, which is treatable with certain medications and/or counseling. A physical disease may have a genetic basis (i.e., tendency to acquire diabetes mellitus), may have an autoimmune disorder basis (i.e., rheumatoid arthritis), or may be caused by germs (pathogens) that could be bacterial, viral, fungal, and so forth. Depending on the type of disease, a medical doctor or other health professional will order medicinal treatment. Even if people have a disease condition (whether mental or physical), they may not always feel unwell or uncomfortable. When people have the flu or a cold, they usually consider themselves ill. The perception of feeling the symptoms of a disease is considered an illness.

Health

What is the meaning of "health"? It appears to be an elusive quality that we seem to cherish, but have difficulty maintaining. In our current world, most health professionals

⌕ *CASE STUDY*

Judy is a 19-year-old college student who has been having unprotected sexual intercourse with her boyfriend, Tom. Unknown to her, Tom has been having unprotected sexual intercourse with another college female who has chlamydia, a bacterial sexually transmitted disease (STD). Tom is having some penile discharge but it is not causing him much discomfort, so he ignores it and continues to have sex with both Judy and the other woman. Judy is one of the 80% to 90% of women who do not show immediate symptoms of chlamydia (e.g., vaginal irritation and redness, swollen labia, vaginal discharge). A couple of months after contracting the STD, Judy began to get an elevated temperature, low pelvic pain, and a discharge. When that occurred, Judy experienced symptoms of the disease and felt ill. At this point, we could say that Judy has the subjective state of illness. An illness is a description of the physical or mental condition of a person who shows symptoms of disease or sickness; an unhealthy state.[3] This event caused Judy to go to a doctor for testing and diagnosis, at which point Judy learned she had the disease called chlamydia.

All of us experience being ill and having a disease at some point in our lives. We will turn to our traditional doctors for diagnosis and treatment; we may seek an alternative practitioner for care; or we may attempt self-care. The reason that we do this is to feel healthy.

Questions:

1. What is good health?
2. Why don't all people experience the same level of health?
3. Do we all seek health for the same reasons? If not, what are those reasons?

view health in a holistic manner, an approach to health care that aims at treating the whole person, both body and mind, rather than focusing solely on a specific set of symptoms. It encompasses the physical, mental, emotional, social, sexual, and spiritual domains. The 2011 Joint Committee on Health Education Terminology[3] has presented several definitions of health.

- A state of complete physical, mental, and social well being, and not merely the absence of disease and infirmity. Source: Preamble to the Constitution of the World Health Organization as adopted by the International Health Conference, New York, 19 June–22 July 1946; signed on 22 July 1946 by the representatives of 61 States (Official Records of the World Health Organization, no. 2, p. 100) and entered into force on 7 April 1948.
- A dynamic state or condition that is multidimensional, a resource for living, and results from a person's interactions with and adaptation to the environment and therefore exists in varying degrees unique to the individual. Adapted from: McKenzie JF, Pinger RR, Kotecki JE. *An Introduction to Community Health.* 7th ed. Burlington, MA: Jones & Bartlett Learning; 2012.
- **Holistic Health**: A concept that concern for health requires a perception of the individual as an integrated system rather than one or more separate parts including physical, mental, spiritual, and emotional. Source: *Mosby's Medical Dictionary.* 8th ed. Elsevier; 2009.

People have potential for achieving their personal, maximal level of good health according to how they adapt to their environment and how they integrate all the dimensions of health. Does this mean that people born with disabling diseases and disorders can live healthy lives? Are individuals who appear extremely healthy really healthy? Do we assign healthy/unhealthy status to individuals when we view them?

Illness-Avoiding Behaviors and Health-Enhancing Behaviors

Health practices can be considered as illness-avoiding or health-enhancing behaviors. Individuals may practice healthy behaviors because they want to avoid getting sick or they may practice healthy behaviors because they want to enhance their health. People who practice health-enhancing behaviors do not live in fear that if they don't practice good health, they will acquire some illness or die. Rather, they practice healthy behaviors because they like the way it makes them feel, function, and look. Health-enhancing behaviors are those that should be practiced over a lifetime. As depicted in **TABLE 1.1**, several major differences exist between illness-avoiding and health-enhancing behaviors. One of the illness-avoiding behaviors, as shown in the table, is setting short-term health-related goals, which is discussed next in the "Informed Consumer: Application of Concepts" section.

🔍 CASE STUDY

Let's contrast the health behaviors of two males, each age 22 years. John has a chronic disease diagnosed as **muscular dystrophy**, which causes progressive weakness and degeneration of the skeletal muscles that control movement. His disease has progressed to the point that he is now confined to a wheelchair. Refer to a photo of John in **FIGURE 1.1**. Matthew is a college baseball player. He is handsome, lean, muscular, and has no known disease condition. See the photo of Matthew in **FIGURE 1.2**. Based on the descriptions provided thus far, who would you say is healthier?

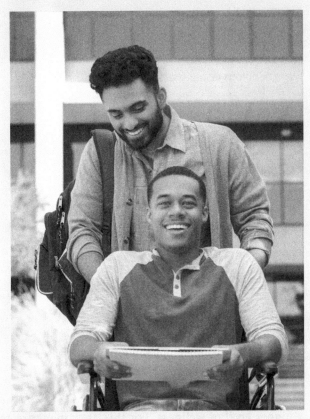

FIGURE 1.1 John.
© Asiseeit/Getty Images

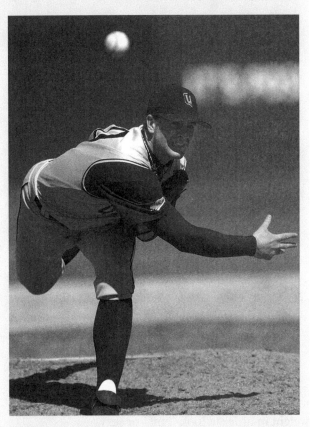

FIGURE 1.2 Matthew.
© Enigma/Alamy Stock Photo

Now let's learn more about each young man. John, who has muscular dystrophy, maximizes his health potential because he follows physicians' medical orders, attends physical therapy sessions, eats a diet appropriate for his health condition, and follows a prescribed exercise regimen. John spends time tutoring at-risk youth at the local high school, has a great sense of humor, and his peers love to be around him.

Matthew, the college athlete, has a less healthy lifestyle and engages in risky health behaviors. He takes steroids, does not eat a healthy diet, drinks heavily on the weekends, drives while drunk, does not use a seatbelt, and practices unsafe sexual practices. He has very few friends because he has an explosive personality and is very egocentric. Based on this description, who do you believe is healthier?

If all individuals could strive to maximize their potential for being healthy, we would see a definite decrease in morbidity (diseases) and mortality (deaths). This case study scenario has demonstrated that a person could have the physical appearance of high quality health but, in actuality, be very unhealthy.

Informed Consumer: Application of Concepts

You are in your junior year of college and the month is January. You and several of your friends are planning a spring break trip to Cancun, Mexico. It has been a stressful year because you have had to take many upper-level science courses (organic chemistry, biology, and physics) and you have been working 20 hours per week. You have been overeating and not exercising like you used to do. Because of this, you have gained 15 pounds and perceive yourself as being fat. You want

TABLE 1.1 Illness-Avoiding Behaviors versus Health-Enhancing Behaviors

Illness-Avoiding Behaviors	Health-Enhancing Behaviors
Avoiding illness is highest priority	High health is highest priority; enjoy healthy behaviors
Motivated by return to health or alleviation of symptoms	Motivated by feeling good, better, best
Minimal goal	Maximal goal
Desire immediate or short-term results	Desire long-term results
Need measurable results	More nebulous results are okay
Time-limited activity	Ongoing activity
Medical-centered motivation	Ego-centric motivation
Authority dominated	Internal control
Fear as motivator	Accomplishment as motivator
External checks mandatory	Few external checks
External rewards	Internal rewards
Specific behaviors	Diffuse behaviors
Reactive (to symptoms or threat of symptoms)	Proactive (don't need that negative force)

to begin a diet and exercise plan so that you will lose weight in order to look "buff" or sexy.

1. What short-term goals should you set?
2. What long-term goals should you set?

You begin your training in January in preparation for the April trip. Lo and behold, the goal is met: you lose weight, acquire some level of muscle mass, and look "leaner" and "sexier."

Questions for Discussion

1. Do you feel better about yourself?
2. What will be your health habits from now on?
3. If your behavior was only practiced to look good for spring break, once it is over, what is the chance that you will continue to eat nutritiously and keep exercising?

We can conclude that people may practice healthy behaviors because they love how it makes them feel or they may practice healthy behaviors because they have a greater fear of becoming ill. The result is that many individuals seek help in achieving a higher level of wellness. For this, they may turn to **conventional medicine, alternative medicine,** or a combination of conventional and alternative approaches to health.

▶ Current Terms and Definitions Regarding Conventional Medicine and Alternative Medicine

Conventional Medicine

Conventional medicine is also known as traditional or orthodox medicine. Conventional medicinal practices include physical examinations, use of x-rays and other such exams to aid in diagnoses or treatments, surgical techniques, prescription drugs, and laboratory tests on blood, urine, and other body excretions. Conventional physicians may be practitioners of either **allopathic medicine** or osteopathic medicine. An **allopathic physician** is also known as a medical doctor (MD). An osteopathic physician has the acronym, DO, which stands for Doctor of Osteopathy. Both have similar academic training and clinical experiences and are the physicians that have been the mainstream of our traditional medical care. Other examples of conventional practitioners are nurses, dentists, social workers, registered dietitians, physical therapists, and health educators. Refer to Chapter 5 for additional information on the training of medical and osteopathic doctors.

Complementary and Alternative Medicine and Integrative Health

Note: Since the first edition of this textbook was published, the National Center for Complementary and Alternative Medicine (NCCAM) changed its name to the National Center for Complementary and Integrative Health (NCCIH).[4] The NCCAM had conducted and reviewed numerous alternative practices throughout the many years it was functioning. Even though the NCCAM has a new name, the main purpose of the newly named agency is essentially the same.

The NCCIH is a center in the National Institutes of Health (NIH) and is the lead agency in the Federal government that conducts and reviews research studies involving complementary and **integrative health** approaches.[5] Its main purpose is to investigate the safety and efficacy of various methodologies and how they may or may not improve health and health care.

- **Complementary**: Complementary practices are considered non-stream, yet are used along with conventional medicine.[5] Such practices might include aromatherapy after surgery, massage to aid a patient with anxiety, and acupuncture to aid addiction recovery.
- **Alternative**: These are practices considered non-stream and are used in place of conventional medicine.[5] This could include using only acupuncture to treat pain or using chiropractic to treat not only back and skeletal/muscle conditions but to treat diseases such as Diabetes. The NCCIH states, however, that true alternative medicine is not used very much as most people seem to use them in conjunction with orthodox or conventional medicine.[4]
- **Integrative health**: Integrative health occurs when there is a coordinated approach to bring alternative medicine and conventional medicine together.[5] Integrative approaches can be used for many conditions such as pain management, stress relief, and symptom management of cancer.[4]

> **BOX 1.1** Conventional Medicine and CAM: Similarities and Differences
>
> - Both conventional medicine and alternative health care embrace holistic health concepts.
> - Alternative practices are generally viewed as unorthodox from the standpoint of scientific medicine as currently taught in medical schools.
> - Alternative health care is more emphatic about the role of the individual in maintaining his or her own health.
> - Practitioners of conventional medicine all must fulfill certain kinds and amounts of training, education, and licensing although many (but not all) alternative practitioners also must fulfill educational requirements and licensing in their field of study.
> - Conventional practitioners tend to treat symptoms of a disease or some other sick or unhealthy state.
> - Alternative health care providers embrace a wide variety of possible practices and emphasize the body's natural self-restoration properties.

Complementary and alternative medicine has in the past been referred to as CAM. We, the authors of this text, will continue to use the CAM acronym but are also making revisions in this second edition to correspond with the NCCIH's current terminology. **BOX 1.1** depicts similarities and differences between conventional and alternative practices.

The NCCIH divides complementary health approaches into two subgroups, mind and body practices and natural products,[5] although the Center acknowledges that other approaches do not fit into those categories. The older website which was the NCCAM had divided CAM therapies into five categories which are preferred by the authors of this text because it helps to distinguish the many practices and systems of alternative medicine. They are: (1) alternative medical systems (**homeopathic medicine**, **naturopathic medicine**, **chiropractic medicine**, **traditional Chinese medicine** (TCM), and **Ayurveda**), (2) mind–body interventions (meditation, prayer, mental healing, art, music, or dance), (3) biologically based therapies (dietary supplements, herbal medicine), (4) manipulative and body-based therapies (chiropractic medicine, osteopathic medicine, massage), and (5) **energy therapies** (qigong, Reiki, Therapeutic Touch, pulsed fields, and magnetic fields). Acupuncture, acupressure, and Tai chi ch'uan are practices used in traditional Chinese medicine. Other examples of CAM therapies include prayer utilized for healing, faith healing, reflexology, yoga, hypnosis, **biofeedback**, and deep breathing exercises. Chapters devoted to more in-depth discussion of alternative therapies are included in this text. Thus far, we have discussed the meaning of health and illness and provided an introduction to orthodox and CAM helping practices. We, the consumers, have to make decisions about the type of health care we want to use and the types of products we want to buy. Let's now explore what being a consumer of health means.

▶ What Does It Mean to Be a Health Consumer?

Americans like "stuff." We like to have as much as possible, right? Stereos, iPods, video gaming systems, computers, clothing, cars, houses, boats . . . We like our stuff, and every time we buy something, we are acting as a consumer. We seek out a product, we purchase that product, we use that product, and, when it is gone or stops working, we throw the product away and replace that product. In other words, we consume the product. Our nation's economy is built on this function, called a material economy, and the economy relies on individuals to keep buying things to keep it healthy.

College students consume health in many ways, and food, needed for good health, is a large part of that consumerism. With newer and healthier student cafeterias on college campuses, many students are eating better. But not all students have meal plans and they remain with economic struggles.

Because we are consumers of goods and services, including health services, we need to make wise and intelligent decisions when spending our money to buy "good health." A major goal in *Healthy People 2020*[7] reads, "Improve the health literacy of the population." Three objectives related to that goal are as follows:

1. Increase the proportion of persons who report their healthcare provider always gave them easy-to-understand instructions about what to do to take care of their illness or health condition.
2. Increase the proportion of persons who report their healthcare provider always asked them to describe how they will follow the instructions.
3. Increase the proportion of persons who report their healthcare providers' office always offered help in filling out a form.

Barrett and colleagues[8] describe consumer health as "encompassing all aspects of the martketplace related to the purchase of health products and services." The health consumer is the one who buys or otherwise acquires, consumes, or makes and then uses services or products intended to promote health. Prior to 1960, there was no history related to protecting the consumer from fraudulent or dangerous products. In 1962, President John F. Kennedy was so concerned about consumer rights that he made it a focus during a speech.[9] President Kennedy outlined four basic rights; later, they were expanded to six basic rights. **BOX 1.2** shows the six basic consumer rights.

BOX 1.2 Consumer Bill of Rights

President John F. Kennedy first conceptualized the Consumer Bill of Rights in 1962. This was professional regulation to serve the public interest. The following are the six basic consumer rights:[11]

- **The right to safety**: To be protected against the marketing of goods that are hazardous to health or to life
- **The right to be informed**: To be protected against fraudulent, deceitful, or grossly misleading information, advertising, labeling, or other practices, and to be given the facts needed to make informed choices
- **The right to choose**: To be assured, wherever possible, access to a variety of products and services at competitive prices; in those industries in which competition is not workable and government regulation is substituted, an assurance of satisfactory quality and service at fair prices
- **The right to be heard**: To be assured that consumer interests will receive full and sympathetic consideration in the formulation of government policy, and fair and expeditious treatment in its administrative tribunal
- **The right to education**: To have access to programs and information that help consumers make better marketplace decisions
- **The right to redress**: To work with established mechanisms to have problems corrected and to receive compensation for poor service or for products that do not function properly

Source: John F. Kennedy Presidential Library and Museum. *Special message to Congress on protecting consumer interest, 15 March 1962.* Digital Identifier JFKPOF-037-028. Available at: http://www.jfklibrary.org/Asset-Viewer/Archives /JFKPOF-037-028.aspx. Accessed June 5, 2018.

According to an article published in *U.S. News & World Report*,[6] a study of 3,000 students at 2- and 4-year colleges in Wisconsin revealed that 71% of the students reported they changed their eating habits and food spending because of lack of money. About 7% of students enrolled in two-year colleges and 5% enrolled in 4-year programs reported that they had gone at least one day without eating because of lack of funds. How does this affect our ideas of health? What are ways of improving college students' lives when they have no funds for the basic necessities such as food?

▶ What Is Consumer Advocacy?

Consumer advocacy reached new levels in 1965 when Ralph Nader[10] published *Unsafe at Any Speed*, a book detailing the manufacturing flaws in the auto industry. Since that time, Nader has been a leading advocate for consumer health and safety. His followers, called Nader's Raiders, have been conducting research and providing advocacy for more than 40 years, spurring the creation and eventual passage into law of a wide range of consumer policy.

We health consumers need to take responsibility for the choices we make. A term for that is *caveat emptor*, which is a warning that means "let the buyer beware." The concept of *caveat emptor* came from the Romans and then became part of English law, the Statute of Frauds, which was enacted by the English Parliament in 1677. It held that a victim of his own mistakes had little or no recourse in the courts. Today, *caveat emptor* is a principle of commerce stating that if no warranty is provided, then a customer buys at his or her own risk. All 50 states in the United States have incorporated this into their laws, and consequentially, it is very difficult to prosecute **fraud**.

A term that places responsibility on the seller is *caveat vendor*. This is a Latin term meaning "let the seller beware." The term implies that it is the seller's responsibility rather than the purchaser's to ensure that the goods or services offered for sale are able to deliver their intended purpose. Again, without a warranty, it is very difficult to get one's money returned for defective products or to prove fraud. Fraud is a deceitful, tricky, or willful act committed to gain an unfair or dishonest advantage or to make a profit (make money off someone else).

To protect the U.S. consumer, the U.S. Department of Health and Human Services, Agency for Healthcare Research and Quality, provides information about getting safer medical care, preventing errors, and getting quality medical care.[11] Several states also have agencies and/or departments that focus on consumer protection. For example, the state of Maryland has an Office of Consumer Protection. An example of service offered by its Office of Consumer Protection is a tip sheet on how to select a health club.[12]Many consumer protection organizations focus on energy and environmental advocacy. An example of Maryland's efforts to protect people's health is establishing the Climate Action Plan, which focuses on reducing greenhouse gas emissions by 80% by the year 2050.[13]

▶ Conclusion

In sum, information in this chapter was intended to provide an introduction to concepts regarding the meaning of health, traditional or orthodox medicine, CAM therapies, and consumer health. To improve and maintain our health, we need to make intelligent decisions and become health-savvy consumers.

Wrap-Up

Key Terms

Acupressure The application of pressure or localized massage to specific sites on the body to control symptoms such as pain or nausea.

Acupuncture A traditional Chinese medicine treatment that uses stainless steel needles at specific points in the body to increase the flow of life energy known as Qi or Chi.

Allopathic medicine The traditional or conventional system of medicine that uses drugs, surgery, or radiation to prevent or treat diseases.

Allopathic physician The medical doctor (MD) or the osteopathic doctor (DO).

Alternative medicine A system of practices not considered to be standard treatments. Examples are chiropractic medicine, Ayurvedic medicine, and traditional Chinese medicine.

Ayurveda A traditional system of medicine of India. The word *Ayurveda* is a Sanskrit word that means science of life or sciences of lifespan.

Biofeedback A technique used to train people to control their own involuntary body processes such as heart rate, respirations, and even brain waves. It requires watching a monitor of some sort in order to change the rate using mental control.

Chiropractic medicine Use of manipulating the spinal vertebra to release subluxations that cause nerve impingement.

Consumer A person who buys and uses goods. In this text, it means the person who buys and uses health-related goods.

Conventional medicine Mainstream medical practices. Also known as orthodox and traditional medicine.

Development assistance for health (DAH) Publicly financed assistance available for underdeveloped countries in the form of financial resources and improved effectiveness of resources.

Energy therapies Practices that increase natural body energy flow known as Chi energy. Examples are Tai Chi Ch'uan and qigong.

Fraud A deceitful, tricky, or willful act committed to gain an unfair or dishonest advantage or to make a profit (make money off someone else).

Holistic health Refers to the physical, emotional, spiritual, social, and mental domains of health. All should be seen as making up the whole person.

Homeopathic medicine Medicines prepared by extreme dilution. The fundamental concept of homeopathic is that "like cures like." Substances in the preparations are thought to stimulate the body's own healing response.

Integrative health Coordinated approach to bring alternative medicine and conventional medicine together.

Muscular dystrophy A genetic disease that is characterized by progressive weakness and degeneration of the skeletal muscles that control movement.

Naturopathic medicine A system of medical practices that relies on more natural healing methods (herbs, massage, exercise). It encompasses a belief in the body's ability to heal itself.

Traditional Chinese medicine The traditional medicine of China. Includes practices such as acupuncture, use of Chinese herbs, and energy therapies.

Suggestions for Class Activities

Select one of the following and present your findings in class.

1. Calculate how much you spend on health-related products or services per week. Consider cost of food, over-the-counter medicines, vitamin supplements, exercise equipment, shoes, massage therapy, and the like.

2. What "illness-avoidance behaviors" do you use? What health-enhancing behaviors do you use?

3. Survey a group of friends to learn whether they have been ripped off when they purchased or used health products or services. Include the action taken and the results. Provide evidence relating it to the *caveat emptor/caveat vendor* concepts.

4. Access your state's Consumer Protection Offices and report on their services.

5. Find a magazine that contains unreliable nutrition information or promotes faddism. Analyze your findings by relating them to health consumer concepts learned in this chapter. Prepare a poster of cutouts from the magazine.

6. Compare and contrast two weight control plans (e.g., Nutrisystem, Weight Watchers, Atkins) to obtain information about procedures used for weight reduction, drugs used, food product prices, costs of service, and related matters. Include your opinions and conclusions.

Review Questions

1. What is the meaning of health and disease?
2. How much is spent annually on health care in the United States?
3. What do the terms "conventional medicine" and "CAM" mean?
4. How do conventional medicine and alternative medicine differ?
5. Why is it important to become an intelligent health consumer?
6. What are the meanings of *caveat emptor* and *caveat vendor*?
7. What are the six basic consumers' rights?

References

1. Dieleman J, Graves C, Johnson E, et al. Sources and focus of health development assistance, 1990–2014. *JAMA*. 2015;313(23):2359-2368.

2. Centers for Disease Control and Prevention. *Gateway to Health Communication & Social Marketing Practice: Preventive Health Care.* Available at: https://www.cdc.gov /healthcommunication/toolstemplates/entertainmented /tips/preventivehealth.html. Updated September 15, 2017. Accessed April 2, 2018.

3. Report of the 2011 Joint Committee on Health Education and Promotion Terminology. *Am J Health Educ.* 2012;43(2):1-25.

4. National Center for Complementary and Integrative Health. *NIH Complementary and Integrative Health Agency Gets New Name.* December 17, 2014. Available at: https://nccih.nih.gov /news/press/12172014. Updated April 15, 2015. Accessed April 2, 2018.

5. National Center for Complementary and Integrative Health. *Complementary, Alternative, or Integrative Health: What's in a Name?* Available at: https://nccih.nih.gov/health/integrative-health. Updated September 24, 2017. Accessed April 2, 2018.

6. Godrick-Rab S, Broton K. To cut costs, college students are going hungry. *U.S. News & World Report*. July 13, 2016. Available at https://www.usnews.com/news/articles/2016-07-13/to-cut-costs-college-students-are-buying-less-food-and-even-going-hungry. Accessed April 2, 2018.

7. HealthyPeople.gov. *Healthy People 2020: Health Communication and Health Information Technology Objectives.* Available at: www.healthypeople.gov/2020/topicsobjectives2020/objectiveslist.aspx?topicId=18. Accessed April 2, 2018.

8. Barrett S, London W, Kroger M, Hall H, Baratz R. *Consumer Health: A guide to Intelligent Decisions*. 9th ed. New York: McGraw-Hill; 2013:1-12.

9. Wikipedia. *Consumer Bill of Rights.* Available at: http://en.wikipedia.org/wiki/Consumer_Bill_of_Rights. Accessed April 2, 2018.

10. Nader R. *Unsafe at any Speed: The Designed-in Dangers of the American Automobile*. New York: Grossman; 1965.

11. U.S. Department of Health and Human Services, Agency for Healthcare Research and Quality. *Advancing Patient Safety*. https://www.ahrq.gov/professionals/quality-patient-safety/patient-safety-resources/resources/advancing-patient-safety/index.html. Published September 2012. Accessed April 2, 2018.

12. Office of Consumer Protection, Montgomery County Government. Available at: http://www.montgomerycountymd.gov/ocp/a_z/health_clubs.html. Accessed April 2, 2018.

13. Office of Consumer Protection, Montgomery County Government. Available at: http://www.montgomerycountymd.gov/OCP/energy/index.html. Accessed April 2, 2018.

CHAPTER 2
Scientific Method

LEARNING OBJECTIVES

As a result of reading this chapter, students will be able to:

1. Explain how to seek adequate information about health products.
2. List and describe six characteristics of scientific testing.
3. Define four types of research design.
4. Identify three main goals of evidenced-based research.
5. Analyze the importance of learning about valid and reliable scientific testing and research practices and their application when attempting to select a health-related product or therapy.

▶ What Are the Characteristics of Scientific Testing?

How many times in our lifetime do we hear someone tell us about a "proven" remedy for some condition or disorder that we may be experiencing? For example, you may have heard this expression: "I heard that cherry juice cures gout." How do we learn whether cherry juice will really cure gout? We need to know if the statement is fact or hearsay. While studying information for personal health consumerism, whether it is part of conventional medicine or complementary and alternative medicine, individuals should learn how to assess whether a treatment modality has been scientifically tested. After reviewing the research results, one could say whether the treatment is legitimate or not. This chapter is intended for those of you who may not yet have had a research course and for those of you who appreciate a review of main concepts. The research procedures to be used should be based on several characteristics:

■ The first characteristic of scientific testing is that the research should be what is called **self-correcting research characteristics**.[1] In other words, if the results of a research study are later found to be false, the research should be conducted again so that the conclusions or results may be modified. When conducting research, the truth is not found in one experiment or study but often requires many studies. An example of how attitudes change based on scientific study is the belief about **acupuncture**, a traditional Chinese medicine (TCM) treatment. For years, many western medical and health professionals believed that acupuncture was a quack procedure. That view is changing due to numerous research studies that show benefit for many conditions. The National Center for Complementary and Integrative Health (**NCCIH**)—formerly the National Center for Complementary and

Alternative Medicine (**NCCAM**)—has conducted and published a review[2,3] of several studies demonstrating the effectiveness of acupuncture and other complementary approaches in treating carpal tunnel pain, back pain, headaches, osteoarthritis of the knee, and more. The results suggest that acupuncture was able to help people manage their back and knee pain.[2,3] Due to the many scientific studies about acupuncture and the millions[2,3] of people who get acupuncture, our U.S. medical physicians are becoming trained in this practice[4] (**BOX 2.1**). Again, for sound research, we emphasize that many studies are needed to find the truth.

■ The second characteristic of scientific testing requires objectivity.[1] The findings must not be derived from a **biased research**, which means that there should not be any bias based on the researcher's personal beliefs, perceptions, values, or emotions. When planning the study, the researcher must develop rules and procedures for the research (such as formulating specific **hypotheses** or **research questions** and setting **significance levels**). Quantitative research methods are those in which a value, score, or scale is used. For example, the research project might involve using a pen and paper or Internet survey. **Objectivity in research** is met fairly easily because the researcher is working with numbers. **Qualitative research** might have more difficulty maintaining objectivity because of the nature of the research. For instance, if researchers were to measure the degree to which individuals liked or disliked television advertisements, they could record the number of times (quantitative research) the subjects changed the channel. However, if they attempted to base the level at which individuals liked or disliked television advertisements by the looks on subjects' faces (qualitative research), the results would more than likely not be objective. Most qualitative research involve more strategies than just given, but this example was used to show a point.

■ A third characteristic is that the findings must be made public.[1] Most researchers attempt to publish their findings in peer-reviewed professional journals. Certainly, findings may be made public by mass media (television, Internet, radio), but **peer review** is essential.

■ A fourth characteristic is that the experiments must be reproducible by other scientists at later time.[1] This requires other scientists to replicate the same research process using the same **research design** and methodology.

■ A fifth characteristic is that the experiment must be **empirical**,[1,5] a word derived from the Greek word for experience or observation. If the research is **experimental**, the researcher may manipulate a variable and then observe the results. Qualitative research, however, often entails observing without manipulating any variables. An example of the latter is Jane Goodall's studies of chimpanzees (**FIGURE 2.1**) from the 1960s to the 1990s, when she observed and recorded them in their native environment, the Gombe Stream National Park, located in Tanzania in southeastern Africa.[6] Jane Goodall watched and observed but did not try to interact with the chimpanzees in any way. In other words, she did not manipulate the variables (the chimpanzees) that could have biased her research.

■ A sixth characteristic is that science should be predictive.[1] Such predictions are demonstrated in scientific theories that arise as a result of research studies. The predictions allow for further research that tests the theories. At times, such theories are found not to be true, and more research and theories are subsequently conducted and planned.

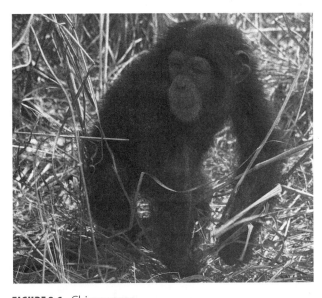

FIGURE 2.1 Chimpanzee.
© Dana Ward/Shutterstock

🔍 CASE STUDY

Abbey is a college student in her senior year. Her major is health education, and she believes it is important to practice healthy behaviors, but she has had many rigorous courses over the past two years and has been working 30 hours per week. As a result, Abbey has not had time to exercise, and she has not eaten very nutritiously. Abbey perceives that she is overweight and out of shape. One day she is watching a 20-minute infomercial on television promoting a fat-burning product. She is impressed by the before-and-after results of three individuals who recounted their experiences using this "wonder" drug and how their lives had changed due to all the weight they had lost. Even though the product is very expensive, Abbey is seriously considering buying it.

Questions:
1. How can Abbey learn whether the product has been scientifically tested?
2. What steps are taken to conduct scientific testing of drugs and products?
3. Do you believe that a drug will be the answer to Abbey's problems? Why or why not?

It is true that scientific testing takes much time and money just to prove that a product or treatment will work. To identify effective health or medical treatments, however, the research must require exemplary scientific testing characteristics, and the researchers have to plan an appropriate research design depending on what is to be tested.

The next section will give you a brief overview of what is involved in scientific testing, starting with information about research design.

▶ What Are the Types of Research Designs?

Research design can be described and defined in many ways. Some design studies are identified as cross-sectional, retrospective, prospective, and longitudinal.[7,8]

- **Cross-sectional.** This is a study of a group of people at a given point in time. It could be carried out by administering a survey on a particular date in a given year.
- **Retrospective.** This is a study involving past records of a group or groups over a long period of time (years) to assess risk factors of a disease such as lung cancer.
- **Prospective.** This could involve studying a group over a long period of time (years) to assess risk for getting a disease sometime in the future such as diseases as a result of smoking cigarettes.
- **Longitudinal.** This is a study of the same individuals (cohort group) over a long period of time on the same health variables and risk factors.

Research design may also be defined as descriptive or analytical.[7,8]

- **Descriptive design** may include surveys (quantitative) or qualitative studies.[7,8] Surveys are used to obtain information about health behaviors or other topics by asking groups of individuals to complete a pen and pencil, computer, Internet, telephone or person-to-person set of questions. Qualitative studies are another way to learn about health behaviors or other topics and the perceptions of each member of a group by conducting personal interviews.[7] Usually, this interview study involves a smaller group than survey studies.
- **Analytical studies** are quantitative and are classified as observational, experimental, and **quasi-experimental** type studies.[7,8,9]
  - *Observational studies* assess a hypothesis and are conducted by using cohort groups, cross-sectional groups and case-control studies.[9,10,11]
  - *Experimental studies* involve randomly selecting subjects and then randomly assigning them into either a treatment or a control (comparison) group.
  - *Quasi-experimental studies* involve comparison groups that are not randomly selected, and many factors may cloud (or confound) the findings. Confounding factors (variables) may relate to both the cause and effect or outcome. An example of how quasi-experimental research results can be misleading due to confounding factors follows. A researcher studies the relationship of ice cream sales and heat stroke. The results of the study showed that ice cream sales and heat stroke are highly positively correlated (related). That researcher could determine that eating ice cream causes heat stroke.

The confounding factor, of course, is the summer season. More people eat ice cream in the summer and the summer weather is a factor in causing heat stroke. A research study may be valuable, but confounding factors need to be accounted for.

Research design may involve the use of various types of statistical techniques such as correlation and prediction. Correlation statistics (correlational studies) are used to assess the relationship of one or more variables to one or more other variables. An example might be to assess a group's eating and exercise habits to weight and blood pressure.

Predictive statistics—also called **inference** studies—assess the cause and effect of variables. An example of a prediction study is the following: A team of researchers want to assess if college students who eat their meals on campus at dining halls offering healthy food choices will at some point in time (i.e., six months later) have gained less weight and made less visits to the student health center for illness conditions. Their aim is to show cause and effect. The research design would also include random sampling and comparing/contrasting their experimental group with a **control group**: students in the same age groups with similar body health assessments but who eat off campus. If there is a significant difference in the experimental group from the start to the end of the study and a significant difference between the experimental and control group, the researchers could infer that students who eat on campus gain less weight and are healthier than students who eat off campus. They likely would generalize their results to other colleges similar in size with similar student populations.

An important question to ask is "What could be the confounding factors in a research study?" As shown, research studies are conducted in a variety of ways, ranging from pen and paper survey studies to group interviews.[1,8,9,10] Studies may involve researching historical facts from archived materials. They may involve analyzing data from large populations over a span of years. They may involve conducting case studies on a limited number of individuals. Most importantly, researchers must carefully select the type of research design most appropriate for the particular study and determine the type of data to be collected. We, as health **consumers**, should become knowledgeable about the steps taken when conducting scientific research so we can determine if a health product or service is one that we should purchase. **BOX 2.2** gives an overview of several types of methods used when conducting research studies.

BOX 2.2 Methods Used to Conduct Research Studies (not an exhaustive list)

- **Case studies:** Observation of people plus interviews.
- **Laboratory experiments:** Conducted in a controlled environment
- **Epidemiological studies:** Analyze data from various population groups over a point in time or for years.
- **Controlled clinical trials:** May involve a number of people using an experimental group and a control group
- **Surveys:** Pen and pencil, computer, telephone, face-to-face, Internet
- **Data collection:** Collecting data from archived records

▶ What Are the Types of Data Collected?

Numerous types of data may be collected. Blood or other body fluids may be drawn and examined in laboratory experiments. **Morbidity** and **mortality** statistics and historical data may be sought from local, state, or national databases. Surveys may be used to collect **demographic**, knowledge, attitude, and behavioral information (via telephone, Internet, computer, personal interview, or paper and pencil). Perceptions and beliefs of individuals may be obtained during personal interviews. These are examples of some, but not all, types of data that can be collected.

▶ What Is Evidence-Based Research?

Evidence-based research is especially important for clinical practices whether it is medicine, nursing, psychology, speech-language-and-hearing or the many alternative practices offered today (such as acupuncture, massage, chiropractic, etc.).[11,12] It means that the study evidence or result is integrated with clinical expertise and patient values when making decisions about patient care.[12] Integration of best research practices, interests and values of patients, and clinical skills are the primary goals of evidence-based research.[11,12,13] Bridge theory suggests there is a gap between the research results and the application of that research to effect a positive change or growth within the environment of professionals involved in a particular practice.[12] Four main steps are identified: Framing the clinical question, Finding the evidence, Assessing the evidence and Making the clinical decision.[12] You may want to assess if specific conventional and/or alternative therapies have been thoroughly researched and meet evidence-based science guidelines the next time you engage in using one of them either as a professional or a user. Next presented are the steps in scientific research.

▶ What Are the Steps in Scientific Research?

Depending on the type of research study, the scientific process may be somewhat different, but the steps listed here are very appropriate for health professionals. The first step involves assessing health problems and conducting a literature review. A **needs assessment**[14,15] may be one of the first steps completed so that a researcher can identify health or health behavioral problems existing in a community, county, or state. It is beneficial if the researcher can use findings from fairly current needs assessments because it saves a great deal of time. Usually, several health and health behavioral problems are identified within needs assessments; therefore, the researcher is able to determine which health problem/s will be researched.

For example, a county (parish) needs assessment may reveal high rates of diabetes, heart disease, hypertension (high blood pressure), lung cancer, sexually transmitted diseases, tobacco use, and teen pregnancy. The researcher cannot investigate all these problems at one time, but needs to select one or two for further investigation. The researcher might develop an educational program that would be tested for effectiveness (teen pregnancy) or the researcher might investigate the reasons (variables) related to a particular disease (e.g., relationship of tobacco use to lung cancer).

A literature review is important because the researcher can identify studies that could be replicated or used as a guide. The literature review may include researching library databases such as ERIC (educational studies), Medline (medical studies), Sociofile (sociology database), or PsychInfo (psychology-behavioral database). Most of the journal articles found in the databases will have been peer-reviewed and accepted by the professional journals. A review of dissertations or theses written during the past few years may also be accessed. The researcher could conduct Internet searches from sources such as PubMed and NCCIH Internet websites.

The research study should now be carefully planned. First, the researcher will develop the hypotheses or research questions, the basis of the study. Next, the researcher will plan the research design including methodology and set the statistical level of significance. The researcher has to determine if this type of research requires being 95% confident about the results (<0.05) or whether the results should be 99% (<0.01) certain. Once the research questions, design and methodology are set, it's time to collect the data. Data could comprise demographic information, physical measurements, blood pressure, bodily liquids (blood, urine, semen, etc.), archival information, knowledge & attitude levels about a health topic, and health behaviors. If the researcher has planned an educational program, a pre and post pen and paper test may be given to assess gains in knowledge and changes in attitudes and behaviors. No matter what the data is composed of, the results are carefully recorded and analyzed. The researcher will subsequently write the study results in a formal manuscript. The manuscript is then sent to professional journals to be peer reviewed, accepted and published. It is important for the findings to be peer reviewed because it is a means to validate the study design, methodology and results.[1] Results of the study may also be presented at professional conferences and/or seminars. The steps in scientific research are summarized for in **BOX 2.3**.

BOX 2.3 Steps in Scientific Research

1. Identify a problem (needs assessment).
2. Review existing research based on the problem (literature review).
3. Develop either hypotheses or research questions.
4. Plan the research design and methodology (complete with the type of statistics to be used and the statistical level of evaluation).
5. Collect and analyze the data.
6. Describe the results of each hypothesis or research question.
7. Publicize the results in peer-reviewed journals and/or professional conferences.
8. Other researchers may subsequently replicate the study.

📄 *IN THE NEWS*

A news article written by Niki Bezzant[16] for *Lifestyle* posted on January 22, 2017, featured turmeric, a spice said to have many health benefits such as anti-inflammatory and antioxidant properties. The spice has been said to have anti-cancer properties, anti-aging properties, and to lessen the symptoms of arthritis. It has also been used for centuries in countries such as India in their foods and medicines. The outcome is that people are jumping on the "turmeric bandwagon" by marketing turmeric lattes and pills in order to make money, and people are buying the product in order to obtain better health. The *Journal of Medicinal Chemistry*,[17] however, published a review of studies on curcumin, a main ingredient in turmeric and found no evidence to support purported therapeutic benefits. The authors of the study[17] do admit that even though their findings of a review of previous studies showed no specific benefits, it could be possible that turmeric does have some beneficial effects.

Questions:

1. If people read this account, what might be their consumer behavior/s?
2. What might be some factors that could make the study results confounding?
3. Do you think this could be probable? Why or why not?

▶ Could You Apply What You Have Learned?

You are taking a basic research class at the undergraduate or graduate level and you have been asked to conduct a study. Your professor has told you that the study has to be a survey to assess knowledge, attitudes, and behaviors about a health topic. Because you are interested in learning more about herbal supplements, you decide that will become your health topic.

Preliminary Information

Your professor has suggested that you use college students as your subjects because they are available and would reduce time and expenses.

Of benefit to you, a health needs assessment was conducted at your university and it revealed several health problems: a large percentage of college students were overweight, did not regularly exercise, felt stressed out, were not eating nutritiously, and were not sleeping well.

Your Task

Using the needs assessment results and the steps in conducting research, describe how you would set up this study. You need to determine what you want to learn about herbal supplement use.

Step 1: Use one or more of the problems identified from the college needs assessment.

Step 2: Identify two or more databases you would use to learn about related studies.

Step 3: Formulate three research questions.

Step 4: Plan your research design.

- What would be the best way to collect your data?
- How many participants do you want to include in your study?
- Could you do a study to investigate if herbal supplement use is related to one or more health problems identified from the college needs assessment?
- Can you think of any confounding factors that would bias your research?

When the steps in scientific research are followed, although it seems to be a slow and precise process, we can usually trust that the findings are the truth. Researchers have to be careful, however, when interpreting and publishing research results because people can become confused about the meaning of those results.

We as health consumers need to research information about health, medicine, and various therapies, but we must be careful not to misinterpret what we read and hear. We are also bombarded with mega amounts of information such as all the television advertisements for prescription drugs and medical devices. This often causes uncertainty when attempting to make a rational decision about what product, medicine, treatment, and/or therapy we should buy and use. Because there are many problems with health information, as listed in **BOX 2.4**, health consumers need to be able to find accurate sources.

BOX 2.4 Problems with Health Information

- Sources not reliable
- Nonprofessionals or pretend scientists promoting products
- Some medical professionals promoting products for their own financial gain
- Media hype on certain products and drugs or supplements

▶ Where Can We Find Valid, Reliable, and Evidence-Based Health Information?

We should have faith in a claim if the source demonstrates that the treatment, product, or medicine is the result of scientifically sound, valid and reliable, research. **Validity** is the extent to which the test predicts the outcome it is supposed to predict, and a test is said to have **reliability** if it yields consistent results.[1,7] For example, a procedure to use stents in carotid arteries has recently been tested and approved to lessen the probability that a person will experience a stroke. The researchers would have posed a research question such as, "Will carotid artery stents lessen the probability of stroke?" The ensuing research demonstrated that the stents did lessen the probability of stroke. Moreover, after a longer period in time, it became evident across a wide population at risk for stroke that the stents were effective. The researchers could make the claim that this treatment was indeed valid and reliable. A red flag should go up, however, when we hear or read promises from sources touting untested or unusual remedies for chronic or incurable diseases. If there is a question about the validity of health information, there are several ways to investigate.

1. Check for verification of the product or drug, such as a peer-reviewed article or report.
2. Investigate safety research on products and side effects of medicines/drugs.
3. Don't rely on the results of one study. Remember that several studies are often required.
4. If you read a report, investigate the origin of the report. Find out if it was from a peer-reviewed study or medical institution. If not, be wary.
5. Ask your doctor.

BOX 2.5 Trustworthy Internet Sources

U.S. National Library of Medicine: MedlinePlus
medlineplus.gov
National Institutes of Health's Senior Health
nihseniorhealth.gov
National Cancer Institute
www.cancer.gov
Harvard Health Publications
www.health.harvard.edu/
National Institutes of Health: National Center for Complementary and Integrative Health
nccih.nih.gov/
The Institute for Healthcare Consumerism
www.linkedin.com/company/the-institute-for-healthcare-consumerism

6. Read reliable magazines and newsletters, such as the following:
   a. *FDA Consumer*
   b. *Consumer Reports on Health*
   c. *Tufts University Diet and Nutrition Letter*
7. Obtain information from **reputable** sources, including:
   a. Governmental agencies such as the Food and Drug Administration (FDA)
   b. American Medical Association
   c. Volunteer agencies (e.g., American Cancer Society, American Heart Association)
   d. Foundations (e.g., Arthritis Foundation)
   e. U.S. Department of Health and Human Services (Office of Public Health and Sciences)
   f. Trusted consumer health publications and Internet websites.

Some trustworthy Internet websites are listed in **BOX 2.5**.

▶ Conclusion

This chapter was intended to raise your awareness of the importance of scientific research and its application in your life as a health consumer. We need to be cautious about what we read and hear, especially on the Internet and from television infomercials. To be optimal health consumers, we need to learn the important steps of scientific research, and we need to learn how to find valid and reliable information.

Wrap-Up

Key Terms

Acupuncture A traditional Chinese medicine treatment that uses stainless steel needles at specific points in the body to increase the flow of life energy known as qi, or chi .

Biased research Errors in research during the selection of subjects, the measurements used, or the treatment process (intervention).

Control group This is the population group used as a standard for comparison to the experimental group.

Consumer A person who buys and uses goods. In this text, it means the person who buys and uses health-related goods.

Demographic A single vital or social statistic of a human population, such as the number of births or deaths.

Evidence-based research Study evidence or result is integrated with clinical expertise and patient values when making decisions about patient care.

Empirical A word derived from the Greek word for experience or observation.

Experimental Subjects are randomly selected or assigned into a treatment or control group.

Hypothesis A research statement or proposal that the subsequent study will find truthful or not.

Inference The ability of the researcher to infer what could happen in the future depending on the significance of a predictive type of research study.

Morbidity Refers to illness or disease.

Mortality Refers to deaths.

NCCAM: National Center for Complementary and Alternative Medicine; former center in the National Institutes of Health. Name has been changed to National Center for Complementary and Integrative Health (NCCIH).

NCCIH: National Center for Complementary and Integrative Health. Current name of the NIH center that conducts research to prove the effectiveness of complementary and alternative therapies.

Needs assessment Investigation to determine health needs. May investigate at the community, county, state, or national level.

Objectivity in research Findings must not be biased by personal beliefs, perceptions, biases, values, or emotions of the researcher.

Peer review Peers review the study usually when it is submitted for publication. It is a means to validate the study design, methodology, and results.

Predictive statistics The researcher makes a guess or prediction about the research problem based on the probability that the prediction is accurate. The study tests the prediction using specialized statistical techniques.

Qualitative research Research that seeks to provide understanding of human experience, perceptions, motivations, intentions, and behaviors. It requires observation and personal interaction with subjects rather than the use of a survey instrument.

Quasi-experimental Comparison groups in a study are not randomly selected, and many things may cloud (or confound) the findings.

Reliability The consistency of a measurement, or the degree to which an instrument measures the same way each time it is used under the same condition with the same subjects. It refers to the repeatability of a measurement.

Reputable Considered to be respectable or acceptable.

Research design A design that may be experimental or quasi-experimental.

Research questions Rather than a statement or statements found in hypotheses, research questions are formulated. The study tests each research question for truth or not.

Self-correcting If results of a previous research study are later found to be false, the research should be conducted again so that the conclusions or results may be modified.

Significance levels The levels set before a research study is begun. If the level is not met for a particular hypothesis or research question studied, the research is said to be non-significant and is rejected.

Validity The strength of conclusions, inferences, or propositions. Validity is the extent to which the test predicts the outcome it is supposed to predict.

Suggestions for Class Activities

Select one of the two.

1. Find a website that deals with health issues or the sale of health products and evaluate it for reliability and scientific soundness. Website evaluation forms are available. Here is a link to aid you in finding a tool: www.hon.ch /HealthEvaluationTool/

TABLE 2.1 Exercise Equipment Rating Form

Note: The pieces of equipment listed below are heavily advertised and many are used in fitness gyms. On a scale of 1 to 5, with 5 being the highest and best number, please rate each item's effect according to fitness level, strength, muscle endurance, and cardiorespiratory endurance. Also rate how each would affect specific body parts. Research the average cost of each. Place your number in the appropriate box and total your points. The items listed below are only samples. You may use them or find different types of exercise equipment.

F = fitness level, **S** = strength, **ME** = muscle endurance, **CRE** = cardiorespiratory endurance

Scale: 1 = Poor; 2 = Fair; 3 = Average; 4 = Good; 5 = Excellent

Equipment	Benefits				Body Parts Affected					Cost	Total Points
	F	S	ME	CRE	Arm	Leg	Shoulder	Back	Core		
Shake weight											
Inversion table											
Exercise bike											
Elliptical machine											
Treadmill											
Fitness balls											
Ab circle pro											

Discussion Questions:

1. After quantifying each of the types of exercise equipment that you chose, were you surprised at your findings? Why?
2. What advice would you offer your friends or family if they were thinking about purchasing a piece of exercise equipment that has been heavily advertised?

2. Exercise.
   a. Analyze four types of exercise equipment using the Exercise Equipment Rating form provided in **TABLE 2.1**. In order to do the analysis, necessary articles for information regarding the particular piece of equipment. Provide a reference list.
   b. Answer the two discussion questions found on the form.

Review Questions

1. How are facts determined?
2. What are the characteristics of scientific testing?
3. What are four types of research design?
4. What is evidence-based scientific research?
5. What steps are involved in conducting scientific research?
6. What are confounding factors?
7. What is the meaning of "validity" and "reliability"? Where can valid, reliable, and/or evidence-based information be found?
8. To what extent should people believe what they read and hear about health matters?

References

1. Perrin K. *Principles of Evaluation and Research for Health Care Programs.* Burlington, MA: Jones & Bartlett Learning; 2015.
2. National Institutes of Health, National Center for Complementary and Integrative Health. *Acupuncture.* Available at: https://nccih.nih.gov/health/acupuncture. Updated September 24, 2017. Accessed April 2, 2018.

3. Nahin R, Boineau R, Khalsa P, Stussman B, Weber W. Evidence-based evaluation of complementary health approaches for pain management in the United States. *Mayo Clin Proc.* 2016 Sep;91(9f):1292-1306.

4. Sierpina V, Frenkel A. Acupuncture: A clinical review. *South Med J.* 2005;98(3):330-337.

5. PennState University Libraries. *Empirical Research in Education and the Behavioral/Social Sciences.* Available at: http://guides.libraries.psu.edu/emp. Updated February 26, 2018. Accessed April 2, 2018.

6. The Jane Goodall Institute. *Our Story. Timeline.* Available at: http://www.janegoodall.org/our-story/timeline. Accessed April 2, 2018.

7. UNITE for Sight. Module 2: Study design and sampling. In: *Module in Research Methodology Course.* Available at http://www.uniteforsight.org/research-methodology/module2. Accessed April 2, 2018.

8. Centre for Evidence-Based Medicine (CEBM). *Study Designs.* Available at http://www.cebm.net/study-designs/. Accessed April 2, 2018.

9. Public Health Social Work, Maternal and Child Health Leadership Training Program. *Types of Observational Studies.* Available at: https://ssw.unc.edu/mch/node/216. Accessed April 2, 2018.

10. PubMed Health Glossary. NIH-National Cancer Institute. *Observational Study.* Available at: https://www.ncbi.nlm.nih.gov/pubmedhealth/PMHT0025839/. Accessed April 2, 2018.

11. Association of Faculties of Medicine of Canada (AFMC). Chapter 5 Assessing evidence and information. In: *AFMC Primer on Population Health.* Available at: https://afmc.ca/AFMCPrimer.pdf?ver=1.1. Accessed April 2, 2018.

12. American Speech-Language-Hearing Association. *Evidence-Based Practice (EBP).* Available at: http://www.asha.org/Research/EBP/. Accessed April 2, 2018.

13. Rebar C, Gersch C. *Understanding Research for Evidence-Based Practice.* 4th ed. Philadelphia, PA: Wolters Kluwer Health/Lippincott Williams & Wilkins; 2015.

14. Sharma A, Lanum M, Suarez-Balcazar Y. *A Community Needs Assessment Guide: A Brief Guide on How to Conduct a Needs Assessment.* Chicago: Center for Urban Research and Learning and the Department of Psychology, Loyola University; 2000. Available at: https://cyfar.org/sites/default/files/Sharma%202000.pdf. Accessed April 2, 2018.

15. Aschengrau A, Seage III G. *Essentials of Epidemiology in Public Health.* 3rd ed. Burlington, MA: Jones & Bartlett Learning; 2014.

16. Bezzant N. A turmeric latte won't prevent cancer. *The New Zealand Herald, Lifestyle.* January 22, 2017. Available at http://www.nzherald.co.nz/lifestyle/news/article.cfm?c_id=6&objectid=11784288. Accessed April 2, 2018.

17. Nelson K, Dahlin J, Bisson J, et al. The essential medicinal chemistry of curcumin. *J Med Chem.* 2017;60(5):1620-1637.

CHAPTER 3

Advertising Health Products

LEARNING OBJECTIVES

As a result of reading this chapter, students will be able to:

1. Explain the ways in which consumers are influenced by product advertising.
2. Describe the principles behind direct-to-consumer (DTC) marketing.
3. Illustrate the more common advertising techniques used to influence consumers.
4. Describe the constructs used in the VALS™ system.
5. Analyze the pros and cons of DTC marketing.

▶ Advertising in America

Without **advertising**, consumers would have no idea what products, services, and options are available to them. Advertising is an absolute necessity. But advertising is also an art form. Language can be used to attract, persuade, and convince consumers that one product or service is better than another. And advertisers know that Americans can be influenced.

The most common source of health communication in advertising is for pharmaceutical products. One source states that Americans see ads for pharmaceutical products on more than 70% of commercial breaks during the most popular hours of television viewing. In 2016, pharmaceutical companies spent more than $6 billion in **direct-to-consumer** (DTC) advertising, up 62% from 2012![1]

The challenge for consumers is weeding though the language used in advertising in an effort to determine which products may be of value to them. It is important to note that laws have existed for a long time to protect the consumer from false or misleading

advertising. More than 100 years ago, the Pure Food and Drug Act was passed, followed shortly thereafter by the **Sherley Amendment** of that Act. Both efforts prohibited companies from making fraudulent claims about their products, or advertising those claims to the general public. Over the last 20 years, advertising of health products, pharmaceuticals in particular, has been a topic of significant debate.

▶ What Is Direct-to-Consumer Marketing?

For most of the 20th century, the marketing of health products was limited to "indirect" means. If a company wanted consumers to purchase that company's version of an antianxiety medicine instead of a direct reference to the medicine, the advertisement would try to build consumer confidence in the company's name. This way, drug companies would attempt to get the consumer to ask for a specific company's products for whatever ailed them. It was not until the mid-1980s that consumers began to hear the names of specific products in an advertisement. When an advertisement makes a pitch for a specific product, it is referred to as DTC marketing.

While the law allowing DTC advertising was formally passed in the mid-1980s, it was a 1997 governmental regulation change that loosened the regulatory limitation on advertising. By 2011, marketing drugs directly to consumers was the most common form of health communication in the United States.[2] While DTC advertising refers to the marketing of any and all health products, it is the pharmaceutical industry that is most discussed and the most controversial. Advertising is still regulated by the Food and Drug Administration, and ads generally fall into one of three categories: product claim ads, reminder ads, and help-seeking ads. Ventola[2] provides a summary of the claim types:

- **Product claim advertising** includes the product name and the ailment that the product is designed to address. They also make claims about how safe the product is. As a result, the FDA requires advertisements to explain both benefits and risks (a practice referred to as fair balance), and provide a summary of the risk factors associated with using the product.
- **Reminder advertising** mentions the product's name, how it is administered, and maybe how much it costs, but they do not discuss the ailment it is used for. Because they do not really make any claims about the product, they do not have to discuss risks or side effects of the product. The FDA does not allow drugs with serious potential side effects to use this form of advertising.
- **Help-seeking advertising** only describes the ailment and encourage people to seek medical attention. Because no specific drugs or outcomes are mentioned, there are fewer regulations to follow.

A 2007 analysis of prescription drug advertising[1] on television indicated that most ads were of the product claim variety. Almost all ads made some sort of emotional appeal (positive and/or negative), nearly one-third used humor and one in four ads used fantasy to make the product appealing. The greatest challenge appears to be in attaining the *fair balance* criteria, where companies are supposed to do an adequate job of explaining both the effectiveness of a product and explaining its risks. A 2016 content analysis of ads for pharmaceuticals found that there were 179 notifications sent from the FDA to companies for violating the fair balance principle, with most of the notices indicating the drug company played down the risks of the drug, or overstated the efficacy of the drug.[3] This sort of challenge, among other issues, has prompted the American Medical Association to propose a complete ban on direct marketing of prescription drugs.[4]

▶ How Can Marketing Influence My Decisions?

More than 40 years ago, Jeffrey Schrank wrote about the most common approaches[5] in advertising used to sway consumer feelings about purchasing a product. Following are the more common approaches seen in advertising health products and services. Details in a tabulated format can be found in **TABLE 3.1**.

- **The Weasel Claim:** A weasel claim uses terms that make a product sound great, but in reality say nothing about the product. It is a hollow claim. For instance, if you read, "Using Product X will practically eliminate your cough," the term "practically" is the weasel. Consumers will think that "practically" must mean the cough medicine does a lot, but it may not. It does not claim to eliminate your cough, only that it will affect it by some degree. Popular weasel words make the consumer feel as though the product can do magic. "Virtually everyone who used Product Y had improved function." The words "virtually" and "improved" imply success, but in reality tell the consumer nothing about the effectiveness of the product.
- **The "Water Is Wet" Claim:** This claim makes a statement that is true to all products like it. Antibacterial soap is a simple example of this. By labeling itself "antibacterial," the soap company helps make consumer think it is a new or better or special product. The reality is that all soaps are antibacterial. They are soap! The term "antibacterial" does not set the product apart from any of the others like it.
- **The "So What?" Claim:** The statements made in these advertisements are essentially true, but really do not mean anything related to the use of or benefit from the product. Statistical references are common in this group. "Product R has 25% more potassium than a banana!" OK, this may be true, but so what? Does that make the product better for you? Or safe? Or does it actually indicate how much 75% is? A banana has approximately 400 mg of potassium. Does 500 mg make a big difference? Consumers need to be cautious of these types of claims—they sound great, but might mean very little.

TABLE 3.1 Examples of Advertising Techniques

Claim Type	Description	Example
The weasel claim	Claims that appear to be substantial, but in the end are empty.	Use of treadmill X will help control your weight.
The unfinished claim	Claims that a product has more of something or is better, but does not say what the comparison is.	Using weight loss product X will make you lose more weight!
The "we are different and unique" claim	Claims that no other product on the market is like it.	Only product Z has Alpha-PQX.
The "water is wet" claim	The claim made for this ad can be said of any other product like it.	Hospital X will bill your insurance, so you do not have to.
The "so what?" claim	Makes a claim, but there is no real indication if it has significance.	Our vitamins have twice the vitamin D as our competitor.
The vague claim	The intent or meaning of the claim is unclear, subjective, and cannot be proven.	Product X will make you feel good again.
The endorsement	Someone famous pitches the claim.	I use product Z to test my diabetes and you should too.
The scientific claim	Claim includes data or testing results.	Product Y burns 27% more fat when used daily.
The compliment the consumers claim	Claim uses flattery to entice the consumer.	You take great care of your children and that is why you feed them product X.
The rhetorical claim	Claim asks a question to entice an answer from the consumer.	You want to feel like the "old you" again, right?

Source: Summarized from Schrank J. *The Language of Advertising Claims: Teaching About Doublespeak.* Urbana, IL: National Council of Teachers of English; 1976.

In 1937, Edward Filene founded the Institute of Propaganda Analysis.[6] His goal was to inform Americans about the techniques used to influence the way Americans think. Many of the techniques he identified in 1937 (actually used in World War I and II propaganda) are still prevalent in American advertising today. Two in particular are **testimonials** and **bandwagon**.

■ **Testimonials:** This technique is used to associate a product or service with someone famous or trusted by the public, and in turn gets consumers to want to "think like" that spokesperson. This technique has been used to sell everything from cars to razor blades to, yes, health products. Today, weight loss and diet programs and products rely heavily on high profile public figures to influence the public. The message is simple: "I believe this can work for you." If the spokesperson is popular enough or influential enough, consumers will want to be like them. Consumers should initially ask themselves what makes this spokesperson qualified to talk about the product.

Are they getting paid to speak the words? The consumer also needs to consider if the spokesperson has actually used the product, and if so, whether the circumstances under which the spokesperson used the product are similar to their own. Make sure you actually look at the product and its benefits, risk, costs, and whether it is really for you, instead of just looking at who promotes the product.

■ **Bandwagon:** Bandwagon advertising tries to convince the consumer to follow the crowd; to join in based on some common feature (race, religion, age, political affiliation, etc.). If everyone else is doing "it," should you not be doing "it" too? What you might hear in the advertisement would be: "How could 6,000 men a day be wrong? You should try Product M too!" Or, it could be as simple as: "Every college student needs a Product M. You do not want to be the last one to own a Product M, do you? Get yours today." The big question here for the consumer to ask is, "Why?" Let us say you choose not to hop on the bandwagon. What happens then? Is it possible that the crowd running along with the bandwagon has missed something about the product?

▶ What Else Can Affect My Health Purchasing Decisions?

There are numerous things that play a role in the decisions young adults make regarding their health, their behavior, and products they choose. A few of the more common ones are optimistic bias, humor, attraction/distraction, and emotion.

- **Optimistic Bias:** If you have ever had the thought, "That can't happen to me" or "That happens to other people who aren't careful," you have been influenced by optimistic bias. *Optimistic bias* is the tendency for people to believe that others are at a greater risk for a particular health outcome than they are. In a 2016 study, Masiero and colleagues found that young adult smokers were more likely to believe others were at more risk than themselves when discussing health issues, particularly cancer and cardiovascular disease.[7] Those beliefs made those studied more likely to continue with negative health behaviors such as smoking and alcohol use. It is always good to have optimism, but as a health consumer this can lead to choosing sketchy products or services with the belief they will be more effective than realistically so. As it relates to our previous discussion on prescription medication and advertising, consumers are more likely to "tune in" to the positive effects of a drug commercial and "tune out" the section on risk factors and adverse effects.[8,9]

- **Humor:** The use of humor in DTC advertising appears to influence consumers in two particular ways. First, a 2015 study[10] found that when consumers with a high fear of negative social appraisal viewed ads utilizing humor, they were more likely to take action on their health issues; particularly when those health issues were sensitive in nature (such as medicines for sexually related issues or mental illness). Limbu and Huhmann[11] did not find that humor directly influenced behavioral *action*, but consumers did have greater *recall* of products when humor was used in the advertising.

- **Attraction and Distraction:** Never underestimate the power of a smile! DTC advertisers are certainly aware of this as well. Consumers can only make good decisions about prescription drugs if they fully understand both the benefits and risks of the drugs being advertised. However, a 2017 study found that advertisements use more smiling faces during the *health risk* sections of their commercials.[12] The study went on to find that, through eye-tracking technology, "happy faces" impacted the consumers' ability to objectively understand the risk information being shared in the commercial.

- **Emotion:** Psychological research on the impact of emotions on personality, mood, and attitude is abundant.[13] Research is used, and even conducted, by advertising firms to determine just what emotions motivate spending. Consider a television advertisement for a drug to lower the risk of heart attack. If the company simply stated that the drug was effective and you should use it, it would not elicit much of an emotional response from the consumer. However, if the ads reference emotional scenarios such as the following, people might be more motivated to watch the commercial and ask their doctor to prescribe the product:
  - *Scenario one*: A television ad shows a person missing a daughter's wedding or a grandchild's graduation because of a heart attack. The ad then plays serene music in the background and shows visuals of how happy the family is if that person is present for the wedding or grandchild's graduation.
  - *Scenario two*: Consider an ad for depression medication. Almost universally, the ad will begin with a visual of a person suffering with depression, and by the end of the commercial, show them happy, more functional, and content. This is done with great purpose—to create in the viewer a sense that the medicine being advertised can make the viewing consumer feel like the actor in the commercial.

Decision-Making and Advertising Influence

According to the *Principles of Advertising: A Global Perspective*,[14] consumers go through five steps in making a decision about whether to purchase a product: need recognition, information search, alternative evaluation, purchase, and evaluation. Advertisers play to each of these levels of processing in their advertisements. Take, for example, **TABLE 3.2** regarding the purchase of a treadmill.

TABLE 3.2 Stages of Decision-Making and Advertising Influence

Stage	Consumer Behavior	Advertising Approach
Need recognition	Issue: Purchase of a treadmill; may or may not realize the need for a product.	For those who already see the need, the advertiser tells how its product can address the need. For those who do not see the need, the advertiser asks rhetorical questions (Do you feel …?)
Information search	Gathers information from self (memory), advertisement, friends, relatives, mail, and salespeople.	Descriptive ads and mailings, comparisons to other similar products.
Alternative evaluation	Determines the best option based on personal needs and potential end result.	Rational and emotional appeal.
Purchase	Buyer closes the deal: what to buy, from whom, what cost, and so on.	Similar to alternative evaluation; designed to prevent consumers from changing their mind.
Evaluation	Consumer needs to feel as though it has been a good investment and that the product will give the intended results.	Designed to overcome the dissonance between wanting the product and spending the money to obtain it (buyer's remorse).

Source: Staging and descriptions summarized from Lee M, Johnson C. *Principles of Advertising: a Global Perspective.* 2nd ed. New York, NY: Hawthorne; 2005.

Beyond the process of choosing, there are certain factors that influence the decisions people make. Lee and Johnson[14] discuss three primary factors that have an influence on whether a person is swayed by advertising. First, personal factors are things unique to each person such as age, sex, education and income. Second, psychological influences also play a role, primarily perception, motivation, attitude, and lifestyle. Finally, social factors such as cultural background, present and perceived importance of social status, and the peer group the individual affiliates with will influence decision-making. Clearly, it is a complicated process, and advertisers may develop several approaches to promote the same product in an effort to appeal to a broad base of people.

▶ Who Makes Sure Advertisers Are Telling the Truth?

Federal agencies are responsible for monitoring product quality and information accuracy. The Federal Trade Commission and the U.S. Postal Inspection Service are two agencies that play a role in this effort. The Federal Trade Commission has the ultimate authority to create laws regarding advertising in the United States. It establishes the standards for what is deceptive, dishonest, or misleading, and is responsible for enforcing the law with people or companies who violate those standards.[15] The U.S. Postal Inspection Service primarily focuses on the use of the postal service to defraud consumers through faulty advertising of jobs and products.

For the most part, the advertising industry tries to maintain its position as a self-regulated industry, minimizing governmental oversight.

There are private organizations that monitor the accuracy and legitimacy of advertising. One such group is the Advertising Self-Regulatory Council (ASRC). The ASRC develops the policies used by the advertising industry, and oversees several branches, including National Advertising Division (NAD), Children's Advertising Review Unit (CARU), **National Advertising Review Board (NARB)**, Electronic Retailing Self-Regulation Program (ERSP) and Online Interest-Based Advertising Accountability Program (Accountability Program).[16] One criticism of the group, particularly the NARB, is that it is predominantly composed of advertising agencies and professionals, with a small number of academic or former public sector professionals. The risk for bias in situations like this is great. Because of the potential for bias, organizations align themselves with groups known for their impartiality; in this case, the NARB functions under the watch of the Council of Better Business Bureaus. There are many agencies that watch out for the general well-being of the consumer. These are discussed more thoroughly in Chapter 17.

The Internet has proven to be a fertile ground for advertising; however, because advertising online is also a self-regulated industry, it has created a new dynamic in consumer protection. Two primary issues of concern are consumer privacy and **behavioral advertising**. The Federal Trade Commission made several suggestions to online advertisers (who, like their alternate media counterparts, would like to remain as unregulated as possible), to enhance the protection of consumer private information when it testified before the Congress in 2014.[17] The FTC addressed tracking methods for the accumulation of names, contact information, credit card numbers, personal health information, and health histories, as these can be at risk for distribution if the company collecting the information does not act in an ethical fashion. The Commission also provided guidelines on consumer choice in downloading programs to their computers or phones and protecting against malicious ads that put consumer security at risk.

The second concern of online advertising that does not exist in print, radio, or television is called *behavioral advertising*. It is defined by the Interactive Advertising Bureau (IAB) as "the collection of data online from a particular computer or device regarding Web viewing behaviors over time and across non-affiliate websites for the purpose of using such data to predict user preferences or interests to deliver advertising to that computer or device based on the preferences or interests inferred from such Web viewing behaviors."[18] In other words, websites, retailers, and marketing firms can track your pattern of online use. When you visit a site online, or use a search engine, make a purchase online, or just kill a couple of hours surfing the web, your history can be tracked and, in some cases, sold to other websites. Marketing firms can then make certain you see products in the form of pop-up ads or sidebar ads that might interest you, based on your usage pattern. The IAB guidelines encourage online businesses to educate the consumer about behavioral advertising, clearly disclose that they are collecting data, allow consumer choice in the collection of personal data, enhance security and protect sensitive information and obtain consent from the consumer if practices change.[18]

▶ How Do Advertisers Know Whom to Target?

In 1978, SRI International released the original **VALS**™ system.[19] VALS™ (not an acronym, although it looks like one), originally used in the business arena, uses individual lifestyles and attitudes as predictors of consumer behavior. Over time, the system evolved and is now focused on psychological traits, as opposed to social norms and shared values. It is owned and operated as a consulting business by an SRI Incorporated spin-off, Strategic Business Insights. VALS™ categorizes consumers into eight different groups based on what motivates them in their decision-making. Each group is motivated by one of three primary factors: ideals, achievement, or self-expression (**TABLE 3.3**), and is additionally impacted by the degree to which they have access to resources.

■ *Believers* and *Thinkers* **are motivated by ideals.** For believers, those ideals are rooted in history and tradition. As consumers have fewer resources, they tend to be conservative, be loyal to a particular product, and have predictable trends in consumer choices. Believers tend to follow doctors' orders with little questioning. Thinkers' ideals still reflect a conservative trend, but these individuals are better educated, more well-off financially, and they want to have thorough and accurate information. Where believers tend to reject change, thinkers are more likely to keep the doors to

TABLE 3.3 VALS™ System		
Motivating Factors	**VALS™ Types**	**Resource Level**
Ideals, achievement, and self-expression	*Innovators*	Very high
Ideals	*Thinkers*	High
	Believers	Low
Achievement	*Achievers*	High
	Strivers	Low
Self-expression	*Experiencers*	High
	Makers	Low
Immediate needs	*Survivors*	Very low

Source: Modified from SRI Business Insights.

change open, if that change seems valuable and functional.

- *Strivers* and *Achievers* **are driven by achievement.** Strivers, on the lower end of the resource spectrum, have to be not only careful about covering basic needs, but can also be impulsive consumers. The opinion of others is a major motivator, because strivers want to be seen as higher on the social order than they actually are. A high percentage of strivers smoke and suffer later in life because of it. Achievers have made their mark, and because of that want to demonstrate that they have made it. Purchasing tends to be of established names, image-related products, and products that save time. Products and services that promote predictability and stability would be desired.

- *Makers* **and** *Experiencers* **are motivated by self-expression.** For makers, self-expression is a function of building things. They value the practical and are not impressed with wealth or status. Products and services must show value, and promote self-sufficiency. Makers pride themselves on being strong and may be more likely to avoid medical care, thinking they can "tough it out." Experiencers are young and impulsive, and value looking good and having a good time. If the product is new and cutting edge, they want it, but as soon as the fad wanes, they are done with it and moving on.

- *Survivors* **and** *Innovators* **are two special categories in the VALS™ system.** Survivors have few resources available to them. They may fall in the lower socioeconomic divisions of the economy, may be retired and living on a fixed income, or may live in a region that has little access to resources. Thirty-two percent of survivors are widowed. Because resources are scarce, the decisions made by these people are based on what they really need to have, not necessarily what they would like to have. Their focus on immediate needs may limit their ability to plan for the future. Health decisions in this group are high on the priority list. Innovators have plentiful resources and as such are motivated by all three of the primary motivators: image, achievement, and self-expression. Image matters, but serves as a function of expressing individuality and personality, not as a means to gain approval from others. Innovators will try anything cutting edge and new, if it fits their lifestyle and allows a free expression of self. Alternative care practices would be intriguing to an innovator. They are quick to do their own medical research and are likely to ask many questions of their health professional. VALS™ helps medical marketers connect target groups with a specific illness or disorder to a specific product or service. In addition to providing insight into the lifestyles of the different VALS™ subgroups, the system also explains the different communication styles of each group so the marketer can tailor its message more effectively.

How Did the Infomercial Begin?

For people born after 1990, **infomercials** may seem like they have always been on television. The truth is that they are a relatively new phenomenon. In the beginning of television, companies quickly figured out that a TV audience was a captive audience. Slowly but surely, program sponsors began placing more and more commercial material into the television programs they were sponsoring. Eventually, in the early 1950s, laws were passed regulating the number of minutes acceptable for commercials during a program. Those rules stayed in place until the **deregulation** of the cable television industry in 1984 by the then-President Ronald Reagan. Within weeks, 30-, 60-, and 90-minute programs for health products such as Herb-a-Life and Soloflex were on the air.[21] Many of the original infomercials were get-rich-quick schemes, but a significant proportion focused on fitness and weight loss. Today, infomercials can be found on just about every cable network, at just about any time of day. Because many infomercials are low-budget endeavors, companies can actually spend less in advertising by taking this approach. Cowan[9] states that as the economy struggled between 2007 and 2010, the number of infomercials increased 18% even as corporate advertising budgets were shrinking. See **BOX 3.1** for special guidelines for marketing aimed at children.

What Are the Advertising Practices in the Field of Health Care?

You will find that advertisers of healthcare products and services use many of the same approaches to influence consumer choice as advertisers of any other product or service. And consumers are utilizing the Internet at an accelerated rate to gain healthcare information. In fact, a Pew Charitable Trust survey[22] indicated the following:

BOX 3.1 How Are Children Protected from Advertising of Unhealthy Foods?

Advertising to children is a relatively new phenomenon, initiating with the introduction of television and exploding with the expansion of the Internet. The American Psychological Association reports that children are highly influenced in their product preferences when exposed to advertising, and that influence not only creates parent-child conflict when the parent denies a child's request, but also usually ends with children making poor nutritional choices after being exposed to advertising.

In 2006, the Council of Better Business Bureaus initiated the Children's Food and Beverage Advertising Initiative (CFBAI). By January 2014, the Initiative had established a comprehensive list of voluntary guidelines for advertising food products to children under the age of 12. The initiative was designed to change the quality of food products advertised to kids in an effort to reduce rates of obesity and encourage healthier lifestyles in children. Under the guidelines, companies that agree to participate commit to the following:[20]

- Devote 100% of their child-directed advertising to better-for-you foods, or to not engage in such advertising.
- Follow the CFBAI category-specific uniform nutrition criteria to govern what foods they may advertise to children.
- Limit the use of third-party licensed characters, celebrities and movie tie-ins in child-directed advertising consistent with the company's advertising commitment.
- Not pay for or actively seek to place their food and beverage products in the program/editorial content of any medium that is child-directed for the purpose of promoting the sale of those products.
- Include only the company's better-for-you foods or healthy dietary choices in interactive games that incorporate a company's food products, and
- Not advertise their branded foods to children in elementary schools (this limitation does not apply to charitable fundraising, displays of food products, public service messaging or items given to school administrators).

The guidelines apply to television, radio, print media, Internet, social and online media, and video games. To date, 18 companies have agreed to the principles—12 companies agreeing to advertise only those products that meet the dietary guidelines during television shows and electronic activities where more than 35% of viewers are under 12 years old, and six companies agreeing to eliminate all advertising to children under 12. These 18 companies account for over 80% of all food advertising to children.

Source: Cowan J. The return of the infomercial. *Can Bus.* 2010; 83(15):19.

- Over 30% of American adults used online sources to try and determine a diagnosis for a medical condition.
- Three of four Internet users say they searched online for health information during the past 12 months.
- Nearly half of Internet users used online sources to gain information about specific health professionals.
- More than one-third of Internet users reviewed hospital references online.
- The most commonly researched topics are specific diseases or conditions; treatments or procedures; and doctors or other health professionals.

A 2007 study of hospital advertising[23] reviewed the most common appeals marketers used for the top 17 hospitals in the nation. More than 61% of all advertisements made some sort of emotional appeal, focusing on hope, fear, happiness, anxiety, or sympathy. Sixty percent of the advertisements reviewed made specific reference to a hospital's status, levels of prestige, or awards received. More than half of the advertisements reviewed made specific reference to a disease or its symptoms. In contrast, less than 10% of the same reviewed advertisements indicated there would be less pain

after the service, indicated minimal invasiveness of the procedure, used statistics to indicate successes, referred to safety, or mentioned cost.

What this study reveals is that hospitals, when competing for patients, use emotional and status-oriented appeals far more regularly than providing information about the services or the hospital. Consumers motivated by status, image, or appearance will be greatly influenced by this type of advertisement, yet may make a decision based on that image as opposed to the services themselves or the track record of the hospital.

▸ What Is the Cost and Effect of Direct-to-Consumer Advertising?

The bulk of research related to health advertising practices focuses on the DTC marketing of pharmaceutical products. In short, it is big business, and pharmaceutical companies make a great deal of money through DTC advertising. One study determined that for every dollar spent on DTC marketing, pharmaceutical companies made $4.20 in profit.[24] More than 39 million people each year report that a DTC advertisement led them to ask their medical professional about a specific drug. Because of the positive impact on sales, pharmaceutical companies now have more than 1,000 lobbyists in Washington, D.C., and spend more than $150 million to influence politicians on regulatory matters.[25] It is big business!

With that much time, energy, and resources being guided toward advertising, a great deal of emphasis has been placed on the outcomes of such an effort. Simply stated, the results are mixed. Pro-Con.org[26] summarizes the arguments both for and against advertising pharmaceutical products directly to the consumer.

■ **Supporters claim:**
  · Consumers are encouraged to seek medical advice from health professionals.
  · Information helps consumers make educated decisions.
  · Advertising encourages patient compliance with treatment plans.
  · Diseases and medical conditions are more likely to be treated.
  · Advertising reduces stigma associated with disease or conditions.
  · Advertising creates revenue, which goes back into research and development.
  · Advertising is protected free speech.

■ **Detractors claim:**
  · DTC advertising misinforms patients.
  · Advertising is promotional and not educational, generally promoting products before long-term efficacy is known.
  · Advertising increases demand for name-brand products instead of less expensive generic options.
  · DTC advertising encourages overmedicating consumers.
  · Advertising "medicalizes" normal human conditions.
  · Advertising promotes brand preference and interferes with physician expertise and decision-making.
  · DTC advertising increases healthcare costs.
  · DTC advertising is banned everywhere except in the United States and New Zealand.

Of course, not everyone reacts the same way to a pharmaceutical advertisement. Several things can influence this reaction, including the degree of existing illness, history, emotional state, personal experience, and existing knowledge of the illness promoted

in the ad. A study completed in 2013[27] shows the complexity of the impact of DTC advertising through the eyes of physicians. In the study, more than two-thirds of physicians believe that DTC advertising encourages consumers to see their physician, but only 20% believe it improves the consumer-physician relationship. Nearly two-thirds of physicians believe DTC advertising promotes patient-clinician dialogue, but less than half think the consumer is actually more educated about the issue when they speak. And finally, while more than half the physicians (52%) believe DTC advertising reduces the stigma associated with disease so that patients will seek help, nearly two-thirds believe the patient is misinformed, and three-quarters believe the patient overestimates the benefits of a drug without fully understanding the risks. Clearly, the relationship between DTC advertising, the consumer, and the clinician is a complicated one.

When all is taken into consideration, the key to success seems to be how the ads balance risk information with benefit information. When consumers have balanced information, they can make choices in their best interest and can initiate dialogue with their physician in an appropriate fashion, as opposed to showing up and demanding a particular drug.

▶ How Should We Analyze Advertising?

Experts suggest advertising should address a series of questions to help consumers make appropriate choices regarding pharmaceutical decisions. Consumers can use these suggestions to determine whether the company has provided enough information on a product to warrant a conversation with their personal physician. The following are guidelines suggested by Frosch and colleagues[28]:

When a product provides information on an illness the consumer has not yet had diagnosed, and the consumer has no symptoms, the advertisement should explain the name of the condition, how prevalent the condition is, what risk factors exist for the condition (including family history, race and ethnicity, and other confounding illnesses), and lifestyle issues that might promote the illness' development. When a product provides information on a disorder, and the consumer *is* experiencing symptoms, the ad should describe the name of the condition and its prevalence, what symptoms the consumer might be experiencing, and the consequences of the condition if it

🔍 CASE STUDY

Following are the transcripts from two hospital advertisements. Identify as many advertising techniques as you can for both of these.

Transcript for a new hospital opening in California:

Person in Ad: This is about making health care better.

Announcer: The extraordinary new Sharp Memorial Hospital is opening in January.

Person in Ad: They've thought of everything to make the nurses' jobs easier, the patient more comfortable, the family more welcome.

Announcer: It's the first hospital in San Diego where every room is a private room.

Person in Ad: And there's even a pull-out couch where family members are welcome to spend the night.

Announcer: For all that Sharp has to offer, call 1-800-82-SHARP or visit Sharp.com.

Person in Ad: You can feel the difference in these rooms.

Transcript for a children's hospital advertisement:

Kids don't use the word "impossible," so neither do we.

I guess having 50 surgical specialists performing 9,000 procedures a year might seem "impossible."

But "impossible" gets no respect around here.

And if one of those surgeries involves your child? You don't want to hear the word "impossible" either.

Our kids don't talk about impossible, so neither do we.

Children's Hospital Central California—amazing people, incredible care.

---

were to go unaddressed. If the consumer has already been diagnosed with a condition, an advertisement should make sure it specifically states the name of the disorder.

Frosch and colleagues[28] recommend that all pharmaceutical advertising address the benefits and potential risks of the drug. Benefit information should include how significant a reduction in symptoms a person should expect, how long treatment will last to get that benefit, how the medicine's benefit compares to a placebo or to lifestyle change benefit, research results of medical trials, and whether a generic alternative exists. When describing risks associated with the drug, information should be contained in a block of text distinct from the rest of the ad, narrated without distractions of noise or picture, and at a pace the consumer can understand.

When these criteria are met, the consumer can make informed decisions about choosing a drug. It then makes sense to have conversations with one's physician to determine whether the drug is the correct choice for the ailment, or if symptoms warrant testing and diagnosis related to the disorder.

▶ Conclusion

Advertising has a powerful effect on consumer decision-making. It is imperative that the consumer recognizes this influence and make every effort to "read through" the approach taken in the advertisement, and see whether the product can have real benefit. In this way, consumers can make legitimate choices regarding their personal health and well-being.

Wrap-Up

Key Terms

Advertising The act or practice of calling public attention to a product or service.

Bandwagon Advertising technique where mass appeal is used to attract customers.

Behavioral advertising Tracking a consumer's pattern of Internet use in an effort to display specific types of advertising that might appeal to those use patterns.

Deregulation To remove governmental regulations and control.

Direct-to-consumer Advertising sent directly to the consumer, not through a third-party provider.

Infomercial A product commercial of significant length designed to look like a television show.

National Advertising Review Board (NARB) A group of advertising professionals organized to self-regulate the advertising industry.

Product claim advertising A form of DTC advertising that reveals the product name and full disclosure of the product uses and side effects.

Reminder advertising A form of DTC marketing that only provides the product name without including details about its use or side effects.

Sherley Amendment The section of the Pure Food and Drugs Act specifically designed to limit the amount of time commercials can be shown during a television program.

Testimonial An advertising technique in which an individual client is used to share with consumers how a product or service worked for them.

VALS™ Marketing model used to design advertising to appeal to a particular group of consumers.

Suggestions for Classroom Activities

1. Track the type of product and frequency of advertising during three different time frames on three different TV stations: midday, evening news and primetime. Compare and discuss the rationale for the differences in what is advertised and at what time of day.

2. Use the VALS™ system categories, and determine (a) what types of advertising techniques would be most effective with each group and (b) which influences in decision-making would be most relevant for.

Review Questions

1. How much money did pharmaceutical companies spend on marketing in 2016?

2. What was the purpose of the Pure Food and Drug Act and the Sherley Amendment?

3. Describe the three primary types of product claims. What is the principle of fair balance?

4. Describe four marketing approaches commonly used in advertising.

5. Describe the stages a consumer goes through when deciding to purchase a product.

6. What is behavioral advertising?

7. Write a five-sentence advertisement for a health product that makes an emotional appeal.

8. Describe the difference between *Thinkers* and *Believers* in the VALS™ system.

9. Describe the difference between *Strivers* and *Achievers* in the VALS™ system.

10. How do innovators and survivors fit into the VALS™ model?

11. What are the advantages of providing DTC marketing for health products?

12. What are the challenges to providing DTC marketing for health products?

13. If you already have been diagnosed with a disease, what should you look for when trying to determine whether an ad is telling you the "whole story" regarding its product? What if you have not been diagnosed yet?

References

1. Horowitz B, Appleby J. Prescription drug costs are up; So are TV ads promoting them. Available at: https://www.usatoday.com/story/money/2017/03/16/prescription-drug-costs-up-tv-ads/99203878/. Accessed April 2, 2018.

2. Ventola CL. Direct-to-consumer pharmaceutical advertising: Therapeutic or toxic? *Pharm Ther*. 2011;36(10):669-684.

3. Kim H. Trouble spots in online direct-to-consumer prescription drug promotion: A content analysis of FDA warning letters. *Int J Health Policy Manag*. 2015;4(12):813-821.

4. American Medical Association. *AMA calls for ban on DTC ads for prescription drugs and medical devices*. Available at: https://www.ama-assn.org/content/ama-calls-ban-direct-consumer-advertising-prescription-drugs-and-medical-devices. Accessed April 2, 2018.

5. Schrank J. *The Language of Advertising Claims: Teaching about Doublespeak*. Urbana, IL: National Council of Teachers of English; 1976.

6. The Propaganda Critic. *Propaganda*. Available at: http://www.propagandacritic.com/articles/index.html. Updated February 28, 2011. Accessed April 2, 2018.

7. Masiero M, Riva S, Oliveri S, Fioretti C, Pravettoni G. Optimistic bias in young adults for cancer, cardiovascular and respiratory diseases: A pilot study on smokers and drinkers. *J Health Psych*. 2018;23(5):645-656.

8. Park JS, Ahn A, Haley E. Optimistic bias, advertising skepticism, and consumer intentions for seeking information about the health risks of prescription medicine. *Health Mark Q*. 2017;34(2):81-96.

9. Ahn H, Park J, Haley E. Consumers' optimism bias and responses to risk disclosures in direct-to-consumer (DTC) prescription drug advertising: The moderating role of subjective health literacy. *J Consum Aff*. 2014;48(1):175-194.

10. Yoon HJ. Humor effects in shame-inducing health issue advertising: The moderating effects of fear of negative evaluation. *J Advert*. 2015;44(2):126-139.

11. Limbu YB, Huhmann BA. Summary brief: Are humor and endorsers effective for direct-to-consumer advertising? Society for Marketing Advances Proceedings, 204-205.

12. Russell CA, Swasy JL, Russell DW, Engel L. Eye-tracking evidence that happy faces impair verbal message comprehension: The case of health warnings in direct-to-consumer pharmaceutical television commercials. *Int J Advert*. 2017;36(1):82-106.

13. Hansen F, Christensen SR. *Emotions, Advertising, and Consumer Choice*. Copenhagen, Denmark: Narayana Press; 2007.

14. Lee M, Johnson C. *Principles of Advertising: A Global Perspective*. 2nd ed. New York, NY: Hawthorne; 2005.

15. Federal Trade Commission. What We Do. Available at: https://www.ftc.gov/about-ftc/what-we-do. Accessed April 2, 2018.

16. Advertising Self-Regulatory Council. Home. Available at: http://www.asrcreviews.org/. Accessed April 2, 2018.

17. Federal Trade Commission. *FTC Outlines Recommendations for Online Advertising in Testimony Before Senate Homeland Security Subcommittee*. Available at: https://www.ftc.gov/news-events/press-releases/2014/05/ftc-outlines-recommendations-online-advertising-testimony-senate. Accessed April 2, 2018.

18. Interactive Advertising Bureau. *Self-Regulatory Principles for Online Behavioral Advertising*. Available at: https://www.iab.com/wp-content/uploads/2015/05/ven-principles-07-01-09.pdf. Accessed April 2, 2018.

19. Strategic Business Insights. *US Framework and VALS™ Types*. Available at: http://www.strategicbusinessinsights.com/vals/ustypes.shtml. Accessed April 2, 2018.

20. Council of Better Business Bureau. *The National Partner Program: About the Initiative*. Available at: https://bbbprograms.org/programs/national-partner/. Accessed April 2, 2018.

21. Cowan J. The return of the infomercial. *Can Bus.* 2010;83(15):19.

22. Lockard P. 5 Healthcare Trends to Watch in 2017. *DMN3*. Available at: https://www.dmn3.com/dmn3-blog/5-healthcare-marketing-trends-you-should-know-about. Accessed April 2, 2018.

23. Larson RJ, Schwartz LM, Woloshin S, Welch HG. Advertising by academic medical centers. *Arch Intern Med.* 2005;165:645-651.

24. Porter, D. Direct-to-consumer (DTC) pharmaceutical marketing: Impacts and policy implications. *SPNHA Review*, 2011;7(1).

25. Government Accountability Office. *Prescription Drugs: Improvements Needed in FDA's Oversight of Direct-to-Consumer Advertising*. Washington, DC: GAO; 2006. GAO-07-54.

26. Should prescription drugs be advertised directly to consumers? ProCon.org. Available at: https://prescriptiondrugs.procon.org/. Accessed April 2, 2018.

27. Communications Media, Inc. CMI/Compas Study on doctors' views of direct-to-consumer drug advertising. Available at: http://worldofdtcmarketing.com/majority-of-physicians-believe-dtc-ads-should-be-cut-back/prescription-drug-dtc-marketing/. Accessed April 2, 2018.

28. Frosch D, Grande D, Tarn D, Kravitz R. A decade of controversy: Balancing policy with evidence in the regulation of prescription drug advertising. *Am J Public Health.* 2010;100(1):24-32.

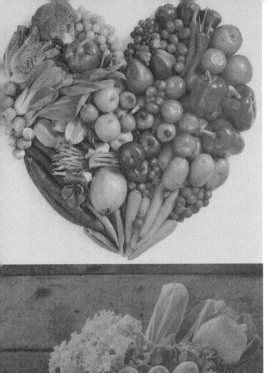

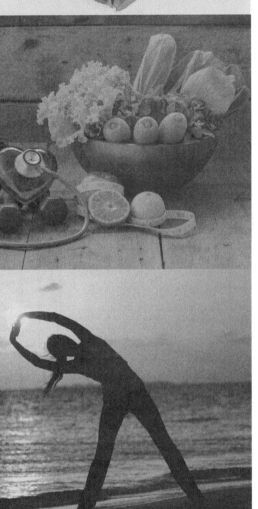

PART 2

Conventional Medicine and Health Care

CHAPTER 4

Cost of Health Care in the United States

LEARNING OBJECTIVES

As a result of reading this chapter, students will be able to:

1. Research the cost of health spending in the United States for the latest year data available.
2. Name and explain three reasons for the high cost of health care.
3. Discuss several ways in which health care may be made more affordable without limiting access to necessary care.
4. Summarize past practices that have increased healthcare costs.
5. Analyze what health consumers can do to decrease healthcare costs.

▶ Is the Cost of Health Care Spiraling Out of Control?

Healthcare costs have risen dramatically over the past 30 years. Costs rose from $253 billion in 1980 to $2.5 trillion in 2009,[1] and as of 2015, it was a massive $3.2 trillion, which is approximately $10,000 per person.[1,2] The Centers for Medicare & Medicaid Services' (CMS) 2015 report reveals that "of the share of the **gross domestic product (GDP)**, health spending accounted for 17.8%,"[2] more than twice the average of countries similar to the United States. **FIGURE 4.1** shows where the 2015 dollars came from and where the national health expenditures went.[2]

By the year 2025, the CMS estimates that projected national health expenditures will rise from 17.8% to 19.9%.[3] This growth is estimated at a rate of 5.6% per year and 4.7% per person per year.[4] National health spending increases will be due to increased spending by Medicare, Medicaid, private health insurance, out-of-pocket spending, hospitals, physician and clinical services, and prescription drug use.[3]

Elizabeth Rosenthal, MD, wrote an eye-opening book,[5] *An American Sickness* (2017), in which she breaks down and exposes the hypocrisy of the American medical system, a system intended to spread health care to all, but which is now referred to by many as "a medical-industrial complex"[5] or big business. Rosenthal proposes that "insurers, hospitals, doctors, manufacturers, politicians, regulators, charities, and more"[5] have contributed to the high cost of health care. She has a lot of advice for us, the health consumers, about what we can do to help bring costs down. Rosenthal's economic rules of the dysfunctional medical market are as follows[5]:

1. More treatment is always better. Default to the most expensive option.

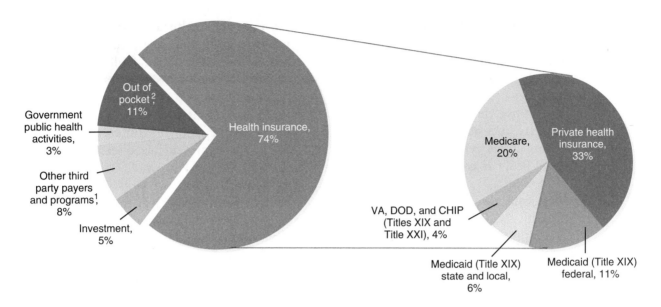

[1]Includes worksite health care, other private revenues, Indian health service, workers' compensation, general assistance, maternal gand child health, vocational rehabilitation, substance abuse and mental health services administration, school health, and other federal and state local programs.

[2]Includes co-payments, deductibles, and any amounts not covered by health insurance.

Note: Sum of pieces may not equal 100% due to rounding.

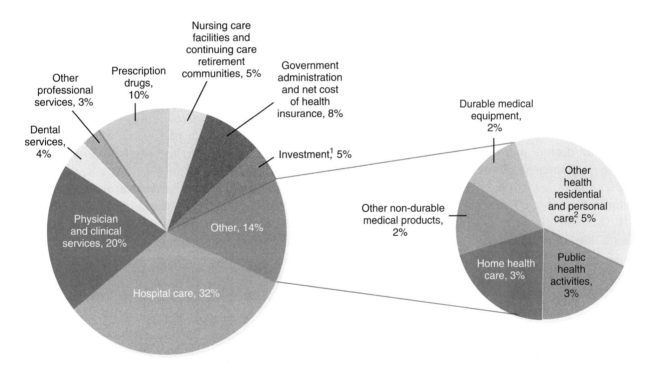

[1]Includes Noncommercial research (2%) and Structures and equipment (3%).

[2]Includes expenditures for residential care facilities, ambulance providers, medical care delivered in non-traditional settings (such as community centers, senior citizens centers, schools, and military field stations), and expenditures for Home and Community Waiver programs under Medicaid.

Note: Sum of pieces may not equal 100% due to rounding.

FIGURE 4.1 The Nation's Health Dollar ($3.2 Trillion), Calendar Year 2015. Where It Went and Where It Came From.

Centers for Medicare & Medicaid Services, Office of the Actuary, National Health Statistics Group.

2. A lifetime of treatment is preferable to a cure.
3. Amenities and marketing matter more than good care.
4. As technologies age, prices can rise rather than fall.
5. There is no free choice. Patients are stuck. And they are stuck buying American.
6. More competitors vying for business does not mean better prices; it can drive prices up, not down.
7. Economies of scale do not translate to lower prices. With their market power, big providers can simply demand more.
8. There is no such thing as a fixed price for a procedure or test. And the uninsured pay the highest price of all.
9. There are no standards for billing. There is money to be made in billing for anything and everything.
10. Prices will rise to whatever the market will bear.

Excerpt from *An American Sickness: How Healthcare Became Big Business and How You Can Take It Back* by Elisabeth Rosenthal, copyright © 2017 by Elisabeth Rosenthal. Used by permission of Penguin Press, an imprint of Penguin Publishing Group, a division of Penguin Random House LLC. All rights reserved.

▸ What Are the Reasons for Rising Healthcare Costs?

There is no dispute that the cost of health care has risen to monumental proportions. The reasons are complex and varied, but in order to maintain a stable economy, the United States must control healthcare costs. The ballooning of healthcare costs in the United States is due to many reasons:

- **Waste in the healthcare system**: A PricewaterhouseCoopers study analyzed the waste in our healthcare system. Their findings contend that $1.2 trillion was excessive or wasteful healthcare spending.[6] The top three areas identified were inefficient claims processing, wasted spending on defensive medicine (unneeded tests), and spending on preventable diseases or disorders such as obesity.[6] An American news and opinion website[7] ran a story on hospital waste. After patients were discharged, the reporter for this article observed personnel in hospital departments discarding unopened boxes of medical supplies such as feeding bags, syringes, diabetes supplies, ostomy kits and more thrown out. The price estimate of hospital discarded supplies amounts to millions or billions of dollars.[7] The impact is that healthcare costs sequentially increase because more supplies must be bought to replace discarded materials.

- **Unhealthy lifestyle**: We, the consumers, drive up healthcare costs when we choose to engage in unhealthy lifestyles[8] such as smoking, regularly overindulging in alcohol drinking, consuming illegal drugs, eating poorly, not exercising, not practicing stress relief techniques, and not attempting to get enough sleep at night. For example, not eating properly could result in obesity. That alone reportedly results in $147 billion in U.S. healthcare costs each year.[9] Tobacco use and smoking-related illness costs approximately $300 billion each year, partly for direct medical care ($170 billion) and partly for loss in productivity (156 billion).[10]

- **Uneducated personal healthcare choices**: Some individuals may get the sniffles and, rather than treating themselves, rush to the doctor's office or to the emergency room (ER). This raises healthcare

🔍 CASE STUDY

Robert, age 48, is a long distance runner who has participated in many marathons in various states in the United States. He takes pride in eating a nutritious diet and having a body that is slender and muscular. He just completed a marathon in New York State and bested his own personal record. When he was running this marathon, he did feel some left arm tingling and numbness just as he had during his last few training runs. Robert ignores these symptoms, believing that he may have a pinched nerve in his neck. He vows that one of these days, he will take the time to get a checkup, but right now, he just does not have time. Robert is trying to maintain his training runs in preparation for the Hawaii marathon, and he has been under a lot of stress at work and needs to pour in some long hours into a new project. In addition, he and his wife have just had twin sons.

Questions:
1. What could be some possible scenarios as Robert continues to do all and be all?
2. What will be the impact on his future healthcare costs?
3. How will those healthcare costs affect his family?

costs. Others may not go to the doctor until they get a life-threatening condition or illness.

■ **Social determinants**: In the United States, the medical system is a proponent of the medical model, or disease model. This model embraces the view that many social problems such as alcoholism, obesity, drug taking, and other addictions (e.g., shopaholic, hypersexuality, gambling problems) are conditions that require medical treatment, a concept called the "medicalization of society."[11] Whether one agrees with this view or not, these treatments drive up healthcare costs.

■ **Our desire for the latest treatments and specialized hospital equipment**: Today, many treatments, including prescription drugs, are advertised on television. In response, we often go to our doctors and demand that they prescribe the medicine for us. Or, pharmaceutical representatives will visit doctors' offices and will market new drugs to the physicians who, in turn, will prescribe them to their patients. These new drugs may or may not be better than the less costly older or generic drugs. Wherein an X-ray of a body part is warranted, often the more expensive **magnetic resonance imaging (MRI)** replaces it. An MRI machine creates a strong magnetic field and combines with radio waves to form a three-dimensional image helpful in showing digital pictures of the brain, nerves, muscles, ligaments, bones, and other soft tissue areas of the body; but it is very expensive, especially when individuals do not have health insurance.[12]

■ **Consumer ignorance of healthcare costs**: Most people who have health insurance do not know the cost of visiting their doctor, going to an ER, or being admitted to the hospital for medical care or surgery. We pay the copay or deductible, and then do not bother to learn what the actual bill is until it is sent to us. Would we have had that knee cartilage repair if we had known what it would cost, or would we have attempted rest and physical therapy to correct the knee problem?

■ **Government mandates**: Federal and state legislation require that specific benefits or services, known as mandated benefits, be added to all health insurance plans. As a result, premiums increase. One federal mandate, the Health Insurance Portability and Accountability Act (HIPAA), although important to protect patients, nonetheless costs millions of dollars to implement.[13] As of May 2017, many changes are being proposed to eliminate some of these mandates in the existing **Patient Protection and Affordable Care Act (ACA)** or eliminated if the ACA is repealed and replaced by a completely new type of health bill. Stay tuned people!

■ **Aging population**: Medical care can get very expensive as people age. Recent estimates are that

📄 IN THE NEWS

A *60 Minutes* news feature shown in 2009 discussed the high cost of health care.[17] One example of the high cost of the last weeks before dying was exemplified by a woman, age 71 years, who was suffering from the complications of colon surgery and a hospital-acquired infection. She was unconscious in the intensive care unit at Dartmouth-Hitchcock Medical Center in Lebanon, New Hampshire, for the better part of a week. Her doctor told a *60 Minutes* correspondent that it costs $10,000 a day to maintain her.

Also reported on this same program was the following case[17]:

Dorothy Glas was a former nurse who had signed a living will expressing her wishes that no extraordinary measures be taken to keep her alive. But that did not stop a legion of doctors from conducting batteries of tests. "I can't tell you all the tests they took. But I do know that she saw over 13 specialists."[14] ". . . Neurological, gastroenterologists. She even saw a psychiatrist because they said she was depressed. And she told the psychiatrist, 'Of course, I'm depressed. I'm dying.'" When we reviewed the medical records, we discovered that there were not just 13 specialists who attended to her mother: there were 25, each of whom billed Medicare separately. The hospital told *60 Minutes* that all the tests were appropriate, and an independent physician said this case was fairly typical. Among the tests conducted was a pap smear, which is generally only recommended for much younger women, not an octogenarian who was already dying of liver and heart disease.

Questions:
1. What do you think is the reason that all those tests were performed?
2. What do you believe is the impact on the cost of health care?
3. What do you believe is the impact on the cost of health insurance?

Sources: (1) De Nardi M, French E, Jones JB, McCauley J. Medical Spending of the U.S. Elderly. National Bureau of Economic Research Working Paper No. 21270; June 2015. Available at: http://www.nber.org/papers/w21270.pdf. Accessed July 15, 2018. (2) CBS News. The cost of dying. *60 Minutes*. Available at: http://www.cbsnews.com/stories/2009/11/19/60minutes/main5711689_page2.shtml?tag=contentMain;contentBody. Accessed April 3, 2018.

between the ages of 70 and 90, medical expenses more than double.[14] About 33% of Medicare spending in 2011 was for people between the ages of 80 and 90 (24% of the Medicare population).[15] People between the ages of 65 and 69 comprised 26% of Medicare, but only 15% of Medicare spending. Part of the Medicare expense is due to nursing home, skilled care expenses, hospital care and hospice care. Arcadia Healthcare Solutions estimates that the cost associated with people who die in the hospital is about seven times the amount of dying at home.[16] The breakdown of their cost estimated associated where people die is as follows [16]:

- Home: $4,760
- Hospital: $32,379
- Hospice: $17,845
- Nursing Facility: $21,221
- Emergency Room: $7,969

As explained earlier in this chapter, there are many complex reasons for the rise in healthcare costs. We, the consumers, must help by attempting to keep ourselves healthy and practicing disease prevention activities such as eating nutritiously, exercising, getting enough sleep, and obtaining health screening tests. When we do get sick, we should obtain information about treating minor conditions rather than running to the ER or the doctor's office. It will require all of us to help solve the healthcare cost crisis.

▶ What Are Our Major Healthcare Expenditures?

Physicians' services, hospital care, dental care, and eye care comprise the bulk of our healthcare expenditures. As people get older, home **health care**, assisted living homes, and skilled nursing care become added financial problems. The next section describes how each adds to the cost of our health care.

Physicians' Services

In the United States, physicians and surgeons held about 708,300 jobs in 2014.[18] Primary care physicians have a median annual income of $241,773[18] and those practicing in medical specialties earned a median annual income of $411,852.[18] The salaries vary according to their number of years in practice, the state or geographic region where they are practicing, and their professional reputation. Self-employed physicians have to provide for their own health insurance and retirement pensions, and this can amount to great sums of money.

As was shown in Figure 4.1, physician/clinical services comprise 20% of healthcare costs.[1,2] Remember that total healthcare costs were $3.2 trillion in 2015 and 20% of $3.2 trillion is $640 billion. An astounding sum, isn't it? We all realize that national health expenditures have risen since 2015, and new graphs and charts will be published when the data are analyzed.

If physicians decide to increase their income, they may charge more for office calls and/or recommend more services per patient (e.g., lab work, blood workups, etc.). A physician fee schedule is used for reimbursement or payment from insurance companies, and **Current Procedural Terminology (CPT) codes** are guides for setting physician fees. Medicare uses a different physician fee schedule than insurance companies and mandated significant annual physician payment cuts for the last 10 years, which has forced many physicians to refuse patients who are on Medicare. The entire 2016 final Medicare Physician Fee Schedule for 2017 can be accessed online.[19] Physician fee schedules not only have served to keep physician fees fairly consistent, but also have caused conflict between physician groups, insurance companies, and the government. Physicians' practices depend on getting paid for services rendered, and their best chance of that is when their patients are insured.

At times, patients may decide to select a physician or hospital that is outside their contracted insurance network. When that happens, there is no set agreement, and doctors (providers) may charge what they want for services incurred. The insurance company, however, may not pay what the provider bills, and patients are expected to pay the difference out of pocket.

Insurance companies that are medical **preferred provider organizations (PPOs)**, **point of service (POS) plans**, **high-deductible health plans (HDHP)**, or the dental PPO plans base their amount of reimbursement on a scheduled fee basis or the **usual, customary, and reasonable (UCR)** schedule, also known as reasonable and customary (R&C). "Usual" refers to the physician's own fees, "customary" to the range of fees charged by all physicians in a given region, and "reasonable" to a fee within a given region or area that falls below the 19th percentile of the customary charges. For non-network claims, the UCR application comes first, and then coinsurance is applied. Individuals can end up paying hefty sums of money if they go out of network for treatment.[20] Doctors also may not get the reimbursement they would ordinarily receive from an insurance company.

Physicians sometimes look for other ways to supplement their income. One of those is investing in a hospital or other type of medical facility. For example,

🔍 CASE STUDY

Claudia resides in Manhattan and is a professional concert pianist. In April 2012, she had cervical spine surgery. She did her homework and made sure that the neurosurgeon was in her network. The hospital website confirmed that the doctor accepted her insurance company. She gave her insurance card to the surgeon's office manager and asked about copayment. The office manager replied that they would bill the insurance company directly. Claudia thought that was unusual but did not question it because she had done her prior research about the doctor. One month later, Claudia received a check from her insurance company for $66,891.78. She called her insurance company and learned that the doctor had dropped her insurance company many years before that. She was told to endorse the check and turn it over to the doctor's office. Two weeks later, Claudia received a bill from the doctor's office for $34,433.22 and was asked to sign a letter stating that she would continue to appeal to her insurance company for more money, which she did. Several weeks later, the insurance company sent her a letter stating that the initial processing of her insurance claim was done incorrectly. They would only cover $3,510.19 of the original bill and was asked to send back the $66,891.78. Claudia then begged the doctor's office to return the money and they would not. Now Claudia owed $97,489.81.

Questions:

1. What have you learned about the high cost of getting a physician who is not in the network?
2. Why do you think the physician and office manager lied about their being in Claudia's network?
3. What lesson have you learned after reading this case study?

Good news: After months of stress and litigation plus much letter and then writing directly to the Director of the Department of Financial Services and to the Office of the Attorney General, Claudia found financial relief. They leaned on her insurance company, which finally took her out of collections and her debt was forgiven. The neurosurgeon, however, never returned any of the money he received.

Question:

1. What do you think should happen to a surgeon and office staff, all of whom were evasive or simply not truthful?

---

some physicians not only own their own medical practice, but also may own a hospital, a laboratory, and/or a physical therapy practice. The Anti-Referral Law[21] (also known as the **Stark Law** after the Congressman who sponsored it) is supposed to prohibit physicians from referring Medicare and Medicaid patients to a healthcare provider or facility with which they have a financial relationship. There are exceptions to the law, such as if a physician has an ownership interest in the entire facility rather than his or her personal specialty area (e.g., a neurologist having a financial interest in the neurology wing of the hospital). The second exception to the Stark Law is that physicians can refer their patients to the hospital if they are active members of the hospital's medical staff. Critics use the argument that physicians who own hospitals may use poor judgment when making medical decisions. The practice may give doctors the incentive to handpick patients who are the least sick or those who have good insurance plans and/or to prescribe unnecessary procedures.

Physicians do have high costs to maintain their practice. Malpractice insurance is one example. The cost, however, is lower than some estimates. David Belk, MD, states that his malpractice is less than $5,000 per year and contends that it is similar to many other physicians.[24] Belk does contend that specialty doctors do pay more but not the hundred or more thousand dollars that people think malpractice costs are. He cites the following 2015 year amount of some specialties:

- Emergency Room Physician: $11,000–$12,000
- Pulmonologist: $6,342
- Anesthesiologists: $12,000–$14,000
- Surgeons: $20,000–$22,000
- Obstetrician/Gynecologist: $34,000

Besides malpractice insurance, physicians are required to take continuing education credits that may require travel to conferences (airfare, hotel, and food expenses). They pay a lot of money to rent office space (if they do not own their own building), mortgage payments (if they do own their own building), maintenance of the building, salaries of nurses and other staff, office equipment and furniture, and simple laboratory equipment (e.g., sphygmomanometers, stethoscopes, scales, etc.).

Along with the high cost of operating physician practices and decreasing reimbursement from insurance companies and Medicare, there has been an increase in physician fraud that is thought to increase health costs by tens of billions dollars each year.[25]

⌕ CASE STUDY

Lydia, age 80 years, has gone to her doctor because of a middle ear infection. She is experiencing pain in her right ear, a feeling of fullness, and some loss of hearing. While in the doctor's office, Lydia also tells the doctor that she is having quite a lot of discomfort in her left hip and has been experiencing difficulty walking, especially on cold, rainy days. Dr. Brown has a major investment interest in the hospital that is attached to her office building. As treatment for Lydia's ear, Dr. Brown prescribes antibiotic ear drops and some pain medicine. She then has Lydia wheeled down the hall and over to the attached hospital to get an MRI on her "bad" left hip. There are two other hospitals in this large city.

Questions:

1. Do you feel that Dr. Brown should have discussed Lydia's options to choose where she would get her MRI procedure done?
2. How would you feel about it if the hospital had been the only one in a small community that had never before been able to raise funds for additional hospitals?

Some estimates are $60 billion yearly. The False Claims Act was enacted so that citizens can now sue on behalf of the government to recover financial damages against people who filed a false claim for medical products and services.[26] It is also known as the whistle blower act or the *qui tam* actions (*qui tam* comes from the Latin phrase *qui tam pro domino rege quam pro se ipso in hac parte sequitur*, meaning "he who brings the action as well for the king as for himself"). Some overcharge the government for products sold or bill the government for services never provided. Still others cheat the government by contract fraud, defense contractor fraud, Medicare fraud, Medicaid fraud, or other public benefit fraud.[26]

Most of the fraud cases are identified as Medicare billing fraud. The definition of "fraud" has expanded to include unnecessary services, ineffective services, or noncompliance by physicians regarding Medicare requirements. Although most physicians who have patients on Medicare give them high quality care and bill only for the services provided, there are physicians who have taken advantage of a poorly regulated Medicare system. The Centers for Medicare and Medicaid Services (CMS), and state and federal governmental agencies (FBI, Department of Justice, Department of Health and Human Services, Office of the Inspector General) are involved in stopping Medicare fraud.

As presented, physician services are valuable, needed, and costly. Physicians incur high costs to maintain their practices, pay office personnel salaries, and pay for malpractice insurance. There are some systems in place to curtail the cost of physician Medicare and insurance reimbursement. Much conflict, however, exists regarding ways to be fair to physicians and to healthcare consumers. The next section presents another major healthcare expenditure: hospital services.

Hospital Services

Hospitals can be classified according to the types of services they provide. For example, a hospital could be known as a trauma hospital, a women's health hospital, a military hospital, a medical school-based hospital, and so forth. Some hospitals are classified by size, based on the number of licensed beds they have. Hospitals could have from 10 beds to more than 1,500 beds. Hospitals may also be classified according to their financial base as a for-profit or nonprofit hospital. Large corporations may own some for-profit hospitals, so those hospitals have to pay back a percentage of their profits to the owners (investors). And as presented earlier, some doctors own for-profit hospitals. Other hospitals are funded largely by community taxes.

As was shown in Figure 4.1, 32% of the $3.2 trillion spent on health care in 2015 was on hospital care. That is a whopping $1.024 trillion. One of the reasons for high hospital costs is the cost of labor. According to the American Hospital Association (AHA), wages and benefits are about 60% of hospital costs. AHA reports also that the cost of electronic health records from 2010 to 2014 have cost yearly about $40,000.[27] Workforce shortages create pressure on hospitals to offer higher salaries for nurses, pharmacists, medical technicians, and other clinicians. The AHA reports that other hospital costs are prescription drugs (6.9%), other products such as food, medical instruments (14.1%), professional fees (9.1%), professional liability insurance (1.2%), and other services (19.8%).[27]

High hospital costs are also due to the specialty medical machines. The following list describes some of these:

- **Computerized axial tomography (CAT):** Provides detailed pictures of the body in order to help physicians more easily diagnose cancers, cardiovascular diseases, and other diseases. CAT scanning requires specialized X-ray equipment, and the scans are computerized so the pictures can be placed on a CD or printed.[28] The pictures show cross-sectional images of body parts. Depending on the model and type of machine, the selling price ranges from $50,000 to over $1 million. Operating costs may annually total $500,000.

- **Positron emission tomography (PET)**: A machine that injects a small radiopharmaceutical, FDG (a glucose analog), into the body in order to study the quality of blood flow to the heart or other tissues and to more easily detect malignancies. The machine costs between $95,000 to over $550,000,[28] and has very high yearly operating costs.

- **Magnetic resonance imaging (MRI)**: An MRI uses magnetic signals and radio waves to produce several planes, image slices, or cross-sections that can aid physicians in diagnosing certain diseases earlier than other imaging techniques. MRI machines can cost between $150,000 and to well over $400,000,[12,28] but that is just the cost of the machine. By the time installation is completed with costs of the tables, cables, amps, and ramps, plus trained technicians, the cost rises to between $1 million and $3 million.[12,28] Not only does the hospital or clinic have to consider the

cost of the machine, but also it has to have a room in which to house it and to provide all the electrical setup. Construction of the suites can cost $500,000.[12,28] If an extremity MRI machine is purchased, this adds $300,000 to the cost and is only used to scan hands, feet, and knees. It also costs an average of $800,000 per year to operate the scanner. The cost of hiring employees to operate these machines is high, as is the cost of repairing them when they break down. Wow! Who knew that technology could be so costly? The unfortunate thing about all this expensive (and valuable) equipment is that it becomes outdated and then needs to be replaced. Hospitals need them to attract doctors. No doctors, no patients, and then no revenue.

Facility expansion is another reason for high hospital costs. Hospitals and clinics expand by building wings onto existing buildings or constructing new buildings on the grounds of the hospital. This cost can range in the millions of dollars. We, the consumers, eventually end up paying for these new buildings and services.

To decrease hospital costs, Medicare devised a method that hospitals have to follow when billing patients for services. It is dependent on physicians' diagnoses called Diagnosis Related Groups (DRGs). Payment is set so that there is consistency for all Medicare patients. The CMS has now converted the DRG system to a more specific group set

🔍 CASE STUDY

The following is an excerpt of an account of a failing hospital in Michigan.[22]

North Oakland Medical Centers has been underwater financially, suffering an operating loss of $13.4 million in 2007. According to Standard & Poor's, it had only 18 days' cash on hand at the end of the year and missed a payment earlier this year on $38 million in bonds issued under a lease agreement with the city of Pontiac. The Pontiac City Council has now agreed to sell the hospital property to Oakland Physicians Medical Center, an LLC formed by a consortium of physicians. The physicians expect to invest as much as $6 million toward the $11-odd million deal, and the hospital's owner, McLaren Healthcare Corp., will need to kick in $5 million.

The Michigan hospital could have closed if the Physicians Medical Center group had not taken over part of the hospital financing. Six million dollars seems like a large sum of money. Why do you suppose that the medical group put up the money? How soon do you think the group will recoup its investment? Do you believe it will eventually make money off this investment? Do you believe that the community will profit from this business venture? Why or why not?

On March 23, 2010, the practice of physician ownership in hospitals was curtailed. The Patient Protection and Affordable Care Act (the Act) was signed into law by President Obama to immediately prohibit future physician investment and caps existing physician investment in hospitals, as of the date of the Act's signing. This new piece of legislation restricts the current Stark law exception that allowed physician ownership in a hospital (the entire hospital, not just a wing of the hospital). The new legislation also states that the physicians who currently own an interest in a hospital cannot increase their interest (e.g., from 20% ownership to 30% ownership).[23]

Source: Zieger A. Case study: Midwest physicians seek hospital ownership deals. August 6, 2008. Available at: http://www.fiercehealthcare.com/story/case-study-midwest-physicians-seek-hospital-ownership-deals/2008-08-06?utm_medium=rss&utm_source=rss&cmp-id=OTC-RSS-FH0. Accessed July 7, 2010.

based on the severity of the diagnosis known as Medicare Severity-DRGs (MS-DRGs).[29] Now, Medicare can split a single DRG with complications into two MS-DRGs: (1) for major complications (MCC), and (2) for regular complications (CC). Payment is then adjusted accordingly. The rationale for this system is that Medicare can pay less for cases that are not major complicated cases. Hospitals will have to review cases that are complicated and the hospital procedures in order to provide good care and to eliminate procedures that increase costs and patients' length of stay.[29]

Over the past 20 years, patients' length of stay in hospitals has decreased. Health insurance companies have initiated this to keep their costs down—patients go home when insurance will not cover costs. Although insurance companies' costs have decreased, patient care also has decreased. Many are forced to recuperate at home rather than in the hospital, and then suffer complications. Hospitals have lost the revenue and are forced to find other ways to make money such as operating health promotion and education centers, mobile X-ray units, and ambulatory care centers.

Knowing that there are various types of hospitals and that hospital services are expensive, how can people select the right hospital? The CMS[30] provides a booklet that can be obtained free of cost online in which it provides tips for selecting the right hospital and even offers a hospital compare worksheet. The booklet contains national surveys of recently discharged patients, specific hospitals' compared to national rates on readmission and 30-day mortality rates. It reports Medicare procedures or treatments given at hospitals and the amount that Medicare pays a hospital.

Thus far, we have identified physician and hospital services as contributing to the high cost of health care. Dental services, nursing home care, in-home care, and other professional services also contribute.

Dental Services

Dental services account for 4% of healthcare costs.[2,3] The costs of oral surgery and techniques for dealing with periodontal disease have contributed to dental care costs. Dentists also must abide by UCR fees. Sometimes, people who have dental bills submit a claim to their insurance company only to get a letter in return stating that the charge submitted was in excess of their UCR fees. One of the reasons is that dentists' fees vary according to geographic area of the country. Some dentists have higher expenses and charge more. Besides the UCR fees, individuals have different dental plans, and some cover more expenses than others.

Nursing Home Care

As was shown in Figure 4.1, nursing home care accounts for 5% of healthcare expenditures. Nursing homes may be identified as assisted living facilities or skilled nursing homes. People who do not require constant care but who can no longer live by themselves qualify for admission to an assisted living facility. Here, they are helped (assisted) with daily care such as eating, bathing, dressing, laundry, medications, and housekeeping. They do not receive much medical care, but they can live independently until they have to be admitted to a skilled nursing facility. In 2016, for a shared room in a skilled facility, the national daily average was $225[31] per day, which amounts to over $80,000 per year. The amount is higher for private rooms, and costs vary according to states. Southeastern or Midwest states have lower costs, but costs are much higher in the Northeast, Alaska and Hawaii. For example, in Louisiana, the average cost per day is $160 ($58,400 per year) compared to Connecticut where the average cost per day is $407 ($148,000 per year).[31]

A skilled nursing home must have registered nurses who can provide 24-hour care, and a licensed physician must supervise each patient's care. Many nursing homes provide custodial care in addition to skilled medical care. Custodial care means personal care: helping residents/patients bathe, dress, and eat. Residents may be living in a skilled nursing home temporarily if they are there for rehabilitation. After a course of treatment, they may return to their assisted living facility or home.

Home Health Care

Even caring for loved ones in the home can be expensive, although depending on the circumstances the costs may not be as high as skilled nursing care or assisted living facilities. As shown in Figure 4.1, home health care accounts for 3% of healthcare expenditures. Medicare does not pay for 24 hours a day care at home, although it will pay for physical therapy, speech-language pathology services, occupational services and intermittent skilled nursing care.[32] The national average for a home health aid is $23 per hour.[33] You can access this site[33] to determine the cost of home health care aid fees for your state. If care is required 24 hours per day, the sum can get very high, and can match a nursing home's cost. If care is only needed for daytime hours, it may be the least expensive solution.

📄 *IN THE NEWS*

Out-of-Pocket Healthcare Spending

PR Newswire printed a story by Kalorama Information[35] online about the amount of out-of-pocket spending in the United States. The amount is a staggering $416 billion. And with a growth rate of 8%, it is expected to reach $608 billion by 2019. Three categories are defined as expenses:

1. Directly on expenditures
2. Copays as part of office and hospital visits and drug purchases
3. Premiums (highest amount)

Questions:

1. Do you think that people can continue to support out-of-pocket expenses?
2. Should insurance companies be required to lower premium amounts?
3. What suggestions could you give to help solve the cost of health care in the United States?

Source: Kalorama Information. Report: U.S. out –of-pocket healthcare spending reaches $416 billion. PR Newswire. May 28, 2015. Available at: http://www.prnewswire.com/news-releases/report-us-out-of-pocket-healthcare-spending-reaches-416-billion-300089701.html Accessed May 3, 2017.

Other Professional Expenses

These services include therapists, chiropractors, optometrists, and podiatrists. According to the CMS, expenditures for these services reached $101.2 billion in 2008,[32] and do not include individuals' out of pocket expenses. The 2013 National Health Expenditure Accounts study reported that $339.4 billion was spent for out of pocket expenses.[34] A second report estimates $416 billion for out of pocket expenses in 2015.[35]

Thus far, we have identified how most of the healthcare expenditures in the United States are spent. The major question to be answered is: In what ways could we control costs? A lot of very intelligent governmental agencies and private citizens are attempting to answer this question, but the solutions are not easy.

▶ How Can We Control Healthcare Costs?

There are many recommendations regarding how to control healthcare costs. The former administration (that of President Barack Obama) had called for a greater emphasis on prevention of diseases, better management of chronic diseases, payment reforms to pay providers on the basis of outcomes, and research on comparative effectiveness to identify preferred diagnostic and treatment options. A new administration (that of Donald J. Trump) is now in office. New and different attempts to control healthcare costs may be implemented, and time will determine how those plans may affect health care, for better or for worse, in the United States.

Many U.S. citizens were in favor of a single payer system (publicly funded and privately administered)[36] as a part of the healthcare reform, and although that did not happen, in 2010 a Democrat-controlled Congress passed healthcare reform legislation called the Patient Protection and Affordable Care Act (ACA). The hope was that the ACA would help decrease costs, but due to high-risk populations' more than healthy people in the insurance exchange pools, copays and deductibles increased and became non-affordable for many. Insurance companies left the exchanges because they contended they were losing money and this worsened the situation as many people subsequently did not have insurance choices. As of May 2017, the Republican-held Congress has not yet passed new health legislation to replace the ACA.

Even though insurance companies did lose some income, an investigative report by Consumer Affairs[37] reveals that many large insurance companies have actually had record profits. For example, UnitedHealth had a record-breaking year in 2015 and even better in 2016. July 2016 quarter revenues totaled $46.5 billion, and $10 billion over the 2015 year.[37] Clearly, large insurance companies have made huge profits. Pharmaceutical companies also have grossed billions of dollars. Many complaints are made about overpriced drugs. Big pharmaceuticals answer that they have to charge more because of all their expenses on research and development (R&D). Several studies have proven that even with R&D costs accounted for, their companies are making huge profits.[38,39] More troubling is that pharmaceutical companies charge extremely high prices for drugs sold in the United States, but charge much lower prices on the same drugs sold in the global market.[40]

Certainly, people should take self-responsibility in decreasing healthcare costs. Some tips from the Blue

---

📄 *IN THE NEWS*

A July 2010 article in the *Baltimore Sun* written by Dr. James Burdick, a Johns Hopkins surgeon,[41] discussed healthcare reform. He made positive comments about the appointment of Dr. Donald Berwick as the administrator of CMS. As of spring 2017, Dr. Berwick had just resigned from this position. But his views are worth thinking about. Burdick was hopeful about the ACA, describing it as open enough at present so that doctors can give input on how to decrease costs and create national treatment standards. Burdick's solutions for decreasing costs are to decrease the amount of red tape that doctors are faced with, form teams of collaborating professionals who communicate with each other, and increase electronic health records so there will eventually be a user-friendly and national record system that can send information to the CMS. He does say that the new law is not complete, and it leaves doctors and patients relying on "insufficiently tamed private health insurance." And yet, he says it is a start to improving coverage and quality of care for millions.

Burdick J. A leader for health care reform [Baltimore Sun website]. July 11, 2010. Available at: http://articles.baltimoresun.com/2010-07-11/news/bs-ed-berwick-medicare-20100711_1_affordable-care-act-health-care-improvement-dr-donald-berwick Accessed July 20, 2010 and May 3, 2017.

Cross Blue Shield of Illinois[42] and Minnesota websites[43] include the following:

- Use doctors and pharmacies in your network.
- Use your preventive care benefits.
- Shop for high-value care.
- Choose the right type of care.
- Ask your doctor for generic drugs.
- Use your health plan's wellness programs.
- Take care of yourself.
- Keep an eye on costs. Review your own medical bills and explanations of benefits.
- Know your physician. Good communication with a physician you know will help prevent medical errors.
- Avoid unnecessary trips to the ER. This tip needs no explanation.
- Step up activity. Exercise is one of those prevention of disease strategies that will decrease healthcare needs, thereby decreasing healthcare costs.
- Take an ounce of prevention. Use seat belts, wear bike helmets, and use other safety equipment whether at work or play.
- Plan a balanced diet. Eating nutritiously will prevent becoming overweight or obese and will aid in disease prevention such as cardiovascular diseases and diabetes.

Using alternative healthcare providers such as physician assistants and nurse practitioners could decrease costs. Regionalizing health services so that hospitals could share expensive equipment such as MRI and CAT scan machines also could help decrease costs. In the past, some thought that managed health care in the form of **health maintenance organizations (HMO)** and the like would be the answer to decreasing healthcare costs. However, although HMOs have decreased users' personal costs, they have not decreased overall healthcare costs. HMOs that offer community-based exercise programs, however, have reduced healthcare costs within the community. More detailed information about various insurance plans is described in a later chapter.

▶ Conclusion

This chapter has presented information regarding the rising cost of health care, reasons for the cost, and some suggestions to decrease healthcare costs. The most important message is that all of us should take responsibility in decreasing costs while doing our part as knowledgeable health consumers.

Wrap-Up

Key Terms

Computerized axial tomography (CAT) An X-ray procedure aided by a computer so that cross-sectional views are obtained. Many X-ray images are taken at various bodily angles.

Current procedural terminology (CPT) codes Guides for setting physician fees.

Gross domestic product (GDP) This is a measure of a country's overall economic output. It is the market value of all final goods and services made within the borders of a country in a year.

High-deductible health plan (HDHP) A type of insurance plan that is typically cheaper than the other health plans, but has a much higher deductible (between \$1,500 and \$5,000). There is no coinsurance, so once the deductible is paid, the remaining expenses are covered 100%.

Healthcare A system that offers, provides, or delivers health care to individuals.

Health Care Refers to care given to a patient by medical or health professionals.

Health maintenance organization (HMO) A type of health insurance provided at a lower rate and less copay. It requires consumers to go to a doctor in the network or expenses will not be covered.

Magnetic resonance imaging (MRI) This machine creates a strong magnetic field and combines with radio waves to form a three-dimensional image helpful in viewing the brain and other soft tissue.

Patient Protection and Affordable Care Act (ACA) A health care reform law intended to expand coverage to millions of people and move the country toward a more primary care-based healthcare system.

Point of service (POS) plan A POS plan is similar to an HMO and PPO. Usually it requires designating a primary care physician who is needed to make referrals to specialists, and the services may include preventative care. The plan may require co-payments and an annual deductible.

Preferred provider organization (PPO) A PPO is a type of health insurance that provides a lower rate wherein people can use an in-network provider or pay somewhat more for an out-of-network provider, but the cost may be higher than the HMO. A primary care physician does not need to be selected., and people may see specialists without a referral.

Stark Law Named after the individual who sponsored it. It is supposed to prohibit physicians from referring Medicare and Medicaid patients to a healthcare provider or facility with which they have a financial relationship.

Usual, customary, and reasonable (UCR) Used by the insurance industry to control costs. It began by reimbursing doctors 98% of the fee, and then went to 95%, 90%, 85%, 80%, and even lower.

Suggestions for Class Activities

1. Determine the average cost of a surgical procedure. You can obtain this information from a hospital, a physician's office, or an insurance company.
2. Write a short descriptive passage about a visit to the doctor or to the ER (could be your visit, a relative's, or a friend's). Include the cost of the ER visit.
3. Visit a local nursing home and talk to the administrator. Inquire about services offered and cost per month for the typical patient in skilled nursing and in assisted living. Ask what percentage of Medicare residents are accepted by the nursing home.

Review Questions

1. What is the 2015 healthcare cost in the United States?
2. Name where the nation's health dollars went and where it came from.
3. Give three of ten Rosenthal economic rules of the dysfunctional medical market.
4. What are the four reasons for the rise in healthcare spending?
5. Analyze the impact of physician Medicare fraud on the cost of health care.
6. What can be done to curtail hospital waste practices?
7. How can health care be made more affordable without limiting access to necessary care?
8. What role should the government play in controlling increases in the cost of care and the cost of health coverage?
9. Should individuals be responsible for the cost of their own care?
10. What is the impact of out-of-pocket expenses faced by many individuals?
11. Name four tips offered by the Blue Cross Blue Shield to lessen healthcare costs.

References

1. Kaiser Family Foundation. Health Spending Explorer. *U.S. health expenditures 1960–2015*. Available at: http://kff.org/health-costs/. Accessed April 3, 2018.
2. The Centers for Medicare & Medicaid Services. *Office of the Actuary, National Health Statistics Group*. Available at: https://www.cms.gov/Research-Statistics-Data-and-Systems/Statistics-Trends-and-Reports/NationalHealthExpendData/Downloads/PieChartSourcesExpenditures2015.pdf. Accessed April 3, 2018.
3. Centers for Medicare and Medicaid Services. *National Health Expenditures Projections 2016–2025*. Available at: https://www.cms.gov/Research-Statistics-Data-and-Systems/Statistics-Trends-and-Reports/NationalHealthExpendData/Downloads/proj2016.pdf. Accessed April 3, 2018.
4. Centers for Medicare and Medicaid Services. *NHE Fact Sheet*. Available at: https://www.cms.gov/research-statistics-data-and-systems/statistics-trends-and-reports/nationalhealthexpenddata/nhe-fact-sheet.html. Accessed April 3, 2018.
5. Rosenthal E. *An American Sickness: How Healthcare Became Big Business and How You Can Take It Back*. New York, NY: Penguin Press; 2017.
6. PricewaterhouseCoopers. *The Price of Excess: Identifying Waste in Healthcare Spending*. Available at: http://www.pwc.com/us/en/healthcare/publications/the-price-of-excess.jhtml. Accessed April 3, 2018.

7. Allen M. *What Hospitals Waste: Why is the Nation's Health Care Tab Sky-High?* (originally published in Propublica SALON). March 14, 2017. Available at: http://www.salon.com/2017/03/14/what-hospitals-waste-why-is-the-nations-health-care-tab-sky-high_partner/. Accessed April 3, 2018.

8. U.S. Department of Health and Human Services. *Healthy People 2020. Leading Health Indicators.* Available at: https://www.healthypeople.gov/2020/Leading-Health-Indicators. Accessed April 3, 2018.

9. Centers for Disease Control and Prevention. *Adult Obesity Causes & Consequences.* Available at: https://www.cdc.gov/obesity/adult/causes.html. Accessed April 3, 2018.

10. Centers for Disease Control and Prevention. *Economic Trends in Tobacco.* Available at: https://www.cdc.gov/tobacco/data_statistics/fact_sheets/economics/econ_facts/. Accessed April 3, 2018.

11. Conrad P. *The Medicalization of Society: On the Transformation of Human Conditions Into Treatable Disorders.* Baltimore, MD: The John Hopkins University Press; 2007:204.

12. Block Imaging. *Your Guide to Medical Imaging Equipment: MRI Machine Cost and Price Guide [2017 Update].* Available at: https://info.blockimaging.com/bid/92623/MRI-Machine-Cost-and-Price-Guide. Accessed April 3, 2018.

13. Securitymetrics Blog. *How Much Does HIPAA Compliance Cost?* Available at: http://blog.securitymetrics.com/2015/04/how-much-does-hipaa-cost.html. Accessed April 3, 2018.

14. DeNardi M, French E, Jones J, McCauley J. *Medical Spending of the U.S. Elderly.* Cambridge, MA: National Bureau of Economic Research. NBER Working Paper No. 21270. Issued June 2015. Available at: http://www.nber.org/papers/w21270.pdf. Accessed April 3, 2018.

15. Neuman T, Cubanski J, Huang J, Damico A. *The Rising Cost of Living Longer: Analysis of Medicare Spending by Age for Beneficiaries in Traditional Medicare.* Menlo Park, CA: The Henry J. Kaiser Family Foundation; 2015. Available at: http://kff.org/medicare/report/the-rising-cost-of-living-longer-analysis-of-medicare-spending-by-age-for-beneficiaries-in-traditional-medicare/. Accessed April 3, 2018.

16. Kodjak A. Dying in a hospital means more procedures, tests and costs. *Shots: Health News from NPR.* June 15, 2016. Available at: http://www.npr.org/sections/health-shots/2016/06/15/481992191/dying-in-a-hospital-means-more-procedures-tests-and-costs. Accessed April 3, 2018.

17. CBS News. The cost of dying. *60 Minutes.* Available at: http://www.cbsnews.com/stories/2009/11/19/60minutes/main5711689_page2.shtml?tag=contentMain;contentBody. Accessed April 3, 2018.

18. Bureau of Labor Statistics, U.S. Department of Labor. *Occupational Outlook Handbook, 2016–2017 Edition, Physicians and Surgeons.* Available at: https://www.bls.gov/ooh/healthcare/physicians-and-surgeons.htm#tab-5. Accessed April 3, 2018.

19. Centers for Medicare and Medicaid Services. *CY 2017 Revisions to Payment Policies under the Physician Fee Schedule and Other Revisions to Part B.* Available at: https://www.cms.gov/Medicare/Medicare-Fee-for-Service-Payment/PhysicianFeeSched/PFS-Federal-Regulation-Notices-Items/CMS-1654-F.html. Accessed April 3, 2018.

20. Consumers Union. *New Yorkers Speak Out About Surprise Medical Bills: Consumer Stories About Medical Bill Shock.* March 24, 2013. Available at: https://stopsurprisemedicalbills.files.wordpress.com/2014/05/surprise-bills-consumer-stories.pdf. Accessed April 3, 2018.

21. Stark Law. *Information on Penalties, Legal Practices, Latest News and Advice.* Available at: http://starklaw.org. Accessed April 3, 2018.

22. Zieger A. *Case study: Midwest physicians seek hospital ownership deals.* August 6, 2008. Available at: http://www.fiercehealthcare.com/story/case-study-midwest-physicians-seek-hospital-ownership-deals/2008-08-06?utm_medium=rss&utm_source=rss&cmp-id=OTC-RSS-FH0. Accessed April 3, 2018.

23. Conway C. *Physician Ownership of Hospitals Significantly Impacted by Health Care Reform Legislation.* Available at: https://www.law.uh.edu/healthlaw/perspectives/2010/(CC)%20Stark.pdf. Accessed April 3, 2018.

24. Belk D. Medical malpractice: Myths and realities. *True Cost of Health-Care.* Available at: http://truecostofhealthcare.net/malpractice/. Accessed April 3, 2018.

25. National Health Care Anti-Fraud Association. *The Challenge of Health Care Fraud.* Available at: https://www.nhcaa.org/resources/health-care-anti-fraud-resources/the-challenge-of-health-care-fraud.aspx. Accessed April 3, 2018.

26. False Claims Act Resource Center. *Federal False Claims Act.* Available at: https://www.falseclaimsact.com/federal-false-claims-act. Accessed April 3, 2018.

27. American Hospital Association. *The Cost of Caring Data Brief, February 2017.* Available at: http://www.aha.org/content/17/costofcaringfactsheet.pdf. Accessed April 3, 2018.

28. Block Imaging. *Your Guide to Medical Imaging Equipment.* Available at: https://info.blockimaging.com/bid/84432/CT-Scanner-Price-Guide. Accessed April 3, 2018.

29. Center for Medicare and Medicaid Services. *Defining the Medicare Severity Diagnosis Related Groups (MS-DRGs), Version 34.0.* Available at: https://www.cms.gov/ICD10Manual/version34-fullcode-cms/fullcode_cms/Defining_the_Medicare_Severity_Diagnosis_Related_Groups_(MS-DRGs)_PBL-038.pdf. Accessed April 3, 2018.

30. Centers for Medicare & Medicaid Services. *Guide to Choosing a Hospital.* Available at: https://www.medicare.gov/Pubs/pdf/10181-Guide-Choosing-Hospital.pdf. Accessed April 3, 2018.

31. Paying for Senior Care. *How to Pay for Nursing Home Care.* Available at: https://www.payingforseniorcare.com/longtermcare/paying-for-nursing-homes.html. Updated October 2017. Accessed April 3, 2018.

32. Centers for Medicare and Medicaid Services. *Is my test, item, or service covered?* Available at: https://www.medicare.gov/coverage/home-health-services.html. Accessed April 3, 2018.

33. Nelson MK. The states where home health aides cost the most. *Home Health Care News.* February 15, 2017. Available at: http://homehealthcarenews.com/2017/02/the-states-where-home-health-aides-cost-the-most/. Accessed April 3, 2018.

34. Health Pocket. *Out-Of-Pocket Costs.* Available at: https://www.healthpocket.com/individual-health-insurance/out-of-pocket-costs/#.WRIxncm1tBw. Accessed April 3, 2018.

35. Kalorama Information. Report: U.S. out-of-pocket healthcare spending reaches $416 billion. *PR Newswire.* May 28, 2015. Available at: http://www.prnewswire.com/news-releases/report-us-out-of-pocket-healthcare-spending-reaches-416-billion-300089701.html. Accessed April 3, 2018.

36. Mahr P. Single payer healthcare only way to control costs. *Lund Report.* June 10, 2009. Available at: https://www.thelundreport.org/content/single-payer-healthcare-only-way-control-costs. Accessed April 6, 2018.

37. Martin A. Health insurance industry rakes in billions while blaming Obamacare for losses. *Consumer Affairs*. November 1, 2016. Available at: https://www.consumeraffairs.com/news/health-insurance-industry-rakes-in-billions-while-blaming-obamacare-for-losses-110116.html. Accessed April 3, 2018.

38. Anderson A. Pharmaceutical industry gets high on fat profits. *BBC News*. November 6, 2014. Available at: http://www.bbc.com/news/business-28212223. Accessed April 3, 2018.

39. Speights K. 12 Big pharma stats that will blow you away. *Motley Fool*. July 31, 2016. Available at: https://www.fool.com/investing/2016/07/31/12-big-pharma-stats-that-will-blow-you-away.aspx. Accessed April 3, 2018.

40. Yu N, Helms Z, Bach P. R&D costs for pharmaceutical companies do not explain elevated US drug prices. *Health Affairs Blog*. March 7, 2017. Available at: http://healthaffairs.org/blog/2017/03/07/rd-costs-for-pharmaceutical-companies-do-not-explain-elevated-us-drug-prices/. Accessed April 3, 2018.

41. Burdick J. A leader for health care reform. *Baltimore Sun*. July 11, 2010. Available at: http://articles.baltimoresun.com/2010-07-11/news/bs-ed-berwick-medicare-20100711_1_affordable-care-act-health-care-improvement-dr-donald-berwick. Accessed April 3, 2018.

42. BlueCross BlueShield of Illinois. Bringing health care costs under control. Available at: https://www.bcbsil.com/leggett/control_cost.html. Accessed April 3, 2018.

43. BlueCross Blue Shield of Minnesota. 7 Ways to save on health care. Available at: https://www.bluecrossmn.com/healthy/public/personal/home/shopplans/shop-individual-family-plans/shop-7-ways-to-save. Accessed April 3, 2018.

examples of...

traditional therapy: Accupuncture
    non-traditional:
Reflexology: Foot, hand, ear; correspond to
    diff. points of the body
Herbal supp.: plants for internal use; garlic

CHAPTER 5

Conventional Medical and Health Care

▶ Where Do We Begin?

As the cost of visiting the doctor continues to rise, practicing **self-care** at home is often a welcome option. For college students, a lack of disposable income, significant distance from their physician, and the generally hectic nature of college life make self-care a necessity! In fact, a 2008 study in the *Journal of American College Health*[1] indicated that 74% of college students used some form of **over-the-counter (OTC) medicine** in the prior 12 months. With that the case, consumers need to then know what to do, how to do it, and when to act. The best technique to use for self-care is to try not to get sick in the first place. Hundreds of resources exist on preventive approaches to lifestyle and how to make positive choices for a healthy life.

▶ How Can I Prevent Illness in the First Place?

The Centers for Disease Control and Prevention (CDC) has summarized much of this information into a short list of general prevention it calls "Tips for College Health and Safety."[2]

- **Eat healthy and be physically active**: This includes a diet with a variety of fruits, vegetables, and whole grains daily; limiting calories, sugar, salt, fat, and alcohol; maintaining a healthy weight; and to consider including 2.5 hours of activity that increases the heart rate each week.
- **Stay safe**: The CDC includes the following suggestions. Manage your stress levels by (1) getting

enough sleep, (2) avoiding the overuse of alcohol, (3) building social supports while retaining time for yourself, and (4) seeking the necessary help if struggling with depression or suicidal thoughts. Advice in this group also includes being aware of and keeping safe from sexual assault. Know your rights and know who to contact if you or an acquaintance is a victim of sexual abuse or violence.

- **Prevent the spread of infectious disease**: Half of all new sexually transmitted infections occur in people under the age of 25. Get tested and know your status. College students, in particular, should ensure their immunizations are up to date (**FIGURE 5.1**).[3]
- **Avoid substance abuse**: Understand the impact of binge drinking and how it contributes to poor decision-making, puts students in risky situations, and is often involved in injury or violence. Do not smoke and avoid illicit drug use.

To be successful in self-care, you must know your own body. When you have taken note of your own physical tendencies, you will more readily know when something odd is occurring. To know your body also means to have an idea of things like your normal blood pressure, cholesterol levels, and family medical history. If there is a dramatic change in your health status or if you begin to exhibit symptoms of an ailment commonly identified in your family, you will have a much better idea of how and when to begin addressing the situation.

You will also need to monitor your symptoms. Symptoms help determine what the cause is and what approach or medicine could be used to help. Choosing an approach to address your situation will require that you accurately describe your symptoms, including the nature of the symptoms you experienced, when the symptoms started, how long they have lasted, and their severity. Knowing this information will allow you to discuss the situation with a physician, if necessary.

▶ What Medicines Are Available to Me Over the Counter?

One trip to the local drug store or pharmacy and it is clear that the consumer has hundreds of choices of OTC medications for virtually every ailment possible. Unfortunately, because anyone can walk up to the counter and buy them, consumers sometimes forget there are potential dangers associated with OTCs, and that they are medications to be used in accordance with accepted guidelines.

The **Food and Drug Administration (FDA)** is responsible for the monitoring and approval of OTC drugs, and states that a drug will become available OTC under the following circumstances:

- The drug's benefits outweigh the drug's risks.
- The potential for misuse and abuse is low.
- The consumer can use them for self-diagnosed conditions.
- The drug can be adequately labeled.
- Health practitioners are not needed for the safe and effective use of the product.[4]

Of common interest are those drugs related to relieving symptoms of pain, cold, and flu. It is vital that the consumer know what they are taking and what each medication is designed to do.

Pain Relievers

Pain relievers, or **analgesics**, come in two forms—acetaminophen and **nonsteroidal anti-inflammatory drugs (NSAIDs)**. Acetaminophen, marketed as Tylenol (**FIGURE 5.2**), for example, is found in over 600 products according to the FDA. Acetaminophen reduces the sensation of pain by blocking pain receptors in the brain and spinal cord.

NSAIDs, in contrast, actually slow the production of enzymes that, in turn, slow the production of **prostaglandins**.[5] Prostaglandins are responsible for swelling and pain production when the body has suffered an injury. By reducing the amount produced by the body, NSAIDs reduce swelling and pain.

There are many different types of NSAIDs in the market today. Although each acts similarly in the body, it is important to remember that each of these forms of NSAID has different dosing requirements. The following are NSAID dosing guidelines approved by the FDA and published by the Agency for Healthcare Research and Quality[6]:

- **Aspirin**: The oldest of the NSAIDs, found in items such as St. Joseph's Aspirin and Bayer. Aspirin also has an added benefit of reducing blood clots and is often recommended for individuals at risk for their development. Product dosing is unique to the product, so follow the product guidelines for dosing.
- **Ibuprofen**: Found in products such as Motrin and Advil (**FIGURE 5.3**). Can be taken in dosages from 200–800 mg, three or four times each day. The maximum daily dose is 3,200 mg.
- **Ketoprofen**: Found in products like Orudis. Each dose is 25–75 mg, taken three or four times per day. The maximum daily dose is 300 mg.

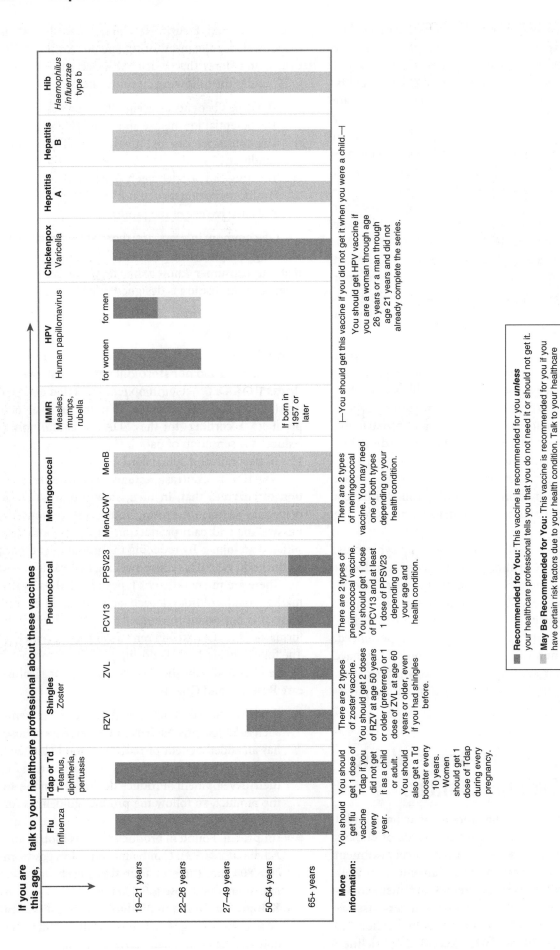

FIGURE 5.1 Recommended immunizations chart.

Source: Centers for Disease Control and Prevention (CDC). https://www.cdc.gov/vaccines/schedules/downloads/adult/adult-schedule-easy-read.pdf

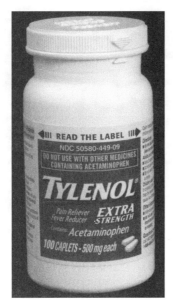

FIGURE 5.2 Tylenol contains acetaminophen.

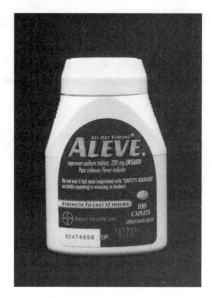

FIGURE 5.4 Aleve is the most common OTC drug with naproxen.

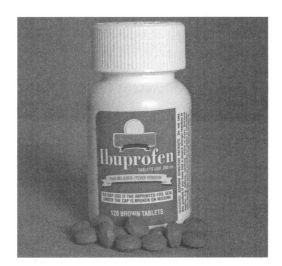

FIGURE 5.3 This product contains ibuprofen.

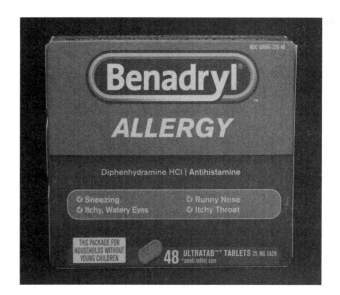

FIGURE 5.5 Benadryl is an antihistamine.

- **Naproxin**: Found in products such as Aleve (**FIGURE 5.4**). Although naproxen comes in many varieties, the most common OTC dosage is 250–500 mg, with a maximum of 1,250 mg per day.

Allergy Medicine

Antihistamines counteract the symptoms associated with an allergic reaction. When the body responds in a negative fashion to a common item, like grass or a cat, a person is said to have an allergy. When the body senses this foreign agent, it releases a substance called **histamine** to defend itself. Histamine causes an individual to experience runny nose, sneezing, and scratchy eyes and throat. There

are more than 30 antihistamines approved for OTC purchase and use that can counter the effects of histamine. First-generation antihistamines are found in some very commonly identified products. Brompheniramine (Dimetapp), chlorpheniramine (Actifed, Contac), doxylamine (Alka-Seltzer Plus), and diphenhydramine (Benadryl; **FIGURE 5.5**) are examples of currently available antihistamines. A new, second generation of antihistamine reduces the degree of tiredness people often feel after using an antihistamine, but they are no more effective than the first generation. They include Cetirizine, Loratadine, and Alavert.[7]

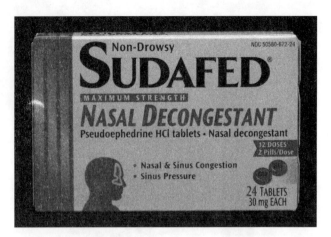

FIGURE 5.6 Pseudoephedrine in products like this was removed from the market because of its drug-making capacity.

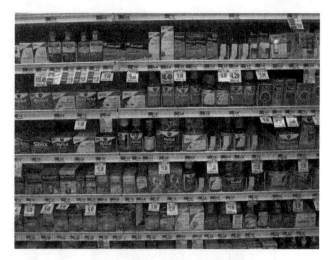

FIGURE 5.7 Hundreds of products are available to treat cough and cold.

Medicines for the Common Cold

If symptoms include stuffy nose and difficulty breathing, a **decongestant** is the medication needed. Currently, there are few oral decongestants approved by the FDA, primarily **pseudoephedrine** and phenylephrine. There are also a few that can be used topically. A decongestant works by reducing the blood flow to the nasal capillaries, thereby reducing the swelling of the tissues in the nose. This opens the air passages for easier breathing.[8]

In 2006, President George W. Bush signed a revised version of The Patriot Act, a portion of which directed that products containing pseudoephedrine (**FIGURE 5.6**) be pulled from availability as an OTC drug due to the substance's use in the making of methamphetamine. **Methamphetamine** is a highly addictive, quickly destructive amphetamine that uses pseudoephedrine as its main ingredient. Currently, 38 states in the United States have laws restricting the availability of pseudoephedrine, most of which limit the amount you can buy, indicate that purchase must come directly from a pharmacist (not OTC), or that a signature documenting receipt of the drug is required.

Medicines for a Nagging Cough

A common physical symptom of illness is a cough and several products are available in the market for treating it (**FIGURE 5.7**). However, not all coughs are the same, and because of that, medicines to treat cough symptoms also vary. Generally, coughs are caused by excess phlegm (a gooey substance in the throat) or dryness causing a cough reflex. Medicines designed to stop the cough reflex are called **antitussives**. They work by reducing the sensations in the nerves that tell the brain to cough.

Dextromethorphan is by far the most common antitussive on the market today, and is found in nearly all OTC cough suppressants. A cough associated with significant phlegm requires the use of an expectorant. An **expectorant** thins and loosens the phlegm so the cough is more "productive," allowing the phlegm's removal. Guaifenesin is the only approved OTC expectorant on the market. Simply stated, the medicine you should choose for your cough, depends on the cough.

▶ What Non-Medicine Options Do I Have?

Medicines you buy OTC are not curing your cold or flu, of course; they are simply easing the symptoms associated with those afflictions. If you prefer not to take something from the pharmacy or you have a preference for a more natural approach, here are some simple ways to get some potential relief:

- **Rest**: It seems to be the last thing people do when they get sick; but the fact is your body only heals while at rest. Thin out your schedule (at a minimum) and allow your body to heal itself.
- **Warm salt water gargle**: Simple and effective. For a stuffy nose, warm salt water can relax nasal passages and allow for better breathing. Warm salt water can also temporarily ease sore throat pain.
- **A hot, steamy shower**: Heat and steam will, again, temporarily help loosen up stuffed nasal passages, and relax sore muscles.

Also, see Chapter 12 on "Aromatherapy" for suggestions on methods to manage a cough.

▶ When Is the Right Time to Go to the Doctor?

So far, we have focused on how to manage illness yourself. There will be times, however, when you should choose to see your physician. *Essentia Health*[9] makes the following suggestions when trying to decide whether you should treat yourself or make an appointment with your doctor.

- **You should treat yourself when:**
  - The illness is minor, such as a cold, influenza, diarrhea, stomachaches, headaches, and skin rashes or fungal infections. Rest and OTC medications can be effective in these situations.
  - You are not on medication for a chronic illness.
  - Your symptoms are mild and familiar (you have experienced them before).
  - Your symptoms do not last very long or are not recurring (coming and going over time).
  - Your pharmacist has given advice on an OTC medication to take.

- **You should see a doctor when:**
  - You have a chronic illness and are unsure if this illness is related.
  - Your symptoms continue or get worse even with rest and the use OTC meds.
  - You are experiencing something new and it has you concerned.
  - You think you may need an antibiotic.
  - You experience diarrhea or constipation for longer than a week, or you notice blood or mucus in your diarrhea.
  - You have feelings of worthlessness or helplessness that last for at least 2 weeks.
  - You are injured and cannot self-treat.

▶ Who Provides the Care?

Physician: Primary Care Provider and Specialists

A variety of health professionals provide primary care, nursing care, and specialty care. The primary care provider is the person first seen for checkups and health problems. This person may be a medical doctor (MD) or a **doctor of osteopathic medicine (DO)**. Both may specialize in internal medicine or family practice. In addition to primary care specialists, some physicians specialize in an advanced practice, for example, a pediatrician specializes in the care of children and an obstetrician or gynecologist specializes in women's

health care and prenatal care. Physicians may specialize in surgery or in neurology. Some may become ophthalmologists (eye doctors) or podiatrists (foot care doctors). There are also nonphysician healthcare providers, which are identified next.

Nonphysician Healthcare Providers

A **nurse practitioner (NP)** is a registered nurse who has obtained advanced education and clinical training; these days, most obtain graduate education that results in a Master's Degree.[10] The NP may work independently or collaboratively on a healthcare team and provides preventative and acute care. The NP may specialize in family medicine, geriatrics, or other areas. NPs take health histories and provide complete physical examinations, diagnose and treat many common acute and chronic problems, interpret laboratory results and X-rays, prescribe and manage medications, and perform other therapies.[10] They may provide health teaching and counseling to support healthy lifestyle behaviors and prevent illness, and are expected to refer patients to other health professionals as needed.

Another type of healthcare provider is the **physician assistant (PA)**, who can also provide many services and works under the guidance of a physician. A typical course of training would be a 33-month graduate curriculum in "pathology, human anatomy, physiology, clinical medicine, pharmacology, physical diagnosis, and medical ethics."[11] Students first complete a bachelor's degree as well as a set of program prerequisites. PAs may be the principal care providers in rural or inner city clinics where a physician is present for only 1 or 2 days each week. In such cases, the PA confers with the supervising physician and other medical professionals as needed and as required by law. Just as with the NP, the PA may provide diagnostic, therapeutic, and preventive healthcare services, as may have been delegated by a physician. They may take medical histories, examine and treat patients, order and interpret laboratory tests and X-rays, and make diagnoses.[11] They also treat minor injuries by suturing, splinting, and casting. Physician assistants also may prescribe certain medications.

▶ Who Are the Orthodox or Conventional Physicians?

Allopathic Physician

The **allopathic physician** is considered the conventional MD. The training of MDs takes many years.[12] Prospective MDs must first get an undergraduate BS or BA degree, usually in biology, chemistry, or physics, while maintaining at least a 3.5 GPA. They usually take the Medical College Admissions Test (MCAT) examination before graduating from college. Based on the old version of the MCAT, to be considered for medical schools, students need a score of 27 or above to be accepted by any school and 30 to be accepted by most schools. The new MCAT has a different scoring process, with 472 being the minimum score and 528 the maximum. The average score that would gain entrance into most schools is 500.[13] There are only 141 accredited 4-year medical schools in the United States, so the process to get accepted into one of them is quite rigorous.

Medical school includes 4 years of preclinical and clinical aspects. After medical school, graduates enter a residency program (graduate medical education). The residency may be from 3 to 7 years or more, depending on the specialty area. For example, family practice, pediatrics, and internal medicine require 3-year residencies, whereas general surgery requires a 5-year residency. According to Study.com,[12] the first year of residency may be considered an internship, although the term is no longer used. After medical school and residency, doctors then have to obtain a license to practice, which requires completing a series of exams. Most physicians will then opt to become board certified in their specialty areas. Moreover, physicians who desire to become more highly specialized in an area may complete a fellowship that could take 1–3 additional years. The learning does not stop there. Even after all the years of training, while in practice, physicians are required to obtain continuing medical education credits every year. Although the figure changes each year, currently, there are approximately 854,000 active MD physicians.[14]

Osteopathic Physician

DOs practice a "whole person" approach to health care by not just treating specific symptoms. Osteopathic physicians are also considered conventional physicians. Osteopathic physicians understand how all the body's systems are interconnected and how each one affects the others. They believe that the musculoskeletal system reflects and influences the condition of all other body systems and believe that disease and its symptoms may be caused by disturbances of bones, muscles, or ligaments.[15]

Andrew Taylor Still was an MD who founded osteopathic medicine in 1874. He was antagonistic toward drug and surgical practices of his day. He was especially disillusioned with bloodletting practices. Dr. Still believed that adequate functioning of the body depends on uninterrupted nerve and blood

supply to tissues; so, he began to use spinal manipulation to remove interference. Thus began the practice of osteopathy, and in 1892, the American School of Osteopathy at Kirksville, Missouri, was founded. Currently, there are 33 colleges of osteopathic medicine in the United States.[16]

To become a doctor of osteopathy, individuals must complete a 4-year undergraduate degree, including specific science courses. Just as applicants for medical schools must do, applicants for osteopathy schools must take the MCAT. In addition, osteopathic medical schools typically require applicants to participate in a personal interview. The curriculum at osteopathic medical schools consists of 4 years of academic and clinical studies, and emphasizes preventive medicine and comprehensive patient care. Clinical studies concentrate on teaching doctoral students how to use osteopathic principles and osteopathic manipulative treatment to diagnose and treat patients. After completing osteopathic medical college, DOs obtain graduate medical education through internships, residencies, and fellowships that range from 3 to 8 years of training. During this time, DOs may specialize in any area of medicine, the same as a MD (e.g., family medicine, general internal medicine and pediatrics, or specialized disciplines such as surgery, radiology, oncology, psychiatry, and sports medicine).[15]

Although many people are not familiar with the educational background and requirements of osteopathic physicians, they are fully trained physicians who prescribe drugs, perform surgery and use accepted methods to maintain and restore health. Currently, there are approximately 100,000 licensed DOs in the United States, and about 60% of them practice as primary care doctors.[15]

▸ What Is the Flexner Report?

We know that MDs go through several years of rigorous training, but what is the foundation for that education? Who decided what should be taught, and is everyone taught the same things? In 1906, Abraham Flexner was commissioned by the Carnegie Foundation and the American Medical Association's Council on Medical Education to review 155 medical schools and their educational curriculum.[17] Flexner was not a doctor; he was a secondary school teacher and principal for 19 years in Louisville, Kentucky. His report was published in 1910 and is known as the Flexner Report.[17,18] Flexner found discrepancies among medical schools in terms of length of program and types of courses. Some medical students had never attended college. The Flexner Report rank ordered the medical schools and triggered much-needed reforms in their standards, organization, and curriculum. As a result of the study, certain schools closed and others were reorganized and restructured. By 1926, the AMA had a monopoly over the education and licensing of physicians.[19] Thereafter, all medical schools in the United States were based at universities and the curriculum became consistent and rigorous among all medical schools.

▶ How Should I Choose or Fire a Physician?

Thus far in this chapter, we have discussed medical self-care and identified several health professionals and physicians you can access if you need a physician. Now, let us discuss how to choose a physician and, if necessary, how to fire one. Finding a good physician is one of the most important health consumer functions that individuals and families need to perform.

Finding and Selecting a Physician

People want to find a doctor with whom they can develop trust and faith; therefore, identifying a potential doctor may take some research. Whatever methods you use to find a physician, the most important step is determining which criteria are important (e.g., clinical training, experience, and board certification, plus interests and expertise in a specialized area). For some people, the age and sex of the physician are important. For many people, it is also important to choose a physician whose philosophy of care is consistent with their own.

As you attempt to select a physician, you might want to consider the setting of the physician's office. Determine if you would like a small, more intimate setting or if you would be agreeable to seeing a physician whose practice is within a large clinic setting. The location of the office is another important criterion. If you live in a large city (e.g., Chicago or Houston), you might want to select a physician whose office is close to your home or work.

Now that you have determined certain important criteria, there are other factors that need to be considered. For instance, if the doctor or clinic accepts your insurance plan, a list of physicians associated with that particular plan is identified—called a physician network. Those physicians listed have agreed to accept a specific payment level from the insurance company for providing services. It is important to note that if you choose to see a provider who is "outside" the network, you can pay significantly more out of pocket to see that provider. With traditional insurance plans and preferred provider organization (PPO) health insurance, a wider physician network is offered than with a more conservative health maintenance organization (HMO) plan. Nonetheless, choices are available.

Some people rely on the recommendation of a physician by an acquaintance or friend. This is a moderately good way for you to select a physician, if your expectations are the same as the person recommending the doctor. Others try researching the physician online—another good method of narrowing your search. Most physicians today have a personal website or one maintained by the hospital or clinic with which the physician is associated. These sites will give you a general idea of the doctor's philosophy, education, and clinical expertise. Another database you could examine is the American Board of Medical Specialties' (ABMS) Certification Matters website to determine if the doctor you are interested in is board certified in their specialty.[20] Most communities and cities have an online Directory of Medical Specialists[21] where people can obtain information about all physicians in the area. You could also check the American Medical Association's online Doctor Finder Directory.[22]

🔍 CASE STUDY

Ann has lived all of her life in a large city in Illinois. She has just graduated from college and has accepted a job in a neighboring state. Ann has moved to a large, strange city where she knows no one, although she met a few people when she interviewed for the job. One of the major tasks that Ann wants to do is to find a family doctor and a gynecologist.

Questions:
1. What steps must Ann take to find competent physicians?
2. How can Ann verify that the physicians she selects have adequate medical training and years of experience?
3. If Ann's doctors do not provide adequate care for her, what options does she have?

As you can see, it is not an easy job to select a physician. You have to decide which personal criteria are important and then make a responsible choice. It is wonderful that today many helpful databases are available—but only if we take the time to access them.

Firing a Physician

There are times when you might encounter problems with your physician. Perhaps, you have to wait a long period of time before getting in to see the doctor. Perhaps, the doctor seemed rushed and eager to get out of the examination room. Perhaps, the doctor did not take time to adequately answer your questions. Perhaps, he or she refused your right to get a second opinion. The main point to consider is that if you have one isolated incident, keep your doctor. But if you have consistent problems, it is your right to find another physician. Start the search using many of the techniques discussed in the previous section. Ask a friend or other healthcare provider. Check credentials. Look for a board-certified physician. When you have selected your new physician, ask in writing to have your records transferred to your new doctor. As shown, to find a doctor that you will be comfortable with, you must conduct a careful and thoughtful research process.

▶ What Institutions Are Caring for the Sick?

However you find your physician, it is important to check to determine whether a prospective doctor is affiliated with a hospital accredited by the Joint Commission. The Joint Commission accredits approximately 4,023 general children's, long-term acute, psychiatric, rehabilitation and specialty hospitals, and 366 critical access hospitals through an accreditation program.[23] Approximately, 88% of the nation's hospitals are currently accredited by the Joint Commission. Also, check the American Hospital Association's *AHA Guide®*,[24] which is an encyclopedic hospital directory of health care and hospital systems profiles.

Hospitals

When people get sick, need surgery, or need mental health services, they usually go to hospitals. Some hospitals are public (nonprofit) and some private (for-profit). A public hospital is owned by the government and receives government funding.

TABLE 5.1 U.S. Hospitals, February 2018

Total number of U.S. registered* hospitals	5,534
Number of U.S. community hospitals**	4,840
Number of nongovernment not-for-profit community hospitals	2,849
Number of investor-owned (for-profit) community hospitals	1,035
Number of state and local government community hospitals	956
Number of federal government hospitals	209
Number of nonfederal psychiatric hospitals	397
Other hospitals	88

Note:
*Registered hospitals meet AHA's criteria for registration as a hospital facility.
**Community hospitals defined as all nonfederal, short-term general, and other special hospitals (obstetrics and gynecology; eye, ear, nose, and throat; rehabilitation; orthopedic; and other specialty services.

© Used with permission of American Hospital Association. Fast Facts on US Hospitals. Available at: https://www.aha.org/system/files/2018-02/2018-aha-hospital-fast-facts.pdf. Accessed April 23, 2018.

People may receive care free of charge. In 2016, of the roughly 5,534 nonfederal, short-term, acute care community hospitals in the United States, approximately 2,849 (51%) were nonprofit.[25] Nonprofit hospitals are often affiliated with a religious denomination and have a charitable purpose. See **TABLE 5.1** for a list of the different types of hospitals in existence as of February 2018 based on data taken in the 2016 American Hospital Association Annual Survey.

Major Medical Centers

Many large cities not only have several hospitals, but also have major medical centers. Those associated with a medical school are often part of a conglomerate of healthcare services. **Healthcare conglomerates** are composed of hospitals, clinics, and research facilities that either include or are affiliated to a medical school. Major medical centers are considered the crown jewels of health care in the United States. See **BOX 5.1** for a sample list of major medical centers. Medical centers vary greatly in their organization, the services they provide, and their ownership and operation.

BOX 5.1 Major U.S. Medical Centers

- Cleveland Clinic
- Mayo Clinic
- Texas Medical Center
- University of Pennsylvania Health System
- Massachusetts General
- New York Presbyterian Hospital
- University of California, San Francisco Medical Center
- Ronald Reagan UCLA Medical Center
- Duke University Health System
- Johns Hopkins Hospital

▶ What Are Our Rights as Patients?

Patients do have the right to be competently cared for, and many patients' bills of rights have been formulated. For example, there are mental health bills of rights, hospice patients' bills of rights, insurance plan bills of rights, and so forth. The most current version of a Patients' Bill of Rights[25] was released by the Obama Administration in 2010 as a component of the Patient Protection and Affordable Care Act. That document declared the following as the rights of U.S. citizens in their relationship to the healthcare system:

- Ensuring coverage for those people with preexisting conditions
- Ensuring the right to choose your doctor
- Ensuring fair treatment when you need emergency care
- Making sure your policy cannot be canceled unfairly
- Ending annual and lifetime limits
- Enhancing access to preventative services
- Ensuring your right to appeal health plan decisions
- Ensuring young adult coverage under their parents' plan

The provisions under the Patient Protection and Affordable Care Act demonstrate that we do have rights as consumers of health care, but when necessary, we must choose to exercise our rights. If our rights are taken from us, one option is to sue the hospital or physician. The problem is that often people instigate malpractice lawsuits that are not necessary and are started for financial gain.

▶ What Is Medical Malpractice and How Has It Impacted Insurance Costs?

Medical malpractice, as noted in Chapter 4, is professional negligence by act or omission by a healthcare provider in which care provided deviates from accepted standards of practice in the medical community and causes injury or death to the patient.[26] There are many legitimate reasons for medical malpractice suits. Doctors may fail to diagnose a disease, misdiagnose it, or do something to cause a patient's death (e.g., medication error). Doctors may make a mistake when conducting surgery or delivering a baby. The consequence is that doctors may find themselves in court.

Statistically, in 2016, the National Practitioner Data Bank reported $3.8 billion in medical malpractice payouts. This was actually the first decrease in payouts since 2012. The most common allegation in lawsuits was based on diagnosis (34%), followed by surgery (24%) and treatment (18%) complications. The most common outcome as the basis of the suit was patient death, nearly one-third of all lawsuits, followed by significant and major permanent injury.[27]

One recent analysis of 42,000 claims indicated 72% of liability claims against doctors were dropped, withdrawn, or dismissed without payment.[27] A significant issue is that those cases cost physicians an average $47,000 to defend in 2010, up 62% since 2001. Of the cases that go to trial, over 90% found that physicians were not negligent. Of all the cases that went to trial in 2010, less than 1% were decided in favor of the patient.[28]

Doctors are not the only ones sued for malpractice. It could be a practicing nurse working at a retirement home or any healthcare professional who does not treat according to the standards of their field. Just because a suit has been started does not mean that the doctor or healthcare professional is guilty as charged. Malpractice has to be proven in court, and many times the cases are settled before they ever reach court. In fact, it has been estimated that 9 out of 10 cases are settled out of court.[27]

It could be that some health professionals and doctors are at fault. Perhaps, they have a history of either poor care or poor doctoring. It could be a failure of state boards to weed them out. However, it could be that many cases were started out of pure greed by patients or lawyers. Frivolous cases (cases without merit) cause the cost of malpractice insurance to explode and have also caused a shortage of doctors in specialty areas that seem to get many lawsuits such as obstetrics and gynecology.

▶ The Informed Consumer: Applying the Concepts Learned to Your Daily Life

Now that you have learned some facts about U.S. health care and the professionals who are available, how can you apply these concepts to your daily life?

You will be graduating from college and will find it necessary to use the healthcare system. Perhaps, you will get married and have a family. It will be important to find a family physician, and if you are a female, a gynecologist. If you get pregnant, you will need to find an obstetrician. How will you get insurance? Will your employer provide insurance or will you have to go on the free market to find it? What would be the criteria that you would use to find your physicians? Would you use an MD or a DO? If you moved from one state to another, what means would you use to locate a competent doctor? You will one day be faced with decisions like these; therefore, now is the time to begin thinking about what you would do. Good luck with all your future decisions.

▶ Conclusion

As shown in this chapter, taking care of yourself and managing the healthcare system is complex. There are many professionals who can give us care, and we have defined who the conventional physicians are. We have a huge responsibility to select our physicians with care and to know when to fire our doctors. It is up to us. Are you up to the challenge?

Wrap-Up

Key Terms

Allopathic physician A conventional or orthodox physician who is an MD.

Analgesic Any member of a group of drugs used to relieve pain.

Antihistamine Drug used to counteract the physiological effects of histamine production in allergic reactions and colds.

Antitussive Capable of relieving or suppressing coughing.

Decongestant Medication or treatment that breaks up congestion, as of the sinuses, by reducing swelling.

Expectorant Promoting or facilitating the secretion or expulsion of phlegm, mucus or other matter from the respiratory tract.

Food and Drug Administration (FDA) A division of the U.S. Department of Health and Human Services that protects the public against impure and unsafe foods, drugs, and cosmetics.

Healthcare conglomerates Comprised of hospitals, clinics, and research facilities that either include or are affiliated to a medical school.

Histamine Stimulates gastric secretion and causes dilation of capillaries, constriction of bronchial smooth muscle and decreased blood pressure.

Methamphetamine Used as a stimulant to the nervous system and as an appetite suppressant, and illicitly as a recreational drug.

Nonsteroidal anti-inflammatory drug (NSAID) Used for reducing inflammation and pain.

Nurse practitioner (NP) A registered nurse who has obtained advanced education and clinical training. Most obtain a master's or doctorate degree in nursing practice studies.

Doctor of osteopathic medicine (DO) A conventional or orthodox physician who has similar training as the MD but who has advanced studies in the interconnection of the muscles, bones, and nerves.

Over-the-counter (OTC) medicine Medicine sold without a prescription.

Physician assistant (PA) A professional who can also provide many healthcare services and works under the guidance of a physician.

Prostaglandin Any member of a group of lipid compounds that sensitize the body to pain.

Pseudoephedrine Drug similar in action to ephedrine; used extensively as a decongestant or illicitly to produce methamphetamine.

Self-care Personal health maintenance.

Suggestions for Class Activities

1. Discuss a newspaper report about an incompetent physician or dentist and the appropriateness of the disciplinary action taken. (You could find this on the Internet or access newspaper archives.)
2. Interview one or two physicians about their philosophy regarding healthcare costs and malpractice. What would they do to solve healthcare delivery problems? Prepare a written summary.
3. Interview one or two physicians or nurses and ask their view about any potential movement for a nationalized health insurance program. Prepare a written summary.

Review Questions

1. What is an over-the-counter medicine?
2. What is an analgesic?
3. Name three common antihistamines.
4. What is the difference between an antitussive and an expectorant?
5. What is an allopathic doctor?
6. What is the main difference in the academic preparation of an allopathic versus an osteopathic physician?
7. What is the philosophy of an osteopathic physician?
8. In what ways did the Flexner Report change the training of MDs?
9. As learned in this chapter, how would you proceed if you wanted to find and select a physician?
10. What reasons would lead you to fire your physician?
11. What are three patients' rights?
12. How have malpractice suits impacted healthcare costs?

References

1. Stasio MJ, Curry K, Sutton-Skinner KM, Glassman DM. Over-the-counter medication or dietary supplement use in college: Dose frequency and relationship of self-reported distress. *J Am Coll Health*. 2008;56:535-547.
2. Centers for Disease Control and Prevention. *Tips for College Health and Safety*. Available at: https://www.cdc.gov/features/collegehealth/index.html. Updated August 8, 2016. Accessed April 6, 2018.
3. Centers for Disease Control and Prevention. *2017 Recommended Immunizations for Adults: By Age*. Available at: https://www.cdc.gov/vaccines/schedules/downloads/adult/adult-schedule-easy-read.pdf. Accessed April 6, 2018.
4. U.S. Food and Drug Administration. *Regulation of Nonprescription Products*. Available at: https://www.fda.gov/AboutFDA/CentersOffices/OfficeofMedicalProductsandTobacco/CDER/ucm093452.htm. Updated March 29, 2018. Accessed April 6, 2018.
5. WebMD. How NSAIDs Work. Updated February 2, 2018. Available at: http://www.webmd.boots.com/osteoarthritis/guide/how-anti-inflammatory-medicines-work. Accessed April 6, 2018.
6. Chou R, Helfand M, Peterson K, Dana T, Roberts C. Appendix C Comparable NSAID Dose Levels. In: *Comparative Effectiveness and Safety of Analgesics for Osteoarthritis. Comparative Effectiveness Review No. 4*. Rockville, MD: Agency for Healthcare Research and Quality. September 2006. Available at: https://www.ncbi.nlm.nih.gov/books/NBK42997/. Accessed April 6, 2018.
7. Healthline. Popular Over-the-Counter Oral Antihistamine Brands. Available at: https://www.healthline.com/health/allergies/antihistamine-brands. Accessed April 6, 2018.
8. Stöppler MC. OTC Cold and Cough Medications. *MedicineNet*. Updated January 18, 2018. Available at: https://www.medicinenet.com/otc_cold_and_cough_medications/views.htm. Accessed April 6, 2018.
9. Essentia Health. *Self-Treat? Or See a Doctor?* Available at: http://www.essentiahealth.org/Main/Health-Library1/SelfTreat-Or-See-a-Doctor-43207.aspx. Accessed April 6, 2018.
10. Mayo Clinic School of Health Science. *Nurse Practitioner*. Available at: http://www.mayo.edu/mayo-clinic-school-of-health-sciences/careers/nurse-practitioner. Accessed April 6, 2018.
11. U.S. Department of Labor, Bureau of Labor Statistics. *Physician Assistants*. Available at: https://www.bls.gov/ooh/healthcare/physician-assistants.htm#tab-4. Updated January 30, 2018. Accessed April 6, 2018.
12. Study.com. *Requirements to Become a Doctor in the U.S*. Available at: http://study.com/requirements_to_become_a_doctor.html. Accessed April 6, 2018.
13. Association of American Medical Colleges. *MCAT Scores for Medical School Admissions*. Available at: https://www.mcat-prep.com/mcat-scores/. Accessed April 6, 2018.
14. Statista. *Statistics & Facts on U.S. Physicians/Doctors*. Available at: https://www.statista.com/topics/1244/physicians/. Accessed April 6, 2018.
15. American Osteopathic Association. *Osteopathic Medicine*. Available at: http://doctorsthatdo.org/. Accessed April 6, 2018.
16. American Association of Colleges of Osteopathic Medicine. *A Brief History of Osteopathic Medicine*. Available at: http://www.aacom.org/become-a-doctor/about-om/history. Accessed April 6, 2018.
17. MedicineNet.com. *Flexner Report . . . Birth of Modern Medical Education*. Updated August 5, 2002 Available at: http://www.medicinenet.com/script/main/art.asp?articlekey=8795. Accessed April 6, 2018.
18. Carnegie Foundation for the Advancement of Teaching. *Medical Education in the United States and Canada Bulletin Number Four (The Flexner Report)*. Available at: http://www.carnegiefoundation.org/publications/medical-education-united-states-and-canada-bulletin-number-four-flexner-report-0. Accessed April 6, 2018.
19. Olakanmi O. *The AMA, NMA, and the Flexner Report of 1910*. Available at: https://californiacollegeofmidwives.org

/ama-nma-flexner-report-1910-ololade-olakanmi/. Accessed April 6, 2018.

20. American Board of Medical Specialties (ABMS). *Certification Matters.* Available at: http://www.certificationmatters.org/. Accessed April 6, 2018.

21. American Board of Medical Specialties (ABMS). The official ABMS directory. Available at: https://www.abmsdirectory.com/abms/static/home.htm. Accessed April 6, 2018.

22. American Medical Association. *DoctorFinder.* Available at: https://apps.ama-assn.org/doctorfinder. Accessed April 6, 2018.

23. The Joint Commission. *Facts About Hospital Accreditation.* Available at: https://www.jointcommission.org/accreditation/accreditation_main.aspx. Updated September 18, 2017. Accessed April 6, 2018.

24. American Hospital Association. *AHA Guide®.* Available at: http://www.ahadata.com/aha-guide/. Accessed April 6, 2018.

25. Families USA. *The Affordable Care Act: Patient Bill of Rights and Other Protections.* April 2011. Available at: http://familiesusa.org/sites/default/files/product_documents/Patients-Bill-of-Rights.pdf. Accessed April 6, 2018.

26. Wikipedia. *Medical malpractice in the United States.* Available at: https://en.wikipedia.org/wiki/Medical_malpractice_in_the_United_States. Accessed April 6, 2018.

27. Diederich Healthcare. *2017 Medical Malpractice Payout Analysis.* February 27, 2017. Available at: https://www.diederichhealthcare.com/the-standard/2017-medical-malpractice-payout-analysis/. Accessed April 6, 2018.

28. Lewis M Jr. Medical malpractice costs continue to climb. *ModernMedicine Network: Medical Economics®.* January 11, 2012. Available at: http://medicaleconomics.modernmedicine.com/medical-economics/news/clinical/practice-management/medical-malpractice-costs-continue-climb. Accessed April 6, 2018.

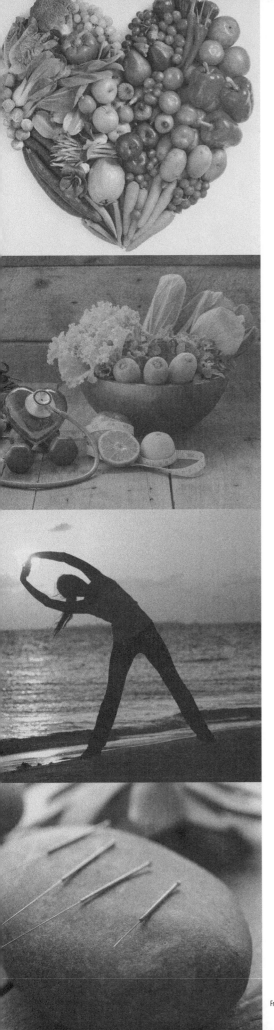

PART 3

Complementary and Alternative Medicine and Health Care

CHAPTER 6

CAM, Integrative Medicine and Health, and Early Pioneers

LEARNING OBJECTIVES

As a result of reading this chapter, students will be able to:

1. Describe the prevalence of complementary and alternative medicine (CAM) use and identify the amount of money spent on CAM products or practices.
2. Identify several barriers to CAM use.
3. Define the term "integrative medicine and health" and assess the impact of integrative medicine on health care in the United States.
4. Name several early pioneers of integrated medicine and health and describe their contribution to the movement.
5. Describe the role of the health consumer in taking self-responsibility for integrative medicine and health care choices.

▶ Introduction

This chapter is intended to familiarize you with information regarding the various populations using **complementary and alternative medicine (CAM)** and the types of CAM modalities used. You will learn how integrative medicine and integrative health have been incorporated into mainstream medicine and how early U.S. pioneers supported and promoted the union of Eastern and Western medicine.

▶ What Is the Prevalence of CAM Use?

The annual National Health Interview Survey (NHIS) is administered by the Centers for Disease Control and Prevention (CDC) and the National Center for Health Statistics (NCHS). The National Center for Complementary and Integrative Health (NCCIH) and the NHIS developed questions addressing complementary health approaches and this section was administered in the 2002, 2007, and 2012 surveys.[1,2] Data were collected from 88,962 adults ages 18 and over who were representative of the civilian U.S. population. The analysis also included assessing differences or similarities in CAM use at the time of the surveys in 2002, 2007, and 2012.[2] A summary of results are as follows:

- The most commonly used were nonvitamin, nonmineral dietary supplements that have stayed fairly consistent: 18.9% in 2002; and 17.7% in 2007 and 2012.
- Deep breathing used independently or as an adjunct to other approaches was second in use: 11.6% in 2002; 12.7% in 2007; and 10.9% in 2012.

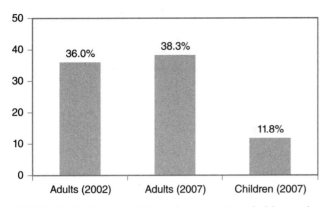

FIGURE 6.1 CAM use by U.S. adults, ages 18 and older, and children.

Source: Barnes PM, Bloom B, Nahin RL. Complementary and alternative medicine use among adults and children: United States, 2007. National health statistics reports; no 12. Hyattsville, MD: National Center for Health Statistics. 2008.

National Center for Complementary and Integrative Health, NIH, DHHS.

- Yoga, tai chi, and qigong ranked third (and all increased yoga the most) in use: 5.8% in 2002; 6.7% in 2007; and 10.1% in 2012.
- The fourth highest use was of chiropractic and osteopathic manipulation: 7.5% in 2001; 8.6% in 2007; and 8.4% in 2012.
- Meditation: 7.6% in 2002; and 8% in 2007 and 2012.
- In addition, **Homeopathic medicine**, **acupuncture**, and **naturopathic medicine** each increased in use to a significant level.
- **Ayurveda**, **biofeedback**, guided imagery hypnosis, and energy healing had no significant change and remained fairly low in use during the three time periods.

Among the adults surveyed, those stating they had used any complementary health method during the past 12 months increased over the three time periods

from 32.3% in 2002 to 35.5% in 2007 and down to 33.2% in 2012.[1] The complete data set for adults consists of 237 pages showing tables for all questions asked in this survey and is open for public viewing. See reference list for the website.[2] See **FIGURE 6.1** for CAM use by U.S. adults and children for 2002 and 2007.

The American Association for Retired Persons (AARP) conducted a study to assess the use of CAM among people ages 50 years and over.[3] About 53% of 1,013 individuals responding to the survey reported using CAM at some time during their lifetime, and 47% had used some form of CAM during the past 12 months. Dietary supplements/herbals were used most, while massage and chiropractic manipulations were next. **FIGURE 6.2** shows the type of CAM that users chose and **FIGURE 6.3** shows the educational level of those users.

Several CAM studies have involved college students. A study at Columbia University revealed that of the 6,482 students, nearly 82% reported they had used at least one CAM approach during the last 12 months. Nonvitamin, nonmineral products, massage, meditation, yoga, and deep breathing were most used.[4] A 2006 study of 506 undergraduates at a large Southeastern school revealed that 58% of students had used at least one CAM therapy and 79% of students had used at least one herbal substance in the last year.[5] A third study involved 997 students participating in a southern university survey study regarding CAM use.[6] About 53% reported knowledge of CAM therapies and 50% of students reported employing at least one CAM therapy in the last year. More females and older students used CAM. The most commonly used CAM therapies in this study were massage (30.9%), herbal

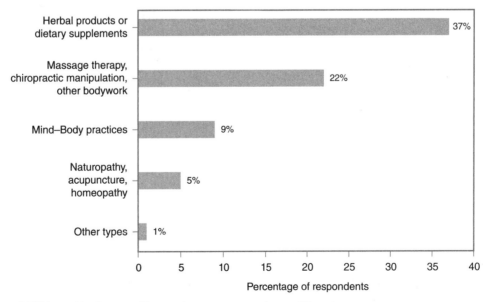

FIGURE 6.2 Type of CAM used in the past 12 months among people age 50+.

Source: AARP/NCCAM (NCCIH) Survey of U.S. Adults 50+, 2010. National Center for Complementary and Integrative Health.

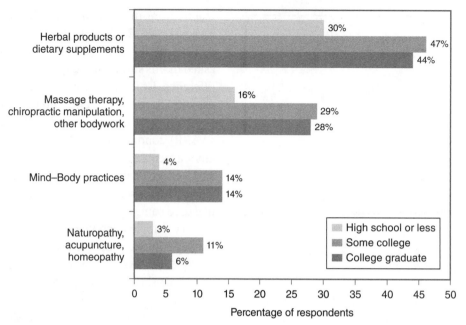

FIGURE 6.3 Education level and type of CAM used in the past 12 months.

Source: AARP/NCCAM (NCCIH) Survey of U.S. Adults 50+, 2010. National Center for Complementary and Integrative Health.

supplements (19.6%), yoga (16.2%), aromatherapy (14.9%), meditation (14.2%), and chiropractic (14.1%). A small percentage used faith healing (5.5%) and reflexology (2.9%).[5] The most commonly used herbal supplements were creatine (12.8%), protein bars (12.8%), Metabolife (7.6%), Xenadrine (7.4%), ginseng (7.3%), gingko biloba (6.4%), Hydroxycut (4.6%), echinacea (2.2%), calcium (2.4%), Stacker 2 & 3 (2%), valerian (1.9%), St. John's wort (1.5%), kava kava (1.3%), herbal teas (1.2%), several types of vitamins and minerals, and 103 other supplements with percentages ranging from 0.2% to 0.7%. Most were bodybuilding supplements, immune boosters, and herbs to treat anxiety or insomnia.[6]

Several studies assessed CAM knowledge and use among nurses. A 2010 publication[7] reported that clinical nurse specialists at a large Midwestern academic medical center used several CAM therapies personally and professionally, including humor, massage, spirituality/prayer, healing touch, acupuncture, and music therapy. After reading the results of these studies, we can ascertain that CAM is used by a wide variety of populations.

▶ How Much Money Has Been Spent on CAM?

Using alternative therapies is not inexpensive. According to the 2012 CDC/NHIS survey,[2] approximately 59 million Americans spent $30.2 billion out

of pocket on CAM.[8] The mean out of pocket expense was $510 per person. About $14.7 billion was spent on complementary practitioners. About $12.8 billion was spent on natural product supplements, and about $2.7 billion was spent on self-care approaches such as homeopathic medicine and books or CDs related to complementary therapies.[8] Based on the usage reports and the amount of money that people are spending on CAM, we can assume that in the future there will be an increase in CAM use and costs.

▶ Why Do People Seek Alternative Forms of Medical Care?

Several reasons why people seek alternative forms of medical care have been proposed. They may be dissatisfied with conventional treatment as expensive, impersonal, and ineffective.[9] Alternative forms of treatment may be compatible with users' own values and spiritual beliefs regarding the nature of their illness. People may desire a greater sense of control over their own treatment and seek out a doctor who will allow them choices about their own health care.[9] Many individuals who use CAM tend to be innovative and at the cutting edge of cultural change. They are very interested in the environment and the world and possess a great sense of spirituality.

Kaptchuk and Eisenberg[10] wrote about the persuasive appeal of CAM and identified four major elements. The first element is the association of CAM with *nature*, a metaphor for many alternative medicines or therapies. For example, food that is labeled as organic rather than processed is desirable. CAM therapies are supposedly more natural than artificial and pure rather than synthetic. Terms such as "pure" versus "synthetic" comprise the language. Organic rather than processed foods are bought and consumed. As a result, stores that sell herbal supplements and organic food supplies have proliferated into the thousands and can be found in most cities (e.g., Whole Foods stores). The result is that a nationwide government study, co-funded by NCCIH, found that in 2007, $34 billion[4] was spent to seek "natural" means to good health. About two-thirds of that money was spent on self-care.

The second element identified was vitalism,[10] the body's capacity to heal itself. The enhancement or balancing of life forces, **qi (chi)**, or psychic energy is a main theme and belief in the concept of vitalism. These life forces are not a physical force but are related to energy within the body that is capable of healing. For patients, there is intuitive appeal in this noninvasive notion of healing from within.

The third element identified was science.[10] Alternative medicine's scientific process may match the steps of biomedical scientific techniques, but it depends greatly on observation. Alternative medicine is a more person-friendly science that embraces the concept of holism (connectedness of physical, mental, spiritual, emotional health). Sickness is viewed as a result of a weakened body that has fallen into an unbalanced condition. As such, it is remedied by overall strengthening of the body's natural resistance to disease. The human experience becomes the central element of CAM science rather than being marginalized. A person would not be told that their condition is "all in their head." In other words, the person is treated, not just the symptom or the disease.

The fourth element was the aspect of spirituality.[10] Spirituality does not refer particularly to religiosity, although for some, it may. Religion or spiritual experiences become important as people view health, illness, and healing. CAM offers a satisfying unification of the physical and spiritual because it bridges the gap between the domain of medical science and religion or spirituality, and the patient is allowed to make connections with nature and the universe.

Several theories have also been posed regarding underlying motives for using CAM. One of these is that patients using CAM may be essentially neurotic, and therefore, are drawn toward the touching/talking approach of many therapies. Because CAM practitioners mainly see people with **chronic** diseases, it could be likely that neurosis levels are high in their patients. It could also be that people with high levels of stress (e.g., stress from having cancer) may seek out CAM practitioners. Another underlying motive is that people who have a better understanding of the workings of the human body are attracted to CAM therapists because diagnosis and treatment involve them more in the process. Some individuals may believe their condition is not serious enough to make an appointment to see their medical doctor (MD) and, therefore, see an alternative practitioner. Some individuals may seek out an alternative practitioner if they fear the side effects of traditional medical treatments.

Despite the limitations of the existing literature on the motives for CAM use, a few consistent findings have emerged. It is clear that, in general, CAM does not replace conventional medicine. Rather, it serves as a substitute in some particular situations and as an adjunct in others. Some individuals simply will not use an alternative therapy when not considered appropriate for the condition in question.

📰 IN THE NEWS

Several news articles described the increased use of pesticides as a contributing factor to the increase in ADHD in children. A 2015 study published in *HealthDay*[11] portrays the main points of several studies. An association or link (not cause and effect) has been found between the use of household pesticides containing pyrethroid and attention deficit hyperactivity disorder (ADHD). In fact, boys showing detectable 3-PBA (a chemical indicator of exposure to pyrethroids) in their urine were three times more likely to have ADHD. Some foods that may contain pesticides are blueberries, strawberries, and celery. All should be washed with cold water before eating. This is a reason that people are drawn to buying foods that are 100% organically grown.

Source: Preidt R. Pesticides linked to ADHD, study says. HealthDay. Available at: http://www.webmd.com/add-adhd/childhood-adhd/news/20150603/pesticides-linked-to-adhd-study-says. Accessed May 17, 2017.

🔍 CASE STUDY

Amy was raised in a small city in Indiana and has had a traditional MD who served as her physician since she was a young girl. She is now 27 years old and has moved to another state. The MD that she saw in this new city seemed cold and impersonal. He gave her little time in the office and did not ask her how she felt about taking medicine that he prescribed for her health problems. A friend convinced Amy to go see a more holistic doctor, a naturopathic physician. Amy made an appointment and went to the new physician the next week. He spent a lot of time with Amy getting to know her and to diagnose her health problems. In addition, the naturopathic physician gave her several treatment options. Rather than being perceived as impersonal and ineffective, Amy felt the naturopathic physician was warm and understanding, and she liked feeling empowered to make treatment choices.

Questions:

1. Are the qualities of being warm and understanding ones that you would treasure in a doctor?
2. Do you like the idea of being given treatment choices or options? Why or why not?

▶ What Are the Barriers to CAM Use?

Several barriers to CAM use have been identified. Although insurance coverage is increasing for CAM therapies, there are still many that are not covered by insurance companies; therefore, expense is a barrier. Another barrier is lack of knowledge. Many people do not have knowledge of alternative practices and are skeptical about their efficacy. They may also fear that alternative therapies are harmful. Even though a lot of people use herbal supplements, many are confused as to why research does not show positive results. One of the reasons is that many herbals contain several ingredients that give synergistic effects, but only one ingredient is researched at one time, and therefore, does not account for the entire supplement.[12]

In sum, we have determined that a lot of people are using CAM and that, without insurance, it is costly. People have varying reasons for using alternative medicine, and certainly there are barriers preventing CAM usage. It seems that people who use CAM want to be a part of the healing process.

▶ What Is Integrative Medicine and Health Care?

Integrative medicine and health units are being implemented into hospitals all over the nation. Many people, however, remain uncertain about the definitions of integrative medicine and integrative health. The NCCIH defines **integrative medicine or integrative health care** as "bringing conventional and complementary approaches together in a coordinated way."[13] Dr. Andrew Weil, MD, is a Harvard-trained doctor and a botanist who has incorporated alternative medicine into his medical practice for years (more about him later in this chapter). Dr. Weil has a wonderful explanation for integrative medicine:

> Integrative medicine is healing-oriented medicine that takes account of the whole person (body, mind, and spirit), including all aspects of lifestyle. It emphasizes the therapeutic relationship and makes use of all appropriate therapies, both conventional and alternative.[14]

The knowledge and use of CAM is an important aspect of integrative medicine and health that helps attain a more in-depth understanding of the nature of illness, healing, and wellness. Integrative medicine has been described by Snyderman and Weil[15] as a movement driven by consumers who sought alternative healing methods. Eventually, integrative medicine gained the attention of academic health centers. In May 2004, an outcome of the integrative medicine and alternative health care movement was the formation of a national consortium, the Academic Consortium for Integrative Medicine & Health.[16] The membership consists of 57 highly reputable academic centers and is supported by membership dues and grants from partners such as the **Bravewell Collaborative**. See **BOX 6.1** for full list of U.S. members. In this table, asterisks indicate that a particular member is a health system and not an academic institution.

Another outcome of the integrative medicine movement was a national summit convened by the Bravewell Collaborative and the Institute of Medicine

BOX 6.1 Academic Consortium for Integrative Medicine & Health

Arizona
University of Arizona
http://integrativemedicine.arizona.edu/education/index.html

California
Scripps Center for Integrative Medicine*
http://www.scripps.org/services/integrative-medicine
Stanford University School of Medicine
http://stanfordhospital.org/clinicsmedServices/clinics/complementaryMedicine/
Sutter Health, Institute for Health & Healing*
http://www.sutterpacific.org/services/integrative/
University of California, Irvine
http://www.sscim.uci.edu
University of California, Los Angeles
http://cewm.med.ucla.edu
University of California, San Diego
http://cim.ucsd.edu
University of California, San Francisco
http://www.osher.ucsf.edu
University of Southern California
http://integrativehealth.usc.edu/

Colorado
University of Colorado School of Medicine, Denver
http://www.uch.edu/integrativemed

Connecticut
University of Connecticut Health Center
http://picim.uchc.edu
Yale University School of Medicine
http://cam.yale.edu

District of Columbia
George Washington University
https://smhs.gwu.edu/integrative-medicine/
Georgetown University School of Medicine
http://cam.georgetown.edu
Veterans Health Administration*
http://www.va.gov/health/

Florida
University of Miami
http://cim.med.miami.edu

Georgia
Emory University School of Medicine
http://med.emory.edu/index.html

Hawaii
University of Hawaii at Mānoa
http://jabsom.hawaii.edu/departments/cim/

Illinois
Northwestern University Feinberg School of Medicine
http://www.feinberg.northwestern.edu/sites/ocim/index.html

University of Chicago Pritzker School of Medicine
http://www.northshore.org/integrative

Kansas
University of Kansas Medical Center
http://integrativemed.kumc.edu/

Kentucky
University of Kentucky Integrative Medicine and Health
http://ukhealthcare.uky.edu/IM/

Maine
Central Maine Healthcare*
https://secure.cmmc.org/

Maryland
Johns Hopkins University School of Medicine
http://www.hopkinsmedicine.org/cam
MedStar Health*
http://www.medstarmontgomery.org/our-services/integrative-medicine/#q={}
University of Maryland
http://www.cim.umaryland.edu

Massachusetts
Boston University School of Medicine
http://www.bu.edu/integrativemed/
Harvard Medical School
http://www.osher.hms.harvard.edu
Tufts University School of Medicine
http://www.tufts.edu/med/
University of Massachusetts Medical School
http://www.umassmed.edu/cfm/index.aspx

Michigan
Beaumont Health*
http://www.beaumont.edu/
University of Michigan
http://www.med.umich.edu/umim

Minnesota
Allina Health, Abbott Northwestern Hospital*
http://www.allinahealth.org
Mayo Clinic
http://mayoresearch.mayo.edu/mayo/research/cimp/
University of Minnesota
http://www.csh.umn.edu

New Jersey
Hackensack Meridian Health*
https://www.meridianhealth.com/index.aspx
Rutgers Biomedical and Health Sciences
http://www.shrp.rutgers.edu/dept/primary_care/ICAM

New Mexico
University of New Mexico, School of Medicine
http://unmmg.org/clinics/cfl/

(continues)

BOX 6.1 *(continued)*

New York
Albert Einstein College of Medicine of Yeshiva
    University
    https://www.einstein.yu.edu/features/stories/802
    /integrative-medicine-at-einstein/
Columbia University Medical Center
    http://www.cumc.columbia.edu/
Icahn School of Medicine at Mount Sinai
    http://www.healthandhealingny.org/Institute
    /educational-programs/default.aspx
Memorial Sloan Kettering*
    https://www.mskcc.org/cancer-care/treatments
    /symptom-management/integrative-medicine
NYU Langone Health
    https://nyulangone.org/
Weill Cornell Medicine
    https://weillcornell.org/integrative
    -health-program

North Carolina
Duke University
    http://www.dukeintegrativemedicine.org
University of North Carolina at Chapel Hill
    http://pim.med.unc.edu
Wake Forest® Baptist Health, Center for Integrative
    Medicine
    http://www.wakehealth.edu/Center-for-Integrative
    -Medicine/

Ohio
Cleveland Clinic
    http://my.clevelandclinic.org/services/wellness
    /integrative-medicine
The Ohio State University
    http://wexnermedical.osu.edu/patient-care/healthcare
    -services/integrative-complementary-medicine
UH Connor Integrative Health Network*
    http://www.uhhospitals.org/services/integrative
    -medicine
University of Cincinnati College of Medicine
    http://www.med.uc.edu/integrativehealth

Oregon
Oregon Health & Science University
    http://www.ohsu.edu/xd/health/services/women
    /services/complementary-medicine.cfm

Pennsylvania
Milton S. Hershey Medical Center
    http://www.pennstatehershey.org/web/guest/home
Temple University School of Medicine
    http://www.temple.edu/medicine/education
    /mdprograms/medical_education/curriculum
    _overview.htm
Thomas Jefferson University, Marcus Institute of
    Integrative Health
    http://marcusinstitute.jeffersonhealth.org/about.html
University of Pennsylvania
    http://www.med.upenn.edu
University of Pittsburgh
    http://www.upmc.com/Services/integrative
    -medicine/Pages/experts.aspx

Tennessee
Vanderbilt University
    http://www.vanderbilthealth.com/osher/

Texas
Texas Tech University Health Sciences Center
    http://www.ttuhsc.edu/som/fammed/divisions
    /integrativemed.aspx
The University of Texas MD Anderson Cancer Cente
    http://www.mdanderson.org/integrativemed
University of Texas Medical Branch
    http://cim.utmb.edu

Utah
University of Utah
    http://www.utah.edu/

Vermont
University of Vermont Larner College of Medicine
    http://www.uvm.edu/medicine/pih/

Washington
University of Washington: UW Integrative Health Program
    http://www.uwmedicine.org/

Wisconsin
Aurora Health Care*
    https://medicalprofessionals.aurorahealthcare.org
    /meded/index.asp
University of Wisconsin-Madison
    http://www.fammed.wisc.edu/integrative

*Member is a health system and is not an academic institution.

Source: Academic Consortium for Integrative Medicine & Health. Member Listing. Available at: http://www.imconsortium.org/members/members.cfm. Accessed May 18, 2017.

in February 2009 to explore integrative medicine's potential to improve the U.S. healthcare system.[17] A quote from the summit chair, Ralph Snyderman, MD, Chancellor Emeritus of Duke University School of Medicine, describes how he views integrative medicine: "The integrative approach flips the healthcare system on its head and puts the patient at the center, addressing not just symptoms, but the real causes of illness. It is care that is preventive, predictive and personalized."[17]

As described, integrated medicine and integrative health care may be bringing a change to how medical professionals and individuals view health and the treatment of illness. Now that the meaning of

🔍 CASE STUDY

Tom lives in Madison, Wisconsin, and is a graduate student in business at the University of Wisconsin. Over spring break, Tom went skiing at a ski resort in the Upper Peninsula of Michigan. He fell while skiing and is now experiencing a great amount of lower back pain and muscle spasms. Tom went to health services on campus and was seen by the university physician. A series of X-rays and an MRI was done. No spinal disc injury was apparent by X-ray, so the doctor diagnosed Tom with spinal **facet joint** injury. Facet joints are the bony projections on the back of the spine. The doctor told Tom that his injury would require rest, heat, and nonsteroidal anti-inflammatory drugs. Furthermore, the doctor told Tom that the university had an Integrative Medicine unit where he could seek some sort of alternative therapy that might help with the muscle spasms and pain. The doctor recommended that Tom see an acupuncturist or the campus chiropractor. Acupuncture is a Chinese technique that involves placing very tiny needles in certain areas of the body to decrease pain from an injury. Tom does not know that much about either therapy and is somewhat apprehensive about them.

Questions:
1. Where could Tom acquire information about both therapies, including results of scientific research studies?
2. What could Tom's doctor say to alleviate Tom's concerns?
3. Where could Tom gain more information about the campus Integrative Medicine clinic?

integrative medicine and integrative health has been introduced, where does one go to get integrated medical care and what are the integrated medicine organizational structures?

▶ What Is the Organizational Structure of Integrated Medicine and Health?

Most integrative medicine and health clinics are located in a hospital setting. Integrative health care, however, may be implemented at doctor's offices or clinics. Some doctors set up an integrative medicine network within a community as they refer their own patients to alternative practitioners (e.g., chiropractors, acupuncturists, massage therapists). Integrative medicine and health structural models have some common characteristics. They embrace the best of both scientific-based medicine and evidence-validated alternative methods. They aim for a patient-centered and interdisciplinary mix of traditional and alternative medical treatments. They may involve individual case management of patients while using several types of healing practitioners. For example, an integrative medicine clinic in Sweden involved a senior researcher, a doctoral student, a general practitioner, and eight complementary therapy providers—massage therapists, **naprapath** (treats connective tissue disorders), shiatsu therapists (Japanese massage and bodywork), an acupuncturist, and a **qigong** therapist (energy healing).[18]

▶ Who Were the Early Pioneers Promoting Integrative Medicine and Health?

Several key **biomedical physicians (or biomedical scientists)** have paved the way for the acceptance of several CAM therapies. A few early pioneers are described in the following sections.

Herbert Benson, MD

The first is Dr. Herbert Benson, a cardiologist and professor at Harvard Medical School (**FIGURE 6.4**). In the late 1960s, Dr. Benson conducted research using monkeys that linked stress to physical health. At that time, this idea was contrary to existing medical thought.[19] Later, Dr. Benson and a colleague, Robert Wallace, researched the effects of **Transcendental Meditation® (TM)** on blood pressure. Benson and Wallace found that subjects who practiced TM, and who were able to change thought patterns, experienced decreases in their metabolism, rate of breathing, and heart rate, and had slower brain waves. They believed the technique was useful for treating conditions such as insomnia, anxiety, hypertension, and chronic pain. Dr. Benson studied other meditative techniques (e.g., diaphragmatic breathing, repetitive prayer, qigong, tai chi, yoga, progressive muscle relaxation, jogging, and even knitting) that he found also produced a relaxed state. He labeled it the "relaxation response," which is the foundation of mind–body medicine.

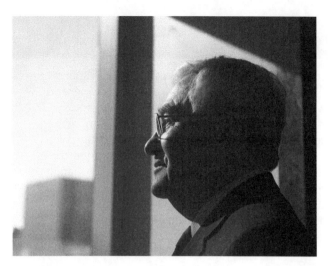

FIGURE 6.4 Herbert Benson, MD.
© Suzanne Kreiter/The Boston Globe/Getty Images

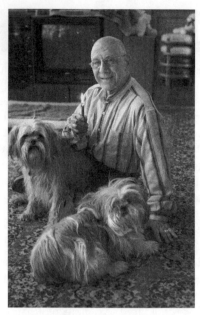

FIGURE 6.5 Bernard (Bernie) Siegel, MD.
With permission from Dr. Bernard Siegel

In 1975, Dr. Benson published a book, *The Relaxation Response*, and since then has published 10 other books focusing on the mind–body connection. Dr. Benson is the founder of the Benson-Henry Institute (BHI) for Mind/Body Medicine at Massachusetts General Hospital. He was formerly the director of BHI and an associate professor of Medicine, Harvard Medical School and remains active in giving live workshops on mind–body medicine.

David Eisenberg, MD

Another key individual is Dr. David Eisenberg, who was the first U.S. medical exchange student to the People's Republic of China. There, he mastered Chinese and attended the Beijing College of Traditional Chinese Medicine while learning Eastern healing modalities (e.g., acupuncture, tai chi). In 1993, he was the medical advisor to the PBS series *Healing and the Mind* with Bill Moyers. Dr. Eisenberg became an MD specializing in internal medicine and joined the faculty at Harvard. He directed two large national U.S. surveys on the use of CAM therapies; wrote a text *Encounters with Qi*; and has published many scientific data-based research studies. Currently, Dr. Eisenberg is the director of Harvard Medical School's Osher Research Center and is the program director of Integrative Medicine at Brigham and Women's Hospital in Boston, Massachusetts.[20]

Bernard Siegel, MD

An early pioneer is Dr. Bernard (Bernie) Siegel (**FIGURE 6.5**), a physician who graduated with honors from Cornell University Medical College. Dr. Siegel practiced medicine for many years and was a general and pediatric surgeon until he retired. He spent much of his life teaching techniques to help cancer patients use their own body energy to help in the healing process, techniques such as meditation and positive imagery. He also believes in using humor as a healing technique. To further his belief in patients' self-healing power, he founded ECaP (Exceptional Cancer Patients) a type of individual and group therapy support that uses drawings, dreams, positive imagery, and other holistic methods. Dr. Siegel has published several best-selling books promoting holistic healing methods, including *Love, Medicine and Miracles*; *Peace, Love & Healing*; and *How to Live Between Office Visits*.[21]

Andrew Weil, MD

Perhaps, one of the best-known key pioneers is Andrew Weil, MD, a Harvard-trained physician (**FIGURE 6.6**). Dr. Weil became a clinical professor at the University of Arizona Medical Center in 1983. While there, he established the Foundation for Integrative Medicine, and in 1994, Dr. Weil founded the Program in Integrative Medicine. Now, it is known as the Arizona Center for Integrative Medicine, and Dr. Weil is the program director.[22] Through his speeches, television appearances, and writings by way of news articles and texts, Dr. Weil's views about CAM therapies and integrative medicine have gained widespread acceptance. His website features "Ask Dr. Weil," a popular venue accessed by individuals wanting information about CAM therapies, including **botanicals**.

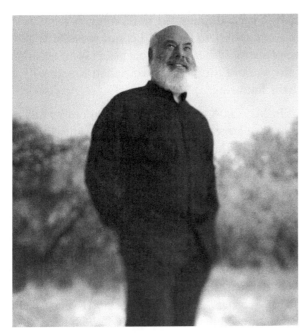

FIGURE 6.6 Andrew Weil, MD.

Courtesy of Weil Lifestyle, LLC

Deepak Chopra, MD

Dr. Deepak Chopra (**FIGURE 6.7**) has done much to promote integrative medicine and is well known and respected worldwide. Dr. Chopra is an Indian-trained biomedical physician, who also completed an internship and several residencies and fellowships at university-affiliated medical centers in Boston.[23] He is cofounder of the Chopra Center for Wellbeing, where he serves as the director of education.[23] The Chopra Center offers training programs in physical, emotional, and spiritual healing. Dr. Chopra gives workshops utilizing Ayurveda medicine modalities and practical tools of mind–body healing such as energy healing, guided meditation, visualization, and writing

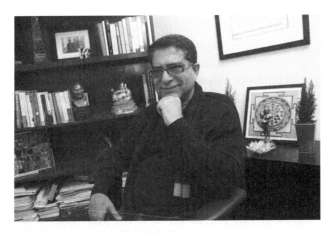

FIGURE 6.7 Deepak Chopra, MD.

© Diane Bondareff/AP Photos

◫ *IN THE NEWS*

Dr. Deepak Chopra, along with special guest, Dr. Andrew Weil were featured in a news article promoting a workshop titled "Journey into Healing: What Are You Hungry For?" The workshop was held from March 6 to March 9, 2013, in Carlsbad, California, at the Omni La Costa Resort. The workshop was based on a mind-body-spirit approach for those wanting to lose weight and get healthier in mind and spirit.[24]

Source: PRWeb News Center. Deepak Chopra and Andrew Weil to lead "Journey into healing: What are you hungry for?" workshop this March at the Omni La Costa Resort in Carlsbad, CA. Available at: http://www.prweb.com/releases/journeyintohealing/chopraandweil/prweb11370230.htm. Accessed May 24, 2017.

exercises.[23] Dr. Chopra is the author of more than 50 books and more than 100 audio, video, and CD-ROM titles. He has been published on every continent and in dozens of languages.

Because of these reputable and respected individuals, integrative medicine programs have been established at dozens of institutions (refer to Table 6.1). The medical profession seems to be selectively embracing CAM in the clinical setting, which has benefited patients by increasing access to many forms of alternative therapies/medicine. An additional potential benefit is that patients going to orthodox physicians will be more likely to disclose the CAM therapies that they are using, especially herbal medicines that could potentially interact with prescription drugs.

▸ What Are the Historical Milestones of Integrative Medicine and Health?

Development of Wellness Programs

The journey to integrative medicine began with the development of wellness programs in which people became more proactive about preventing diseases and taking responsibility for their own health. During the 1950s, there were only a few wellness programs. Halbert Dunn was one of the first to develop employee wellness programs in the 1950s.[25] Several wellness programs were developed during the 1960s and 1970s, and "wellness" became a buzzword as people became aware of the benefits of exercise and nutrition in preventing high cholesterol levels, heart attacks, and stroke.

During the 1980s, additional wellness programs were being developed, such as the 1982 "wellness awareness" training program developed by Teamster leaders in Orange County, Florida, so that they could decrease the cost of their union's health insurance program.

During the 1990s, even more companies began to develop wellness programs as an incentive to their employees to lose excess pounds and to quit smoking.

Development of Health Promotion Programs

A 1990 study by Dean Ornish, MD, showed that lifestyle changes can eventually reverse heart disease.[26] This study gave legitimacy to wellness programs, and they proliferated in the 1990s and 2000s. By this time, the programs began to be called "health promotion programs," because many more strategies than educational programs were being incorporated into the programming (e.g., use of media, health fairs, laws, etc.). In addition to worksites, schools, universities, medical centers, hospitals, community health departments, and state health departments were implementing health promotion programs. The importance of wellness and health promotion programs is that people began to be enthusiastic about the value and benefits of a healthy lifestyle. People began to investigate ways to make themselves feel better through rest, stress management, exercise, and better eating habits. All of this paved the way for a natural progression of examining other treatment modalities, many of which came from European and Eastern countries.

At the governmental level, two extremely important developments occurred: the establishment of the NCCIH and the formation of the White House Commission on Complementary and Alternative Medicine Policy.

Establishment of the National Center for Complementary and Integrative Health

The establishment of the NCCIH, is one of the most important milestones that give scientific credence to select CAM practices. The NCCIH was first created in 1992, but began as the Office of Alternative Medicine (OAM). At that time, the U.S. Congress passed legislation (Public Law 102-170) to provide $2 million to establish the OAM to assess the worth of promising unconventional medical practices. By 1999, Congress updated the status of the OAM to become the National Center for Complementary and Alternative Medicine (NCCAM). In 2014, the NCCAM became the present day NCCIH.[27] Even though the name has

changed several times, the main mission remains the same and that is to fund and conduct research about complementary health approaches.[28] Some examples of the work of the NCCIH from their timeline[29] page are the following:

- In May 2004, the NCCAM announced its findings from a large national survey about Americans' use of CAM. This was a part of the 2002 NHIS.
- In December 2008, the NCCAM released data regarding children's use of CAM and assessed trends in adult CAM use.
- In July 2009, the NCCAM revealed the results of a 2007 national study regarding the amount of money Americans spend on CAM annually: nearly $34 billion out of the pocket, of which about two-thirds was for self-care.
- In February, 2015, the NCCIH and NCHS announced the 2012 findings of the NHIS.

▶ The White House Commission on Complementary and Alternative Medicine Policy

In March 2000, President Clinton appointed 20 people (physicians, registered nurses, PhDs, CAM practitioners) to the White House Commission on Complementary and Alternative Medicine Policy.[30] The commission was to make legislative and administrative recommendations to aid public policy in ensuring the safety of products and practices that had been, or might be, labeled "CAM" and to identify potential benefits for the public. After 18 months of reviewing a thousand papers on CAM use and listening to over 700 testimonies about CAM, several recommendations about the role of the federal government emerged.[30] They are summarized as follows:

The federal government should disclose research findings; ensure the safety of products; help assess the appropriate levels of training of various CAM practitioners and the research regarding their practice; aid in evaluating the different ways that states are regulating CAM practitioners; and facilitate dialogue among CAM and conventional providers, scientists, and the public. The report also emphasized that states can take a leadership role in the regulation of CAM practitioners and orthodox practitioners who incorporate CAM into their practices.

What Changes Have Occurred in Medical Care and Education?

The White House Commission on Complementary and Alternative Medicine Policy is advocating that the education and training of conventional health professionals should include CAM and that the training of CAM practitioners should include conventional health care.[30] Medical schools throughout the country have ongoing initiatives in integrative medicine. As previously discussed, 57 medical centers and agencies formed the Consortium of Academic Health Centers for Integrative Medicine.

Cowen and Cyr[31] analyzed the curriculum of 130 U.S. medical schools and found that half of the schools offered at least one CAM course. **TABLE 6.1** lists their findings.[31]

Several health professionals have outlined CAM educational curricula needs: (1) focus on critical thinking and critical reading of the literature; (2) identify thematic content and express topics in clear language; (3) formulate concise learning objectives; (4) include an experiential component; (5) promote a willingness to communicate professionally with CAM clinicians; and (6) teach students to talk with patients about alternative therapies. Brokaw and colleagues.[32] advocate that CAM studies should emphasize a critical evaluation of the scientific literature, should enlist the involvement of basic science departments, and should avoid advocacy of unproven therapies. Furthermore, the Society of General Internal Medicine (SGIM) has outlined its view of what CAM education should be in a position paper published in 2008.[33] The SGIM laid out primary goals for physicians regarding CAM practices so that they could better understand the basic theories, benefits, risks, evidence basis for therapies, and how to adopt a nonjudgmental attitude about CAM to enhance their patient–doctor relationships. Secondary goals of the SGIM were to help patients integrate CAM and conventional therapies at appropriate times.

▶ How Do Practicing Physicians View CAM?

A sign that physicians are more accepting of CAM therapies is that many are referring their patients to alternative practitioners such as chiropractors, massage therapists, acupuncturists, and other types of alternative practitioners. Over 50% of conventional physicians in the United States use or refer patients for some CAM treatments.[34,35,36] Other

TABLE 6.1 Topics Included in Medical School Courses

Topic	Number of Courses Containing Topic	Percentage
CAM	40	31.5
Traditional medicine	25	19.7
Acupuncture	22	17.3
Meditation	21	16.5
Spirituality	18	14.2
Herbs	17	13.4
Massage	14	11.0
Energy medicine	14	11.0
Chiropractic	10	7.9
Osteopath	10	7.9
Yoga	9	7.1
Biofeedback	7	4.7
Hypnosis	5	3.9
Creative arts therapies*	5	1.6
Tai Chi	2	3.9
Naturopathy	2	1.6

*Reference to music or dance therapy, fine arts, poetry, or writing was indicated in the course topics.

Abbreviations: CAM, complementary and alternative medicine.

Source: Cowen V, Cyr V. Complementary and alternative medicine in US medical schools. *Adv Med Educ Pract.* 2015; 6:113-117. Available at: https://www.dovepress.com/complementary-and-alternative-medicine-in-us-medical-schools-peer-reviewed-article-AMEP. Accessed July 15, 2018.

professions (e.g., psychotherapy) are also beginning to incorporate certain alternative therapies within the treatment regimen. Most perceive them as having efficacy,[35] are interested in learning more about the therapies, and have generally positive attitudes toward alternative medical practices.[35] The American Medical Association has issued a proclamation to all members encouraging them to become involved in the scientific evaluation of alternative medicine.

Historically, the traditional or conventional field of medicine (i.e., **biomedicine**) rigorously opposed and ridiculed many CAM therapies.[34] A part of the opposition may have stemmed from the belief that the client's (patient's) role was to be compliant, to not question, and to be accepting of what the doctor prescribed. The physician's role was to be the authoritative and all-knowing figure in the client–doctor relationship. Disease was only considered to be the result of a **pathogen** entering the body, and treatments of disease consisted mainly of treating the symptoms with medications (e.g., antibiotics for bacterial infections) and surgery. Doctors did not typically sit with patients and explain ways in which they could help themselves in the healing process.

The acquisition and the healing of diseases, however, is a complicated process and often requires more than traditional therapies.[37] Many alternative health practices help an individual to self-heal (e.g., meditation, biofeedback, imagery, and more). Healing requires a harmony of the mind, body, and spirit and a healthy lifestyle (good nutrition, physical exercise, stress management, restful sleep, etc.). Positive health practices will aid the person who does get ill and will help them achieve a higher level of wellness faster. One of the most important concepts to understand is that people heal in different ways, that is, what works well for one person may not work for another.

▶ What Changes Have Occurred in Insurance Coverage for CAM or Integrated Health Care?

The Affordable Care Act mandates that certain licensed health care practitioners such as massage therapist and acupuncturists should not be discriminated against, but the Act does not require that the insurance company is mandated to cover the payment. Some health plans cover chiropractic, acupuncture, traditional Chinese medicine, homeopathy (provided by a licensed physician), naturopathy, and massage, whereas others offer only chiropractic care.[38] Additionally, many state legislatures have begun to mandate insurance coverage (e.g., Washington State mandates chiropractic coverage). Insurance companies do recognize that more people are seeking out alternative practitioners and are responding to that by offering health insurance.

A program that Medicare agreed to cover is Dr. Dean Ornish's lifestyle program. His many years of clinical research demonstrated that comprehensive lifestyle changes (e.g., exercise, nutrition) may begin to reverse even severe coronary heart disease without using drugs or surgery.[39] Dr. Ornish conducted a more recent **randomized controlled study** that demonstrated how comprehensive lifestyle changes may stop or reverse the progression of prostate cancer. His explanation is that comprehensive lifestyle changes affect gene expression—"turning on" disease-preventing genes and "turning off" genes that promote cancer and heart disease.

If you are unsure about coverage, you should contact your insurance company and ask. Some insurance companies require a referral from an MD and you should request that information. Some other details that you should obtain are as follows:

- Do you need to co-pay?
- Do you have to meet a deductible?
- How many visits can you make or are you limited?
- Do you have to stick with practitioners in your local network?

It is true that a large percentage of individuals are seeking CAM practitioners and would like health insurance coverage, but is it cost effective? A study presented at a conference in the Netherlands[36] found that integrated medicine was cost effective. Two U.S. studies of economic evaluations of CAM also found some positive results,[40,41,42] but much more research needs to be conducted before declaring that integrated medicine is cost effective.

Although the government-sponsored Medicare program is quite selective about CAM funding, private insurance companies more than likely will compete if there is evidence of profitability. Companies want to be sure that they will save money on use of complementary therapies relative to conventional therapies. Meanwhile, a benefit of potential increased insurance coverage may motivate CAM practitioners to standardize their diagnostics and treatments in order to receive reimbursement.

▶ What Is the Future of Integrative Medicine?

The term "integrative medicine" is catching on in medical circles, and medical schools are integrating CAM courses into their curricula. MDs and other health care professionals are learning more about holistic ways of healing and holistic lifestyles. Physicians are learning much more about traditional Chinese medicine and how to incorporate acupuncture into their practices. New kinds of health institutes are being built such as healing centers (hybrids between spas and clinics) that address lifestyle issues. Centers for the practice of meditation are proliferating. There is broader insurance coverage for CAM practices and more innovative research. Lay people as well as physicians are learning more about botanicals—their functions and effects.

- University of Arizona
- Bastyr University
- University of North Carolina, Chapel Hill
- Harvard Medical School
- Morgan State University
- Oregon Health & Science University
- Pennington Biomedical Research Center
- University of California, San Francisco
- University of Virginia
- Weill Cornell Medical College

National Center for Complementary and Integrative Health. NCCIH-funded Ruth L. Kirschstein National Research Service Award (NRSA) Institutional Training Grant Programs (T32s). Available at: https://nccih.nih.gov/training/t32. Accessed July 24, 2018.

Postdoctoral fellowships are being instituted. The Bravewell Collaborative, the National Institute of Nursing Research, and the National Institutes of Health Clinical Center sponsored a BNC Fellowship for research in integrative medicine in 2006, 2008, and 2010.[43] Fellows attended the University of Arizona's Program in Integrative Medicine and were involved in an integrative medicine–related research project at the NIH campus in Bethesda, Maryland. The Osher Center for Integrative Medicine at Northwestern University offers postdoctoral fellowship in integrative medicine.[44] The NCCIH funds postdoc programs through the Ruth L Kirschstein National Research Service Award institutional training grant programs.[45] Universities collaborating with this program are listed in **BOX 6.2**.

New and innovative proposals related to integrative medicine are being formulated. One proposal is that a new NIH institute be formed: a National Institute of Healing. This type of institute or center could investigate all healing phenomena, spontaneous remissions of cancer, and other diseases. Some are proposing that a National Registry of Healing, classified by disease, should be developed. The future of integrative medicine appears to be bright. We all should hope that whatever occurs, integrative medicine will be evidence-based and truly used in ways that optimize health.

▶ What Should Consumers Keep in Mind When Using Alternative Modalities?

We have determined that a lot of people are using CAM and that, without insurance, it is costly. People have varying reasons for using alternative medicine, and certainly there are barriers preventing CAM usage. Here, in the United States, our MDs are beginning to engage in CAM educational classes, are conducting research studies of CAM therapies, and are becoming skilled in selective CAM modalities (e.g., acupuncture). Integrative medicine and health clinics are being implemented in many hospitals and universities across the nation. We should be responsible consumers of our health care when making decisions while selecting alternative health care therapies. We can do much to advance safe integrative medicine practices by researching a particular integrative medicine clinic. Certainly, the number and type of traditional and alternative practitioners should be identified. We should learn the academic background of each individual. Often, the backgrounds of all physicians and therapists may be obtained online or in brochures or pamphlets produced by the clinic.

It is our responsibility to also research all the "natural and holistic approaches" to health and healing offered by the site. Certainly, anyone who uses herbal supplements, or is engaging in an alternative therapy, should inform their family physician. If you believe that you will use, or are using an alternative therapy, you should ask your health insurance company if it covers any alternative therapies. Most of all, you should be an informed **consumer** of both traditional and alternative therapies.

▶ The Informed Consumer: Applying the Concepts Learned to Your Daily Life

Thus far, you have received some information regarding the meaning of integrative medicine and some of the past resistance to it.

- Do you feel that this resistance was legitimate? Why or why not?
- If you are asked to be a student member of a committee at your university to explore the viability of developing an integrative medicine clinic, what advice would you offer to fellow committee members?
- Do you think the university group healthcare plans should cover integrative medicine practices?
- What information could you give committee members about the NCCIH?
- Do you think that faculty, staff, and students at your university would be accepting of an integrative medicine clinic? Why or why not?

▶ Conclusion

This chapter was intended to raise your awareness and knowledge about CAM use, integrative medicine, the development of integrative medicine and health clinics, and the early pioneers who advocated for alternative medicine. A historical timeline of events leading to a more holistic type of health care was also presented. Hopefully, you will become a responsible consumer of your own health care when the time comes for you to select your physicians and other health care providers.

Wrap-Up

Key Terms

Acupuncture A traditional Chinese medicine treatment that uses stainless steel needles at specific points in the body to increase the flow of life energy known as Qi or Chi.

Ayurveda A traditional system of medicine of India. The word *Ayurveda* is a Sanskrit word that means science of life or sciences of lifespan.

Biofeedback The technique used to train people to control their own involuntary body processes such as heart rate, respirations, and even brain waves. It requires watching a monitor of some sort in order to change the rate using mental control.

Biomedical physician (or biomedical scientist) These physicians apply research in many fields related to life sciences or body processes (anatomy and physiology, biology, pathology). They research the process of disease causation and attempt to find new treatment modalities.

Biomedicine The application of the principles of the natural sciences, especially biology and physiology, to clinical medicine.

Botanicals Substances obtained from plants.

Bravewell Collaborative Founded in 2002 by a small group of leading philanthropists dedicated to transforming the culture and delivery of health care and improving the health of the public through integrative medicine.

Chronic Refers to an illness or medical condition that is characterized by long duration or frequent recurrence.

Complementary and alternative medicine (CAM) A group of diverse medical and healthcare systems, practices, and products that are not generally considered to be part of conventional medicine (NCCIH definition).

Consumer A person who buys and uses goods. In this text, it means the person who buys and uses health-related goods.

Facet joints These are synovial joints that help support the weight and control movement between individual vertebrae of the spine. Facet joints are at the back on either side of the spinal column, between the discs and the vertebral bodies. The bony prominences of each vertebra form a joint with the vertebrae above and below. The role of the facet joints is to limit excessive movement and provide stability for the spine.

Homeopathic medicine Medicines prepared by extreme dilution. The fundamental concept of homeopathic is that "like cures like." Substances in the preparations are thought to stimulate the body's own healing response.

Integrative medicine or integrative health care Combines treatments from conventional medicine and CAM for which there is evidence of safety and effectiveness. Bringing conventional and complementary approaches together in a coordinated way is the healing-oriented medicine that takes account of the whole person (body, mind, and spirit), including all aspects of lifestyle.

Naturopathic medicine A system of medical practices that relies on more natural healing methods (herbs, massage, exercise). It encompasses a belief in the body's ability to heal itself.

Naprapath A person who treats connective tissue disorders

Pathogen A disease-causing germ such as bacteria, virus, or fungus. A disease-producing agent such as a virus, bacterium, or other microorganism.

Qi (chi) According to traditional Chinese medicine, qi is a bodily energy that flows through unseen channels in the body called meridians. Illness is believed to occur when qi is blocked.

Qigong A type of energy therapy that uses movement, breathing techniques, and meditation to enhance and move Qi throughout the body. This is purported to improve health and overall life energy.

Randomized controlled study A study in which the people involved are randomly drawn from a population and then assigned to a treatment protocol by a random draw.

Transcendental A belief in the supernatural; a belief in miracles; a belief in the spiritual.

Transcendental Meditation® (TM) A technique wherein people repeat a phrase to help themselves relax during medication.

Suggestions for Class Activities

1. Research your county (parish) or several cities in your county (parish) to assess if there are any established integrative medicine clinics.
2. Visit an integrative medicine clinic and report on your findings.
3. Conduct a short knowledge and attitude survey on your campus related to integrative medicine and report the findings to your class.

Review Questions

1. What are the numbers of CAM users and what demographic population uses CAM?
2. Name and explain several barriers to using CAM?
3. How much money is spent out of pocket on CAM
4. What is the definition of integrative medicine?
5. What are integrative medicine clinics?
6. What have been the reasons for past resistance to alternative medicine and integrated care?
7. Who were the early pioneers promoting CAM and integrative medicine?
8. List and describe three historical milestones of integrative medicine?
9. Do you believe the Presidential Commission and/or the establishment of the NCCIH helped to expand CAM therapies? If so, how?
10. What changes have been made in medical care and medical education related to CAM?
11. How has insurance coverage for CAM care changed through the last 20 years?
12. What is the future of integrative medicine?
13. Should we, as health consumers (or patients), take responsibility regarding alternative health care? If yes, what should we be responsible for?
14. Is it correct to say that CAM users are "shopping for health"?
15. What is the name of the national CAM research center?

References

1. Clarke T, Black L, Stussman B, Barnes P, Nahin R. *National Health Statistics Reports, no. 79. Trends in the Use of Complementary Health Approaches Among Adults: United States, 2002–2012.* Hyattsville, MD: National Center for Health Statistics; 2015. Available at: https://www.cdc.gov/nchs/data/nhsr/nhsr079.pdf. Accessed April 9, 2018.
2. Centers for Disease Control and Prevention. *2012 National Health Interview Survey (NHIS): Adult Complementary and Alternative Medicine Public Use File (ALT).* Available at: ftp://ftp.cdc.gov/pub/Health_Statistics/NCHS/Dataset_Documentation/NHIS/2012/althealt_freq.pdf. Accessed April 9, 2018.
3. AARP Inc., National Center for Complementary and Integrative Health. *CAM Use. AARP/NCCAM Survey of U.S. Adults 50+, 2010.* Available at: https://nccih.nih.gov/news/camstats/2010/findings1.htm. Published April 13, 2010. Accessed April 9, 2018.
4. Nowak A, Daugherty A, O'Keefe R, Seward Jr S, Setty S, Tang F. Prevalence and predictors of complementary and alternative medicine (CAM) use among ivy league college students: Implications for student health services. *J Am Coll Health.* 2015;6(63):362-372.
5. Johnson S, Blanchard A. Alternative medicine and herbal use among university students. *J Am Coll Health.* 2006;55(3):163-168.
6. Synovitz L, Gillan W, Wood R, Nordness M, Kelly J. An exploration of college students' complementary and alternative medicine use: Relationship to health locus of control and spirituality level. *Am J Health Educ.* 2006;37(2):84-93.
7. Cutshal S, Derscheid D, Miers A, et al. Knowledge, attitudes, and use of complementary and alternative therapies among clinical nurse specialists in an academic medical center. *Clin Nurs Spec.* 2010;24(3):125-131.
8. National Center for Complementary and Integrative Health. *Americans Spend $30 Billion a Year Out-of-Pocket on Complementary Health Approaches.* Available at: https://nccih.nih.gov/research/results/spotlight/americans-spend-billions. Published June 22, 2016. Accessed April 9, 2018.
9. Astin J. Why patients use alternative medicine. *JAMA.* 1998;279(19):1548-1553.
10. Kaptchuk T, Eisenberg D. The persuasive appeal of alternative medicine. *Ann Intern Med.* 1998;129(12):1061-1065.
11. Preidt R. Pesticides linked to ADHD, study says. *HealthDay News.* June 3, 2015. Available at: http://www.webmd.com/add-adhd/childhood-adhd/news/20150603/pesticides-linked-to-adhd-study-says. Accessed April 9, 2018.
12. Fonta A. Patient perspectives: Barriers to complementary and alternative medicine therapies create problems for patients and survivors. *Integr Cancer Ther.* 2007;6(3):297-300.
13. National Center for Complementary and Integrative Health. *Complementary, Alternative or Integrative Health: What's In a Name?* Available at: https://nccih.nih.gov/health/integrative-health. Updated June 2016. Accessed April 9, 2018.
14. Weil A. What is integrative medicine? DrWeil.com. Available at: https://www.drweil.com/health-wellness/balanced-living/meet-dr-weil/what-is-integrative-medicine/. Accessed April 9, 2018.
15. Snyderman R, Weil AT. Integrative medicine: Bringing medicine back to its roots. *Arch Intern Med.* 2002;162(4):395-397.
16. Academic Consortium for Integrative Medicine & Health. *Member Listing.* Available at: http://www.imconsortium.org/members/members.cfm. Accessed April 9, 2018.
17. Bravewell Collaborative. The Summit on Integrative Medicine and the Health of the Public. February 2009. Available at: http://www.bravewell.org/transforming_healthcare/national_summit. Accessed April 9, 2018.
18. Sundberg T, Halpin J, Warenmark A, Falkenberg T. Towards a model for integrative medicine in Swedish primary care. *BMC Health Serv Res.* 2007;7:107.
19. Benson-Henry Institute for Mind Body Medicine. *About the Benson-Henry Institute for Mind Body Medicine.* Available at: http://www.massgeneral.org/bhi/. Accessed April 9, 2018.

20. Harvard TH Chan School of Public Health. Faculty and Research Directory; David Eisenberg. Available at: https://www.hsph.harvard.edu/david-eisenberg/. Accessed April 9, 2018.

21. Siegel B. *Accept, Retreat & Surrender: How to Heal Yourself.* Available at: http://www.shareguide.com/Siegel.html. Accessed April 9, 2018.

22. Arizona Center for Integrative Medicine. About the Center: Andrew Weil, MD. Available at: https://integrativemedicine.arizona.edu/about/directors/weil. Accessed April 9, 2018.

23. The Chopra Center. Deepak Chopra, MD: Co-founder of the Chopra Center for Wellbeing. Available at: https://www.chopra.com/bios/deepak-chopra. Accessed April 9, 2018.

24. Prweb News Center. Deepak Chopra and Andrew Weil to lead "Journey into healing: What are you hungry for?" workshop this March at the Omni La Costa Resort in Carlsbad, CA. Available at: http://www.prweb.com/releases/journeyintohealing/chopraandweil/prweb11370230.htm. Accessed April 9, 2018.

25. Global Wellness Institute. The History of Wellness. Available at: https://www.globalwellnessinstitute.org/history-of-wellness/. Accessed April 9, 2018.

26. Ornish D, Brown SE, Scherwitz LW, et al. Can lifestyle changes reverse coronary heart disease? The lifestyle heart trial. *Lancet.* 1990;336(8708):129-133.

27. National Center for Complementary and Integrative Health. *NIH Complementary and Integrative Health Agency Gets New Name.* Available at: https://nccih.nih.gov/news/press/12172014. Published December 17, 2014. Accessed April 9, 2018.

28. National Center for Complementary and Integrative Health. *About NCCIH: Mission.* Available at: https://nccih.nih.gov/about. Accessed April 9, 2018.

29. National Center for Complementary and Integrative Health. *NCCIH Timeline.* Available at: https://nccih.nih.gov/about/nccih-timeline. Accessed April 9, 2018.

30. White House Commission on Complementary and Alternative Medicine Policy. *Chapter 4: Education and Training of Health Care Practitioners.* Available at: http://govinfo.library.unt.edu/whccamp/pdfs/fr2002_document.pdf. Published March 2002. Accessed April 9, 2018.

31. Cowen V, Cyr V. Complementary and alternative medicine in US medical schools. *Adv Med Educ Pract.* 2015;6:113-117.

32. Brokaw JJ, Tunnicliff G, Raess BU, Saxon DW. The teaching of complementary and alternative medicine in U.S. medical schools: A survey of course directors. *Acad Med.* 2002;77(9):876-881.

33. SGIM CAM Interest Group. *Position Statement on CAM Education.* July 5, 2008. Available at: https://www.sgim.org/File%20Library/SGIM/Communities/Education/Resources/SGIM-CAM-Statement-7-5-08.pdf. Accessed April 9, 2018.

34. Levine M, Weber-Levine M, Mayberry R. Complementary and alternative medical practices: Training, experience, and attitudes of a primary care medical school faculty. *J Am Board Fam Pract.* 2003;16(4):318-326.

35. Boucher T, Lenz S. An organizational survey of physicians' attitudes about and practice of complementary and alternative medicine. *Altern Ther Health Med.* 1998;4(6):59-65.

36. Baer H. *Toward an Integrative Medicine: Merging Alternative Therapies with Biomedicine.* Walnut Creek, CA: AltaMira Press; 2004.

37. Eliopoulos C. *Integrating Conventional and Alternative Therapies: Holistic Care for Chronic Conditions.* St. Louis, MO: Mosby; 1999.

38. Renter E. Does your health insurance cover alternative medicine? *U.S. News Health Care.* March 9, 2015. Available at: http://health.usnews.com/health-news/health-insurance/articles/2015/03/09/does-your-health-insurance-cover-alternative-medicine. Accessed April 9, 2018.

39. Healthways. *Ornish Lifestyle Medicine™.* Available at: http://www.healthways.com/intensivecardiacrehab. Accessed April 9, 2018.

40. Baars EW. Cost-effectiveness and efficiency of CAM. Paper presented at: Complementary and Alternative Medicine-An investment in health; June 27, 2013. Brussels, Belgium. Available at: http://www.icmart.org/files/presentation_baars.pdf. Accessed April 9, 2018.

41. Herman P, Poindexter B, Witt C, Eisenberg D. Are complementary therapies and integrative care cost-effective? A systematic review of economic evaluations. *BMJ Open* 2012;2(5):e001046.

42. Tais S, Zoberg E. The economic evaluation of complementary and alternative medicine. *Nat Med J.* 2013;(5):2.

43. Bravewell Collaborative. The Bravewell Fellowship Program. Available at: http://www.bravewell.org/transforming_healthcare/models_for_change/bravewell_fellowship/. Accessed April 9, 2018.

44. Northwestern Medicine Feinberg School of Medicine. *Osher Center for Integrative Medicine at Northwestern University.* Available at: http://www.feinberg.northwestern.edu/sites/ocim/research/post-doctoral-fellowship.html. Accessed April 9, 2018.

45. National Center for Complementary and Integrative Health. *NCCIH-Funded Ruth L. Kirschstein National Research Service Award (NRSA) Institutional Training Grant Programs (T32s).* Available at: https://nccih.nih.gov/training/t32. Accessed April 9, 2018.

CHAPTER 7

Complementary and Alternative Health Care: Historical Foundations of Holistic Healing

▶ Introduction

Many people in the United States remain skeptical about Eastern and European medical practices, even though practitioners, doctors, and people in China, India, Korea, Greece, Italy, England, and other countries have used innumerable methodologies for centuries. To give you a glimpse into the past, a historical account is presented in this chapter preceded by the concepts of the healing process and the role of the healer. The chapter ends with a discussion of CAM as scientifically legitimate or not.

▶ What Is Healing and What Is the Healer's Role?

There is a distinction between the word "healing" and the word "cure." People with chronic illnesses may realize that they cannot be cured of the disease, but they want to feel as well as they possibly can, given the limitations of the disease. They consider factors other than the "elimination" of the disease, such as the kinds of adjustments they need to make in order to live with the disease. Healing means to use the mind, body, and spirit to control disease, promote a sense of well-being, and enhance the quality of life. A sense of well-being, comfort, and an integration of the body–mind–spirit are important characteristics of the healing process.

On the other hand, the healer role is an important aspect. The healer is the one who restores health or makes a person whole again. Compassion, empathy, touch, and caring are all significant aspects of the healer's role. Scientific knowledge and skill in performing caregiving activities are important foundations to a healing relationship between the healer and the patient. Clinicians and healthcare professionals use various healing approaches such as nurturing and caring, facilitating practices, assisting with transitions, promoting, and restoring balance of mind, and encouraging optimal functioning and quality of life. The healer needs to develop personal attributes in the area of respecting clients, listening, providing time, and trusting intuition. The healer needs to recognize his or her own strengths and limitations. In addition, the healer's role is to model positive health practices and to understand the role of the body, mind, and spirit in the healing process. Finally, the healer must recognize that the quality of self that he or she offers may be more significant to the healing process than the procedures that are performed.

The next portion of this chapter will help you understand some historical aspects of alternative and traditional healing modalities and the progression to current health consumer actions.

▶ What Are the Key Historical Healing Modalities Impacting Current Healing Practices?

Healing methods have been around since ancient times. The following is a historical overview of healing practitioners and methodologies that will include **shamanism**, Greek Asclepion institutions, Chinese medicine, Ayurvedic medicine, and early Christian healing. An overview of key events occurring during the scientific healing revolution and the impact of psychology and **spirituality** on present-day medicine also is presented.

Shamanism

Primitive tribes considered illness the work of evil spirits. The tribes, therefore, selected masters of the healing tradition who were known as medicine men, witch doctors, seers, or shamans.[1] The word "shaman" literally means "he (or she) who knows." To aid healing

of tribe members, early shamans used various types of communication with the spiritual world that included singing, dancing, storytelling, and drawing.[1,2,3] Many achieved altered states of consciousness to assist in their healing rituals. Prehistoric paintings on cave walls and ceilings in France and Spain dating back some 32,000 years are thought by some researchers to have been the work of shamans.[4] David Lewis-Williams, a social anthropologist and art historian at University of Witwatersrand, Johannesburg,[4] has proposed that Cro-Magnon (the earliest modern people in Europe) shamans made some of the paintings. They would enter dark caves and, while in a trance state, paint images of their visions. The paintings were of strange patterns and lines, and later included animals. Lewis-Williams interprets images from a cave in Lascaux, France, as hallucinogenic sequenced experiences.[5] Cave paintings, however, have been found all over the world. For example, the *Cueva de las Manos* in Patagonia, Argentina, is famous for the stenciled outlines of human hands (*Cueva de las Manos* in Spanish means "Cave of the Hands") and also for the many paintings of animals that are found in the region in addition to paintings of hunting scenes (**FIGURE 7.1**).[6] Interestingly, this UNESCO Word Heritage Site is located close to the Pinturas River, with *pinturas* being the Spanish word for paintings.[6]

Anthropological studies have proven that many shamanic cultures used hallucinogenic substances to enter the "Otherworld."[1,2,3] Shamans were thought to be aided in this voyage to the Otherworld by particular animals that were the "spirit guides." Other ways in which shamans entered a trance state were to fast, place themselves in isolation for long periods of time, use sensory deprivation, and even undergo torture. Much of what we read about shamans portrays them as men, but in many cultures, women exceeded the

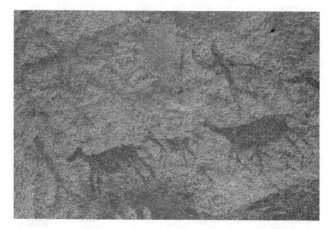

FIGURE 7.1 Cave painting from Patagonia, Argentina.
© Eduardo Rivero/Shutterstock

men in importance. In fact, in certain cultures, images of the time and historical accounts show that female shamans predominated over males.[3] Also interesting to note is that many male shamans wear female clothing or garb as they perform healing rituals.[3]

Shamans are said to act as intermediaries between the world of men and the gods, and have the power to descend into the realms of the dead. The shamans' spirits are believed to journey forth from their bodies, which remain in a state of trance. They describe the long journey in a chant. Sometimes, shamans induce the conditions of ecstasy by beating a drum or by an elaborate and exciting dance.[2,3] Shamans do not separate the body, mind, and soul, but see these parts as an integrated whole. The outcome is that when shamans communicate with the spiritual world, they gain a position of respect and power within their tribes.

In summary, there are three key features of shamanism:

1. Shamans can voluntarily enter altered states of consciousness.
2. In these states, they may experience themselves journeying to other realms.
3. They use these journeys to acquire knowledge or power and to help people in their community.

Even though modern medicine has spread throughout the world, many cultures continue to rely on shamans for healing. In Native American groups, only the shaman has the power to communicate with gods or spirits. The shaman is considered a mystic, a poet, a sage, and a healer. This person is usually extraordinary in appearance and in acting talents. To promote healing and to communicate with the outerworld, the Native American shaman uses drumming, singing, fasting, dancing, spinning, and sweat lodges. The **sweat lodge**, built as a ceremonial sauna, is used for a purification ceremony.[7] Because sweat lodges can be dangerous in terms of dehydration and elevated body temperature, participants are monitored very closely. See **FIGURE 7.2** for a picture of a dome-shaped Native American ceremonial sweat lodge in Monument Valley, Utah.

Greek Asclepions

The **Asclepions** (also spelled Asklepions) were sanctuaries of healing and had their roots in ancient Greece on the island of Kos (also spelled Cos).[8,9] They were named after Asclepius, the Divine Physician, who was worshipped as the god of medicine. Asclepius was said to be the son of Apollo and the Nymph Coronis, and is often shown in pictures as standing with a long

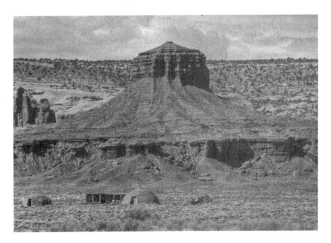

FIGURE 7.2 Native American ceremonial sweat lodge, Monument Valley, Utah.

© Jeffrey T. Kreulen/Shutterstock

wooden staff with a long snake entwined around it.[10] See **FIGURE 7.3** for an image of Asclepius.

Early Asclepions were built in areas of natural beauty throughout Greece. They created a healing environment that addressed the physical, mental, and spiritual aspects of individuals. Before people could enter the Asclepions, they had to undergo Katharsis (catharsis) or purification.[8,9] This consisted of a series

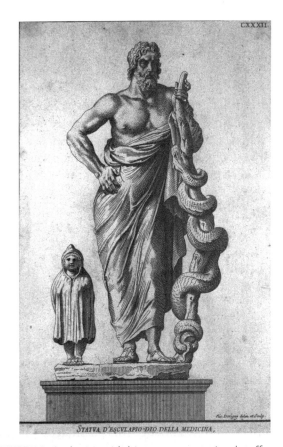

FIGURE 7.3 Asclepius with his serpent-entwined staff.

Courtesy or National Library of Medicine

of cleansing baths and purging, accompanied by a cleansing diet. Purification could last several days. Once admitted to the healing centers, the healers utilized music, dream interpretations, drama, massage, humor, baths, herbs, and rest as treatments.[8,9]

Greek and Roman Influences on Healing

The foundation of modern medicine is thought to come mostly from ancient Greek physicians, although both Greek and Roman physicians had a tremendous influence on medicine. Probably the most famous physician of all is Hippocrates, who lived from 460–377 BCE and is known as the father of modern medicine. He was born on an Aegean island named Cos,[11] and his father was also a physician. Hippocrates spent much of his early years on Cos at a local Asclepion. Hippocrates founded the Hippocratic School of Medicine, and even today, new MDs pledge the Hippocratic oath. From the Greeks came other great physicians such as Galen (great anatomical knowledge), Soranus (study of gynecology), and Dioscorides (books on herbal medicines). The Greeks had an extensive knowledge of herbs and herbal properties and used them when treating illnesses.[11,12] Women also played a major role as healers during early Greek medicine times.[9] They became doctors along with men and many became midwives who assisted in the birthing process.

Greek healing methodologies influenced Roman medicine and Roman methods influenced the Greeks. Because the Romans knew that poor hygiene was linked to disease and death, public bath houses and other similar public hygienic facilities were built and maintained.[13] More influences from the Romans came through their use of surgical tools. Some that were used in ancient Rome were scalpels, hooks (as probes for dissection and raising blood vessels), bone drills, forceps, catheters, vaginal specula, and surgical saws for amputations and surgeries.[13]

Chinese Medicine

At one time, Chinese medicine was thought to have begun during the time of Qin (221–206 BCE), but based on manuscripts excavated in 1973 from Tomb Three of the Mawangdui site at Changsha, Hunan, most of the standardization of Chinese medicine occurred during the Western Han dynasty (206 BCE to 220 AD).[14] Knowledge of healing was recorded in the *Huangdi Neijing* (*The Yellow Emperor's Inner Canon*)[14,15] and knowledge of pharmacology was recorded in the *Shennong Jing* (*Classic of Shennong*) and *Shennong Bencao Jing* (*Herbal Classic of Shennong*). More on the contributions of Shennong, known as the Divine Farmer, follows in a later chapter. A third important medical classic is the *Nanjing* (*Classic of Difficult Issues*), which explains medical theory and practice more clearly than the *Huangdi Neijing*.[15]

In general, herbal medicines and acupuncture therapy are the two aspects most associated with Chinese medicine. Early Chinese medicine physicians recognized the movement of life energy or **qi (chi)**. They believed that illness occurs when energy flow is blocked. Acupuncture and herbal medicines are used to unblock energy so that it can flow more freely through the body. However, acupuncture as we know it today (inserting steel needles into body parts) was not mentioned in the Mawangdui manuscripts and is not believed to have been used before 168 BCE.[15] Chinese doctors did use stone probes to open up boils and abscesses.[14,15] Traditional Chinese medicine (TCM) seems to be increasing in popularity in the United States today.

Ayurvedic Medicine

Ayurvedic medicine is the traditional system of medicine of India. The word "Ayurveda" means the "science of life" or "sciences of lifespan." It is the oldest healing system and may have begun sometime between 5,000 and 10,000 years ago.[16,17] Ayurvedic medicine is a holistic healing system that may have influenced ancient Chinese medicine and the humoral medicine practiced by Hippocrates in Greece. Some call it the "mother of all healing."[17] The early healers of India were known as sages or **seers**, and they were the ones who began to systemize healing after having identified "Veda," the knowledge of how our world works.[16,17] The secrets of sickness and health were communicated to the sages through deep mediation and were written down over 2,000 years ago in the four main Vedas (Rig, Sama, Yajur, and Atharva), which are sacred texts of India. The Rigveda is said to be the oldest surviving book of any Indo-European language.[18] All that the sages learned was organized into the Indian healing system called Ayurveda. The *Charaka Samhita* text was written 2,000 years before the microscope was invented, and yet it listed 20 different microscopic organisms that can cause disease and discussed how disease spreads. The *Sushrutha Samhita* text (300–400 AD) offered information about surgery, surgical equipment, suturing, and the importance of hygiene.[19]

Ayurveda healing techniques promote unity of the mind, body, and spirit. Similar to Chinese medicine, the Ayurveda belief is that when energy fields are blocked, they cause illness; however, in Ayurvedic medicine, the energy fields are identified as chakras.

Ayurvedic medicine went through a period of decline in India during the British rule, but in 1947, when India gained its independence, Ayurveda again grew in importance and new schools of medicine were established. More on Ayurvedic medicine may be found in a later chapter describing various methods of using Ayurveda to treat illness.

Early Christian Healing

The Bible is used as evidence of the spiritual dimension to restore physical health. Jesus Christ was known as a healer and worker of miracles, someone who healed people both physically and spiritually. Early Judean beliefs held that people who had sinned or who were evil became sick, and that health and healing stemmed from repentance and divine forgiveness. (Judea was a kingdom ruled by the Herods and was part of the Roman province of Syria.) To heal the sick, a ceremonial practice called **anointing** was used.[20]

In early biblical times, both laypeople (men and women) and priests used anointing to heal the sick using oils such as frankincense and myrrh. It involved dipping a finger in the oil and touching the person either on the forehead or on another body part. By the middle ages, anointing became used solely by male Catholic priests, and rules were set as to who could and could not anoint. After the Reformation in the 1500s, the use of anointing (laying on of hands) by most of the newer Christian denominations sharply decreased in scope and breadth.[20] Anointing has returned somewhat in the present day. The Roman Catholic Church uses blessed oil for final anointing or at the time of last breath. The Anglican Church allows anointing when visiting the sick, and in the Lutheran tradition, anointing is used after a silent laying on of the hands. The belief that anointing is superstitious is waning, and many groups want to restore the practice as a sign of hope for those suffering spiritually as well as emotionally or physically.[20]

An example of the 1800s Christian healer is Mary Baker Eddy (1821–1910), the founder of **Christian Science**.[21] She had grown up in ill health most of her life. When she was in her early 40s, she became a patient of a New England healer, Phineas Parkhurst Quimby.[21] At the time, Mrs. Eddy was an invalid, but after undergoing one week's treatment by Mr. Quimby, she was "cured." During the ensuing years, Eddy worked with Quimby and began to write and give public lectures on Quimby's healing process. Several years later, Eddy had an accident and almost died.

Quimby himself had died earlier, so she used Quimby's healing methods to heal herself. She called this the "Science of Christianity," and later named it Christian Science, a healing methodology that did not use medicine and that was based on the healing methods of Phineas Quimby. When Mrs. Eddy was 88 years old, she founded the *Christian Science Monitor*.[21] In 1995, Mary Baker Eddy was elected to the National Women's Hall of Fame as the only U.S. woman to found a worldwide religion.

Scientific Healing Revolution

The Scientific Revolution occurred during the 1800s. Physicians and nurses began separating themselves from the early healing practices and moved toward scientific practices. René-Théophile-Hyacinthe Laennec invented the stethoscope in France in 1816, a new technology that helped fight tuberculosis, said to be the single worst disease of the urban landscape. If contracted, the chances of survival were about 60%. Another new technology was the further perfection of the microscope by Carl Zeiss in Germany. Zeiss worked with others to solve disease problems at the cellular level. On a greater scale, the position of Public Health Officer was created and the person assigned or hired to that position, along with civil engineers, worked to improve the deplorable sanitary conditions in major cities.[22]

Cholera was another horrific epidemic. In 1849, approximately 7,000 people died in London from cholera. In 1883, the organism causing cholera (*Vibrio cholerae*, a comma-shaped bacterium) was identified in water by Robert Koch via the microscope and subsequently was contained by public health officials. Great gains also were made during the 1800s in cellular biology and public health. Public health laws were passed in order to protect people from epidemic diseases.[22]

The scientific revolution not only encompassed new technology and new public health laws, but also distinguished some individuals who became notable for saving lives through public health practices. Florence Nightingale was one of those people (**FIGURE 7.4**). She was born to wealthy British parents and named after the city in which she was born—Florence, Italy.[23] Nightingale had to overcome prejudice and convince her wealthy parents to allow her to become a nurse, a practice associated with working class women. In the 1850s, Russia invaded Turkey, and Britain and France went to Turkey's aid (Crimean War). A newspaper in London published stories about typhus, cholera, and dysentery among the servicemen. The government allowed Nightingale to travel to Turkey and to take 30 other nurses with her. They found deplorable,

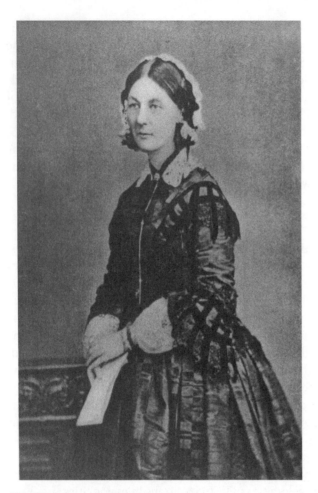

FIGURE 7.4 Florence Nightingale.

Courtesy of Library of Congress, Prints & Photographs Division [reproduction number LC-USZ62-5877].

unsanitary conditions—soldiers in bloody, dirty uniforms and unwashed. Her efforts at sanitizing the service hospitals and aiding the wounded rapidly turned around the death toll in the Crimean War. On the base of the Turkish army barracks that served as British military base and hospital, a Florence Nightingale museum has been established in Istanbul, Turkey.[23] Nightingale will always be remembered as having promoted a holistic approach to caring for the wounded and ill.

Psychology and Spirituality

It is impossible to discuss a history of healing without pointing out the impact of psychology and spirituality. In the 1960s and 1970s, health care began being sensitive about the importance of mind, body, and spirit in healing. Theoretical frameworks began describing various paradigms or theories; the decision of which theory to use was based solely on the unique characteristics and preferences of the clinician. An early holistic psychological theory is Gestalt psychology, meaning "unified whole."[24,25]

Gestalt therapy was founded by Frederick (Fritz) and Laura Perls in the 1940s. It is a theory characterized by the phrase "the whole is greater than the sum of its parts"—hence, "wholistic" or "holistic." In other words, the theory speaks to mental health as being dependent on the rest of the human experience: social, emotional, physical, and sexual. It is most famous for the Gestalt "laws" of perception, which attempted to describe which properties of visual elements make them appear to belong together as an entity.

Currently, holistic psychology builds on Gestalt, transpersonal, and psychosynthesis psychological theory. It involves adopting, adapting, and using techniques to effect personal change, transformation, and healing. It is a psychology that is no longer one-dimensional but reveals a multidimensional, yet unique, individual. It seems to be a psychology that complements our new attention to alternative healing methods. Through the years, many psychology theories have been developed, and clinicians select a model that aligns with their views about mental health (i.e., behavioral, cognitive, developmental, humanist, personality, and social psychology). An example of a personality theory is Freud's psychoanalytical theory. On the other hand, behaviorists align more with behavioral or cognitive behavioral theories.

Spirituality models are being developed and are evolving. Some align spirituality and religion, whereas others show a distinct difference. It has been difficult to assess spirituality because the meaning is different and personal from individual to individual. Attempts have been made to quantify spirituality. For instance, a spirituality scale has been developed for the purpose of testing the spiritual dimension,[26] and future studies using the scale may produce deeper insights about people's spirituality concepts. Kurtz and Ketcham are authors of a book about finding spirituality through the process of storytelling,[27] and some of you may find this an interesting read.

Most theoretical frameworks include the concepts of self-discovery, relationships, and ecoawareness. Self, Others, and God are three key elements found as the result of one literature review.[28] Identified within those three key elements were emerging themes such as meaning, hope, relatedness/connectedness, beliefs/belief systems, and expressions of spirituality.[28] In particular, the nature of God was viewed as taking many forms and essentially is whatever an individual takes to be of highest value in his or her life. The authors concluded that the themes that emerged could be used as a framework for future exploration of the concept

I (Dr. Synovitz) taught the concepts of health and wellness dimensions for many years (physical, emotional, mental, social, and spiritual). I asked my classroom students what spirituality means to them and when do they feel most spiritual. Some students answered that they felt most spiritual when they were sitting in church but others felt spiritual when they were walking on a sandy beach while looking at the ocean. I feel spiritual when I am standing on top of a mountain ready to downhill ski. When and where do you feel most spiritual? What does spirituality mean to you?

of spirituality.[28] See **BOX 7.1** for discussion about the meaning of spirituality.

A look at some historical events that have impacted healing through the ages is important, in that it shows us where we were and helps us assess what the future may bring. As you can see, a holistic approach to healing seems to be valued throughout history and is valued today. Many professional associations exemplify holistic thought by using the word "holistic" in their name (i.e., American Holistic Nurses Association, American Holistic Medical Association, and American Holistic Health Association). All these professional associations have provided high standards and principles of practice. Both alternative medicine and traditional (Western) medicine will continue to complement each other more and more through the coming years. We, the healthcare consumers, need to make careful choices and utilize the best of both.

▶ Is CAM Scientifically Legitimate or Is It Quackery?

CAM as Scientifically Legitimate

Most of the scientific research on selective forms of alternative medicine practices are being conducted at the National Center for Complementary and Integrative Health (NCCIH).[29] At present, the NCCIH funds four research centers: Centers of Excellence for Research on CAM, Centers for Dietary Supplements Research: Botanicals, Developmental Centers for Research on CAM, and International Centers for Research on CAM.[29] Each funds specific research and are presented in **BOX 7.2**.

The NCCIH publishes the results of studies in professional journals and on its website and provides links to research that is ongoing or completed

- **Centers of Excellence for Research on CAM:** Research on acupuncture (Massachusetts), antioxidants (Oregon, North Carolina), botanicals (Montana, South Carolina, Illinois, New York, California), energy medicine (Pennsylvania), mind–body/meditation (California, Wisconsin), and TCM (for alcohol and drug abuse in Massachusetts, arthritis in Maryland, and Chinese herbal therapy in New York).
- **Centers for Dietary Supplements Research:** Research of botanicals in six areas, namely, age-related diseases (Indiana), metabolic syndrome (Louisiana), women's health (Illinois), immuno-modulators (New York), lipids (North Carolina), and dietary supplements (Iowa).
- **Developmental Centers for Research on CAM:** These centers collaborate with CAM schools and conventional biomedical research institutions. Research on acupuncture (Massachusetts), botanical medicine (Minnesota, Washington), chiropractic manipulation (Iowa, Kansas, New York), mind–body medicine (Oregon), and osteopathy (Arizona, Texas).
- **International Centers for Research on CAM:** Research on botanicals (International Center for Indigenous Phytotherapy Studies, HIV/AIDS) and TCM for functional bowel disorders (Massachusetts).

on specific topics. To give one example, the NCCIH provides a link on the use of acupuncture for carpal tunnel pain relief.[29] The NCCIH website also provides links to PubMed CAM research studies that have been published in various scientific journals. NCCIH's website also provides information regarding grants and training programs, plus links to other CAM sites.

CAM research is ongoing. Some results will be promising, some will demonstrate effectiveness, and some will identify CAM practices that are not effective. Every day, we learn something new about CAM, a practice or a medicine (herb or supplement). We need to study the research and then make intelligent choices.

CAM as Quackery

The most publicized source of CAM criticism comes from *Quackwatch*,[32] a website operated by Stephen Barrett, MD. *Quackwatch* reports on its website that

▤ IN THE NEWS

Features on CAM Studies

U.S. News & World Report published a study on yoga as relief for back pain on February 21, 2017.[30] The author, Benjamin W. Friedman, MD, who is an emergency physician, described how his views are changing about helping people with low back pain. His standard methods were to prescribe nonsteroidal anti-inflammatory drugs (NSAIDS) such as Aleve (naproxen) and muscle relaxants such as Flexeril or Valium, and even opioids such as Percocet (oxycodone/acetaminophen). His research over many years led him to the conclusion that the use of the stronger muscle relaxant medications did not improve pain levels any more than the NSAIDS, but even those only help 1 out of 10 patients. Instead, he encourages people to try massage, acupuncture, and yoga and testifies that his happiest patients are the ones who practice stretching and yoga techniques.

A second article published on April 24, 2017 in *U.S. News & World Report* regarded the use and dangers of some supplements.[31] The author, Tamara Duker Freuman, recounts the story of one of her female patients who for years took a high-dose vitamin B$_6$ supplement that her naturopath had recommended, although no testing had been done to show that the patient was deficient in this particular vitamin. The supplement was quite expensive and the dose was 3800% of what is recommended for daily use. She eventually began to experience some nerve symptoms of pain and tingling in her arms and legs. She went to a medical doctor for diagnosis who found that she had irreversible nerve damage from the toxic levels of the vitamin B$_6$ supplement. She should never have been started on the vitamin in the first place because she had no deficiency.

Questions:

1. What have you learned from the two *U.S. News & World Report* stories about making choices when seeking alternative forms of care?
2. What steps could the second patient have taken to prevent herself from harm?

Sources: Friedman BW. Seeking relief for back pain? Reach for a yoga mat, not meds. U.S. News & World Report. February 21, 2017. Available at: http://health.usnews.com/health-care/for-better/articles/2017-02-21/seeking-relief-for-back-pain-reach-for-a-yoga-mat-not-meds. Accessed April 10, 2018. Freuman TD. What your alternative health provider might not tell you about megadosing supplements. U.S. News & World Report. April 24, 2017. Available at: http://health.usnews.com/health-news/blogs/eat-run/articles/2017-04-24/what-your-alternative-health-provider-might-not-tell-you-about-megadosing-supplements. Accessed April 10, 2018.

it is affiliated with the National Council Against Health Fraud, an organization that Dr. Barrett has been a member of for many years. Dr. Barrett and others (e.g., Rosemary Jacobs, William T. Jarvis) hold the view that there is no alternative medicine, only scientifically proven, evidence-based medicine that is supported by data-driven studies. Dr. Barrett writes that the alternative movement is a type of societal trend that is rejecting science as a method of determining truth, and that the movement supports pseudoscience over science.[32] His case in point is a section he wrote on "Science versus Vitalism." As discussed earlier, Chinese traditional medicine and Ayurvedic medicine are based on the principle of vitalism (a life force within the body). Dr. Barrett claims that vitalists pretend to be scientific, but they really reject scientific methods and regard "personal experience, subjective judgment, and emotional satisfaction as preferable to objectivity and hard evidence."[32] One section under *Quackwatch* is titled "Questionable Products, Services and Theories." Over 100 topics are listed alphabetically, from acupuncture to chiropractic, homeopathy, naturopathy, Therapeutic Touch, and so forth, either condemning or questioning each as quackery. In fact, Barrett is so passionately against alternative medicine that he wrote an article in *Quackwatch* pointing out reasons why the NCCIH should be defunded.[32]

After reading the preceding sections on "CAM as Scientifically Legitimate" and "CAM as Quackery," perhaps as a health consumer, you could ponder and answer the following questions:

1. Do you believe that CAM research should continue? If so, why?
2. Do you believe that funding for CAM research at the NCCIH should be withdrawn? If so, why?
3. If funding were withdrawn from the NCCIH and for all those sites across the United States that are conducting CAM research, how would research continue?
4. If Dr. Barrett believes that healing modalities need to be tested scientifically and proven effective (evidence based) and if he is calling upon defunding of our major national research center (NCCIH), how does he expect to learn what really works and what does not?
5. What can you do as a health consumer to advocate for the scientific study of any medical or healing treatment, whether it is labeled alternative or traditional?

▶ Conclusion

Those practices that we "Westerners" call alternative are in actuality healing methods that have been used for centuries. This chapter was intended to give you an historic perspective about CAM and views about CAM as scientifically legitimate practices or practices considered quackery. Concepts about healing and the healer's role were introduced so that you could relate how and why people turn to alternative practitioners. Perhaps, as we study more about CAM practices, we will learn some beneficial information from our predecessors.

Wrap-Up

Key Terms

Anointing Involves dipping a finger in oil and touching a person either on the forehead or on another body part as a part of religious ceremony.

Asclepions Sanctuaries of healing. They had their roots in ancient Greece on the island of Kos.

Ayurvedic medicine A traditional system of medicine of India. The word *Ayurveda* is a Sanskrit word that means science of life or sciences of lifespan.

Christian Science A healing methodology that does not use medicine. Mary Baker-Eddy founded Christian Science and based it on the healing methods of Phineas Quimby.

Qi (chi) According to TCM, Qi is a bodily energy that flows through unseen channels in the body called meridians. Illness is believed to occur when Qi is blocked.

Seer Masters of the healing tradition. A person who knows.

Shamanism An anthropological term referencing a range of beliefs and practices regarding a person (shaman) who is believed to be able to communicate with the spiritual world.

Spirituality A belief in a higher power; a way to find meaning and hope in one's life; awareness of purpose and meaning in life.

Sweat lodge Used for a purification ceremony; a place built as a ceremonial sauna lodge.

Suggestions for Class Activities

1. Research more in-depth one of the historical figures presented. Prepare a report and present it to your classmates.
2. Organize a classroom debate over CAM as scientific or quackery.
3. Research modern day Asclepions. (Where located, services offered, looks of the building and grounds, cost for clients.) Prepare a report and present it to your classmates.

4. Visit a health food store:
   a. Describe the kinds of products sold, product claims (to improve health or intended use), and product prices.
   b. Ask the proprietor and salespeople what their educational background is and what kind of training they received in order to sell products and herbs.
   c. Bring a sample or two back from the health store (if not expensive) and show to your classmates. (Samples could be a food product such as potato chips, an energy bar, or soap.)
   d. Prepare a written report of your findings.

Review Questions

1. What is the definition of "healing"?
2. What are three characteristics of the healer's role?
3. What is the role of the shaman?
4. What main characteristic is similar in shamans all over the world and in various cultures?
5. What is an Asclepion?
6. How have the Greeks and Romans contributed to medicine and healing?
7. How long have Ayurveda and Chinese medicine been practiced?
8. Who was the most revered Judaean early healer?
9. What was Mary Baker Eddy's contribution to healing?
10. Describe how Florence Nightingale impacted healing practices.
11. How have psychology and spirituality impacted healing?
12. What is the name of the national CAM research center?
13. What is the name of the quackery website presented in this chapter?

References

1. Walsh R. *The World of Shamanism: New Views of an Ancient Tradition.* Woodbury, MN: Llewellyn Worldwide; 2007.

2. Ingerman S. *Shamanic Journeying: A Beginner's Guide.* Boulder, CO: Sounds True; 2004.

3. Narby J, Huxley F. *Shamans Through Time: 500 years on the Path to Knowledge.* New York, NY: Jeremy P. Tarcher/Putnam; 2001.

4. Coppens P. Cave paintings: entrancing the otherworld. *Frontier.* 2003;9:6. Available at: http://www.philipcoppens.com/cavepaintings.html. Accessed April 10, 2018.

5. Lewis-Williams D. The mind in the cave: *Consciousness and the Origins of Art.* London, UK: Thames & Hudson; 2004.

6. United Nations Educational, Scientific and Cultural Organization. Cueva de las Manos, Río Pinturas. Available at: https://whc.unesco.org/en/list/936. Accessed April 10, 2018.

7. Wikipedia. Picture of Hupa Sweat House. Available at: http://en.wikipedia.org/wiki/File:Hupa_Sweat_House.jpg. Accessed April 10, 2018.

8. Greek Medicine.net. The Asclepions: Sanctuaries of Healing. Available at: http://www.greekmedicine.net/mythology/asclepions.html. Accessed April 10, 2018.

9. The Role of Women in the Art of Ancient Greece. Ancient Greek Medicine: Index of Ancient Greek medicine. Available at: http://www.rwaag.org/gmed. Accessed April 10, 2018.

10. Asklepion. Picture of Asclepius Purchased from Pixmac at: http://www.pixmac.com/picture/white+marble+classic+statue+of+asclepius+isolated+on+black+background/000061901311. Accessed April 10, 2018.

11. Greek Medicine.net. Hippocrates: Father of Medicine. Available at: http://www.greekmedicine.net/whos_who/Hippocrates.html. Accessed April 10, 2018.

12. Trueman CN. Hippocrates. The History Learning Site. Available at: http://www.historylearningsite.co.uk/a-history-of-medicine/hippocrates/. Published March 17, 2015. Accessed April 10, 2018.

13. Wikipedia. Medicine in ancient Rome. Available at: http://en.wikipedia.org/wiki/Medicine_in_ancient_Rome. Accessed April 10, 2018.

14. Galambos I. *The Origins of Chinese Medicine—The Early Development of Medical Literature in China.* Available at: http://www.zhenjiu.de/Literatur/Fachartikel/englisch/origins-of.htm. Publsihed 1996. Accessed April 10, 2018.

15. Purify Our Mind. History of Traditional Chinese Medicine. Available at: http://www.purifymind.com/HistoryMed.htm. Accessed April 10, 2018.

16. Bruning N, Thomas H. *Ayurveda: The A-Z Guide to Healing Techniques from Ancient India.* New York, NY: Dell Publishing; 1997.

17. JMD. The Wonders of Ayurveda. 10 facts on Ayurveda. Available at: https://www.jmdmedico.com/10-facts-on-ayurveda/ Accessed April 14, 2018.

18. Bradford N, ed. *The One Spirit Encyclopedia of Complementary Health.* London, UK: Hamlyn; 2000.

19. Ambassadors Light. About Ayurveda. Available at: http://ambassadorsoflight.com/ayurveda/. Accessed April 10, 2018.

20. Smith LL. What happened to Christian anointing – How did we lose it in history? *EzineArticles.com.* August 16, 2008. Available at: http://ezinearticles.com/?What-Happened-to-Christian-Anointing—How-Did-We-Lose-it-in-History?&id=1416033. Accessed April 10, 2018.

21. Thomas H, Thomas DL. Mary Baker Eddy–A biographical sketch. Available at: http://marybakereddy.wwwhubs.com/mbe1.html. Accessed April 10, 2018.

22. Picard L. Victorian Britain: Health and hygiene in the 19th century. *British Library.* October 14, 2009. Available at: https://www.bl.uk/victorian-britain/articles/health-and-hygiene-in-the-19th-century. Accessed April 10, 2018.

23. Spartacus Educational. Florence Nightingale. Available at: http://spartacus-educational.com/REnightingale.htm. Accessed April 10, 2018.

24. Yontef G. *Gestalt Therapy: An Introduction. Awareness, Dialogue, and Process.* Gouldsboro, ME: Gestalt Journal Press; 1993.

25. The Gestault Centre. What is Gestalt? Available at: http://gestaltcentre.org.uk/what-is-gestalt/. Accessed April 18, 018.

26. Delaney C. The spirituality scale: Development and psychometric testing of a holistic instrument to assess the human spiritual dimension. *J Holist Nurs.* 2005;23(2):145-167.

27. Kurtz E, Ketcham K. *Experiencing Spirituality: Finding Meaning through Storytelling.* New York, NY: Jeremy P. Tarcher/Penguin; 2016.

28. Dyson J, Cobb M, Forman D. The meaning of spirituality: A literature review. *J Adv Nurs.* 1997;26(6):1183-1188.

29. National Center for Complementary and Integrative Health. Research Results by Date. Available at: https://nccih.nih.gov/research/results/spotlight. Accessed April 10, 2018.

30. Friedman BW. Seeking relief for back pain? Reach for a yoga mat, not meds. *U.S. News & World Report.* February 21, 2017. Available at: http://health.usnews.com/health-care/for-better/articles/2017-02-21/seeking-relief-for-back-pain-reach-for-a-yoga-mat-not-meds. Accessed April 10, 2018.

31. Freuman TD. What your alternative health provider might not tell you about megadosing supplements. *U.S. News & World Report.* April 24, 2017. Available at: http://health.usnews.com/health-news/blogs/eat-run/articles/2017-04-24/what-your-alternative-health-provider-might-not-tell-you-about-megadosing-supplements. Accessed April 10, 2018.

32. Barrett S. Your Guide to Quackery, Health Fraud, and Intelligent Decisions. Quackwatch. Available at: http://www.quackwatch.org. Updated March 16, 2018. Accessed April 10, 2018.

CHAPTER 8

Alternative Medical Systems: Ayurveda and Its Practices

LEARNING OBJECTIVES

As a result of reading this chapter, students will be able to:

1. Explain the foundation of Ayurvedic medicine principles.
2. Name one of the three great Ayurveda classics.
3. Compare and contrast Ayurveda and Western medicine diagnostic methods.
4. Discuss Ayurveda general guidelines for treating dosha imbalances.
5. Analyze what should be the minimum standard for the sale of over-the-counter Ayurvedic medicines.

▶ What Is Ayurveda?

Ayurveda is a Sanskrit word that means "science of life." It is derived from two roots: *Ayur* meaning "life" and *Veda* meaning "knowledge or science." The practice of Ayurveda had its origins in India 5,000–10,000 years ago, making it the oldest healing science known.[1,2,3] Ayurveda healing methods were first taught and passed down orally and were eventually written several thousand years ago, although much of the written material is inaccessible. Ayurveda has three classic texts written in Sanskrit, the classical language of Hinduism in India that is used today in religious and ceremonial events. The *Charaka Samhita* is a text on Ayurveda estimated to have been written about 400–200 BCE. The second classic, *Sushruta Samhita*, was written about 2,000 years ago by the surgeon Sushruta. His text contained details about surgery for various conditions, postmortem dissection, and even plastic surgery, which formed the basis for plastic surgery today.[3] The third, the *Ashtanga Hridayam*, is thought to have been written later than the first two classics by a man named Acharya Vagbhata. The basic philosophies and medicinal practices were first set forth in these ancient texts. Ayurveda places equal emphasis on body, mind, and spirit, and strives to restore the innate harmony of the individual. To promote healing, life stresses must be alleviated and the natural flow of energy within people must be balanced so that the body's immune system will be enhanced, thus able to defend more against disease. The basic life force in the body is **Prana**, and is similar to the Chinese notion of chi. Today, those practicing **Ayurvedic medicine** maintain that it is not a substitute for Western medicine but complements it. Today, Ayurveda focuses on naturalistic healing methods, and surgery is no longer common for Ayurvedic physicians or practitioners, although it was historically.

▶ What Are the Main Ayurveda Principles?

Four main principles are identified in Ayurveda: Principle of Inner Balance, Principle of Universal Cosmos (Five Elements), Principle of Body Energies (Doshas), and Principle of Disease Causation.

Principle of Inner Balance

Ayurvedic principles are based on a holistic view of healing. One of the Ayurvedic principles is to maintain inner balance by placing major emphasis on maintaining health by preventing disease and illness.[1,2,3] Diet, exercise, positive lifestyle, and balancing one's life (physically, mentally, emotionally, and socially) are encouraged. Ayurvedic science holds that each person is unique and has a different pattern of energy that comprises or makes up that person's constitution.[2,4] That constitution stays with the person throughout life.

Both internal and external factors may be responsible for upsetting balance within an individual, thereby upsetting that person's constitution. Examples that may cause imbalance are diet and food choices, differing seasons and weather, social relationships, and work-related stresses. In Ayurveda, the diagnosis needs to focus on finding the source of the interrupted balance, and treatment will strive to bring a person back to his or her original constitution.

Principle of Universal Cosmos: Five Elements

According to Ayurveda, every human being is a creation of the cosmos and universal consciousness.[1,2,3,4,5] The universe consists of **five elements** (or tattwa) that form the sum and substance of the physical universe as well as serve as the building blocks of nature, and they originate from and are composed of an energy called Prana. The five elements are: (1) earth (Prithvi), (2) water (Apa), (3) fire (Tejas), (4) air (Vayu), and (5) ether, or space (Akash).[1,2,3,4] All five elements are thought to be present in all cells of the body. Every substance in our world is made up of a combination of the tattwa, and all substances can be classified according to their predominant element. The tattwa combine to make the **seven tissues (dhatu)** that give the body its structure—plasma, blood, muscle, lipid, bone, and nervous and reproductive systems. Tattwa also make up the different tastes of sweet, salty, sour, pungent, bitter, and astringent.

Prana is the prime moving force in the body and the universe. The word prana is composed of two

parts: *pra* means foreword or before and *ana* means breath.[4] Ayurvedic philosophy holds that there are five pranic forces that govern body movement and function: prana, udana, samana, apana, and vyana.[1,2,4] Prana provides the elements with energy and gives them power to become the building blocks for all bodily functions. The five elements are described in **BOX 8.1**.

Principle of Body Energies (Dosha)

Ayurveda holds that the five elements make up the body's constitution, which is identified as **dosha**. There are three mental doshas and three body doshas.[2,3,4,5] The three body doshas are vata (movement), pitta (transformation), and kapha (structure).[2,3,4,5] Each individual is composed of a combination of the three, although different people have different ratios of the three doshas. Each person's combination of doshas (or body constitution) is established at birth. In males, the energy is called Purusha, choiceless passive awareness. Female energy is called Prakruti, choiceful active

---

BOX 8.1 Definitions of the Five Elements

- **Ether** represents the space or field in which everything happens. At the same time, it is the source of all matter and represents the distance among matter. Sound and nonresistance is a chief characteristic of ether.
- **Air** is matter in a gaseous form. It is moving and dynamic. All energy transfer reactions require oxygen within the body. Air is also required for fire to burn. Air has no form.
- **Fire** is powerful because it can change solids into liquids and gases and back again. Energy (fire) within our bodies binds atoms together and changes food that we eat into fat (stored energy) and muscle. Fire also is responsible for our nervous reactions, our feelings, and even our thought processes. Fire has a form but no substance.
- **Water** is the liquid state and represents change. No living thing can survive without water. The human body is largely composed of water. Bodies contain blood, lymph, and other fluids that circulate throughout the body and in between cells of the body. Those fluids help to carry away waste, regulate body temperature, and carry hormonal information throughout the body. The blood contains our disease protection properties (immune system). Water is seen as a substance but has no stability.
- **Earth** represents the solid state of matter. Earth is represented in our bodies as the bones, teeth, cells, and tissues. Earth is considered a stable substance. It manifests stability, permanence, and rigidity.

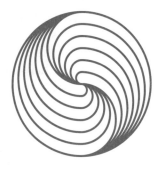

FIGURE 8.1 Vata sign.

consciousness. Most sources do not distinguish the gender energies and use the term Prakruti for both genders. When there is imbalance in the body elements (vata, pitta, or kapha), disease occurs because of a lack of proper cellular function. In Indian terminology, the imbalance is called Vikruti.[3,4]

Vata, pitta, and kapha can exist in varying combinations, but usually one of the three is predominant. According to Ayurveda, there are seven body types: mono (vata, pitta, or kapha predominant), dual (vata-pitta, pitta-kapha, or kapha-vata), and equal (vata, pitta, and kapha in equal proportions). See **BOX 8.2** for examples of combinations. When all of the types are evenly distributed, a person is said to be **tri-doshic**.[6] These individuals are more likely to remain in balance, because the ratio of vata, pitta, and kapha is nearly even. They will tend to have lifelong good health and a good immune system, but because they do not have a "lead" dosha to start with, when they get out of balance, they have to work harder to balance all three doshas.

Characteristics of Vata, Pitta, and Kapha

The characteristics of vata, pitta, and kapha vary quite a bit, and are described in the following sections.

Vata

Vata is composed of space and air. The images found for vata incorporate the sense of air (**FIGURE 8.1**). Vata is the subtle energy associated with movement and is located in the brain, large intestine, pelvic cavity, bones, skin, ears, and thighs.[3,4] Vata governs breathing, blinking muscle and tissue movement, heartbeat, and cellular activity. According to Ayurveda, vata is the most important dosha because it leads the other doshas. More than half of all illnesses are vata disorders. If vata is kept in balance, pitta and kapha will stay in balance. Attributes of vata types are dry, light, cold, rough, subtle, mobile, clear, and astringent[6,7,8] (**TABLE 8.1**).

TABLE 8.1 Vata Qualities and Manifestations in the Body

Qualities	Manifestations in the Body
Dry	Dry skin, hair, lips, and tongue; dry colon, tendency toward constipation; hoarse voice
Light	Light muscles, bones, thin body frame; light, scanty sleep; tendency to be underweight
Cold	Cold hands and feet; poor circulation; hates cold and loves hot; stiffness of muscles
Rough	Rough cracked skin, nails, hair, teeth, hands, and feet; cracking joints
Subtle	Subtle fear, anxiety, and insecurity; fine goose pimples; minute muscle twitching, fine tremors; delicate body
Mobile	Fast walking and talking; doing many things at once; restless eyes, eyebrows, hands, and feet; unstable joints; many dreams; loves traveling but does not stay long at one place; swinging moods, shaky faith, scattered mind
Clear	Clairvoyant; understands immediately and forgets immediately; clear, empty mind; experiences void and loneliness
Astringent	Dry choking sensation in the throat; hiccoughing, burping; loves oily foods and mushy soups; craves sweet, sour, and salty tastes; tendency toward constipation

According to Ayurveda, the body type of vata people tends to be thin, which is somewhat analogous to the Western description of the endomorph body shape. They have a tendency to have cold hands and feet and hate cold weather. A person with a predominant vata personality has a quick mind, and is flexible and creative.[3,4,6,7] Vata types grasp concepts quickly, but then forget them quickly. Vatas are usually "on the move"; their energy vacillates back and forth. They walk, talk, and think fast. Their sleeping patterns are erratic and they seek adventuresome activities. They not only seem to like foods such as salads and raw vegetables, but also balance that by eating foods that are cooked. The tastes best associated with vata are sweet, sour, and salty foods.

In Balance: Vata promotes creativity and flexibility. Vata types have normal sleep patterns.

Out of Balance: Vata types may experience psychological disorders of fear, anxiety, and various phobias. Movements for eating, digestion, and elimination are disturbed. They may have insomnia, or light or interrupted sleep.[3,4]

Common vata disorders include flatulence, tics, twitches, aching joints, dry skin and hair, nerve disorders, constipation, and mental confusion.[1,3,4,7] Vata types tend to have neurological, muscular, and rheumatic diseases. Vata in the body tends to increase with age and is exhibited by the drying and wrinkling of the skin. Vata types should avoid excessive stimulation like drinking caffeine and watching television. Vata people should dress warmly and eat warm, moist, slightly oily, heavy foods.[4] They should attempt to maintain a constant daily schedule and obtain regular sleeping habits and meals.

Pitta

The pitta dosha is made up of fire and water. The image for pitta incorporates this sense. When looking at the image shown in **FIGURE 8.2**, you can see the fire on top and water on the bottom.

FIGURE 8.2 Pitta sign.

Some say the pitta dosha is "digestive fire," or agni. The pitta dosha is located in the small intestine, stomach, sweat glands, blood, skin, and eyes. In Ayurveda, good digestion is the key to good health. When digestion is poor, a substance, ama, is produced, and may not only be seen in the body as a white coating on the tongue, but can also be lining the colon and clogging blood vessels.[2,4,7] Agni, when working normally, will maintain good digestion and ensures that the body's waste products, **malas** (sweat, urine, feces), are working efficiently. Pitta governs digestive functions such as absorption, assimilation, nutrition, metabolism, and body temperature, and also governs the ability to digest ideas and gain an understanding of true reality. A person with a dominant pitta body type usually has a medium build, is strong, has stamina and endurance, and maintains a stable body weight,[8] which is analogous to the Western mesomorph body type. Qualities of the pitta type include hot, sharp, light, sour, oily, spreading, bitter, pungent, red, and yellow[2,4,7] (**TABLE 8.2**).

Pittas are generally very intelligent and quick-witted, but may be overly critical. They tend to possess little patience and a short temper, and may erupt from time to time.[1]

In Balance: Pitta promotes understanding and intelligence. There is strong and complete digestion, healthy facial tone and coloration, and stimulated and open intellect.[8,9,10]

Out of Balance: Pitta arouses anger, hatred, and jealousy. Pittas tend to have incomplete digestion; variable, blotchy skin color; an unhealthy appearance; and cognitive reasoning is impaired.

Likely diseases in pitta types are inflammatory diseases such as boils, abscesses, ulcers, irritable bowels, hemorrhoids, and diarrhea. Pitta people should not push themselves too hard,[8] should avoid artificial stimulants and alcohol, should regularly meditate, and should sleep and work in cooler rooms.

Kapha

Kapha is made of earth and water. The image for kapha incorporates water on the top of the image and earth on the lower half (**FIGURE 8.3**).

Kapha supplies water for all body parts and systems. It lubricates joints, moisturizes skin, and maintains immunity. It is the energy that forms the body structure and provides support for the bones, muscle, and insulating fat.[1,2,3,4,7] It gives people stamina and physical strength. Kapha is located in the chest, lungs, and the spinal fluid surrounding the spinal cord.

TABLE 8.2 Pitta Qualities and Manifestations in the Body

Qualities	Manifestations in the Body
Hot	Good digestive fire; strong appetite; body temperature tends to be higher than average; hates heat; tendency toward grey hair with receding hairline or baldness; soft brown hair on the body and face
Sharp	Sharp teeth, distinct eyes, pointed nose, tapering chin, heart-shaped face; good absorption and digestion; sharp memory and understanding; irritable; probing mind
Light	Light/medium body frame; does not tolerate bright light; fair shiny skin, bright eyes
Oily	Soft oily skin, hair, and feces; sensitive to deep-fried foods (which may cause headache)
Liquid	Loose liquid stools; soft delicate muscles; excess urine, sweat, and thirst
Spreading	Rashes, hives, acne, inflammation all over the body or in certain areas; wants to spread his or her name and fame all over the country
Sour	Sour acid stomach, acidic pH; sensitive teeth; excess salivation
Bitter	Bitter taste in the mouth; nausea; vomiting; repulsion toward bitter taste; cynical
Pungent	Heartburn, burning sensations in general; strong feelings of anger and hate
Red	Red flushed skin, eyes, cheeks, and nose; red color aggravates
Yellow	Yellow eyes, skin, urine, and feces; jaundice; overproduction of bile; yellow color aggravates

Kapha people have heavy bones, muscles, and fat. The body type is analogous to the Western ectomorph body type. Their tendency is to be overweight, and they have slow metabolism and digestion. The skin may be cool and clammy, the eyes big and liquid looking, and their hair thick and wavy. Qualities of kapha are heavy, slow, cool, oily, liquid, hard, soft, dense, static, viscous, cloudy, slimy, sweet, and salty[3,4,7] (**TABLE 8.3**).

Kaphas are slow to pick up new ideas but have great long-term memories. They are slow to start new projects. They tend to be slow at everything they do,

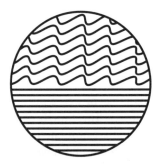

FIGURE 8.3 Kapha sign.

contrary to vatas who are always on the run. They move slowly, eat slowly, act slowly, think slowly, and are slow to anger. Kaphas tend to be forgiving, loving, and compassionate. A person with a dominant kapha metabolic body type is easygoing, laid back, and relaxed.

In Balance: This is expressed as love, calmness, and forgiveness. They appear strong and calm.

Out of Balance: This may lead to attachment, greed, and envy. They appear dull and lethargic.

Likely diseases in kapha people include respiratory, asthma, allergy, and sinusitis problems. Kapha people need stimulation such as physical activity and new life experiences. They need to avoid sweet and heavy foods, but need hot and spicy foods.[6,7,8]

If you are interested in finding out what your dosha is, please complete a dosha questionnaire, like the one found in **FIGURE 8.4**.[9] A second suggestion is to access a dosha quiz found at www.JoyfulBelly.com.[10] Since there are many to be found on the Internet, you may find it fun to do an Internet search for a dosha quiz that appears interesting to you.

TABLE 8.3	Kapha Qualities and Manifestations in the Body
Qualities	**Manifestations in the Body**
Heavy	Heavy bones and muscles; large body frame; tends to be overweight; grounded; deep, heavy voice
Slow	Walks and talks slowly; steady appetite and thirst with slow metabolism and digestion
Cold	Cold clammy skin; repeated colds, congestion, and cough; desire for sweets and cold drinks
Oily	Oily skin, hair, and feces; lubricated, unctuous joints and other organs
Liquid	Congestive disorders; edema; excessive salivation; mucus
Hard	Firmness and solidity of muscles; compact, condensed tissues
Smooth	Smooth skin; gentle, calm nature; smoothness of organs; smooth, gentle mind
Dense	Dense pads of fat; thick skin, hair, nails, and feces
Soft	Soft pleasing look; love, care, compassion, kindness, and forgiveness
Static	Loves sitting, sleeping, and doing nothing
Viscous	Viscous, sticky, cohesive quality causes compactness, firmness of joints, muscles, tissues, and organs; loves to hug; is deeply attached in love and relationships
Cloudy	Mind is cloudy and foggy in the morning; often desires coffee as a stimulant to start the day
Slimy	Excess salivation; slow digestion; attachment
Sweet	Anabolic action of sweet taste stimulates sperm formation, increasing quantity of semen; craving for sweets
Salty	Helps digestion and growth; gives energy; maintains osmotic condition; craving for salt; water retention

Subdoshas

Each of the doshas has five subdoshas. See **TABLE 8.4** for the subdoshas and their function.[11] The concept of doshas and their subdoshas has been scientifically tested. Alex Hankey[12,13,14] tested the concepts by conducting a statistical (factor) analysis of the results of completed prakriti (Ayurveda body type) questionnaires. He found that dosha qualities and functions describe individual differences in physiology. Hankey used a different approach to test for regulatory functions of the organs and found they were equated with the three doshas. He also used an electrophysiological approach that indicated that dosha differences influence fundamental cellular functions and, ultimately, tissue function.

As previously stated, according to Ayurveda, health exists when all aspects of the body are in proper balance; disease occurs when that balance is disturbed. According to Ayurveda philosophy, out of balance doshas or subdoshas lead to disease conditions. Excess vata, for example, might lead to arthritis, anxiety, and fatigue. Excess kapha, on the other hand, is said to cause obesity and diabetes.

Principle of Disease Causation

Besides the belief that an imbalance in the dosha causes body dysfunction and disease, Ayurveda identifies four main causes of disease: mental factors, lifestyle habits, dosha imbalance, and metabolic toxins.[2,8] Mental factors begin with an emotional imbalance or stress in an individual. If individuals are stressed, it will lead to unhealthy lifestyles and worsening mental stresses. Lifestyle habits include lack of exercise, substance-taking habits, poor dietary behaviors, poor sleep patterns, and unsafe sexual practices. Previously discussed was the concept of dosha imbalance (imbalance of vata, pitta, kapha, or one of the combinations). The fourth cause of disease is metabolic toxins that accumulate in the body because of the by-products of metabolism and presence of other toxins. Treatment is based on the cause of the disease and is discussed later in this chapter.

Discover Your Dosha

This quiz gathers information about your basic nature—the way you were as a child and the basic patterns that have been true for most of your life. If you developed an illness in childhood or as an adult, think of how things were for you before that illness. If more than one quality is applicable in each characteristic, choose the one that applies the most.

For fairly objective physical traits, your choice will usually be obvious. Because mental traits and behavior tend to be more subjective, you should answer according to how you have felt and acted most of your life, or at least in the past few years. Check the appropriate boxes in each column for all the parameters and place the total in the last row of each column. The column with the highest total is your predominant dosha.

Frame	☐ I am thin, lanky, and slender with prominent joints and thin muscles.	☐ I have a medium, symmetrical build with good muscle development.	☐ I have a large, round or stocky build. My frame is broad, stout or thick.
Weight	☐ Low; I may forget to eat or have a tendency to lose weight.	☐ Moderate; it is easy for me to gain or lose weight if I put my mind to it.	☐ Heavy; I gain weight easily and have difficulty losing it.
Eyes	☐ My eyes are small and active.	☐ I have a penetrating gaze.	☐ I have large pleasant eyes.
Complexion	☐ My skin is dry, rough or thin.	☐ My skin is warm, reddish in color and prone to irritation.	☐ My skin is, thick, moist, and smooth.
Hair	☐ My hair is dry, brittle or frizzy.	☐ My hair is fine with a tendency towards early thinning or graying.	☐ I have abundant, thick and oily hair.
Joints	☐ My joints are thin and prominent and have a tendency to crack.	☐ My joints are loose and flexible.	☐ My joints are large, well-knit and padded.
Sleep Pattern	☐ I am a light sleeper with a tendency to awaken easily.	☐ I am a moderately sound sleeper, usually needing less than eight hours to feel rested.	☐ My sleep is deep and long. I tend to awaken slowly in the morning.
Body Temperature	☐ My hands and feet are usually cold and I prefer warm environments.	☐ I am usually warm, regardless of the season, and prefer cooler environments.	☐ I am adaptable to most temperatures but do not like cold, wet days.
Temperament	☐ I am lively and enthusiastic by nature. I like to change.	☐ I am purposeful and intense. I like to convince.	☐ I am easy going and accepting. I like to support.
Under Stress	☐ I become anxious and/or worried.	☐ I become irritable and/or aggressive.	☐ I become withdrawn and/or reclusive.
Total	Vata _____	Pitta_____	Kapha _____

FIGURE 8.4 Naturally Healthy with Ayurveda Dosha Questionnaire

Courtesy of The Chopra Center https://shop.chopra.com/dosha-quiz/

TABLE 8.4 Subdoshas and Their Function

Subdoshas	Location	Direction	Function
Vata Subdoshas			
Prana Vata	Brain, heart, respiratory system	Inward and downward	Respiration, swallowing, perception of senses
Udana Vata	Throat to top of head	Upward	Speech, self expression, health of throat
Samana Vata	Stomach, small and large intestines	Balancing and equalizing	Digestion, intestinal peristalsis
Vyana Vata	Heart, circulatory system, whole body	Pervasive, entire body, circular	Circulation, sweating, walking, gait
Apana Vata	Pelvis, colon	Downward and outward	Urination, elimination, menstruation, ejaculation

(continues)

TABLE 8.4 *(continued)*

Subdoshas	Location	Direction	Function
Pitta Subdoshas			
Sadhaka Pitta	Heart, brain, mind	Inward	Emotions, memory, intellect, learning
Alochaka Pitta	Eyes	Upward	Visual perception, eye color
Pachaka Pitta	Stomach, small intestine	Equalizing	Digestion, absorption, governs agni
Bhrajaka Pitta	Skin	Outward	Complexion, skin color, pigmentation, temperature
Ranjaka Pitta	Liver, gall bladder, spleen, blood	Downward	Formation and color of blood cells, produces bile and liver enzymes
Kapha Subdoshas			
Tarpaka Kapha	Head, sinus, cerebrospinal fluid	Inward	Thought, emotions, knowledge
Bodhaka Kapha	Tongue, mouth, throat	Upward	Perception of six tastes, lubrication of oral cavity with saliva
Kledaka Kapha	Stomach, digestive tract	Balancing	Liquefies food
Sleshaka Kapha	Joints	Outward	Lubrication of all joints
Avalambhaka Kapha	Lungs, heart, back	Downward	Heart, lungs, chest, exchange of lung gases

▶ What Types of Diagnostic Methods Are Used in Ayurveda?

Determination of Dosha Type

First, Ayurvedic physicians will determine body dosha type by administering a dosha questionnaire or orally asking selective questions to determine dosha. Next, they may administer a test to determine dosha balance (**prakriti**) or imbalance (**vikruiti**).

Health and Family History and Physical Examination

Once the dosha and either balance or imbalance have been established, Ayurvedic physicians or practitioners complete health and family histories.[2,15,16,17] They will conduct physical examinations such as palpating the body or listening to the heart, lungs, and intestines with a stethoscope. They will conduct systemic examinations of body systems (digestive system, respiratory system, heart and circulatory system, nervous system, urinary system, musculoskeletal system, reproductive system, skin and hair, and eyes). Ayurvedic physicians

utilize observation more than laboratory testing, but will utilize blood, stool, and urine laboratory testing.

Ayurvedic physicians will, however, continue the examination much differently than Western physicians by examining in detail the pulse, tongue, lips, eyes, and nails to aid in diagnosing wellness or illness. The following gives an overview of pulse, tongue, facial, nail, lip, and eye diagnoses. Note: Researchers have assessed many of the following Ayurvedic diagnostic techniques for reliability (consistency among doctors examining patients) and have found them lacking.[18] The authors of the study conclude that Ayurvedic medical institutions should provide more standardized diagnostic techniques and that future reliability studies should become more rigorous.[18]

Pulse Diagnostic Technique

Ayurvedic physicians use the pulse to describe the balance (or imbalance) of the three doshas and to diagnose body illnesses such as heart disorders. The Ayurvedic technique of **pulse taking** may have been derived from the Chinese medical theory. A radial artery pulse is felt with the first three fingers, the index, middle, and ring fingers, and the pulse is taken from both wrists.[16] There are three aspects to the pulse:

- **Snake pulse (Vata):** The position of the index finger denotes the vata dosha. When vata is strong in the constitution, the index finger will feel the pulse strongly. The pulse will be irregular and thin, moving in waves like the motion of a serpent.
- **Frog pulse (Pitta):** The middle finger denotes the pulse corresponding to the pitta dosha. When the person has a predominant pitta constitution, the pulse under the middle finger will be stronger. Ayurveda describes this pulse as "active, excited, and moves like the jumping of a frog."
- **Swan pulse (Kapha):** When the throbbing of the pulse under the ring finger is most noticeable, it is a sign of a kapha constitution. The pulse feels strong and its movement resembles the floating of a swan. Hence, this pulse is called swan pulse.

Tongue Diagnostic Technique

Ayurvedic physicians examine the size, shape, surface, margins, and color of the tongue. The tongue is mapped much like the feet in zone therapy, that is, different areas of the tongue are thought to correspond to different organs of the body[17] (**FIGURE 8.5**).

A blemish, discoloration, or coating on some part of the tongue is used to indicate a body problem.[17]

- **Pale tongue:** Anemic condition or lack of blood in the body.
- **Blue tongue:** Indication of heart disease.
- **Whitish tongue:** Indication of kapha imbalance and mucus accumulation.
- **Red or yellow-green tongue:** Indication of pitta imbalance.
- **Black or brown tongue:** Indication of vata imbalance.
- **Coating on the tongue:** Indication of toxins in the stomach, or small or large intestine (**FIGURE 8.6**).

Facial Diagnostic Technique

Ayurveda holds that the face mirrors the mind and that disorders and/or disease may be indicated by wrinkle pattern, looks of the eyelids and eyes, appearance and shape of the nose, and appearance of the lips.[2,15,19] The following gives an indication of facial characteristics

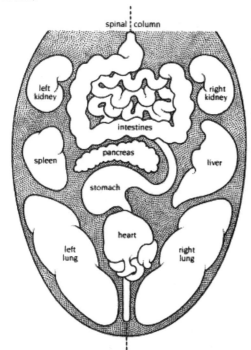

Diagram 6
Tongue Diagnosis (Jihva)

CONDITIONS: A discoloration and/or sensitivity of a particular area of the tongue indicates a disorder in the organ corresponding to that area (see diagram). A whitish tongue indicates *Kapha* derangement and mucus accumulation; a red or yellow-green tongue indicates *Pitta* derangement; and a black-to-brown coloration indicates *Vata* derangement. A dehydrated tongue is symptomatic of a decrease in the *dhatu Rasa* (plasma), while a pale tongue indicates a decrease in the *dhatu Rakta* (red blood cells).

Note: *This diagram is used to look at one's own tongue in a mirror. It is a mirror image.*

FIGURE 8.5 Tongue mapping.

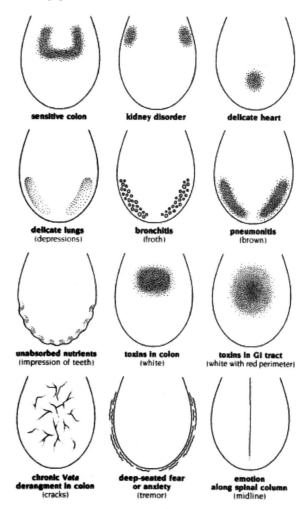

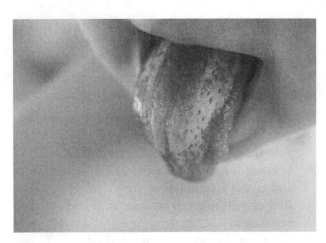

FIGURE 8.6 Coated tongue.

© Victoria 1/Shutterstock

that may be associated with certain bodily disorders. Please note:

- **Wrinkles:**
  - *Horizontal wrinkles on forehead*: Indicate deep-seated anxiety and worry.
- **Eyelids and eyes:**
  - *Lower eyelid fullness*: Indicates impaired kidneys.
  - *Excessive blinking*: Indicates nervousness, anxiety, or fear and is vata imbalance.
  - *Drooping upper eyelid*: Indicates sense of insecurity, fear, or lack of confidence and is vata imbalance.
  - *Prominent eye*: Indicates thyroid gland dysfunction.
  - *Yellow conjunctiva*: Indicates a weak liver.
  - *Small iris*: Indicates weak joints.
  - *White ring around the iris*: Indicates an excessive intake of salt or sugar.
  - *Prominent white ring*: Indicates joint degeneration with potential for arthritis and joint pain.
- **Nose:**
  - *Butterfly-like nose discoloration*: Indicates malabsorption of iron or folic acid and may indicate a digestive disorder.
  - *Shape of the nose*: Indicates the dosha. Sharp nose is pitta, crooked nose is vata, and blunt nose is kapha.
- **Lips:**
  - *Dry and rough lips*: Indicate dehydration or vata imbalance.
  - *Pale lips*: Indicate anemia.
  - *Repeated attacks of inflammatory patches along the margins of the lips*: Indicate the presence of herpes and a chronic pitta derangement.
  - *Multiple pale brown spots on the lips*: Indicate poor digestion or worms in the colon.

- *Yellow lips*: Indicate jaundice.
- *Blue lips*: Indicate or may signal heart problems.[2,15]

Once a diagnosis has been established, Ayurvedic physicians will recommend therapy or treatment.

▶ What Are the Major Ayurvedic Therapies?

Several types of treatment are recommended in Ayurveda. Treatment is usually comprehensive and customized. The health program is based on maintaining Prakruti (balanced dosha constitution) and focuses on healing Vikruti (imbalanced dosha constitution).

General Guidelines for Balancing Vata, Pitta, and Kapha

See **BOXES 8.3**, **8.4**, and **8.5** for vata, pitta, and kapha balancing guidelines, respectively, and see **BOX 8.6** for overall Ayurveda treatments.[1,2]

BOX 8.3 General Guidelines for Balancing Vata

- Keep warm
- Keep calm
- Avoid cold, frozen, or raw foods
- Avoid extreme cold
- Eat warm foods and spices
- Keep a regular routine
- Get plenty of rest

BOX 8.4 General Guidelines for Balancing Pitta

- Avoid excessive heat
- Avoid excessive oil
- Avoid excessive steam
- Limit salt intake
- Eat cooling, nonspicy foods
- Exercise during the cooler part of the day

BOX 8.5 General Guidelines for Balancing Kapha

- Get plenty of exercise
- Avoid heavy foods
- Keep active
- Avoid dairy
- Avoid iced food or drinks
- Vary your routine
- Avoid fatty, oily foods
- Eat light, dry food
- No daytime naps

BOX 8.6 Ayurveda Treatments: General Summary

- A dosha-specific natural diet custom suited for you
- Therapeutic nutritional supplements
- Healing botanical herbs and spices
- Detoxification of accumulated toxins
- Ayurvedic bodywork and massage
- Rejuvenation therapy to delay aging and promote energy
- Yoga
- Daily routines
- Understanding of a healthy lifestyle

Ayurvedic treatments are categorized into six major treatment concepts[2,20,21]:

1. **Shodhanam**: Cleansing
2. **Shamanam**: Balancing
3. **Pathya vyavastha**: Prescription of diet and activity
4. **Nidan parivarjan**: Avoidance of disease-causing and aggravating factors
5. **Rasayana**: Rejuvenation
6. **Satvajaya**: Mental hygiene/psychotherapy

Before Shodhanam therapy begins, Ayurveda recommends precleansing procedures called purva-karma,[20] which prepare the body for Shodhanam.

Purva-Karma Therapy

Two main treatments are utilized to carry out purva-karma: Snehan and Swedan. **Snehan treatment** is given both internally and externally. In internal Snehan, patients are given medicated edible oil or medicated edible butter in a dose prescribed by the Ayurvedic therapist (e.g., two spoonfuls). Nothing else is taken in on that day.[2,20,21] The mixture is called **ghee** or sneha and is best if made from cow's milk. The intention of internal Snehan is to enhance later Pancha karma procedures in order to rid the body of impurities. External Snehan is carried out by medicated ghee body massage, given every few days for a week or more. Ghee is also known as clarified butter, and is prepared by simmering unsalted butter until all water is evaporated. It will become a clear, golden liquid. The liquid may then be mixed with herbs. The skin absorbs part of the medicated oil and carries it to the bloodstream.[20,21] See **FIGURE 8.7** of a person receiving body massage with ghee.

The second **purva-karma treatment** is Swedana therapy or Swedan. **Swedan treatment** is the use of dry or wet fomentation or heat therapy to facilitate sweating. It can be given in many ways: sunbathing, in a sweat box, pouring warm water on the body, a steam

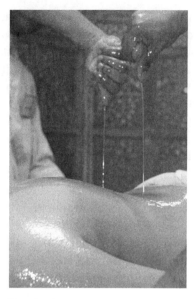

FIGURE 8.7 Ghee body massage.
© iStockphoto/Thinkstock

bath, or sitting in a tub of warm water. The water may contain milk, herbs, or medicated oil. According to individual needs, Swedan can be whole body therapy or just focus on a diseased part of the body. Swedan reportedly liquefies toxins and increases the movement of toxins into the gastrointestinal tract.[20,21] Once purva-karma procedures are completed, Shodhanam therapy begins.

Shodhanam Therapy

Shodhanam therapy involves five procedures grouped under a term called **Panchakarma treatment**.[20,21,22,23] Pancha in Sanskrit stands for five and Karma stands for therapeutic measures, so Panchakarma means five types of therapeutic measures. Panchakarma is a comprehensive system of knowledge and practices to purify the body of toxins and restore it to balance with the laws of Mother Nature.[22,23,24,25] The therapies are intended to balance the doshas, relieve stress, and rid the body of toxins. A recommendation is that while a person is undergoing Panchakarma treatment they should also be on a special diet that is monitored by a doctor.[4,22,25] The following describes the five procedures intended to rid the body of toxins:

- **Vamana**: First is forced vomiting. It is intended to remove kapha toxins collected in the body and respiratory tract. It is given to people with a kapha imbalance by a daily treatment that is supposed to loosen and mobilize toxins.
- **Virechana**: Second is forced purging. This therapy is intended to remove pitta toxins that accumulate in the liver and gallbladder by completely cleansing the gastrointestinal tract. Benefits of

Virechana include helping to root out chronic fever, diabetes, asthma, skin disorders such as herpes, paraplegia, hemiplegia, joint disorders, digestive disorders, constipation, hyperacidity, vitiligo, psoriasis, headaches, elephantiasis, and gynecological disorders.[23,24,25]

- **Basti**: Third is medicated enema or colonic irrigation. Basti is intended to eliminate loosened vata dosha, which is predominantly located in the colon and bones, but also supposedly cleanses the body of toxins from all three doshas.[22,23,24,25] The treatment involves the introduction of medicinal substances, such as herbal oils and decoctions in a liquid medium, into the rectum of the person. Medicated oil or ghee and a herbal decoction are given as enema to cleanse the colon and increase the muscle tone. This procedure is usually applied for 8–30 days, based on the medical condition of a person. It reportedly benefits hemiplegia, paraplegia, colitis, cervical spondylosis, irritable bowel syndrome, constipation, digestive disorders, backache and sciatica, hepatomegaly and splenomegaly, obesity, hemmorhoids, sexual arousal problems, and infertility.[22,23,24]

- **Nasya**: Fourth is nose or sinus cleaning. Nasya treatment is intended to cleanse kapha toxins from the head and neck region. Some use a **neti pot** to pour salt water through the nose to combat chronic sinus problems (water irrigation). Medicated oil may also be administered through the nose for up to 30 days, depending on the medical condition of a person. Nasya reportedly benefits trigeminal neuralgia, Bell's palsy, memory, eyesight, insomnia, elimination of excess mucus, hyperpigmentation in the face, premature graying of hair, clarity of voice, headaches of various origin, hemiplegia, loss of smell and taste, frozen shoulder, migraine, stiffness of the neck, nasal allergies, nasal polyps, neurological dysfunctions, paraplegia, and sinusitis.[2,4,23,25]

- **Raktamokshana**: Fifth are procedures to detoxify the blood. This may include bloodletting or the use of certain herbs to cleanse the blood. It is not advisable during general Panchakarma, and most Ayurveda centers do not offer Raktamokshana due to the high risk of infection involved in blood cleansing.[22,23,24]

A study at the Institute of Science, Technology and Public Policy at Maharishi University of Management in Fairfield, Iowa, in collaboration with a special laboratory at Colorado University, demonstrated that classical Panchakarma treatment eliminated up to 50% of the detectable toxins in the blood.[26] This particular study found that PCB and DDE are entering the food chain, causing high levels of these chemicals to appear in the blood in the general population. With the Panchakarma treatments, a large proportion of these fat-soluble toxins were reported to be eliminated from the body.[26]

As shown, Shodhanam therapy requires quite a lot of time. First, there is a week of pre-preparation called purva-karma, and then, depending on individual needs, panchakarma therapy could last a week or more. In addition, Shodhanam therapy could be harsh on the body because it is intended to be a thorough cleansing. The purpose is to drive imbalanced doshas out of the body. The next therapy discussed in this chapter, Shamana, is much milder.

Shamana Therapy

Shamana therapy is intended to achieve a balanced state in the body and to alleviate symptoms of disease.[4,22] This intervention focuses on the spiritual dimensions of healing,[2,3] and is much milder than Shodhan therapy; however, according to Ayurvedic thought, it is not as long lasting. Kulkarni[24] describes seven Shamana procedures:

1. **Deepan (creating appetite)**: Consuming food or mild medicines that help in empowering agni (digestive fire or digestive enzymes). This includes consuming ghee, oil, spices, hot drinks, and warm food. Improving deepan helps achieve dosha balance.

2. **Pachan (digesting)**: Pachan is an aid to digest toxins (ama). This is a preferred treatment in digestive disorders. People are encouraged to eat foods such as dry ginger and sweet kernel, which help digestion when eaten after lunch or dinner.

3. **Kshudha-nigrah (hunger control/fasting)**: This is a treatment for dosha imbalance and involves total, partial, or selective fasting. Avoiding food for a period of time or changing lifestyle can provide rest to the digestive tract.

4. **Trushna-nigrah (thirst control)**: This treatment helps when water retention is a problem. In the case of generalized edema or ascites, if water intake is monitored, the urinary tract gets an opportunity to clear the accumulated fluid from the body.

5. **Vyayam (exercises)**: This is the prescribed treatment in conditions like obesity and diabetes. It helps to reestablish balance without medicines or with the lowest possible dose.

6. **Atap-seva (sun bath)**: This is a preferred treatment in vata disorders. It is recommended for

many skin disorders and uses solar energy as a medicine. This treatment also works well in cases of arthritis pain and rheumatic conditions.

7. **Marut-seva (consumption of fresh air):** This is the prescribed treatment for tuberculosis, asthma, and other lung conditions. Breathing fresh air helps lung function and provides energy within the respiratory system. (Known as sitting in the wind/breathing exercises—pranayama.)

Pathya Vyavastha Therapy

This treatment is a prescription of diet and activity.[2,4,7] Patients might be encouraged and taught yoga; all forms of physical activity are recommended in order to enhance the effects of therapeutic measures. A nutritious diet is prescribed in order to stimulate agni and optimize digestion. In our society, we identify certain foods as healthy and others as unhealthy. In Ayurveda, what is good for one person is bad for another and vice versa. For example, a person tending toward an excess of vata might be advised to avoid raw vegetables but consume nuts and seeds in abundance. Someone with an excess of kapha would be given the opposite recommendation. The foods recommended may also change depending on the season. In Ayurvedic medicine, individuals are given specific details about the optimal ways to prepare and consume foods.[7]

Nidan Parivarjan Therapy

This treatment focuses on helping individuals change their lifestyles to avoid known disease-causing factors (e.g., smoking, alcohol and other drug use, diet).[2,3]

Rasayana Therapy

In Ayurveda, Rasayana means that, which nourishes the body and boosts immunity. It is also called rejuvenation therapy,[27] and focuses on promoting strength and vitality. It may involve the use of herbs or drugs, diet, and a changed lifestyle. One source refers to Rasayana therapy as the use of Panchakarma techniques.[27,28] Although we found no scientific documentation, Ayurveda purports that the benefits of Rasayana are many (e.g., more youthful skin, higher resistance to disease, improved intelligence, improved attitude about life, better sense of well-being).

Satvajaya Therapy

Satvajaya treatment is psychotherapy or mental health counseling for those needing it. It might involve helping people to restrain from overindulging in alcohol or other drugs, or it might involve helping people to improve their memory or gain self-concept and self-esteem. One of its therapies is the use of meditation.[28,29]

Thus far, most of the Ayurveda therapeutic modalities have been very holistic, in that the body and mind are addressed in the treatment plan. Shodhanam (Panchakarma) could be challenging, and if not monitored well, could be harmful because of dehydration or electrolyte imbalances. The other treatments are certainly utilized in Western as well as Ayurvedic medicine.

▶ What Herbs or Plants Are Used in Ayurvedic Medicine?

According to a 2004 survey conducted by the National Center for Health Statistics (NCHS) and National Center for Complementary and Integrative Health (NCCIH),[30] more than 750,000 people in the United States had used Ayurvedic medicine in the previous year. But, are Ayurvedic medicines safe? More than 600 herbal formulas and 250 single-plant drugs[30] are used in Ayurvedic medicine. Ayurvedic pharmaceuticals form a branch of Ayurveda that deals with the collection and selection of drugs. The practice studies the preparation, preservation, mode of administration, and dosage specifications. Many processing techniques of crude drugs are carried out and tested, much like Western pharmaceutical companies do. For example, trituration (reducing to a powder or diluting a medicinal powder) is used. Some crude drugs are treated by heating them or placing them in liquid. Some are preserved (stored) in various types of containers, and the effect of using various types of containers is tested. Drugs are also formulated in various ways, including distillations, ointments, powders, pills, medicated oils, and so forth. The drugs are scientifically tested. There is a preclinical stage of testing a drug, after which comes a drug development period that is composed of four phases of clinical studies.[31] After Phase III, the drug is either approved for safety and efficacy or rejected. Phase IV and V studies are conducted while the drug is being marketed.

Some Ayurvedic medicines have been scientifically tested according to Western standards, but many have not. There have been concerns about toxicity, formulations, interactions, and evidence of scientific testing on these medicines. One study found that nearly 21% of Ayurvedic medicines tested had detectable levels of lead (most common), mercury, or arsenic.

Some over-the-counter drugs manufactured in South Asia use fillers for some of these herbs that may contain lead, mercury, and/or arsenic.[32,33,34] Adverse drug reactions to other Ayurvedic medicines have been reported, but may be due to inadequate preparation of the drug. The NCCIH reports that health officials in India and other countries have taken steps to address these concerns.

On the other hand, scientific testing here in the United States has shown favorable results for **turmeric** (curcumin)[35,36] and *Salvia lavandulaefolia* (Spanish sage).[37,38] For example, positive results were revealed in a study to assess the use of curcumin to lessen the effects of radiation dermatitis.[36] The participants were 30 adult females with breast cancer who received no chemotherapy, only radiation therapy. There was a significant reduction in radiation dermatitis in patients who received 6 grams of curcumin per day compared to those getting placebo during treatment.

Turmeric has been used for thousands of years to treat many different illnesses.[35,39] The plant is related to ginger and is grown in Asia, India, and Central America. It is a common spice and is used as food coloring. It gives Indian curry its color and flavor. It is also used in mustard, butter, and cheese to enhance the yellow color. Turmeric is used as an anti-inflammatory, to treat digestive and liver problems, and stimulate the production of bile by the gallbladder, but it does have adverse effects so should be used wisely. It could make gallbladder disease worse, might slow blood clotting, might decrease blood sugar in diabetes, might make gastroesophageal reflux disease (GERD) worse, and might lower testosterone levels in men. It is likely safe during pregnancy if taken in amounts found in food but not safe to take in larger prescribed medicinal amounts. There is not enough scientific evidence to support its use during breast feeding. See **FIGURE 8.8** for a photograph of a turmeric plant and root.

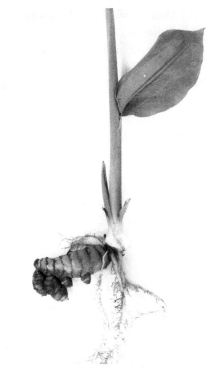

FIGURE 8.8 Turmeric plant and roots.
© Anan Kaewkhammul/Shutterstock

Salvia too has been assessed in many studies.[37,38] A recent 2017 review study of the effects of *Salvia* (sage)[38] confirm earlier reports that *Salvia* influences many biological functions that seem to impact both neurological and cognitive function.

BOX 8.7 has examples of plants and herbs associated with Ayurvedic medicine and their intended uses.[39,40,41] We, the authors of this text, are neither recommending nor condemning these plants and herbs for medicinal use. We do recommend that if you want to try an herb to treat yourself for any condition that you may have, please do so after researching scientific studies of those plants and under the guidance of your doctor/s.

🔍 CASE STUDY

You live in a large city on the West Coast of the United States. You have learned information regarding some of the Chinese medicine healing practices such as acupuncture and have participated in some energy work (tai chi). Since your 20s, you have suffered with digestive disorder problems and have been diagnosed with irritable bowel syndrome, a condition that causes you a lot of abdominal pain after eating. A friend suggested that you go see an Ayurvedic medicine doctor or practitioner for treatment.

Questions:
1. Where would you find the credentials of an Ayurvedic medicine doctor or practitioner?
2. If the doctor suggested that you undergo Shodhanam treatment, which of the five would you agree to?
3. What could be some therapeutic synd/or ill effects from Shodhanam treatment?
4. Which of the Shamana therapy treatments would you want prescribed and why?

BOX 8.7 Ayurvedic Plants/Herbs and Their Uses

Amalaki (Ami) is an herb made from the Indian gooseberry (*Embilica officinalis* or *Phyllanthus emblica*). It is usually used in juice form and is supposed to help promote longevity. Some test tube studies suggest that it has antioxidant, antibacterial, and anti-inflammatory properties. It is used in Ayurvedic medicine to rebuild and maintain new tissues and increase red blood cell count. It is considered helpful in cleansing the mouth, strengthening teeth, and nourishing the bones, and is the highest natural source of vitamin C. It is one of the three herbs used in *triphala*, the primary Ayurvedic tonic for maintaining health.

Arjuna (*Terminalia arjuna*, bark extract) is another herb that is supposed to have antioxidant properties. In Ayurveda, it is used as a cardiac tonic, and is traditionally given to support circulation and oxygenation of all tissues. It is often combined with ashwagandha, brahmi, and guggul in heart formulas.

Ashoka is Sanskrit for "without sorrow." The bark, flowers, and seeds of the Ashoka plant are used. It is used in Ayurveda as an aid for heavy menstrual periods due to uterine fibroids. It is also used to help maintain proper function of the female reproductive system.

Ashwagandha means "winter cherry." It is made from a small evergreen perennial shrub that grows to 1.5 meters tall and is found in dry areas of India and as far west as Israel. In Sanskrit, it means "the sweat or smell of a horse" because the roots smell like a horse. It is sometimes referred to as Indian ginseng, making reference to its nervous system tonic actions. In Ayurveda, it is used as an antioxidant, antibacterial, and antianxiety herb. It is purported to have aphrodisiac properties.

Bacopa is said to aid mental acuity and has antianxiety properties. It has also been used to help epilepsy.

Bhringaraj is used on the head to lessen premature graying of hair, balding, and bald spots. The herb is ground into a powder and added to an oil. It is also thought to be a liver tonic that is helpful for chronic hepatitis.

Bibitaki is used as a laxative to cleanse the bowels. It is also used as a gargle for sore throats because of its heating and soothing properties. It is one of three herbs used in *triphala*, the primary Ayurvedic tonic for maintaining health.

Bitter melon is said to regulate the body's ability to process sugars by suppressing the neutral response to the stimuli of sweet tastes.

Boswellia (frankincense) has been used extensively in Ayurveda for its anti-inflammatory effects and joint support such as in rheumatoid arthritis, bursitis, tendonitis, or osteoarthritis.

Brahmi has been used as a tonic for improving memory, relieving stress and anxiety, and increasing mental alertness. It has been used for epilepsy and premature aging. It is considered the primary Ayurvedic nerve and cardiac tonic. It is also available in oil form.

Chitrak is a pungent herb used to support liver function, improve digestion, and remove toxins from the GI tract.

Chyavanprash is a famous herbal jam made from amalaki fruit, one of the highest sources of vitamin C. It is fortified with over 20 herbs to rejuvenate and strengthen the immune system. It is used in Ayurveda as a longevity tonic.

Cilantro and coriander are powerful aids to digestion. They come from the same plant: cilantro comes from the first or vegetative stage of the plant's life cycle and coriander is the dried seed of cilantro. According to Ayurveda, allergies result from improper digestion and an accumulation of ama (toxic substances) in the body. By enhancing digestion, cilantro and coriander work to alleviate the root cause of allergies.

Coleus forskohlii has been a part of Ayurvedic medicine for centuries. An extract from the plant is used to treat hypothyroidism, heart disease, and respiratory disorders.

Cumin is the seed of a small plant and is supposed to aid digestion and help flush toxins out of the body. Sprinkle ground, dry-roasted cumin on fresh yogurt, add salt to taste, and enjoy at lunch.

Dandelion and dandelion root are regarded as a liver tonic. It is used for people who suffer from mild fluid retention, such as may occur in PMS.

Fennel is said to be extremely good for digestion. In India, eating a few fennel seeds after a meal is a common practice. Fennel is a cooling spice.

Garcinia cambogia **extract** is used as an ephedra-free diet aid. It contains biologically active phytochemicals such as hydroxycitric acid and antioxidants. It supports normal appetite levels and metabolism and storage of carbohydrates and fats to maintain normal body weight.

Gokshura has diuretic properties and is useful in renal stones, painful urination, and kidney dysfunction. It is also used to support proper function of the urinary tract and prostate.

Gotu kola is used to promote wound healing and slow the progress of leprosy. It was also reputed to prolong life, increase energy, and enhance sexual potency. The best-documented use of gotu kola is to treat chronic venous insufficiency, a condition closely related to varicose veins.

Guduchi is a bitter tonic that has diuretic properties and is supposed to help remove urinary stones. It is also touted as enhancing immune resistance to diseases and as being protective of liver function.

(continues)

BOX 8.7 *(continued)*

Guggul (also known as guggulu) is made from the sap or gum resin of the mukul myrrh tree. Historically, it was used for its antiseptic and deep penetrating actions in the treatment of elevated blood cholesterol and arthritis. It is often used as a carrier and combined with other herbs to treat several specific conditions. It is traditionally used for arthritis, skin diseases, pains in the nervous system, obesity, digestive problems, infections in the mouth, and menstrual problems.

Gymnema is commonly referred to as "Gurmar, the destroyer of sugar." It is traditionally used in formulas to control blood sugar levels in the body. It is a member of the milkweed family. Leaves of the herb are chewed as a therapy for diabetes mellitus, snakebites (root powder), fever, cough, hemorrhoids, and urinary disorders.

Haritaki is used for many conditions. Topically as a paste, it is used for wounds and hemorrhoids. In a gargle, it is used for oral ulcers and sore throat. It is used internally as a digestive aid and for diarrhea. It is also used to aid coughing and asthma. It is one of three herbs used in triphala, the primary Ayurvedic tonic for maintaining health.

Holy basil is considered a sacred plant by the Hindus in India and is often planted near shrines. It is used for the common cold, asthma, bronchitis, and earache.

Kutki is a bitter and pungent herb used to support proper function of the liver and spleen. One of the chemicals in kutki, picroliv, is in Phase II clinical trials in India to support claims that it is a powerful liver protectant.

Manjista is considered one of the best blood purifying herbs in Ayurveda. It is thought to detox blood and dissolve plaque in the blood. It is used as an immune regulator and has antioxidant properties.

Neem is considered one of the best healing and disinfectant agents for skin diseases and an anti-inflammatory for joint and muscle pain. The neem tree has been called the village pharmacy, because its bark, leaves, sap, fruit, seeds, and twigs have so many diverse uses in the traditional medicine of India. Poets called it "Sarva Roga Nivarini," or The One That Can Cure All Ailments.

Phyllanthus amarus is used to treat jaundice and thought to be effective for treating hepatitis B. Despite numerous test tube and animal studies showing efficacy against the hepatitis B virus, it did not generally do well in human trials.

Phyllanthus embilica is commonly known as Indian gooseberry. It is supposed to decrease blood cholesterol and blood glucose levels.

Shatavari root is traditionally used to support women's health by restoring hormonal balance in women during the menstrual cycle and menopause. It is also used as an aid for stomach ulcers, inflammation, and chronic fevers.

Turmeric is a widely used tropical herb in the ginger family. The active ingredient in turmeric is curcumin. Its stalk is used in both food and medicine, yielding the familiar yellow ingredient that colors and adds flavor to curry. Turmeric is believed to have anti-inflammatory, antiseptic, and antibacterial properties. It is used to strengthen the overall energy of the body, relieve gas, dispel worms, improve digestion, regulate menstruation, dissolve gallstones, and relieve arthritis.

Tylophora indica is a climbing perennial plant indigenous to India, where it grows wild in the southern and eastern regions. The leaves and roots have laxative, emetic, and expectorant properties. It is supposed to be a remedy for asthma (hence the name T. Asthmatica). However, the studies that found it effective were poorly designed and a better designed study found no benefits. It is still recommended for some of its other traditional uses, including hay fever, bronchitis, and the common cold.

▶ What Minerals and Metals Are Used in Ayurvedic Medicine?

Several metals and minerals are purified or refined for use in Ayurvedic medicine.[22,40,41] These include gold, silver, copper, lead, tin, iron, sand (from river banks), lime, red chalk, gems, salts, red arsenic, and mercury. There are references to the uses of rasa (mercury), metals, and gems in the classical Ayurvedic texts, the *Charaka Samhita* and *Sushruta Samhita*. Within the classical texts, all the adverse reactions to medicines when prepared or used inappropriately are described.[34] To gain a brief understanding of the Ayurvedic preparation and use of metals, an explanation of gold follows.

Gold has been used since Ayurvedic medicine began. It supposedly has many purposes, including to promote longevity, combat aging, and treat impotency. It is used in Ayurvedic medicine as a tonic and an anti-infective, combats liver and heart disease, and currently is used for rheumatoid arthritis. The preparation of gold involves several complicated steps described by Mishra.[22] The steps for this are simplified and paraphrased in the following paragraph.

📰 *IN THE NEWS*

An article published in *TopNews*[33] on August 4, 2010 concerned Ayurvedic medicines and lead content. A middle-aged man in Sydney, Australia, took Ayurvedic medicine that was produced in India. After consuming the medicine for several months, he started having pain and vomiting. He was admitted to a hospital, where doctors found high levels of lead (2.3%) in his blood. Also, his blood report showed a significant amount of mercury and arsenic. Although the news article was disconcerting, there was a lot of missing information, including:

- Reason for taking the medication
- Identification of the medication
- Dosage recommended
- Length of time the medication was recommended to be taken
- Whether the individual followed the recommended dosage and length of time
- Whether the individual was under a doctor's care
- The general health of the individual
- Whether the individual was taking other medications

Therefore, it is extremely important that we, as health consumers, analyze and assess what we read in the newspapers, what we read online, and what we hear on television.

Questions:
1. What other information do you think might be missing from this news article?
2. What impact do you think such an article has on Ayurvedic medicine?

Source: Ayurvedic Center. Historical uses of Ayurvedic herbs. Available at: http://www.holheal.com/ayurved4.html. Accessed July 15, 2018.

The leaves of gold are heated, and when red hot, are dipped in a special oil. This process is repeated seven times. The same process is repeated using buttermilk, cow's urine, strongly processed herbs (decoction), rice made into sour gruel, and radish. The leaves are dried by heat. The gold is then carefully measured along with other ingredients and placed in an earthenware container and mixed with another ingredient called latex of *Calotropis gigentea*. The mixture is titrated, made into a paste, and dried in the sunlight. This process is repeated 7–14 times using fresh latex. A portion of the mixture is poured into liquefied metallic gold in a closed earthen pot and heated to above 1,000°C. The mass disintegrates into a red-brown powder, which is collected and becomes the gold drug.

We have given you an account of how one particular metal (gold) is processed into medicine. Again, we are neither promoting nor condemning these medicines, but hopefully, having presented a brief explanation of Ayurvedic medicines, you will become more motivated to explore further and to assess the literature for scientific research that may have been conducted. One study conducted found that all metal-containing products exceeded one or more standards for daily intake, although the American Herbal Products Association showed a lower level of toxic metals.[33] We, the consumer, need to make careful choices when we are selecting and buying our over-the-counter medicines, including Ayurvedic medicines.

There are concerns about the use of silver. For example, colloidal silver, a traditional Ayurvedic remedy, is considered a powerful germicide, but when taken in excessive amounts can be toxic to all human tissue. If taken, only about 50 micrograms can be excreted per day. The rest is deposited under the skin and tissues as silver sulfide and can cause permanent gray-black staining of the skin and mucous membranes. Excess colloidal silver can cause arteriosclerosis and could damage organs.[42] Colloidal silver can react with other drugs and cause even greater side effects. Because of this, the U.S. Food and Drug Administration refuses to approve the use of colloidal silver supplements for medicinal purposes.[42]

▶ What Does the NCCIH Report About Ayurveda?

Proponents of Ayurveda consider it helpful for several conditions such as alleviating side effects of cancer chemotherapy; recovering from the effects of surgery, because it encourages healing; and aiding chronic, metabolic, and stress-related conditions.[2,4] According to the NCCIH,[30] there is not enough scientific evidence to vouch for the effectiveness of Ayurvedic practices, and so it is calling for more rigorous research. Most clinical trials have been small, had research design problems, lacked appropriate control groups, or had other problems.

On the NCCIH[30] website, examples of Ayurvedic medicine research include studies of the following:

- Herbal therapies, including curcuminoids (substances found in turmeric), used for cardiovascular conditions
- A compound from the cowhage plant (*Mucuna pruriens*) used to prevent or lessen the side effects from Parkinson's disease drugs
- Three botanicals (ginger, turmeric, and boswellia) used to treat inflammatory disorders such as arthritis and asthma
- Gotu kola (*Centella asiatica*), an herb used to treat Alzheimer's disease

▶ What Is the National Institute of Ayurvedic Medicine?

The National Institute of Ayurvedic Medicine (NIAM) is located in Brewster, New York. The NIAM was established in 1982 by Scott Gerson, MD, the nation's only medical doctor to hold a PhD in Ayurveda as well as a conventional allopathic medicine degree.[43] Gerson wrote his doctoral paper, *Panchakarma Chikitsa* (detoxification therapy), which was approved in 2003 by both the Pune University and the Tilak Ayurved Mahavidyalaya in Pune, India. Dr. Gerson's medical practice is at the NIAM, where he has combined Ayurveda and conventional medicine for more than 15 years. The institute is the largest holder of Ayurveda data and information in the United States.[43]

One can take a certificate course in Ayurveda at the NIAM, which is a 3-year program. Candidates for the program must have completed 2 years of college or university study and have graduated from a school of medicine, nursing, oriental medicine, nutrition, physical therapy, massage, social work, or other allied health discipline. The following gives more detail about various ways to become an Ayurvedic physician or practitioner.

▶ What Is the Training of an Ayurvedic Medicine Doctor or Practitioner?

In India, the highest degree one can obtain in Ayurveda is a PhD. Students can get a Bachelor of Ayurvedic Medicine and Surgery (BAMS) in a 5½-year program of study. The postgraduate programs lead to the doctorate in Ayurveda. Graduates can get employment as medical officers/doctors at government and private Ayurvedic hospitals or open their own practices.[44]

In 2004, the National Ayurvedic Medical Association established educational standards in the United States. There is no widely accepted licensure for the practice of Ayurvedic medicine in the United States; however, there are several schools that offer extensive training. The types of training programs offered in the United States are as follows:

- **Correspondence programs:** Some include Internet study and others include reading textbooks required by the instructor. Testing and credit hours vary. The National Ayurvedic Medical Association does not recognize correspondence course hours toward national certification.
- **Full-time training programs:** Two examples of this type of program are at the California College of Ayurveda (18-month course) and the Ayurvedic Institute in New Mexico (16-month course).
- **Weekend training program:** There are about 10 weekend training programs; the length varies from 12 weekends to 24 weekends.
- **Short-term seminar courses:** Many of these are introductory courses, although some focus on a specific treatment modality.
- **Internship programs:** Internship programs were started at the California College of Ayurveda, but today several schools offer them. Student interns may simply observe an Ayurvedic practitioner or actually engage in Ayurvedic practices under the direct observation of an Ayurvedic doctor or practitioner.

See **BOX 8.8** for places that provide Ayurveda training in the United States.

BOX 8.8 Ayurveda Training in the United States

The Ayurvedic Institute
11311 Menaul NE, Albuquerque, NM 87112
Phone: 505-291-9698
Website: http://www.ayurveda.com

California College of Ayurveda
1117A East Main Street, Grass Valley, CA 95945
Phone: 530-274-9100
Website: http://www.ayurvedacollege.com

American Institute of Vedic Studies
PO Box 8357, Santa Fe, NM 87504
Phone: 505-983-9385
Website: http://www.vedanet.com

▶ Conclusion

A great deal of information about Ayurvedic medicine has been included in this chapter, but it clearly has offered only a brief summary of its practices. Please keep in mind that because a practice is termed "alternative" does not mean that it is not effective. On the other hand, we should not believe that all alternative practices are, indeed, effective. We, as health consumers, need to be willing to investigate all forms of healing practices and make our decisions about our health and lifestyles based on knowledge of what is safe and efficacious.

Wrap-Up

Key Terms

Ayurveda Sanskrit word that means life science or sciences of life.

Ayurvedic medicine A form of holistic alternative medicine that is the traditional system of medicine of India. It may have influenced ancient Chinese medicine and the humoral medicine practiced by Hippocrates in Greece.

Basti Medicated enema or colonic irrigation.

Constitution According to Ayurvedic medicine, it is a pattern of energy that comprises or makes up a person.

Dosha Five elements (ether, air, fire, water, and earth) make up the body's constitution called dosha; there are three doshas: vata, pitta, and kapha.

Five elements In Ayurveda, they are ether (space), air (vayu), fire (agni), water (apa), and earth (prithvi).

Ghee A mixture also known as sneha made from cow's milk into an edible oil or medicated butter.

Malas Waste products such as urine, feces, or sweat.

Nasya Nose or sinus irrigation.

Neti pot Used to give nose or sinus irrigation, usually using a mild salt solution.

Panchakarma treatment Five types of cleansing therapy (vomiting, purging, colonic cleansing, nose and sinus cleansing, and blood detoxification).

Pathya vyavastha treatment Use of diet and activity.

Prakriti Dosha balance.

Prana Energy.

Pulse taking There are three types of pulses: snake pulse, which denotes vata dosha; frog pulse, which denotes pitta dosha; and swan pulse, which denotes kapha dosha.

Purva-karma treatment Precleansing procedures before shodhanam or shamanam treatment. It involves snehan and swedan treatments.

Raktamoksha Detoxifying the blood by bloodletting or using certain herbs.

Salvia lavandulaefolia Plant known as Spanish sage. Used for healing purposes.

Satvajaya treatment The use of mental hygiene/psychotherapy.

Seven tissues (dhatu) Plasma, blood, muscle, lipid, bone, nervous system, and reproductive system.

Shamanam treatment A balancing treatment.

Shodhanam treatment A cleansing treatment using five procedures called panchakarma treatment.

Snehan treatment Internally it involves ingesting medicated edible oil or butter; externally it is medicated body massage.

Swedan treatment Use of dry or wet fomentation or heat therapy to facilitate sweating.

Tri-doshic Having fairly equal characteristics of vata, pitta, and kapha.

Turmeric A plant that contains curcumin. Used for healing purposes.

Vamana Forced vomiting.

Vikruiti Dosha imbalance.

Virechana Forced purging.

Suggestions for Class Activities

1. With a partner, research five Ayurvedic herbs listed in this chapter to assess whether there are any published scientific studies that show benefits or harmful effects from the herbs.
2. Practice the Ayurvedic method of taking a pulse using three fingers.
3. Take the Dosha questionnaire and, according to Ayurvedic principles, determine the type of dosha you are.

Review Questions

1. What is the meaning of the word "Ayurveda?"
2. What is one of the three great classics written in Sanskrit?
3. From what country does Ayurvedic medicine originate?

4. What are the five elements?
5. What does dosha mean?
6. What are the three doshas? Describe two characteristics of each.
7. What is prana?
8. What is the meaning of agni and ama?
9. What diagnostic methods are used in Ayurveda, and how do they compare with traditional Western diagnostic methods?
10. Compare and contrast shamanam and shodhanam treatments.
11. What is snehan treatment?
12. What is panchakarma treatment? Describe three of the five types of panchakarma.
13. What is the status of scientific research on Ayurvedic medicines?
14. What is the NIAM?
15. What is the academic training of Ayurvedic practitioners, and where in the United States could a person receive Ayurvedic medicine training?

References

1. Lad V. Ayurveda: A Brief Introduction and Guide. Available at: http://www.sahej.com/ayurveda_intro.html. Accessed April 12, 2018.
2. Lad V. *Ayurveda: The Science of Self-Healing. A Practical Guide.* Twin Lakes, WI: Lotus Press; 2009.
3. Lad V. Ayurvedic medicine: An introduction to ayurveda. *Healthy.net.* Available at: http://www.healthy.net/scr/article.aspx?Id=373. Accessed April 12, 2018.
4. Svoboda R. *Prakriti: Your Ayurvedic Constitution.* 2nd ed. Twin Lakes, WI: Lotus Press; 2011.
5. The Chopra Center. Ayurveda: The science of life. Available at: https://chopra.com/articles/what-is-ayurveda. Accessed April 12, 2018.
6. Coffey LM. Tri-doshas. What's your dosha? Available at: http://www.whatsyourdosha.com/trdoshas.html. Accessed April 12, 2018.
7. Tiwari M. *A Life of Balance: The Complete Guide to Ayurvedic Nutrition & Body Types with Recipes.* Rochester, VM: Healing Arts Press; 1995.
8. Bradford N, ed. *The One Spirit Encyclopedia of Complementary Health.* London, UK: Hamlin; 2000.
9. The Chopra Center. Dosha Quiz. Available at: https://shop.chopra.com/dosha-quiz/. Accessed May 17, 2018.
10. Joyful Belly. Find Your Ayurvedic Body Type with this Free Dosha Quiz. Available at: http://www.joyfulbelly.com/Ayurveda/assessment/Dosha. Accessed April 12, 2018.
11. Rafael T. *Ayurveda for the Childbearing Years: A Primer. Table B: The Subdoshas.* Boulder, CO: Terra Rafael; 2009:4.
12. Hankey A. Establishing the scientific validity of tridoshas: Doshas, subdoshas and dosha prakritis. *Anc Sci Life.* 2010;29(3):6-18.
13. Hankey A. A test of the systems analysis underlying the scientific theory of Ayurveda's tridosha. *J Altern Complement Med.* 2005;11(3):385-390.
14. Hankey A. The scientific value of Ayurveda. *J Altern Complement Med.* 2005;11(2):221-225.
15. Planet Ayurveda. Methods of Diagnosis in Ayurveda. Available at: http://www.planetayurveda.com/diagnosis-methods-ayurveda.htm. Accessed April 12, 2018.
16. HolisticOnline.com. Pulse diagnosis. Available at: http://www.holistic-online.com/ayurveda/ayv-diag-pulse.htm. Accessed April 12, 2018.
17. Lad V. Tongue and Corresponding Organ Locations. The Ayurvedic Institute. Available at: http://www.ayurveda.com/resources/articles/tongue-and-corresponding-organ-locations. Accessed April 12, 2018.
18. Kurande VH, Waagepetersen R, Toft E, Prasad R. Reliability studies of diagnostic methods in Indian traditional Ayurveda medicine: An overview. *J Ayurveda Integr Med.* 2013;4(2):67-76.
19. SvasthaAyurveda. Ayurvedic Facial Diagnosis: What are the lines on your face revealing about your health? Published January 23, 2017. Available at: http://svasthaayurveda.com/ayurvedic-facial-diagnosis-what-are-the-lines-on-your-face-revealing-about-your-health/. Accessed April 12, 2018.
20. Kulkarni S. Ashtang-Ayurved: Purva-karma. Health Information Network. Available at: http://www.nzhealth.net.nz/ayurveda/purva-karma.shtml. Accessed April 12, 2018.
21. KeralaAyurvedics.com. Purva Karma Before Panchakarma in Ayurveda. Published March 23, 2007. Available at: http://www.keralaayurvedics.com/diseases-diagnosis-and-treatment/treatments/panchakarma/purva-karma-before-panchakarma-in-ayurveda.html. Accessed April 12, 2018.
22. Mishra L, Singh BB, Dagenais S. Healthcare and disease management in Ayurveda. *Altern Ther Health Med.* 2001;7(2):44-50.
23. IloveIndia.com. Panchakarma Treatment. Available at: http://ayurveda.iloveindia.com/panchakarma/index.html. Accessed April 12, 2018.
24. Kulkarni S. Ayurveda: Shaman. Health Information Network. Available at: http://www.nzhealth.net.nz/ayurveda/shaman.shtml. Accessed April 12, 2018.
25. IndiaNetzone. Shamana Chikitsa, Ayurveda. Available at: http://www.indianetzone.com/6/shamana.htm. Updated June 6, 2013. Accessed April 12, 2018.
26. Herron RE, Fagan JB. Lipophil-mediated reduction of toxicants in humans: An evaluation of an Ayurvedic detoxification procedure. *Altern Ther Health Med.* 2002;8(5):40-51.
27. Ayuskama Ayurveda Clinic & Panchakarma Center. Ayurveda Rasayana Therapy. Available at: http://www.ayuskama.com/ayurveda-rasayana. Accessed April 12, 2018.
28. Prokerala.com. Ayurveda rejuvenation—Rasayana Therapy & Ayurveda Panchakarma. Available at: http://www.prokerala.com/health/ayurveda/rasayana-ayurveda-rejuvenation.htm. Accessed April 12, 2018.
29. Cohen D. Ayurvedic Medicine with Dr. David Cohen. Available at: http://www.doctordavidcohen.org/ayurveda2.html. Accessed April 12, 2018.
30. National Center for Complementary and Integrative Health. Ayurvedic Medicine: In Depth. Available at: https://nccih.nih.gov/health/ayurveda/introduction.htm. Updated April 7, 2016. Accessed April 12, 2018.
31. Lavekar GS. Scientific Validation of Drug Development and Clinical Research in Ayurveda. New Delhi, India: Central Council for Research in Ayurveda and Siddha; AYU No. 5 2006:66-85.
32. Saper RB, Phillips RS, Sehgal A, et al. Lead, mercury, and arsenic in U.S. and Indian-manufactured Ayurvedic medicines sold via the Internet. *JAMA.* 2008;300(8):915-923.

33. Pathania A. Ayurvedic medicine containing lead, causes ill-effect. *TopNews*. August 4, 2010. Available at: http://topnews.us/content/224260-ayurvedic-medicine-containing-lead-causes-ill-effect. Accessed April 12, 2018.

34. Modha J. Adverse drug reaction of Ayurveda medicines. Boloji.com. January 24, 2010. Available at: http://www.boloji.com/ayurveda/av078.html. Accessed April 12, 2018.

35. Kiefer D. Novel turmeric compound delivers much more curcumin to the blood. Life Extension. October 2007. Available at: http://www.encognitive.com/files/Novel%20Turmeric%20Compound%20Delivers%20Much%20More%20Curcumin%20to%20the%20Blood_0.pdf. Accessed April 12, 2018.

36. Ryan J, Heckler C, Ling M, Katz A, Williams J, Pentland A, Morrow G. Curcumin for radiation dermatitis: A randomized, double-blind, placebo-controlled clinical trial of thirty breast cancer patients. *Radiat Res*. 2013;180(1):34-43.

37. Tildesley NT, Kennedy DO, Perry EK, et al. *Salvia lavandulaefolia* (Spanish sage) enhances memory in healthy young volunteers. *Pharmacol Biochem Behav*. 2003;75(3):669-674.

38. Lopresti AL. Salvia (Sage): A review of its potential cognitive-enhancing and protective effects. *Drugs RD*. 2017;171(1):53-64.

39. Aggarwal BB, Sundaram C, Malani N, Ichikawa H. Curcumin: The Indian solid gold. *Adv Exp Med Biol*. 2007;595:1-75.

40. Ayurvedic Center. Historical uses of Ayurvedic herbs. Available at: http://www.holheal.com/ayurved4.html. Accessed April 12, 2018.

41. Premila MS. *Ayurvedic Herbs: A Clinical Guide to the Healing Plants of Traditional Indian Medicine*. New York, NY: Haworth Press; 2006.

42. Valentino S. Colloidal silver side effects. *EzineArticles*. November 9, 2006. Available at: http://ezinearticles.com/?Colloidal-Silver-Side-Effects&id=353791. Accessed April 12, 2018.

43. Vedic Society. The National Institute of Ayurvedic Medicine, New York, USA. Available at: http://www.panchakarma.com/the-national-institute-of-ayurvedic-medicine-new-york-usa-p-342.html. Accessed April 12, 2018.

44. Ponmelil VA. About Ayurveda, medicine higher studies in India. *NewKerala.com*. Available at: http://education.newkerala.com/india-education/About-Ayurveda-Medicine-Higher-Studies-in-India.html. Accessed April 12, 2018.

CHAPTER 9

Alternative Medical Systems: Traditional Chinese Medicine

LEARNING OBJECTIVES

As a result of reading this chapter, students will be able to:

1. Assess why people are skeptical about the efficacy of medical systems different from Western traditional medical practice.
2. Explain how traditional Chinese medicine (TCM) could coexist with and complement Western traditional medicine.
3. Analyze the impact that TCM may have on future U.S. medical practices.
4. Describe four steps that consumers could take in making a decision about whether or not to use TCM treatments.

▶ What Is Traditional Chinese Medicine?

The oldest written records of a Chinese medicine system originated about 2,800 years ago, although evidence of Chinese medical practices such as surgical tools, dietary medicine, and herbal formulas were evident centuries before.[1] In an e-mail conversation (August 21, 2010), S. Dharmananda clarified that during the early period, Chinese medicine was not known as TCM because there was nothing to contrast it to such as modern medicine. It was known as *Zhong Yi*—*Zhong* is short for *Zhong Guo* (central country, meaning China) and *Yi* means medicine.

Ancient TCM was a complex, empirical natural science that was an integral part of the culture of China that is now referred to as Daoism.[1] Around 100 CE (AD), the doctrines of TCM were laid out in the *Huangdi Neijing* (also spelled *Huang Di Nei Jing*), *Yellow Emperor's Canon of Internal Medicine* or *Yellow Emperor's Inner Canon*. It included **physiology**, **pathology**, prevention, **diagnosis**, meridian theory, acupuncture, and other treatments.[2,3]

Western influence caused a decline in TCM, but after the Communists took power in 1949, they sent researchers out to the countryside to interview and learn from the old practitioners. At that time, there were little or no medical services, and TCM was cheaper to use than modern medicine. Thus began the resurgence of TCM not only in China, but also in the West. Modified forms of TCM also are practiced in other parts of the East and Southeast Asia. Today, many Chinese medical doctors and practitioners are trained in TCM as well as Western medical thought and theory.

Rather than focusing on specific parts of the body affected by disease or injury, TCM is based on a **holistic** approach to health care; therefore, remedies are prescribed to treat the entire body. Chinese medicine focuses on treating the root cause of illnesses, not just their symptoms. Acupuncture, acupressure, herbal medicines, **qigong**, **tai chi**, Chinese psychology, massage, dietary therapy, and exercise are mainstream TCM treatment modalities. According to results from the 2012 National Health Interview Survey (NHIS), about 33.2% of U.S. adults reported having used complementary health approaches in the previous year and "there was a small, but linear increase in the use of acupuncture,"[4] up from the 3 million reported in the 2007 NHIS results to 3.5 million in the 2012 NHIS results. Internationally, TCM is widely used in China, Japan, and Korea,[5] and is also becoming popular in Europe and the Americas.

Four main theories constitute the basis of TCM: the theory of **qi (chi)**, meridian theory, the theory of **yin–yang**, and the theory of the **five elements**. The following sections present these theories and their application to medicine.

What Is the Theory of Qi (Chi)?

At the heart of TCM is the concept of a vital energy the Chinese call qi (chi), pronounced chee. Qi is also known as vital breath, vital force, life force, vital power, moving power, and so forth. Qi energy manifests simultaneously on a spiritual as well as on a physical level, and it is in a constant state of change.[6] According to Chinese philosophers, qi is the force that animates humans as well as the entire universe, and it unites the heavens and earth. It flows along the surface of the body and through the body's organs.[5] One of the ways that TCM is used to treat disease is to overcome blockages in the circulation of qi. According to the Chinese, qi takes many forms and functions within the body, and is derived from two main sources: the inherited form we receive from parents prior to birth and the external form from the air we breathe as well as the food we eat.[5] Qi is believed to flow through the body by way of channels or **meridians**, that correspond to particular organs or organ systems. Each organ, in turn, has its own characteristic qi. According to TCM, there is a liver qi, kidney qi, and other forms of qi. For instance, nutritive qi is thought to exist within the body and nourishes it; defensive qi exists more externally (but is still within the body) and serves to protect the body.[6]

What Is the Theory of Meridians?

In TCM, qi is thought to flow throughout the body both externally and internally through channels called meridians. According to Chinese belief, there are 12 major meridians that link to 12 vital organs, plus 6 minor meridians that link to other areas of the body. Six of the major meridians are linked to yin and six are linked to yang. (A discussion of yin–yang follows this section.) The meridians form a network that crisscrosses throughout the body linking organs, skin, flesh, muscles, and bones. The qi circulates through the meridians from internal organs out through major meridian branches to smaller ones. The meridians supposedly go outside the body in the skin and then return to the internal body, transporting energy and blood, much like the pattern of blood vessels and nerves.[7] The meridians can be thought of as rivers of energy with the main purpose of transporting qi throughout the body (**FIGURE 9.1**).

According to TCM, the meridians have a dual role. One is to prevent harmful energies (e.g., bacteria and viruses) from entering the body; the second is to indicate the presence of harmful energy already inside the body, indicated by body symptoms such as aches, pains, heat, or cold. Any type of "disease" is a sign that the energy within the meridian system is out of balance. When a meridian is blocked, one part of the body is getting too much qi and enters a state of excess or overactivity, while another part of the body or organ is getting too little and becomes deficient in qi and appears underactive.[7] Along the meridians are highly charged energy points, which are called pressure points in Western medicine, or tsubo in Japanese. Stimulating different tsubo (e.g., using acupuncture) is supposed to affect qi movement and correct an energy imbalance. Meridian points connected to major organs are the lung meridian, large intestine meridian, spleen meridian, stomach meridian, heart meridian, small intestine meridian, urinary bladder meridian, pericardium (lining over the heart) meridian, liver meridian, gallbladder meridian, and triple heater meridian. The pericardium meridian (yin) is paired with the triple heater meridian (yang). The triple heater meridian heats three sections of the body[7]: the upper section is the head and neck area, the middle section is the chest area, and the bottom section is in the naval area. The triple heater meridian regulates the flow of energy in these three regions.[7]

You may access additional information about meridians and view charts online. Thus far, we have discussed the theory of a particular energy called qi

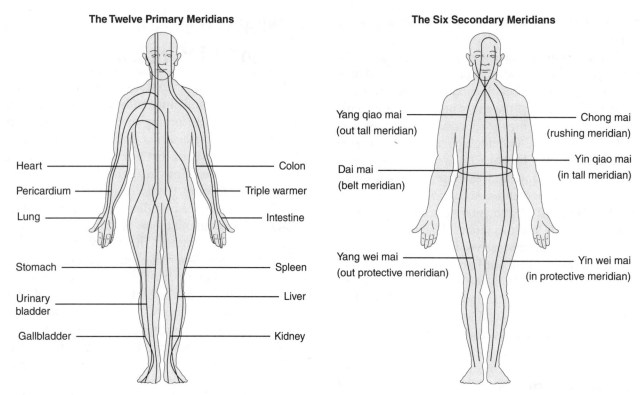

FIGURE 9.1 Twelve primary meridians and six secondary meridians.

that moves within and throughout the body within channels called meridians. When qi is blocked, disease occurs. According to the Chinese philosophers and medical doctors, qi is not the only factor determining wellness and illness. The next theory in the grand scheme of TCM is the theory of yin–yang.

▸ What Is the Theory of Yin and Yang?

The theory of yin and yang is the basis of ancient Chinese philosophy and has been applied to TCM thought and practice. The first references to yin-yang date back to the Zhou dynasty (about 1000–770 BCE).[5] TCM belief is that everything is composed of two opposing but complementary energies—yin and yang. Even though yin and yang are opposite, one cannot exist without the other; therefore, they are never separate. This intertwined relationship is expressed in the classic yin–yang symbol (**FIGURE 9.2**).

The outer circle represents "everything," and the black and white shapes within the circle represent the interaction of two energies called yin (black) and yang (white). They are not completely black or white, just as things in life are not completely black or white, and

they cannot exist without each other. The yin–yang symbol expresses the interaction between these two forces; the two spots denote that each principle contains the seed of its opposite, which it will produce through interacting with its opposite.

Yin and yang are in a constant state of dynamic balance; when one becomes unbalanced, the other changes proportion and achieves a new balance. TCM belief is that there is no absolute yang or absolute yin. Yin and yang are manifested everywhere, and all movement and changes are in between them. The Chinese call these

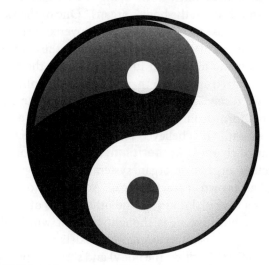

FIGURE 9.2 Yin–yang symbol.

movements life. The designation of yin or yang is said to be relative to, or in comparison with, some other related condition, that is, yin and yang describe relationships.[5] For example, yin originally meant the dark side of the mountain and yang meant the sunny side. On the body, the yang meridians are on the side that is normally in the sun (the back) and the yin meridians are on the shadow side (the front). But, early morning can be said to be yang in comparison to late afternoon, which is more yin. A man is more yang than a woman, but a young woman is more yang than an old woman. See **TABLE 9.1** for yin–yang characteristics.[5]

The theory of yin–yang is reflected in medicine as the opposing yin–yang of human body structures, the opposing yin–yang character of the organs, and the opposing yin–yang symptoms that occur with illness. For example, yin organs are those that store the fluids extracted by yang organs (blood, body fluids, qi). The yin organs are of vital importance for the body, because weakness of the yin organs often leads to death. On the other hand, the yang organs play an important role in digestion and, if necessary, can even be removed without causing death.[5] Every yin organ is related to a yang organ with a similar function (e.g., lung/large intestine for excretion and inhalation; spleen/stomach for storage; kidney/bladder for purifying). The area above the waist is said to be yang and is affected by yang pathogenic factors such as the wind. The area below the waist is said to be yin and affected by yin pathogenic factors such as dampness[5] (**BOX 9.1**).

Another principle holds that yin and yang continue to change and to succeed each other. As each force reaches its extreme, it becomes the other, thus producing a never-ending cycle. For example, as day (yin) progresses, it eventually becomes night (yang), and then the cycle repeats in an eternal cycle of reversal.[5] TCM holds that all phenomena have within them the seeds of their opposite state, that is, sickness has the seeds of health, health contains the seeds of sickness, wealth contains the seeds of poverty, and so on. According to TCM, one is never really healthy because health contains the principle of its opposite, sickness.

The application of qi and yin–yang to medicine is beginning to unfold, but cannot be complete without a discussion of the theory of the five elements.

BOX 9.1 Yin and Yang Organs

Yin Organs	Yang Organs
Lung	Large intestine
Spleen	Stomach
Kidney	Bladder
Heart	Small intestine
Liver	Gallbladder

What Is the Theory of the Five Elements?

The theory of the five elements in TCM is another ancient philosophical concept used to explain the physical universe. The first recorded reference to the five elements dates back to the Warring States Period (476–221 BCE).[5] The theory marked the beginning of Chinese "scientific" medicine, because the healers now observed nature and set out to find patterns within it to apply in interpreting disease states. The five elements are identified as water, fire, wood, metal, and earth; all are found in the natural environment and are used to interpret the relationship between the physiology and pathology of the human body and nature[8] (**FIGURE 9.3**).

In TCM, the five elements have basic qualities. Water moistens downward. Fire flares upwards. Wood can be bent and straightened. Metal can be molded and can harden. Earth permits sowing, growing, and reaping.

TABLE 9.1 Yin–Yang Characteristics

Yin Characteristics	Yang Characteristics
Earth	Heaven
Female	Male
Matter	Energy
Darkness	Light
Shade	Brightness
Cold	Warm
Winter	Summer
Passive	Active
Sweet	Salty

Source: Maciocia G. The foundations of Chinese medicine: A comprehensive text for acupuncturists and herbalists. Philadelphia: Churchill Livingstone; 2005.

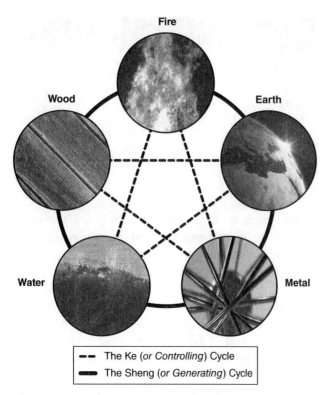

FIGURE 9.3 Five elements symbol.

The five elements are also seen as stages of a seasonal cycle.[8] Wood corresponds to spring and is associated with birth because that is the time for growth. Fire corresponds to summer and is associated with growth, radiating, and flourishing. In late summer (earth) everything is ripening. In autumn (metal), the forces return to the earth. In winter (water) life is directed to the inside and associated with storage.

The five elements are also described as movements. Wood is seen as outward movement in all directions; metal is inward movement; water represents a downward movement; fire represents upward movement; and earth is seen as a neutral movement or stability.

An interrelationship exists among the five elements. In a *generating sequence*, wood generates fire, fire generates earth, earth generates metal, metal generates water, and water generates wood.[5] In a *controlling sequence*, wood controls earth, earth controls water, water controls fire, fire controls metal, and metal controls wood.[6] There also are other documented interrelations, but those mentioned should give an idea regarding interrelationships. When applied to medicine, an example of the five elements during a controlling sequence is spleen controls the kidneys, lungs control the liver, and kidneys control the heart.[5]

The five elements constantly move and change and are dependent on one another. The **visceral organs**,

as well as other body organs, are thought to have similar properties to the five elements and interact physiologically and pathologically just as the five elements do. **TABLE 9.2** shows the categorization of phenomena[8] according to the five elements.

As shown in the table, the five elements are also associated with body shapes.[9]

- **Wood type**: Slender and tall body shape
- **Fire type**: Pointed head and chin, small hands, with curly or a small amount of hair
- **Metal type**: Square and broad shoulders, strong body type, and a triangle-shaped face
- **Earth type**: Large head, larger body and belly, strong legs, and a wide jaw
- **Water type**: Round face and body with a longer than normal torso

From examining Table 9.2 and the relationship of the five elements with body type, one can perceive that the five elements of nature correspond with, among other things, body parts, sensations, and colors. The theory of the five elements reinforces basic concepts in Chinese medicine regarding the wholeness of body, mind, and spirit and the importance of maintaining harmony with nature and balance within the body.

▶ What Are TCM Diagnostic Methods?

Now that we have explored the theories that comprise the basis of Chinese medicine, let us examine several TCM diagnostic methods. Of course, not only are there similarities between TCM and traditional, Western diagnostic methods, but there also are some differences.

Observation of the Patient

Just like traditional physicians, TCM doctors and practitioners observe and examine the body with their eyes and listen to body sounds with a stethoscope. However, they also listen to the voice and the breath, and they note the smell of the breath, skin, secretions, or excretions.[9] The sound of the voice, such as hoarseness or an unusually loud voice, indicates certain body deficiencies or illnesses. Body odors such as **halitosis** might indicate a stomach disorder. **Rancid** odors are supposedly related to liver problems. Scorched or burned odors are related to the heart and **putrid** odors are related to the kidneys.[9]

TABLE 9.2 Five Elements and Yin–Yang Chart					
Yin–Yang	**Wood**	**Fire**	**Earth**	**Metal**	**Water**
Seasons	Spring	Summer	Late summer	Autumn	Winter
Directions	East	South	Center	West	North
Colors	Green	Red	Yellow	White	Black
Tastes	Sour	Bitter	Sweet	Pungent	Salty
Climates	Wind	Heat	Dampness	Dryness	Cold
Zodiac animals	Tiger, rabbit	Snake, horse	Ox, dragon, goat, dog	Monkey, rooster	Pig, rat
Animals	Fish	Birds	Humans	Mammals	Shell-covered
Celestial animals	Dragon	Phoenix	Serpent	Tiger	Tortoise
Grains	Wheat	Beans	Rice	Hemp	Millet
Yin organs	Liver	Heart	Spleen	Lungs	Kidneys
Yang organs	Gallbladder	Small intestine	Stomach	Large intestine	Bladder
Sense organs	Eyes	Tongue	Mouth	Nose	Ears
Emotions	Anger	Joy	Worry	Grief	Fear
Emotional	Hot temper	Hysteria	Depression	Self-pity	Phobias
Form	Tall/rectangular	Angular/pyramid	Flat/square	Round/circular	Irregular/wavy
Sounds	Shouting	Laughing	Singing	Crying	Groaning
Danger	Rot, disease	Conflagration, fire	Collision, falling	Wounding	Flooding
Activity	Creativity, relationships with children	Intellect, schooling, fame	Estate, house, home	Commerce, success, trade	Travel, writing, communication

As part of the physical examination, the entire body appearance is noted and related to one of the five element body types. Other body observations might include noting if a person appears very skinny (emaciated) or very large, the size of their thighs, hair loss, musculoskeletal problems, and any changes in muscles, tendons, blood vessels, skin, and bones. If an abnormality is found, the doctor will determine whether it is due to an excess or deficiency of yin or yang. TCM doctors also observe their patients' spirit, called Shen. The Shen is supposed to exhibit qualities such as vitality and mental, emotional, and spiritual well-being and is thought to show in the eyes, complexion, and state of mind.[9]

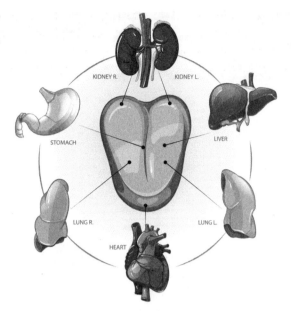

FIGURE 9.4 Chinese tongue diagnosis chart.
© MSSA/Shutterstock

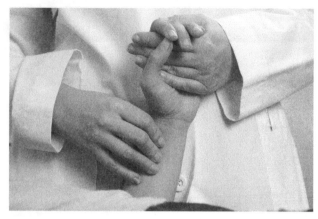

FIGURE 9.5 Pulse taking.
© doglikehorse/Shutterstock

Tongue Diagnosis

As with Ayurvedic medicine, TCM doctors or practitioners will examine the tongue, which aids in their diagnosis. They observe the color (normal is pink or light red), shape, features (texture, spots, numbness, deviated), moisture (dry or wet), coating (white, powder, yellow, gray, black), coat thickness, cracks (short ones, long ones, transverse, irregular), and coat root (rooted coating cannot be scratched off).[9] Again, the doctors will examine the tongue to determine whether there is an excess or deficiency of yin and yang (**FIGURE 9.4**).

Pulse Diagnosis

During the physical examination, TCM doctors or practitioners use pulse diagnosis. Various sources differ, but there are approximately 29 different pulse qualities. Each of the 29 has a designated Chinese name. Pulses are felt on both the left and right wrist at three radial artery sites on each wrist and at three depths (superficial, middle, and deep).[10]

Pulse Taking Practice

To feel a pulse, use the middle three fingers of your left hand to feel the right pulse and vice versa for the left pulse reading. The second finger should rest just below the wrist crease on the thumb side. The other two fingers will rest next to this. Press with all three fingers gently and then deeper until you feel a pulse. What you are trying to do is feel for the quality of the pulse as well as the count. Press hard until you do not feel a pulse, and then ease off until you feel it again. Now, see if the quality has changed. See **FIGURE 9.5** for an image of pulse taking.

As in the other diagnostic methods, general deficiency and excess of yin and yang are identified by the pulse diagnosis. See **BOX 9.2** for main pulse descriptions.[9]

BOX 9.2 Traditional Chinese Medicine Pulse Descriptions

Fu mai (floating, superficial)
Hong mai (surging, flooding)
Ge mai (leathery, drum skin, tympanic, hard)
Kou mai (hollow or scallion stalk, green onion)
Ru mai (soft or soggy)
San mai (scattered)
Xu mai (forceless, empty, deficient)
Chen mai (deep)
Fu mai (hidden)
Lao mai (firm, confined)

Ruo mai (weak)
Chi mai (slow)
Huan mai (slowed down, moderate, or relaxed)
Se mai (choppy, hesitant)
Jie mai (knotted, bound)
Shi mai (excess, full, replete, forceful)
Hua mai (slippery, rolling)
Jin mai (tight, tense)
Chang mai (long)
Xuan mai (wiry, taut)
Wei mai (minute, faint, indistinct)

Xi mai (thready, thin)
Duan mai (short)
Dai mai (regularly intermittent)
Shuo mai (rapid)
Ji mai (racing, swift, hurried)
Cu mai (rapid/irregular, skipping, abrupt)
Dong mai (moving, throbbing, stirring)
Da mai (large, big)

Eight Guiding Principles

The TCM practitioner or doctor may also use the Eight Guiding Principles when making a diagnosis to differentiate energetic imbalances in the body. These consist of the four polar opposites: yin/yang; cold/heat; deficiency or excess energy, blood, or fluids; and interior/exterior.[5] A cold diagnosis would involve a slowed metabolism, low-grade fever, pale skin, and chills, whereas a heat diagnosis would result from a high fever and reddened or flushed skin. Interior means pathogens that enter the body, whereas exterior means pathogens that cause problems on the skin or hair. A lack of blood or other body fluids would cause a deficiency, whereas swelling, because of too much fluid in the body or too much qi energy, would cause an excess diagnosis. If either yin or yang becomes too dominant, the practitioner would attempt to treat that condition.

Medical History

Just as in traditional Western medicine, TCM doctors or practitioners use questioning as a diagnostic tool. They will interview a patient about past medical history, origin of the problem, living and environmental conditions, current and past emotional issues, and eating patterns and diet, and ask specific questions related to all the body systems (e.g., circulatory, respiratory, nervous, etc.).[9]

After all the diagnostics are completed and a diagnosis is made, treatments are prescribed. One TCM source, *The Chinese Medical Sampler*, likened the planning of treatment to a tree. That relationship is paraphrased as[11]:

> The reason that the person goes to the doctor or practitioner is the presenting complaint or problem. That represents one branch of the tree. Other signs and symptoms represent the other branches of the tree. The underlying cause of the illness is represented by the main root of the tree, and factors contributing to the illness are represented by other tree roots. After assessing all the branches and roots, three possible types of treatment are selected.
>
> 1. Treat the branches—making the patient comfortable.
> 2. Treat the root—restoring health.
> 3. Treat both the root and the branches—the branches are interfering to the point that reducing their effects is a high priority.

Just as in Western medicine, Chinese medicine doctors and practitioners have to plan and make priority decisions before starting a treatment program. As mentioned earlier, the treatment modalities used are acupuncture, acupressure, herbal medicines, qigong, tai chi, Chinese psychology, massage, diet, and exercise.

What Are TCM Treatment Modalities?

In TCM, the mainstream treatments are **acupuncture** and acupressure, herbal medicines, diet, and exercise. Because there is a myriad of information regarding each, they will be introduced separately.

▶ What Are Acupuncture and Acupressure?

Acupuncture is the insertion of stainless steel needles into the skin at specific points on the body called acupuncture points to affect the flow of qi (energy) through body channels or meridians.[12,13,14,15] The needles used are sterilized or are sterile, disposable needles. They are about the thickness of a human hair and would fit inside the body of a hypodermic needle used for drawing blood. They range from 0.16 mm to 0.38 mm in thickness, and the tip is conical, allowing it to penetrate tissues separating muscle fiber without causing damage.[13] The shape and size of the needle make the insertion relatively painless (**FIGURE 9.6**).

Acupressure is an ancient healing method that uses a finger to find key points (trigger points) on the surface of the body. As with acupuncture, the object is to promote the flow of qi energy and to stimulate the body's own immune system. Gentle and firm pressure of the hands and even the feet are used to stimulate the trigger points, which are the same points used in

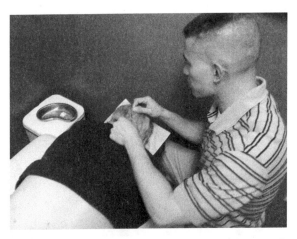

FIGURE 9.6 Scalp acupuncture by Kenneth K. Chow, Dipl OM, DNM, CBP, Baton Rouge, Louisiana.

Kenneth K. Chow, Dipl OM, DNM, CBP–Baton Rouge, LA.

acupuncture. A major difference between acupressure and acupuncture is that people can be taught to apply acupressure on their own bodies. It may be effective in helping to relieve such conditions as headaches, eye-strain, sinus problems, neck pain, muscle aches, and lower backaches.

How Acupuncture Works

How acupuncture works is still not fully known. Although the TCM explanation is that acupuncture affects the flow of qi, some studies from the early 1980s found that it stimulated the release of **endorphins**, the body's natural feel-good chemicals.[14] Others believe that acupuncture stimulates the body's immune system and affords protection against disease.[13,15,16]

Methods of Giving Acupuncture

Besides the needling technique, acupuncture may be given in several other ways[2,14,17,19]:

- **Electroacupuncture**: Mild electrical pulses are relayed via acupuncture needles to various trigger points in the skin (**FIGURE 9.7**).
- **Trigger point acupuncture**: Needles are inserted at a location that is distant from the affected organ or body part. Qi energy is channeled through nerves.
- **Laser acupuncture**: Rays or laser beams are used in place of the acupuncture needles to facilitate the trigger point.
- **Acupuncture point injection**: Sterile syringes are used to inject medication such as vitamins and herbal products into the system via trigger points.
- **Moxibustion**: Heat is used at acupuncture points. The herb *Artemisia*, also known as mugwort,

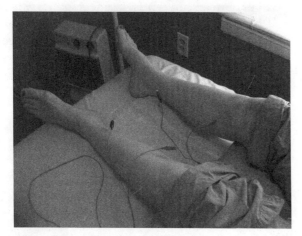

FIGURE 9.7 Electroacupuncture by Kenneth K. Chow, Dipl OM, DNM, CBP, Baton Rouge, Louisiana.
Kenneth K. Chow, Dipl OM, DNM, CBP–Baton Rouge, LA.

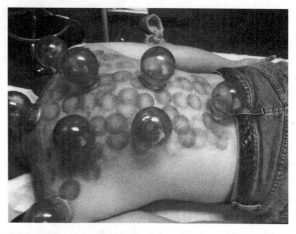

FIGURE 9.8 Cupping by Kenneth K. Chow, Dipl OM, DNM, CBP, Baton Rouge, Louisiana.
Kenneth K. Chow, Dipl OM, DNM, CBP–Baton Rouge, LA.

a type of chrysanthemum, is burned near the body to create heat in the meridian and increase the flow of energy and blood. It may be directly applied on the skin, rolled up and placed on the needle, or used as a stick of moxa that can be held over the desired area to be treated.

- **Cupping**: A round glass cup is heated and kept upside down over an area of the body, creating a vacuum that will keep the cup attached to the skin. The purpose is to promote blood circulation or energy and to open skin pores so that toxins are flushed out (**FIGURE 9.8**).
- **Injection**: Sterile water, saline, procaine, morphine, or vitamins are injected into the meridian points.
- **Earlobe needling**: Needles or staples are used in ear acupuncture points.

The Japanese, Koreans, and Vietnamese have also developed their own forms of acupuncture with modifications such as needleless and trigger point acupuncture, which will be discussed in a later section.

Early Acupuncture Techniques

The earliest acupuncture tools were sharp pieces of bone, stone (bian stone), or flint used to scratch or prick acupuncture points. Bian stone needles were excavated from ruins in China dating back to the New Stone Age (4,000–10,000 years ago).[15] As time went on, early needles were made from bamboo and bone, but those were thicker than modern needles, and more than likely caused discomfort. Metal needles were employed at the advent of the Iron Age and Bronze Age. Early metals used were iron, copper, bronze, silver, and gold. It was not until the 20th century that stainless steel needles were used; these are still in use today.

Wang Weiyi, a famous physician during the Song Dynasty (960–1279) wrote a text, *The Illustrated Manual on Points for Acupuncture and Moxibustion*, in which he identified 657 acupuncture points. He also created two bronze statues to illustrate meridians and acupuncture points.[15] During the Ming Dynasty (1568–1644), new developments in acupuncture occurred. The technique was refined; moxa sticks were used for indirect treatment; and extra points outside the main meridians were identified.

Acupuncture Treatment Process

To give acupuncture, the client is either seated or asked to lie on a cot or table, much as one does when getting a massage. Usually, 3–15 long, thin, solid, sterile disposable or stainless steel needles are placed in various locations on the body according to the meridians, not necessarily at the anatomic site of symptoms. The acupuncturist may insert and remove the needles quickly or leave them in for longer periods of time, often with the application of heat or electrical impulses.[12,16] In order to stimulate qi, the needles are twirled once when placed in the skin and then left in for approximately 20–30 minutes.

Acupuncture Styles

There are several different styles of acupuncture.[17] Although acupuncture originated in China, it has spread to Korea, Japan, Vietnam, Europe, and the Americas; thus, various styles have evolved.

- **Traditional Chinese acupuncture**: This is the most common form studied and practiced in the United States. Traditional Chinese acupuncture uses thicker needles and deeper insertion than the Japanese style. A deep, radiating sensation is sought with each needle. In the hands of master Chinese practitioners, this technique is not very painful, though it can cause soreness.[18]
- **Japanese acupuncture**: The Japanese style of acupuncture uses fewer and thinner needles with less stimulation. Kanshinho is a guiding tube insertion method developed by the famous 17th century blind acupuncturist Waichi Sugiyama. The guiding tube method drastically decreases the pain associated with the initial insertion of the needle and is now used by practitioners worldwide.[19]
- **Five-element acupuncture**: Even though the concept of the five elements exists in all classical forms of acupuncture, five-element acupuncturists focus more on the energetic, spiritual, and emotional components of health. One of the five elements

(fire, earth, metal, water, or wood) is diagnosed as a cause of a patient's disorder. The practitioner analyzes where the energetic blocks are through the use of acupuncture. Five-element acupuncturists generally use thinner needles with more subtle stimulation than TCM practitioners.[20]

- **Korean acupuncture**: Korean acupuncture uses points in the hand that correspond to areas of the body and bodily symptoms. Korean acupuncture placed a great deal of emphasis on the five elements theory and takes into account a person's body type and constitution.[17,18]
- **Auricular acupuncture**: This acupuncture uses points in the ears that correspond to areas of the body and bodily symptoms. It is more commonly used for pain control and drug, alcohol, and nicotine addictions.[17,18] For some people, auricular acupuncture offers a pleasurable alternative to using needles on other parts of the body.[12]
- **Medical acupuncture**: Medical acupuncture is performed by a Western medical doctor. The definition from the American Board of Medical Acupuncture (ABMA) is "Medical acupuncture is a medical discipline having a central core of knowledge embracing the integration of acupuncture from various traditions into contemporary biomedical practice. A Physician Acupuncturist is one who has acquired specialized knowledge and experience related to the integration of acupuncture within a biomedicine practice."[19]
- **Veterinary acupuncture**: This acupuncture is used on animals.[23,24] Some conditions are arthritis and hip dysplasia, back pain and disc disease, **incontinence** and **urinary retention**, some types of nerve damage, and chronic painful conditions.[21]
- **Trigger point therapeutic treatments**: Trigger points are specific areas in the muscles where stabbing pain, weakness, tingling, or aching pain is felt. Pressure is applied at those points or needles may be inserted. Massage therapists and physical therapists as well as acupuncturists may use trigger points.[18]

Side Effects of Acupuncture

In general, adverse reactions to acupuncture are minimal, although case reports of complications do exist. Bleeding rarely occurs. Infection is minimized by most practitioners through the recommended use of sterile disposable needles or the use of Clean Needle Technique (now a requirement for certification). Allergic reaction to the stainless steel needles is also rare. Pain, nausea, dizziness, and fainting vary by patient, and treatment is usually painless or slightly painful. Some patients report that their symptoms temporarily increased rather than decreased after having acupuncture. The possibility of inflammation of the cartilage (**chondritis**) and organ puncture exist, although they are rare.[11]

Acupuncture Research

Some of the diseases that have been treated with acupuncture are headaches, menstrual cramps, dental pain, tennis elbow, fibromyalgia, **osteoarthritis**, stroke rehabilitation, asthma, addiction, postoperative nausea, lower back pain, gynecological problems, gastrointestinal ailments, and carpal tunnel syndrome (CTS). Research is often contradictory. One meta review study found that moxibustion, acupuncture, and **laser acupoint stimulation** were effective with OB-GYN issues, particularly the correction of breech presentation,[22] while a more recent meta analysis[23] on a variety of OB-GYN applications of moxibustion did not yield such support.

Acupuncture research is ongoing in the United States. The National Center for Complementary and Integrative Health (NCCIH) has funded several studies that have shown positive results.

- A review of literature conducted by NCCIH and published in *Mayo Clinic Proceedings* indicated acupuncture showed "more positive than negative results" for the management of back pain and osteoarthritis of the knee.[24] This study reviewed all published work on MEDLINE between the years of 1966 and 2016.
- A review of randomized studies on the use of acupuncture versus a pharmaceutical approach to help symptoms of post-traumatic stress disorder (PTSD) revealed early support for the practice. While researchers were cautious about giving complete support because the number of randomized studies was limited, there seems to be indications that the use of acupuncture for PTSD can be effective.[25]

- A 2016 study of 209 women between the ages of 45 and 60 who were experiencing multiple daily hot flashes revealed acupuncture can be beneficial in the lowering the number and severity of hot flashes. It also supported acupuncture in improving general quality of life, including mood, memory, and sleep.[26]

- A study of 80 patients at six major hospitals and medical centers published in 2017 indicates promising outcomes in the treatment of CTS. The study reviewed the difference in true acupuncture and sham acupuncture treatments in the level of pain experienced by patients. True acupuncture at the hand and the opposing ankle produced measurable improvements in the function of the affected wrist. Interestingly, the study determined through MRI technology that the relationship of brain function and pain sensation related to CTS also improved with true acupuncture.[27]

Other studies utilizing acupuncture for stress management[28] and chronic headaches[29] also showed promising results.

Thus far, the research studies presented have been those that show promising or positive results. There are, however, many other reports that have cast doubt on the effectiveness of acupuncture. One central location for a broad set of analyses related to acupuncture is Cochrane.org. Cochrane is a global network of more than 30,000 health professionals and care providers dedicated to bringing the latest research to light by reviewing evidence-based clinical studies.[30] More than 100 acupuncture-based reviews have been published and stored in the Cochrane Library. The reviews of acupuncture research have concluded that any perceived benefit of acupuncture for the following conditions has been a **placebo** effect: for smokers trying

---

📄 IN THE NEWS

In a *Medical News Today* article titled "Study Shows Why Acupuncture Might Work," Ana Sandoiu describes the research of Dr. Sheng-Xing Ma, lead medical researcher at LA Biomed. Ma's research reviewed how acupuncture might work, and why there is conflicting results in the body of research on the effectiveness of acupuncture. What Ma's group found was that the effectiveness of acupuncture was most likely based on the release of nitric oxide during needling. Nitric oxide creates a sensation of warmness by increasing blood flow to the area of insertion, which, in turn, promotes healing. However, Ma's team noted that the technique used for insertion makes a difference. More gentle insertion, with occasional slow rotation of the needles (acupuncture reinforcement) triggered the warmth and healing response, whereas the more aggressive insertion with rapid rotation of needles (reduction technique) actually created a sensation of coldness in patients. This variance in technique outcomes could explain differences in prior research outcomes on the effectiveness of acupuncture.[31]

Source: Sandoiu, A. Study shows why acupuncture might work. Medical News Today. July 2, 2017.

to quit, cocaine dependence using auricular acupuncture, inducing labor, epilepsy treatment, Bell's palsy, chronic asthma, stroke rehabilitation, breech presentation, depression, CTS, irritable bowel syndrome, and many other conditions.[30] Cochrane also criticized the quality of many of the clinical trial studies. On the positive side, the Cochrane found that there were some conditions in which acupuncture was found to be effective. Some of those are pelvic and back pain during pregnancy, lower back pain, fibromyalgia, headaches, osteoarthritis, postoperative nausea and vomiting, chemotherapy-induced nausea and vomiting, neck disorders, and bedwetting.[30]

Prevalence, Training, Certification, and Licensing of Acupuncturists

As stated earlier, according to the 2012 National Center for Health Statistics report,[4] 3.5 million U.S. adults and 79,000 children received acupuncture treatment in 2012.[4] The number of acupuncturists is rapidly growing, and according to acupuncture.com, there are 18,000 licensed acupuncturists (LAc) in the United States, with an estimated 12,000 in active practice.[32] A variety of clinicians incorporate acupuncture into their practices, including chiropractors, dentists, medical doctors, naturopaths, osteopaths, physical therapists, **podiatrists**, and veterinarians.

Since its inception in 1982, the National Certification Commission for Acupuncture and Oriental Medicine (NCCAOM) has certified close to 21,000 Diplomates in Acupuncture, Chinese Herbology, and Asian Bodywork Therapy. The degrees received vary, including licensed acupuncturists (LAcs), Oriental medical doctors (OMDs), and physician acupuncturists (MDs or DOs).[33,34]

Currently, there are approximately 3,000 acupuncturists with medical degrees practicing in the United States.[35,36] The regulation and licensing of acupuncturists in the United States is state dependent; most states require a health professional degree such as being a medical doctor, doctor of **osteopathy**, chiropractor, dentist, podiatrist, naturopath, physician assistant, or registered nurse. In the United States, there are nonphysician and physician acupuncturists.

Nonphysician Acupuncturists

The education, testing, and licensing of nonphysician acupuncturists varies by state. Most states require that applicants, who are trained in the United States, must have graduated from a program accredited by the Accreditation Commission for Acupuncture and Oriental Medicine (ACAOM). The typical education standard for an acupuncturist is between 2,000 and 3,000 hours of training at an independently accredited master's degree 4-year school. ACAOM's professional requirements are stated in the *ACAOM Accreditation Manual* as follows[33]:

> *1.2.1.* Master's-Level and Master's Degree Programs.
>
> The professional program in acupuncture shall be at least three academic years in length and follow at least two years of accredited postsecondary education. The professional program in Oriental medicine shall be at least four academic years in length and follow at least two years of accredited postsecondary education. The program of study covering acupuncture and herbal medicines covers history; theory (e.g., qi, yin–yang, five elements); acupuncture and point/meridian theory; diagnostic skills; treatment planning; treatment techniques, equipment, and safety; counseling and communication skills; ethics and practice management; biomedical clinical sciences; Oriental herbal studies; and other Oriental medicine modalities (body work, exercise/breathing therapy, diet counseling).[33]

The ACAOM administers a qualifying exam for certification as a Diploma in Acupuncture (Dipl. Ac.), although particular licensing requirements vary by state. Typically, a licensing board will also require that the applicant pass the NCCAOM certification examination. Once certified, acupuncturists can apply for a license. The NCCAOM website includes a chart that outlines how various states use its certification examination in their acupuncturist licensing requirements. This can be viewed at www.nccaom.org /state-licensure.[37] Only a few states require the supervision of a physician for the almost 11,000 practicing nonphysician acupuncturists.

Physician Acupuncturists

Most states recognize acupuncture as being within the scope of practice for licensed physicians, but state regulations vary. Although some states allow physicians to practice acupuncture without additional education, most states require between 200 and 300 hours of specialized training in acupuncture, and in some cases they must pass an examination. The ABMA[36] has published standards set by the **World Health Organization (WHO)** and the World Federation of Acupuncture and Moxibustion Societies (WFAS).

🔍 *CASE STUDY*

Blake is having a great deal of hip and back pain. He used to run a lot and still plays tennis, which he does not want to give up. His private medical doctor has told him that the MRI showed he has a pinched sciatic nerve from a herniated disc. The doctor has suggested that Blake have back surgery to remove the disc and stabilize the vertebrae. He is very concerned about having this done. A friend suggested that Blake should try other means to treat the condition and specifically said he should try acupuncture. Blake has heard about acupuncture but he has a fear of needles.

Questions:

1. What would you suggest Blake could do to learn more about acupuncture as a treatment for back pain?
2. Where would he find a person or doctor who would be a professionally trained acupuncturist?
3. Do insurance companies pay for acupuncture?

4.2.1 For licensed graduates of modern Western medical colleges, who already have had education and training in anatomy, physiology, neurology, and all the other basic and clinical sciences involved in medical diagnosis and treatment, training in acupuncture can be accomplished following a different training pathway for them to master acupuncture as a special medical modality.

The theoretical part and objectives of this acupuncture training are parallel to those described in the complete training section, and the acupuncture core syllabus will be the same. ... The whole course should be devoted to acquiring the knowledge and skill in acupuncture as well as the related basic theory for at least 200 hours of formal training. By the end of the course the participants should be able to integrate acupuncture into their medical practices. The proficiency of training and practice should be evaluated through an official examination by health authorities to ensure safety, competence, and efficacy.

The American Academy of Medical Acupuncture[35] (AAMA) is the only acupuncture society in North America and represents over 1,300 physician acupuncturists, but does accept members from diverse backgrounds. The World Federation of Acupuncture-Moxibustion Societies set the training guidelines and membership requirements.[36] Requirements for admission to the AAMA include possessing an active MD or DO license (or equivalent) to practice medicine under U.S. or Canadian jurisdiction; completion of a minimum of 220 hours of formal training in medical acupuncture (120 hours didactic, 100 hours clinical), or the equivalent in an apprenticeship program acceptable to the Membership Committee.[35]

The ABMA was formally established in 2000 as an independent entity within the AAMA.[36] Its mission is to promote safe, ethical, efficacious medical acupuncture to the public by maintaining high standards for the examination and certification of physician acupuncturists as medical specialists. A physician who desires certification by the ABMA must complete a formal course of study and training designed for physicians that, at a minimum, meets the guidelines and standards set forth by the WHO and the WFAS. Programs must be a minimum of 200 hours of acupuncture-specific training, post–medical school, of which 100 hours should be clinical. Currently, 200 AAMA members have qualified for ABMA Board Certification.

As discussed, becoming an acupuncturist requires knowledge about the body's anatomy and physiology as well as the basic tenets of Chinese medicine. The study of herbal medicine is included within the curriculum of most acupuncture programs. Even though this text includes a separate chapter on herbal medicines, a brief overview of traditional **Chinese herbal medicine (CHM)** is presented next.

▶ What Is Chinese Herbal Medicine Therapy?

Traditional CHM is the study and use of plants and plant parts. In the United States, herbal products are classified as dietary supplements. Different parts of plants are brewed, stewed, and squeezed to make the medicine.[38] For example, the roots of ginseng, Chinese gromwell, and Taiwan Angelica are used. Dried ginger and lily bulb are from the rhizome of plants. Additionally, leaves, flowers, seeds, and even grass and vines are used in making herbal medicines.[39] Before being prescribed, each person is evaluated according to Chinese medicine theory (previously described in this chapter), and then a specialized formula made up of one or several herbs is prescribed for that person.[38]

History

Some say that Chinese usage of herbal medicine dates back to 3494 BCE. The Chinese people say that the founder of herbal medicine is Shen Nong (also spelled Shennong), the legendary emperor who lived during that time. He is also known as the Divine Cultivator/Divine Farmer by the Chinese people because he taught people how to farm.[40] To determine the nature of different herbal medicines, Shen Nong would ingest various kinds of plants to assess how they affected his own body. To find the appropriate herbs for pain or illness, Shen Nong is said to have tasted 100 herbs, including 70 toxic substances in a single day. Because there were no written records, the discoveries of Shen Nong were passed down verbally for 2,000 years from generation to generation.[41] See **FIGURE 9.9** for an image of Shen Nong.

Another pioneer, considered the most famous of China's ancient herbal doctors, was Zhang Zhongjing (or Zhang Ji). His text, *Shang Han Za Bing Lun* (*Treatise on Cold Damage*), contained over 100 effective formulas, many of which are still in use today.[38] An early herbalist, Tao Hongjing, reorganized the *Shen Nong Ben Cao Jing* (the earliest Chinese herbal materia medica). He added 365 new herbs, which brought the total number of herbs to 730, and divided the herbs into categories and "qualities," which he recorded in a book. This early classic greatly impacted the study of herbs in future generations. The earliest Tang dynasty herbal dictionary is thought to be entirely based on it.[38] In other classic texts, there are early written accounts from 180 BCE that describe herbs still used today in Chinese medicine.

Safety Issues

There are approximately 6,000 different medicinal substances listed in the Chinese **pharmacopoeia**; about 600 different herbs are used today.[42] Because herbal medicines are considered dietary supplements, the manufacturer does not have to prove the product's safety and effectiveness before it is marketed.[43] According to federal regulation of dietary supplements, manufacturers are expected to make sure their products are safe by processing them consistently and by meeting quality standards. Current Good Manufacturing Practices (CGMP) regulations went into effect in 2008 for large companies and were phased in for small companies in 2010. CGMP regulations ensure drugs "contain minimum requirements for the methods, facilities, and controls used in manufacturing, processing, and packing of a drug product."[44]

Many Chinese herbs are available over the counter; however, other than remedies for minor ailments, they may not be safe for public use.[43] Chinese herbs should be prescribed by a qualified practitioner who has made a full diagnosis, making the remedies safe for everyone. The problems that have occurred have been because an unqualified practitioner has prescribed the herbs and may have prescribed them in an untraditional way or the herb was made with poor quality control. In rare instances (1 in 10,000 experiences), an allergic reaction from using the herbs might occur (e.g., an herb used for skin diseases).[43] If individuals have poor digestive functions, a more common reaction is a gastrointestinal response, which might include constipation or diarrhea, nausea, or bloating. It could be that the side effect may occur if the herbal formula is not quite right for the needs of the individual.[44] A suggestion is to look for a practitioner who is registered with the Register of Chinese Herbal Medicine.[45] These practitioners are fully informed about herbs and their safe use, and they will follow detailed guidelines and a code of practice produced by the Register.[45] However, keep in mind that even though a Chinese herbal doctor or a practitioner may prescribe the herbs, it is the Chinese herbal pharmacist who prepares and dispenses them, even though he or she is not registered to practice herbal medicine.

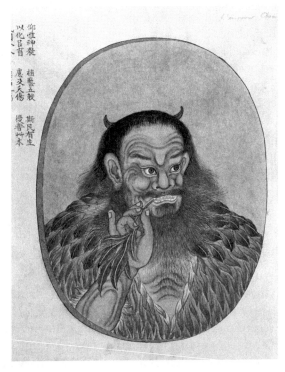

FIGURE 9.9 Shen Nong.
© Chinese School/The Bridgeman Art Library/Getty Images

Herbal Properties and Classification

Many Chinese herbs have been shown to have antibiotic, antifungal, and anticancer properties. In TCM, herbal medicine is used along with acupuncture in treating illnesses and is thought to strengthen people for acupuncture. Herbal medicine is also prescribed to balance the body.[46,47] The classification of herbs is quite varied. They may be classified as upper, middle, and lower. Upper herbs are thought to expel illnesses, but their strength and function are gentle. It might take months or years for these herbs to have an effect. Middle herbs are thought to cure illness. If taken to eliminate suffering, they are to be used quickly, but if taken to increase life span, they should be taken gradually. Lower herbs are used to attack the organism causing the illness and are to be taken short term.[47]

Herbs also may be classified according to direction. There are herbs that work up, down, outward, and inward. Herbal medicines that work from inside out are considered yin (preparations taken internally) and those that work from outside in are yang (e.g., ointments used on the skin).

Herbs also may be classified according to temperature. There are herbs that warm and those that cool. For example, cold herb might be zhi mu or the *Anemarrhena rhizome*, which is used to lower high temperature due to fever; the correct dosage would ensure it is not brought too low.[46,47] Hot herbs are used for severe and often acute internal coldness. Warm herbs are thought to create movement and warmth.[47]

Chinese pharmacists have also categorized and identified herbs based on their taste:

- Sour tasting herbs are indicated for use in prolonged cough, chronic diarrhea, urinary incontinence, and other conditions related to hypometabolism (underperformance).[48,49] In TCM, these diseases are seen as deficiencies or cold patterns.
- Bitter herbs are commonly used for the acute stage of infectious diseases as well as for the patterns of damp-heat or damp-cold, such as in arthritis. They are identified as herbs that descend, dry, and detoxify.[48,49]
- Sweet herbs are thought to tone and harmonize many body systems such as the digestive, respiratory, immune, and endocrine systems. They are thought to promote urination. Sweet tasting herbs inhibit pain due to muscle constriction and are commonly used for treating dry cough and dysfunction of the gastrointestinal tract such as spleen and stomach disharmony.
- Spicy herbs are thought to disperse and circulate qi and have an overall effect of activating and enhancing metabolism. They are thought to vitalize the blood to promote good blood circulation and stimulate the sweat glands to perspire. Spicy herbs are commonly used in the treatment of external patterns (catching a cold).
- Salty herbs detoxify (e.g., sore throat),[48,49] purge, and open the bowels. In addition, salty herbs have the function of softening firm masses and fibrous adhesions; therefore, they are often indicated for sores, inflammatory masses, cysts, and connective tissue proliferation.[48]
- Finally, herbs may be classified as related to yin (sour, bitter, and salty tastes) and yang (acrid, sweet), or as herbs that **tonify** or **stagnate**.[48,49]

Forms of Herbal Preparations

Usually, it is not one herb but a combination of herbs mixed together that achieves the desired effect. A **decoction** (concentrated tea or soup) is the traditional way to prepare herbal medicine. The practitioner weighs out a day's dosage of herbs and combines them in a bag. Enough bags are given for the length of days required. The patient will boil a bag each day for 30–60 minutes and consume it several times during that day.

Herbs also may be given as granulated herbs or highly concentrated powdered extracts. First, the herbs are prepared in the same manner as the decoction, and then they are dehydrated to leave a powder residue. The powders are mixed together for each patient in a custom formula. The patient will take it home and boil it for consumption, in effect, recreating the decoction.[47]

Premade formulas may consist of 4–20 herbs mixed according to a formula, and then delivered as pills, tablets, capsules, powders, alcohol extracts, or water extracts. Some herbs are also made into a paste and applied to the skin.[47] Please see **BOX 9.3** for 15 commonly used Chinese herbs.[47]

Chinese Herbal Medicine Research Results

CHMs have been studied by the NCCIH for use in many health-related issues.[50] The following list presents studies reported by the NCCIH of some of the herbs listed in Box 9.3:

- **Astragalus:** Historically used in Chinese medicine to support and enhance the immune system. There is not an abundance of research, however, regarding astragalus for any health condition because high-quality clinical trials (studies in people) are generally lacking. Some preliminary evidence indicates that astragalus, either alone or in combination with other herbs, may have potential

BOX 9.3 Fifteen Most Commonly Used Chinese Herbals

Astragalus (*huangqi*): The long tap roots of astragalus are, today, the most commonly used herb material in China. Astragalus normalizes immune responses (used for immune deficiency, allergies, and autoimmunity), benefits digestive functions, and treats disorders of the skin from burns to carbuncles. Astragalus is used as a promoter of the functions of several other herbs such as salvia and tang-kuei (mentioned below). It is used in the treatment of AIDS and hepatitis, for chronic colitis, senility, and cardiovascular diseases. Cancer patients who take this herb can often avoid the white blood cell deficiencies (leukopenia) that occur with chemotherapy. The root is rich in polysaccharides and flavonoids that produce the beneficial effects. Astragalus may be used by itself, usually as a liquid extract, or in combination with other herbs in the form of teas, pills, or tablets. Dosage is from 1–60 grams per day, depending on the application and form. *Caution:* Some individuals may experience flatulence and abdominal bloating from use of astragalus.

Atractylodes (*baizhu*): The rhizomes of atractylodes are considered very important to the treatment of digestive disorders and problems of moisture accumulation. The herb helps move moisture (and nutrients) from the digestive tract to the blood, reducing problems of diarrhea, gas, and bloating, and helps move moisture from the body tissues to the bladder for elimination, alleviating edema. The herb is frequently included in tonic prescriptions, and the herb is rarely used by itself. Dosage is from 200 milligrams in capsules and tablets to 15 grams per day in the form of decoction. *Caution:* Persons suffering from a hot and dry condition may experience worsening of those symptoms if large amounts of atractylodes are used.

Bupleurum (*chaihu*): The thin roots of bupleurum are one of the most frequently used herbs in the Japanese practice of Oriental medicine. Doctors in Japan have found it useful in the treatment of liver diseases, skin ailments, arthritis, menopausal syndrome, withdrawal from corticosteroid use, nephritis, stress-induced ulcers, and mental disorders. The roots are rich in saponins that reduce inflammation and regulate hormone levels. The herb is not used by itself, but rather in formulas with about 4–12 ingredients, made as teas, pills, or tablets. Dosage ranges from a few hundred milligrams of powder to about 15 grams in tea per day. *Caution:* Some individuals may experience dizziness or headaches from use of bupleurum.

Cinnamon (*guizhi* and *rougi*): The twigs (guizhi) and bark (rougi) of this large tropical tree are said to warm the body, invigorate the circulation, and harmonize the energy of the upper and lower body. Modern studies demonstrate that cinnamon reduces allergy reactions. Traditionally, cinnamon twig is used when the peripheral circulation is poor and cinnamon bark is used when the entire body is cold. If the upper body is warm and the lower body is cold, then cinnamon will correct the imbalance. Cinnamon is usually cooked together with other herbs to make a warming tea or powdered with other herbs to make a pill or tablet that regulates circulation of blood. Dosage is 0.3–3 grams of bark and up to 9 grams of twig per day. *Caution:* Large amounts of cinnamon are irritating to the liver and should not be used by those with inflammatory liver disorders.

Coptis (*huanglian*): This rhizome (underground stem) is one of the most bitter herbs used in Chinese medicine. It is rich in alkaloids that inhibit infections and calm nervous agitation; it is usually combined with other bitter-tasting herbs, such as phellodendron, scute, and gardenia, to promote these actions. Examples of its many uses include treatment of skin diseases, intestinal infections, hypertension, and insomnia. Coptis is a close relative of an extremely bitter and very useful American herb, goldenseal. Because of its taste, coptis is most often used in the form of pills or tablets. Typical dosage is from a few hundred milligrams of powder to 3 grams in decoction per day. *Caution:* Regular use of coptis in large dosage may cause diarrhea.

Ginger (*jiang*): The fibrous rhizome of this herb is highly spicy and said to benefit digestion, neutralize poisons in food, ventilate the lungs, and warm the circulation to the limbs. Today, ginger is commonly used as a spice in cooking; as a medicine, it has been shown helpful in counteracting nausea from various causes, including morning sickness, motion sickness, and food contamination. Many herbalists use ginger in the treatment of cough (it acts as an expectorant) and common cold. Ginger is used in making teas and the powder is encapsulated for easy consumption. Typical dosage is from a few milligrams used as an assistant in herb formulas to about 3 grams per day in making decoctions. Instant tea granules (sugar or honey base) are available. *Caution:* Persons who suffer from dryness—dry cough, thirst, dry constipation, and more—may find that ginger worsens the condition.

Ginseng (*renshen*): The root has long been cherished as a disease prevention and a life preserver. It calms the spirit, nourishes the viscera, and helps gain wisdom. Modern applications include normalizing blood pressure, regulating blood sugar, resisting fatigue, increasing oxygen utilization, and enhancing immune functions. Traditionally, the root is cooked in a double boiler to make tea, used either alone or with several other herbs. Today, teas can be made quickly from carefully prepared extracts in liquid or dry form; ginseng powder is made into tablets or encapsulated, and ginseng formulas are available in numerous forms for easy consumption. Typical dosage is 0.5–3.0 grams. Higher

(continues)

BOX 9.3 *(continued)*

doses may be used over the short term for specific therapeutic actions; in China, 30 grams is recommended to treat shock (sudden hypotension). *Caution:* Excessive consumption of ginseng can lead to nervousness and may produce hormonal imbalance in women.

Hoelen (*fuling*): This herb is a large fungus that grows on pine roots. It is used to alleviate irritation of the gastrointestinal system and, like atractylodes, it helps transport moisture out of the digestive system into the blood stream and from the various body tissues to the bladder. When bits of the pine root are included in the herb material, it is called fushen; the combination of the fungus and pine produces a mild sedative action. This herb, because it is quite mild, is mostly used in making decoctions or dried decoctions, with a dosage equivalent of about 10–15 grams per day. The herb is nontoxic and rarely causes any adverse effects.

Licorice (*gancao*): These roots have an extremely sweet taste (but are also bitter) and are said to neutralize toxins, relieve inflammation, and enhance digestion. In Europe, a drug has been made from licorice extract that heals gastric ulcers. Licorice is used by Chinese doctors in the treatment of hepatitis, sore throat, muscle spasms, and, when baked with honey, for treatment of hyperthyroidism and heart valve diseases. Traditionally, licorice is thought to enhance the effectiveness of herb formulas and is used to moderate the flavor of herb teas; as a result, it is found in about one-third of all Chinese herb prescriptions. Licorice powder is encapsulated for easy consumption or mixed with other herbs and tableted. Dosage is from very small amounts (a few hundred milligrams) to 15 grams per day in decoction used to treat viral hepatitis. *Caution:* Excessive consumption of licorice over an extended period of time can cause sodium/potassium imbalance with symptoms of tachycardia and/or edema.

Ma-huang (*mahuang*): These stem-like leaves when taken in a dose of several grams stimulate perspiration, open the breathing passages, and invigorate the central nervous system energy. It has been shown that most of these effects are due to two alkaloid components, ephedrine and pseudoephedrine, both of them having been made into modern drugs (for asthma and sinus congestion, respectively). In addition, the stimulating action of ma-huang has led to its use as a metabolic enhancer (burns calories more quickly) for those who are trying to lose weight. Ma-huang also has anti-inflammatory actions useful in treating some cases of arthralgia and myalgia. Ma-huang can be made into a tea or used in extract form; powdered ma-huang is rarely used. Dosage range is 1–9 grams per day, usually in two or three divided doses. *Caution:* The stimulant effect of ma-huang can cause insomnia and agitation; persons with very high blood pressure may find this symptom worsened by use of ma-huang.

Peony (*baishao* and *chihshao*): The root of this common flower is used to regulate the blood. It relaxes the blood vessels, reduces platelet sticking, nourishes the blood, and promotes circulation to the skin and extremities. The roots of both wild and cultivated peonies are used. The wild peony yields "red peony" (chihshao), a fibrous root that is especially used for stimulating blood circulation. The cultivated peony yields "white peony" (baishao), a dense root that nourishes the blood. Peony is often combined with tang-kuei, licorice, or other herbs (mentioned here) to enhance or control their effects. The dosage range is from 0.5–15 grams per day. Peony rarely causes any adverse reactions.

Rehmannia (*dihuang*): The root of this herb is a dark, moist herb that is extensively used to nourish the blood and the hormonal system. It is frequently used in the treatment of problems of aging because of its ability to restore the levels of several declining hormones. There are two forms of the herb that are currently used: one, designated shengdihuang or raw rehmannia, is given to reduce inflammation and is included in many formulas for autoimmune disorders; the other is designated shoudihuang or cooked rehmannia, and is used as a nourishing tonic. Often, the two forms are combined together in equal proportions to address inflammatory problems that are related to the lack of adequate levels of regulating hormones. The herb is mainly used in making decoctions or dried decoctions, with a dosage of 10–30 grams per day. *Caution:* Persons with weak digestion and tendency to experience loose stool or diarrhea may find that this herb, especially cooked rehmannia, worsens those symptoms.

Rhubarb (*dahuang*): This large root was one of the first herbs that the Western world imported from China. It serves as a very reliable laxative, and also has other benefits: enhancing appetite when taken before meals in small amounts, promoting blood circulation and relieving pain in cases of injury or inflammation, and inhibiting intestinal infections. Rhubarb also reduces autoimmune reactions. The impact of rhubarb is influenced by how it is prepared; if it is cooked for a long period of time, the laxative actions are reduced but other actions are retained. Typical dosage is 0.5–3 grams per day. *Caution:* Rhubarb, alone or in formulas, should not be used by those with irritable bowel conditions, as it may cause cramping and diarrhea.

Salvia (*danshen*): The deep red roots of this Chinese sage plant have become an important herb during the past two decades, even though it was used for centuries before that. It is applied in almost all cases where the body tissues have been damaged by disease or injury; thus, it is given for post-stroke syndrome, traumatic injury, chronic inflammation and/or infection, and degenerative diseases. It is best known for its ability to promote circulation in the capillary beds—the so-called microcirculation system. In addition, salvia lowers blood pressure, helps reduce cholesterol, and enhances function of the liver. It may be consumed alone or with other herbs, in wines, teas, pills, or tablets; dosage is 1–20 grams per day. Salvia rarely causes any adverse reactions.

Tang-kuei (*danggui*): This root has long been respected as a blood-nourishing agent. It has its highest rate of use among women because tang-kuei will help to regulate uterine blood flow and contraction, but when employed in complex formulas, it can be used by both men and women to nourish the blood, moisten the intestines, improve the circulation, calm tension, and relieve pain. Tang-kuei is frequently said to have estrogenic effects, but this is not a valid claim. The recommended dosage for tang-kuei is 0.5–9 grams per day. Tang-kuei may be made as a tea or cooked with chicken to make soup (the taste is quite strong), but it is often used today as a powder, encapsulated or made into tablets, alone or with other herbs. *Caution:* Some individuals find that tang-kuei causes nausea or loose stool.

Source: Courtesy of Institute for Traditional Medicine.

benefits for those with kidney issues and viral myocarditis (a heart infection), but the research is not strong. It does not appear that astragalus has a benefit on the effects of fatty liver disease or extending the life of lung cancer patients.

- **Cinnamon** (*guizhi* and *rougi*): The twigs and bark are said to improve circulation, reduce allergy attacks, and harmonize the upper and lower body. There is not much support in the research for the use of cinnamon for health concerns. A 2012 review of 10 randomized trials revealed no improvement in blood sugar levels for diabetics taking cinnamon. NCCIH is currently looking into the effects of cinnamon on the processes involved with multiple sclerosis.

- **Ginger** (*jiang*): Ginger has been used to aid digestion, neutralize poisons in food, and counteract nausea. It has also been used for rheumatoid arthritis, osteoarthritis, and joint and muscle pain. The NCCIH reports that some studies suggest that the short-term use of ginger can safely relieve pregnancy-related nausea and vomiting, and with cancer chemotherapy nausea when used in addition to conventional anti-nausea medications. Results are mixed on whether ginger is effective for nausea caused by motion or surgery. In addition, the studies are unclear as to whether ginger is effective in treating rheumatoid arthritis, osteoarthritis, or joint and muscle pain.

- **Ginseng** (*renshen*): The root has been used for numerous conditions and support for overall health. Modern applications include normalizing blood pressure, regulating blood sugar, resisting fatigue, increasing oxygen utilization, and enhancing immune functions. Studies reported at the NCCIH have shown that Asian ginseng may lower blood glucose, and beneficial effect of

Alaskan ginseng on colorectal cancer cells in lab studies. Evidence is mixed on ginseng effects on Alzheimer's disease. Most evidence is preliminary (based on small clinical trials). Ongoing research is studying the herb's potential role in treating insulin resistance and cancer.

- **Licorice** (*gancao*): Licorice contains a compound called glycyrrhizin (or glycyrrhizic acid). The roots have an extremely sweet taste (but are also bitter) and are said to neutralize toxins, relieve inflammation, enhance digestion, heal gastric ulcers, and treat hepatitis. The NCCIH reports that an injectable form of licorice extract—not available in the United States—has been shown to have beneficial effects against hepatitis C in clinical trials. A topical form of licorice may help with rash and inflammation. One Finnish study showed that the children of mothers who consume licorice during pregnancy have higher risk for behavioral challenges, attentionality challenges, and aggression. The NCCIH reports that research on licorice use for oral and dental issues is mixed.

The following Chinese herbs have been researched and reported in journals and texts other than at the NCCIH website:

- **Atractylodes** (*baizhu*): The rhizomes of atractylodes are considered very important to the treatment of digestive disorders and problems of moisture accumulation. The herb has also been investigated for possible antitumor properties. Laboratory research studies of baizhu indicated that the herb causes apoptosis (programmed cell death) of human leukemia cells,[51] and some rhizomes showed protective properties against liver cancer cells and neuroblastoma cells.[52] Besides *Atractylodes macrocephala*, there are several other

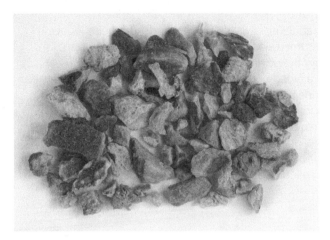

FIGURE 9.10 *Atractylodes macrocephala.*
© ARCO/Diez, O/age fotostock

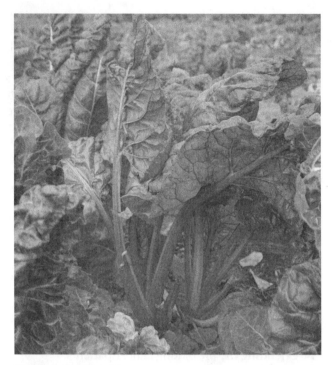

FIGURE 9.11 Rhubarb.
© mikeledray/Shutterstock

species of *Atractylodes*, including *carlinoidses, chinensis, comosa, cuneata, erosodentata, japonica, koreana, ovata,* and *rubra.*[53] Japonica was shown to have hypoglycemic (lowering blood sugar) and anti-inflammatory actions[54,55] (**FIGURE 9.10**).

- **Ma-huang**: Ma-huang is a tall shrub with many branches that grows mostly in the desert. This herb was used in Chinese medicine for 500 years to treat asthma. It contains two alkaloid components, ephedrine and pseudoephedrine, which are used as modern drugs for treating asthma and sinus congestion. The stimulating action of ma-huang led to its use as a metabolic enhancer (burns calories more quickly) for those trying to lose weight. Adverse reactions to ma-huang were heart related: sudden deaths, strokes, ministrokes, rapid heartbeat, and heart attacks. In the year 2000, the FDA issued a warning about the use of ma-huang in dietary supplements, and in 2004 banned the use of *Ephedra sinica* and active ephedrine alkaloids.[56,57] The plant, however, is not banned and certain species of ma-haung may be found in medicines today.[56] There is scientific evidence that ma-huang combined with caffeine is an effective weight loss product (but has dangerous side effects), and has been historically effective for asthma and chronic obstructive pulmonary disease.[57,58]

- **Peony** (*baishao* and *chihshao*): The root of this common flower is used to regulate the blood. It relaxes the blood vessels, reduces platelet sticking, nourishes the blood, and promotes circulation to the skin and extremities. Numerous studies of the effects of the peony root have been conducted, and results show that the white peony root has a strong antispasmodic effect as well as analgesic, sedative, and anticonvulsive effects. A recent study of the red peony indicated that

large doses may have a curative effect on cholestatic hepatitis.[59]

- **Rhubarb** (*dahuang*): The root of the rhubarb plant (**FIGURE 9.11**) has laxative effects, promotes circulation, and inhibits intestinal infections. No U.S. studies were found, but there are Chinese research studies. One analysis of studies on the use of rhubarb indicates there may be positive outcomes for limiting infection of the GI tract, lung and liver caused by sepsis,[60] peri- and postmenopausal symptoms,[61] and hepatitis (liver disease).[62]

- **Salvia** (*danshen*): Chinese sage plant. Proponents of salvia claim it is beneficial when body tissues have been damaged by disease or injury (e.g., post-stroke syndrome, traumatic injury, chronic inflammation and/or infection, and degenerative diseases). It promotes circulation, lowers blood pressure, helps reduce cholesterol, and enhances function of the liver. The research studies on salvia are mixed, mostly due to the research design. Studies over the last decade, however, have shown some support for salvia to help in the treatment of cancer.[63,64] One outcome of studying salvia was establishing the interaction between salvia and warfarin (a drug to prevent blood clotting).[64] Salvia is known to affect blood clotting and could cause hemorrhaging if a patient is taking warfarin and salvia at the same time.[64]

By reviewing the scientific studies of these Chinese herbs, we can discern that Western medical science believes CHM needs much more scientific study. Just because more studies are needed does not, however, mean that these drugs are not effective nor does it mean they are. We have to keep in mind that many of these herbal medicines have been used for hundreds of years, and there must be a good reason that practitioners would continue to make their formulas and use them for people who are ill or injured. If an herb or combination of herbs were found to achieve a desired effect, it would follow that the herb would be used again, and again, and again. To satisfy Western science, however, the future will surely bring more and better research studies of herbal medicines.

We have just explored two of the mainstream TCM treatments, acupuncture and herbal medicines. Massage, diet, and exercise are also important Chinese treatments and are presented next.

▶ What Is Chinese Massage Therapy?

Chinese massage or Oriental body therapy has been used in China for over 2,000 years.[65,66] It is a type of therapeutic bodywork called *tui na* (also spelled **tuina** and pronounced tway-nah), which means "the manipulation and mobilization of soft tissue."[1] The focus of tuina is to stimulate or subdue qi energy in the body and bring the patient's body back into balance. A wrist pulse diagnosis aids the practitioner to find the meridians that need work. The use of hand techniques to massage soft tissue (muscles and tendons) is combined with acupressure to directly affect the flow of qi, and manipulation techniques to realign musculoskeletal and ligament relationships.

The following four styles are taught in the main schools in China:

1. **Rolling method**: The rolling method is used for joint and soft tissue problems, insomnia, migraines, and high blood pressure.
2. **One-finger method**: The one-finger method is similar to a deep tissue work massage called Shiatsu. In the one-finger method, practitioners push points (tsubo) along the meridian with the tip of the thumb or finger. It is supposed to help chronic and internal problems, pediatric patients, and gynecological problems.[1]
3. **Nei gung method**: The *nei gung* method utilizes *nei gong* qi energy exercises and specific massage methods to revitalize depleted energy systems.[65]

BOX 9.4 Tuina Rolling

"A favorite move for a client's leg now is rolling my forearm and wrist. With tui na, I can use my whole arm. The movements are more rapid and can wake the muscles up. Runners love it!"

—Erica Williams, a Western-trained massage therapist who added tuina to her practice

Source: Excerpts from Kovach V. The tui na touch: the intensity of Chinese medicine at your fingertips [Massagetherapy .com]. Available at: http://www.massagetherapy.com/articles/index.php/article_id/The-Tui-Na-Touch. Accessed July 18, 2017. Originally published in Massage & Bodywork magazine, April/May 2003.

4. **Bone-setting method**: The bone-setting method specializes in joint injuries and nerve pain. Manipulative massage is used to realign the musculoskeletal and ligament relationships.

The two tuina methods most used today are the rolling and the one-finger method. The rolling method uses vigorous rolling with the knuckles and the back of the hand on body parts. Along with that could be "scrubbing" with the pinky finger side of the hand, applying elbow pressure, pulling at the back and spine with splayed fingers and interlocked thumbs, and brisk tapping with the cupped hands or edges of the palms.[65] See **BOX 9.4** for more on tuina rolling. It is an extract from an article by Vesna Vuynovich Kovach, originally published in *Massage & Bodywork*.[66]

One-finger massage uses the index finger or thumb to stimulate tsubo points on the meridians. Dependent on the body condition, the tuina practitioner will make a decision about which moves to use (pushing, pulling, nipping, strong pinching, chopping, rubbing, or kneading).[65] Sometimes, walking massage is used with the aid of a steel bar frame that the practitioner hangs onto while walking on the client (legs, back). See **BOX 9.5** for tuina sensations, which is another extract from the Kovach article published in *Massage & Bodywork*.[66]

BOX 9.5 Tuina Sensations

A few moments later, I'm experiencing another set of surreal sensations: the back of my neck is being kneaded and grasped with upward motions that make my whole spinal column feel like it's floating, suspended, above the table.

—Quote online from a person receiving tuina massage

Source: Excerpts from Kovach V. The tui na touch: the intensity of Chinese medicine at your fingertips [Massagetherapy .com]. Available at: http://www.massagetherapy.com/articles/index.php/article_id/The-Tui-Na-Touch. Accessed July 18, 2018. Originally published in Massage & Bodywork magazine, April/May 2003.

Because tuina massage focuses on specific problems rather than being used for generalized massage, it is becoming an excellent adjunct therapy for many joint injuries and muscle strains, and is often used as a complement to traditional Western massage (e.g., Swedish-style massage).[66]

What Is Chinese Diet and Exercise Therapy?

Diet Therapy

The Chinese believe that the diet is one of the sources of qi energy, and is grounded in the five elements and eight guiding principles theory.[42] Rather than emphasizing a balance of protein, carbohydrates, and fats, **Diet therapy** identifies foods as having yin and yang, warming and cooling, and drying and moistening properties. According to the Chinese medicine, if a person presents with a cold or damp condition, they should not eat raw fruits and vegetables (yin foods) because those would cause a further loss of body heat and fluid secretion.[1] They might be encouraged to eat ginger to help with digestion and barley to help with dampness.[67] Dampness is a by-product of eating popular foods such as cheese, yogurt, white flour, and sugar, and the person might present symptoms of sinus-type problems and loose stools or constipation.[67]

On the other hand, a person who has a hot or dry diagnosis would be advised not to eat fried, broiled, high fat, or spicy foods (yang) because they are warming foods and would generate even more heat and stimulate circulation.[1] The Chinese diet is planned to optimize digestion and aid organ function. Foods not found on the menu are cold, raw foods such as salads, iced drinks, and frozen foods because it is difficult for the body to process them.[67] The type of foods selected are built around steamed rice, cooked vegetables, and small quantities of animal protein or beans.

Exercise Therapy (Qigong and Tai Chi Ch'uan)

Qigong Exercise

Exercise in TCM includes qigong, a practice that is supposed to optimize the flow of qi. Qigong exercises are intended to regulate the mind and breathing; therefore, posture, movement, breathing, meditation, and visualization are all incorporated. Qigong can be considered a psychosomatic therapy because it has not only a physical component, but also helps to regulate and balance the mind. It is a practice that works to ease and regulate breathing while storing up energy in the body.[1] Research shows that qigong can help premenstrual pain; head, neck, shoulder, back, and wrist pain; headaches/migraines; and the side effects of chemotherapy.[68] Two types of qigong are practiced: internal and external. **Internal qigong** is used to maintain health by regulating qi and harmonizing the internal energy of the body. Internal qigong movement postures are the most common form of practice today. Certain movements and breath work or visualization gather and circulate qi in the body. **External qigong** is used by the practitioner to transfer qi to another person for healing purposes, and is similar to other bodywork modalities in the West, such as Therapeutic Touch. More about qigong can be found in Chapter 15. An example[68] of a simple qigong arm swinging exercise follows:

> Begin with feet firmly planted, shoulder width apart. Rotate on the heels while turning left to right from the hips. Arms hang limply at the sides, swinging as the lower body turns from side to side. Lead from the hips, not from the shoulders.
>
> *Breathing*: Breathe consciously in and out through the nose. Use deep, low belly breaths from the diaphragm.
> *Repetition*: 10–15 minutes each day morning and evening.
> *Benefits*: Prevents stagnation (or pain) in shoulder, hip, knee and ankle joints, wrists, and back.

Tai Chi Ch'uan Exercise

Tai chi (simplified spelling) is another Chinese medicine exercise that is practiced by millions of Chinese each day and is growing in popularity in the United States. It originates from the martial arts, complete with self-defense applications. Young and old can learn and use it. Tai chi involves very slow movements. Those who practice it are likely to get stronger, improve balance, improve flexibility, and have less anxiety.[69] There are several forms of tai chi, some short (12 movements) and some long (55 movements).[70] One example is the tai chi Form 24 Taiji, also known as Standard 24 Form; as its name suggests, it contains 24 movements[71] (**FIGURE 9.12**).

A video of tai chi Form 24 Taiji can be accessed from the website. Tai Chi instructors say that it is suitable for the young and the old because people are taught stretching and flexing joints, and it reflects

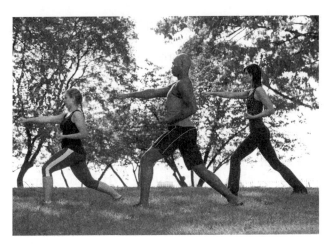

FIGURE 9.12 24 movement tai chi.
© Tyler Olson/Dreamstime.com

qigong can have a positive effect on quality of life, sleep quality, balance, blood pressure, flexibility, and psychological benefits (stress reduction).[72] A 10-year research trial through Harvard, Emory, and Yale Universities published in the *Journal of the American Geriatrics Society* found that tai chi practitioners had overall better balance and reduced their risk of falling by 47.5%.[72] A study by Oh and Kim (2016)[73] found that tai chi practice in individuals recovering from alcohol addiction had increased levels of serotonin, decreased nicotine needs, and lower levels of depression and anger. Comprehensive reviews of randomized controlled studies to assess the health benefits of both qigong and tai chi found a significant number of health benefits.[74]

Chinese traditional philosophy. Tai chi is discussed further in Chapter 15.

Research on Qigong and Tai Chi

Researchers analyzed 19 randomized control studies related to qigong. The studies were published between 2002 and 2016. Their review indicated

▶ Conclusion

This concludes the chapter on TCM. You have been given a bird's-eye view about TCM philosophy, diagnostics, and mainstream treatment methods. Please keep in mind that there is so much more to learn. We hope that you will be motivated to investigate and further explore more TCM concepts and practices.

Wrap-Up

Key Terms

Acupuncture Procedure that increases the flow of qi energy to treat illness or provide local pain relief by the insertion of stainless steel needles at specified sites on the body.

Acupuncture point injection Sterile syringes are used to inject vitamins or herbal products into the system via the trigger points.

Auricular acupuncture Uses points in the ears that correspond to areas of the body and bodily symptoms.

Chinese herbal medicine (CHM) The study and use of plants for medicinal purposes.

Chondritis Inflammation of a cartilage.

Decoction The process of boiling a substance in water to extract its essence.

Diagnosis Identification of a diseased condition.

Diet therapy Prescribed to increase qi energy; it is grounded in the theories of five elements and eight guiding principles.

Electroacupuncture Mild electrical pulses are relayed via acupuncture needles to various trigger points in the skin.

Endorphins Natural pain-killing substances produced in the human body and released by stress or trauma.

External qigong The practice of transferring the practitioner's qi to another person for healing purposes. This form of qigong is similar to other bodywork modalities in the West such as Therapeutic Touch.

Five elements In TCM, they are water, fire, wood, metal, and earth.

Halitosis Offensive odor of the breath.

Holistic A concept in medical practice upholding that all aspects of people's needs, psychological, physical, mental, emotional, and social, should be taken into account and seen as a whole.

Incontinence Inability to control excretion of urine and feces.

Internal qigong Uses certain movements and breath work or visualization to gather and circulate qi in the body.

Japanese acupuncture Uses fewer and thinner needles with less stimulation than traditional Chinese acupuncture.

Korean acupuncture Uses points in the hand that correspond to areas of the body and bodily symptoms.

Laser acupoint stimulation Uses rays or laser beams rather than acupuncture needles to facilitate the trigger point.

Medical acupuncture Acupuncture performed by a Western medical doctor.

Meridians According to traditional Chinese medicine, there are 12 major meridians that link to 12 vital organs, plus six minor meridians that link to other areas of the body.

Moxibustion The stimulation of an acupuncture point by burning herbs called moxa, which are placed at or near the point.

Osteoarthritis A type of arthritis of the joints that leads to joint pain, stiffness, and swelling.

Osteopathy A traditional medical system originally based on the premise that manipulation of the muscles and bones to promote structural integrity could restore or preserve health.

Pathology The science or the study of the origin, nature, and course of diseases.

Pharmacopoeia A pharmaceutical book that contains a list of drugs, their formulas, methods for making medicinal preparations, requirements and tests for their strength and purity, and other related information.

Physiology The functions and activities of the body.

Placebo A substance having no pharmacological effect but administered as a control in testing experimentally or clinically the efficacy of a biologically active preparation.

Podiatrist A person qualified to diagnose and treat foot disorders.

Putrid Having the odor of decaying flesh.

Qi (chi) According to TCM, qi is a bodily energy that flows through unseen channels in the body called meridians. Illness is believed to occur when qi is blocked.

Qigong A type of energy therapy that uses gentle movement to access and redistribute energy surrounding and within the human body. Incorporates posture, movement, breathing, meditation, visualization, and conscious intent in order to move qi energy throughout the body.

Rancid Having a bad smell or taste. Fats and oils when stale become spoiled or rancid.

Stagnate To stop developing, growing, progressing, or advancing.

Tai chi A Chinese exercise system that uses slow, smooth body movements to achieve a state of relaxation of both body and mind.

Tonify Gentle stimulation of an acupuncture point.

Tuina A type of massage to stimulate or subdue qi energy in the body and bring the patient's body back into balance.

Urinary retention Holding urine in the urinary bladder.

Veterinary acupuncture Acupuncture used on animals to treat a variety of conditions (e.g., arthritis and hip problems, back pain and disc disease, incontinence and urinary retention).

Visceral organs Internal organs of the body, specifically those within the chest (as the heart or lungs) or abdomen.

World Health Organization (WHO) The directing and coordinating authority for health within the United Nations system.

Yin–yang Two energies that control different bodily systems but cannot exist without each other.

Suggestions for Class Activities

1. Invite a traditional Chinese medicine doctor to class to discuss TCM philosophy and treatment modalities.
2. Research one or more of the websites listed for acupuncture research. Report your findings to the class.
3. Visit a Chinese pharmacy and note the types of herbals and their forms.
4. Ask a tai chi instructor to engage classmates in tai chi.
5. Invite a Chinese massage therapist to class to demonstrate tuina massage.
6. Go on a field trip to an herbal garden. Take pictures of various herbs.
7. Research the common Chinese herbs and assess if new information is revealed.
8. Research online several meridian charts, including the triple heater meridian points chart.

Review Questions

1. What does TCM stand for?
2. Explain the theory of the meridians and the concept of qi.
3. What is the theory of yin and yang?
4. Name a yin organ and a yang organ.
5. What are the five elements, and how are they applied to TCM?
6. What is different about the TCM observation diagnostic practice compared to traditional Western medicine practice?
7. Explain how TCM utilizes the tongue for diagnosis.
8. Compare and contrast TCM pulse diagnosis with traditional Western medicine's technique.
9. Name five different ways acupuncture may be given.

10. Compare and contrast moxibustion and cupping.
11. Which acupuncture style is used by U.S. medical doctors?
12. What does the research say about acupuncture?
13. What kind of training does a person need to have to become an acupuncturist?
14. Where in the United States can a person go for acupuncture school?
15. Name two properties of herbal medicines.
16. How may herbal plant therapy be classified?
17. What are the five taste classifications of herbal plant therapy?
18. What does the research show about the 15 most commonly used CHMs?
19. Describe what rolling massage and one-finger Chinese massage are.
20. What would the diet prescription be for someone who is considered cold/damp?
21. What is the purpose and function of qigong exercise?
22. From what practice did tai chi originate?
23. How many movements are there in tai chi?
24. What advice would you give to someone considering going to a traditional Chinese medical practitioner or doctor?

References

1. Reller PL. An Historical Perspective in Traditional Chinese Medicine. Available at: http://www.acupunctureintegrated.com/articles/history-of-traditional-chinese-medicine. Updated August 3, 2017. Accessed April 13, 2018.
2. Freeman L, Lawlis G. *Mosby's Complementary and Alternative Medicine: A Research-Based Approach*. St. Louis, MO: Mosby; 2001.
3. Purify Our Mind. History of Traditional Chinese Medicine. Available at: http://www.purifymind.com/HistoryMed.htm. Accessed April 13, 2018.
4. Clarke TC, Black LI, Stussman BJ, Barnes PM, Nahin RL. *National Health Statistics Reports No. 79. Trends in the Use of Complementary Health Approaches Among Adults: United States, 2002-2012*. Hyattsville, MD: National Center for Health Statistics; 2015. Available at: https://www.cdc.gov/nchs/data/nhsr/nhsr079.pdf. Accessed April 13, 2018.
5. Maciocia G. *The Foundations of Chinese Medicine: A Comprehensive Text for Acupuncturists and Herbalists*. Philadelphia, PA: Churchill Livingstone; 2005.
6. Traditional Chinese Medicine Resource Center. What is Qi? Available at: http://www.tcmcentral.com/what-is-qi/. Published November 6, 2008. Accessed April 13, 2018.
7. Natural-health-zone.com. The Body Meridians. Available at: http://www.natural-health-zone.com/body-meridians.html. Accessed April 13, 2018.
8. Shen-Nong. What is the Five Elements Theory? Available at: http://www.shen-nong.com/eng/principles/whatfiveelements.html. Accessed April 13, 2018.
9. Sacred Lotus Chinese Medicine. TCM Diagnosis by Looking (Observation)—One of the 4 Pillars. Available at: https://www.sacredlotus.com/go/diagnosis-chinese-medicine/get/4-pillars-looking-tcm-diagnosis. Accessed April 13, 2018.
10. Yin Yang House. Pulse Diagnosis in TCM Acupuncture Theory. Available at: https://theory.yinyanghouse.com/theory/chinese/pulse_diagnosis#meridiancorrelations. Accessed April 13, 2018.
11. Chinese Medicine Sampler. Risks of Acupuncture. Available at: http://www.chinesemedicinesampler.com/Ac/AcRisks.html. Accessed April 13, 2018.
12. Acupages.com. Acupuncture Styles. Available at: http://www.acupages.com/Acupuncture-Center/Acupuncture-Styles.html. Accessed April 13, 2018.
13. Tiegen R. What is acupuncture? SpineUniverse. Available at: http://www.spineuniverse.com/treatments/alternative/what-acupuncture. Updated January 4, 2018. Accessed April 13, 2018.
14. All4NaturalHealth.com. How is Acupuncture Done? Some Methods Explained. Available at: http://www.all4naturalhealth.com/how-is-acupuncture-done.html. Accessed April 13, 2018.
15. Suvow S. Acupuncture History. Available at: http://www.scottsuvow.com/acupuncture-history/. Accessed April 13, 2018.
16. Russell M. Methods in Acupuncture. *EzineArticles.com*. January 29, 2017. Available at: http://ezinearticles.com/?Methods-in-Acupuncture&id=435536. Accessed April 13, 2018.
17. Fratkin JP. Acupuncture styles. Acupuncture.com. February 2008. Available at: http://www.acupuncture.com/newsletters/m_feb08/Acupuncture%20Styles.htm. Accessed April 13, 2018.
18. Tanaka TH. Acupuncture Styles and Techniques. Available at: http://www.acupuncture-treatment.com/styles.html. Published January 2003; Updated May 2010. Accessed April 13, 2018.
19. Joswick D. What are the different styles of acupuncture? *Acufinder.com*. Available at: http://www.acufinder.com/Acupuncture+Information/Detail/What+are+the+different+styles+of+acupuncture+. Accessed April 13, 2018.
20. Gumenik NR. Classical five-element acupuncture. *Acufinder.com*. Available at: https://www.acufinder.com/Acupuncture+Information/Detail/Classical+Five-Element+Acupuncture. Accessed April 13, 2018.
21. Blue Sky Natural Vet. Veterinary Acupuncture. Available at: http://www.blueskynaturalvet.com/acupuncture.html. Accessed April 13, 2018.
22. Xun L, Hu J, Wang X, Zhang H, Liu J. Moxibustion and other acupuncture point stimulation methods to treat breech presentation: A systematic review of clinical trials. *Chin Med*. 2009;4:4.
23. Ernst E, Lee MS, Choi TY. Acupuncture in obstetrics and gynecology: An overview of systematic reviews. *Am J Chin Med*. 2011;39(3):423-431.
24. Nahin RL, Boineau R, Khalsa PS, Stussman BJ, Weber WJ. Evidence-based evaluation of complementary health approaches for pain management in the United States. *Mayo Clin Proc*. 2016;91(9):1292-1306.
25. Kim YD, Heo I, Shin BC, Crawford C, Kang HW, Lim JH. Acupuncture for posttraumatic stress disorder: A systematic review of randomized controlled trials and prospective clinical trials. *Evid Based Complement Alternat Med*. 2013;2013:615857.

26. Avis NE, Coeytaux RR, Isom S, Prevette K, Morgan T. Acupuncture in menopause (AIM) study: A pragmatic, randomized controlled trial. *Menopause.* 2016;23(6):626-637.

27. Maeda Y, Kim H, Kettner N, et al. Rewiring the primary somatosensory cortex in carpal tunnel syndrome with acupuncture. *Brain.* 2017;140(4):914-927.

28. Eshkevari L, Egan R, Phillips D, et al. Acupuncture at ST36 prevents chronic stress-induced increases in neuropeptide Y in rat. *Exp Biol Med (Maywood).* 2012;237(1):18-23.

29. Vickers AJ, Cronin AM, Maschino AC, et al. Acupuncture for chronic pain: Individual patient data meta-analysis. *Arch Intern Med.* 2012;172(19):1444-1453.

30. About Us. Cochrane.org. Available at: www.cochrane.org. Accessed April 13, 2018.

31. Sandoiu, A. Study shows why acupuncture might work. *Medical News Today.* July 2, 2017. Available at: https://www.medicalnewstoday.com/articles/318209.php. Accessed April 13, 2018.

32. Acupuncture Information. Acupuncture.com. Available at: http://www.acupuncture.com/misc/acuinfo.htm. Accessed April 13, 2018.

33. Accreditation Commission for Acupuncture and Oriental Medicine. ACAOM accreditation standards: Master's and professional doctorate programs in acupuncture and/or oriental medicine. Available at: http://acaom.org/wp-content/uploads/2018/02/ACAOM-Rev-Masters-and-PD-Standards-Apprv-for-Public-Comment.pdf. Published February 16, 2018. Accessed April 13, 2018.

34. National Certification Commission for Acupuncture and Oriental Medicine. History and Overview. Available at: http://www.nccaom.org/about-us/history. Accessed April 13, 2018.

35. American Academy of Medical Acupuncture. Welcome. Available at: http://www.medicalacupuncture.org/. Accessed April 13, 2018.

36. American Board of Medical Acupuncture. Home page. Available at: http://www.dabma.org. Accessed April 13, 2018.

37. National Certification Commission for Acupuncture and Oriental Medicine. State Licensure Requirements Interactive map. Available at: http://www.nccaom.org/state-licensure/. Updated January 1, 2018. Accessed April 13, 2018.

38. Traditional Chinese Medicine Information Page. Herbal Therapy. Available at: http://www.tcmpage.com/herbal_therapy.html. Accessed April 13, 2018.

39. Travel China Guide. Chinese Herbal Medicine. Available at: http://www.travelchinaguide.com/intro/medicine/herbal.htm. Accessed April 13, 2018.

40. Somerville R, ed. *The Alternate Advisor.* Alexandria, VA: Time-Life Books; 1997.

41. Dharmananda S. The Lessons of Shennong: The Basis of Chinese Herb Medicine. Available at: http://www.itmonline.org/arts/shennong.htm. Accessed April 13, 2018.

42. Traditional Chinese Medicine Information Page. Herbal Therapy. Available at: http://www.tcmpage.com/herbal_therapy.html. Accessed April 13, 2018.

43. National Center for Complementary and Integrative Health. Safe use of Complementary Health Products and Practices. Available at: https://nccih.nih.gov/health/safety. Updated September 24, 2017. Accessed April 13, 2018.

44. U.S. Food and Drug Administration. Current Good Manufacturing Practices (CGMP) Regulations. Available at: https://www.fda.gov/drugs/developmentapprovalprocess/manufacturing/ucm090016.htm. Updated March 30, 2018. Accessed April 13, 2018.

45. Register of Chinese Herbal Medicine. Welcome. Available at: http://rchm.co.uk/. Accessed April 13, 2018.

46. Bradford N, ed. *The One-Spirit Encyclopedia of Complementary Health.* London, UK: Octopus; 2000.

47. Dharmananda S. An Introduction to Chinese Herbs. November 1996. Available at: http://www.itmonline.org/arts/herbintro.htm. Accessed April 13, 2018.

48. Huang K. *The Pharmacology of Chinese Herbs.* 2nd ed. Boca Raton, FL: CRC Press; 1996.

49. Oriental Medicine. The Properties of Herbs. Available at: http://www.orientalmedicine.com/properties-herbs. Accessed April 13, 2018.

50. National Center for Complementary and Integrative Health. Herbs at a glance. Available at: https://nccih.nih.gov/health/herbsataglance.htm. Updated September 24, 2017. Accessed April 13, 2018.

51. Huang HL, Chen CC, Yeh CY, Huang RL. Atractylodes reactive oxygen species mediation of baizhu-induced apoptosis in human leukemia cells. *J Ethnopharmacol.* 2005;97(1):21-29.

52. Xu K, Feng ZM, Yang YN, Jiang JS, Zhang PC. Four new C_{10}-polyacetylene glycosides from the rhizomes of Atractylodes lancea. *J Asian Nat Prod Res.* 2017;19(2):121-127.

53. Zhang N, Liu C, Sun TM, Ran XK, Kang TG, Dou DQ. Two new compounds from Atractylodes macrocephala with neuroprotective activity. *J Asian Nat Prod Res.* 2017;19(1):35-41.

54. Park SK, Park SJ, Park SM, et al. Inhibition of acute phase inflammation by *Laminaria japonica* through regulation of iNOS-NF-κB pathway. *Evid Based Complement Alternat Med.* 2013;2013:439498.

55. Dong H, He L, Huang M, Dong Y. Anti-inflammatory components isolated from *Atractylodes macrocephala* Koidz. *Nat Prod Res.* 2008;22(16):1418-1427.

56. National Institutes of Health Office of Dietary Supplements. Health Information: Ephedra. Available at: https://ods.od.nih.gov/Health_Information/Ephedra.aspx. Accessed April 13, 2018.

57. EphedraOutlet. Available at: http://ephedraoutlet.com. Accessed April 13, 2018.

58. National Center for Complementary and Integrative Health. Ephedra. Available at: https://nccih.nih.gov/health/ephedra. Accessed April 13, 2018.

59. Xiao M, Ji W, Xuan H, et al. Large dosage of chishao in formulae for cholestatic hepatitis: A systematic review and meta-analysis. *Evid Based Complement Alternat Med.* 2014;2014:328152.

60. Lai F, Zhang Y, Xie DP, et al. A systematic review of rhubarb (a traditional Chinese medicine) used for the treatment of experimental sepsis. *Evid Based Complement Alternat Med.* 2015;2015:131283.

61. Kaszkin-Bettag M, Beck S, Richardson A, Heger PW, Beer AM. Efficacy of the special extract ERr 731 from the rhapontic rhubarb for menopausal complaints: A 6-month open observational study. *Altern Ther Health Med.* 2008;14(6):32-38.

62. Ding Y, Zhao L, Mei H, et al. Exploration of emodin to treat alpha-naphthylisothiocyanate-induced cholestatic hepatitis via anti-inflammatory pathway. *Eur J Pharmacol.* 2008;590(1-3):377-386.

63. Wang WH, Hsuan KY, Chu LY, Lee CY, Tyan YC, Chen ZS, Tsai WC. Anticancer effects of Salvia miltiorrhiza alcohol extract on oral squamous carcinoma cells. *Evid Based Complement Alternat Med.* 2017;2017:5364010.

64. Wu CF, Bohnert S, Thines E, Efferth T. Cytotoxicity of Salvia miltiorrhiza against multidrug-resistant cancer cells. *Am J Chin Med*. 2016;44(4):871-894.

65. Helm B. Tui na - Chinese bodywork therapy. Acupuncture .com. Available at: http://www.acupuncture.com/qigong_tuina /tuinabodywork.htm. Accessed April 13, 2018.

66. Kovach VV. The tui na touch: The intensity of Chinese medicine at your fingertips. *Massage & Bodywork*. April/May 2003. Available at: http://www.massagetherapy.com/articles /index.php/article_id/60/The-Tui-Na-Touch. Accessed April 13, 2018.

67. Celli M. The Chinese Medicine Diet. Inner Light Wellness Acupuncture. May 1, 2010. Available at: http://innerlight -wellness.net/articles/the-chinese-medicine-diet. Accessed April 13, 2018.

68. Marazita E. Alternative medicine: Qigong: Chinese exercise for better health. Available at: http://www.seattlepi.com /health/288318_altmed12.html. Published October 11, 2006. Accessed April 13, 2018.

69. Idea Health & Fitness Association. Tai Chi: Moving Slow in a Fast World. February 19, 2007. Available at: http://www .ideafit.com/fitness-library/tai-chi-moving-slow-in-a-fast -world. Accessed April 13, 2018.

70. Everyday Tai Chi. Tai Chi from Beijing 24 Teaching Clips. Available at: http://www.everyday-taichi.com/tai-chi-form -beijing-24.html. Accessed April 13, 2018.

71. Garofalo MP. T'ai Chi Chi'uan: National 24 Form. Available at: http://www.egreenway.com/taichichuan/short .htm. Accessed April 13, 2018.

72. Zou L, SasaKi JE, Wang H, Xiao Z, Fang Q, Zhang M. A systematic review and meta-analysis baduanjin qigong for health benefits: Randomized controlled trials. *Evid Based Complement Alternat Med*. 2017;2017:4548706.

73. Oh CU, Kim NN. Effects of Tai Chi on serotonin, nicotine dependency, depression, and anger in hospitalized alcohol-dependent patients. *J Altern Complement Med*. 2016;22(12):957-963.

74. Pelletier K. *The Best Alternative Medicine*. New York, NY: Simon & Schuster; 2000.

CHAPTER 10

Alternative Medical Systems: Naturopathic and Homeopathic Medicine

LEARNING OBJECTIVES

As a result of reading this chapter, students will be able to:

1. Name the founder of Naturopathy in America.
2. List and define five major beliefs of Naturopathy.
3. Name and explain four of six Naturopathic diagnostic methods.
4. Identify and analyze four Naturopathic treatment methods.
5. Name three ways to become a Naturopath or Naturopathic physician.
6. Assess the impact of naturopathy on current medical practices.
7. Explain what homeopathy is.
8. Name the founder of homeopathy.
9. List and describe the three essential principles of homeopathy.
10. Analyze reasons why, or why not, homeopathic substances can be effective.
11. Name four types of licensed professionals who are allowed to employ homeopathy within their practices.

▶ What Is Naturopathic Medicine and How Did It Develop?

Naturopathic medicine is a holistic, whole body health care system based on the belief that the body has the potential to heal itself and that the physician's role is to support the body's efforts.[1,2] The founder of naturopathy in America has been attributed to Dr. Benedict Lust (1872–1945), a German immigrant.[3] He described naturopathy as a system of returning to nature to cure diseases by drinking clean water, getting air and sunlight, by exercising, getting rest and eating a proper diet. Dr. Lust also believed that naturopathy should be a natural therapy used to educate people to live healthier lives and not as a means for treatment for disease.[3] Currently, however, naturopathic medicine employs multidisciplinary means of preventing and treating disease.

Historical Development

The philosophical roots of naturopathic medicine stem from the time of Hippocrates, the Greek father of medicine (about 400 BCE).[4] Hippocrates incorporated natural means such as diet, exercise, manipulative therapies, and **hydrotherapy** into his practice.[5] At that time, other physicians also studied the laws of nature and applied those principles within their medical practices. *Vis medicatrix naturae*, Latin for the healing power of nature, was their code and became the mantra for present-day naturopathic medicine. The practice of naturopathy began as a part of the European nature cure, which evolved during the 18th and 19th centuries.[6] Six **cholera epidemics** occurred during the 19th century in Asia, Europe, North Africa, and the Americas. Paris and London were affected especially hard, with thousands of deaths. In 1842, Chadwick submitted a *Report on the Sanitary Conditions of the Laboring Population of Great Britain* to the English Parliament.[7] In it, Chadwick wrote that the spread of cholera was due to contaminated drinking water from human sewage. Chadwick did not accept germ theory as the cause of cholera. He believed that filth that could be seen by the eyes and smelled by the nose was the main cause of pandemic disease. His solution was to change the urban sanitation **infrastructure** by incorporating garbage collection, toilets with flushing mechanisms, and enclosed sewage systems, therein assuring cleaner drinking water.

In 1848, Arnold Rikli, who was born in Sweden but lived most of his life in Bled, Slovenia, also advocated for the importance of fresh air, sunlight, and swimming in cold water (water cure) in order to cure diseases and remain healthy.[7] He believed that suntanning and walking were also important for health. In sum, rather than scientific medicines, changing the environment (nature) was believed to be the *real* cure for diseases by these early pioneers of natural healing methods.

The term "naturopathy" was coined in 1892 and described a system of natural therapies.[8] The word comes from Greek and Latin and translates to "nature disease."[9] In 1902, Dr. Benedict Lust founded the American School of Naturopathy in New York after having cured himself of **tuberculosis** by a natural means—hydrotherapy (water therapy). Dr. Lust received a degree in 1898 from the Universal Osteopathic College of New York, a degree in Homeopathic medicine in 1902, and a medical degree from the Eclectic Medical College in New York in 1913.[3] Some courses that he taught included herbal medicine, nutrition, physiotherapy, psychology, **homeopathy**, and manipulation techniques.[10] In 1919, Dr. Lust founded the American

Naturopathic Association, which was incorporated in 19 states.[1,2,3] In the ensuing years, however, naturopathic medicine did not become a popular discipline here in the United States. After Dr. Lust's death, there was conflict among the various schools of natural medicine (homeopathy, herbalism, physiomedicalism). Medical technology had advanced, and conventional medicine had consolidated politically and virtually "swamped natural means of medical care."[5] During the 1970s and 1980s, however, a movement of health consciousness began to inspire people to move from the pharmaceutical to a more natural and holistic means of healing, and naturopathic medicine again began to gain in appeal.

▶ What Are the Major Beliefs of Naturopathy?

The following are the five major beliefs of naturopathy:

1. **Disease is a natural part of nature**. Disease is viewed as a natural part of nature and is caused by a violation of nature's laws (e.g., sleeping poorly, eating poorly, irrational thinking patterns, irresponsible alcohol drinking behaviors, unprotected sexual conduct). When healthy functioning is disturbed, the naturopathic belief is that disease will result in humans just as it does in the plant and animal kingdoms.

2. **Promote health and prevent disease**. Prevention of disease is another major belief in naturopathy. Naturopathic practitioners or physicians work on promoting health to prevent disease.[11] They encourage patients to be responsible for their own health by living healthy lifestyles. Good health is seen as a triad: maintaining a balance among the body's structure, its biochemistry, and the emotions.

3. **The body will heal itself**. A major belief of naturopathy is that the body is its own best healer and knows what it needs to get well or heal itself.[12] Symptoms of disease are viewed as a result of the body trying to purify itself. The preferred mode is to allow the body to heal on its own by using positive strategies to strengthen the immune system (diet, fluids, rest). In naturopathy, the cause of the symptoms (problem) is investigated and diagnosed before treatment is prescribed, which would include treating the patient in a holistic and natural fashion.[11-13]

4. **Germs are not the major cause of disease**. Naturopaths invoke a few simplistic theories

to explain the causes of disease. They do not believe that **pathogens** or germs are the main cause of disease. They believe that disease is caused by several other phenomena that could include the actions of "toxins" (accumulation of waste materials and bodily refuse); food allergies; dietary sugar, fat, and gluten; inadequate vitamin and mineral intake; vertebral misalignments; imbalances of qi energy; and a few others.[12,13] Acute (short-acting) diseases such as fevers, measles, childhood chicken pox, colds, and the like are believed to be the body's attempt to get rid of waste products that are interfering with the body's functioning systems. On the other hand, all chronic (long-lasting) diseases are viewed as the result of continued suppression of the same acute diseases or from self-initiated attempts at body cleansing.

5. **First, do no harm**. Finally, a naturopathic medicine belief is to "First, do no harm." Based on this belief, the naturopathic physician uses methods and substances that are as nontoxic and noninvasive as possible.[10,12,13] Naturopathy views the naturopathic physician as a teacher who can educate people about their lifestyle that may be contributing to their present condition. One of their core beliefs is to address each person in a holistic way, body, mind, and spirit.[14]

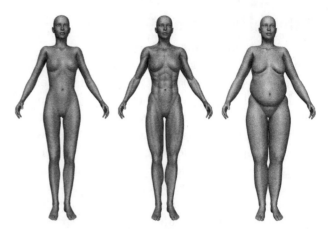

FIGURE 10.1 Biotypes (left to right): Ectomorph, mesomorph, and endomorph.
© Scott Camazine/Alamy Images

has certain characteristics that are related to the risk of acquiring particular diseases. The **biotypes** (**FIGURE 10.1**) are **ectomorph** (long and lean), **mesomorph** (muscular and perhaps stocky), and **endomorph** (soft and round).[17]

Endomorphs may have more gallbladder disorders, whereas ectomorphs are more prone to rheumatoid arthritis and mesomorphs are more inclined to suffer **degenerative arthritis**.[5] The naturopath may use body type as a start in the diagnostic process.

▶ What Are the Naturopathic Diagnostic Methods?

Traditional Diagnostic Methods

Naturopathic practitioners use many of the diagnostic methods of the traditional physician such as observing the overall look of the patient, taking the pulse and blood pressure, listening to the heart and breathing, and so forth. Naturopaths will take a detailed history and will ask questions related to lifestyle and diet. They may order standard blood and urine laboratory tests.[15,16] Naturopaths also may order radiology for diagnostic purposes, although they do not use radiology for treatment purposes.

Biotypes

Besides the traditional diagnostic methods, naturopaths assess biotype or constitution to aid in diagnosis because they believe that each type

Iridology

Iridology is the examination of the iris or colored portion of the eye for markings that supposedly reveal changing conditions of every part and organ of the body. In 1670, a physician, Phillippus Meyens, wrote a book called *Chromatica Medica* in which he wrote about the eye and the relationship of its appearance to the physical body.[18] In the middle of the 19th century, when still a child, Ignatz Von Peczely caught an owl, and as the owl struggled, it accidentally broke its leg. Just after, the boy saw a black line rising in the owl's eye. Later in life, Von Peczely became a physician and began to study the irises of his patients. Because he believed there was a relationship between changes in the body and iris markings, he developed an iris chart.[18,19]

Around the same time, a 14-year-old Swedish boy, Nils Liljequist, became severely ill following a vaccination. He was treated with **quinine** and other potent drugs, after which his iris color changed. His iris color changed again after his ribs were broken years later. He, like Von Peczely, believed there was a relationship between the iris and body injuries and disease. In 1893, Liljequist published over 258 drawings showing the iris/body relationship. His iris maps were very similar to Von Peczely's.[19] Through the years, the iris chart was continually researched and revised. Some of the most widely used maps for iridology were eventually published by Dr. Bernard Jensen in the 1950s. Dr. Jensen was a chiropractor, an entrepreneur, and the author of numerous books and articles on health and healing.

Certain areas of the iris are believed to correspond to organ and body systems and are analyzed to reveal inherent weaknesses and strengths in the organ systems. Those who study the iris (iridologists) do not claim that it will diagnose disease, but believe that the markings on the iris can indicate if an individual has overactivity or underactivity in areas of the body.[20] For example, an underactive pancreas might indicate a diabetic condition. See **FIGURE 10.2** for an iridology chart.

The theory of iridology includes the view that the iris contains four layers that indicate tissue activity: acute changes, subacute changes, chronic changes, and degenerative changes. The color of the iris is also used in assessment. See **BOX 10.1** for differentiation of blue-eyed, mixed, and brown-eyed types.[19]

The markings on the iris are designated as white, yellow-white, yellow, orange, red-brown, brown, and

---

BOX 10.1 Iris Colors Used for Diagnostic Purposes

- **Blue-eyed type**: Supposedly have increased risk for upper respiratory, digestive tract, urogenital tract, lymphatic tissue, joint, kidney, and adrenal gland imbalances.
- **Mixed eye type**: Has discolorations (usually light brown) on top of a blue background. Supposedly has increased risk for liver-related problems, digestive tract problems, and allergies.
- **Brown-eyed type**: Supposedly predisposed to blood disorders and imbalances of minerals. Cautioned to pay attention to the circulatory system, liver, bone marrow, spleen, digestive system, and endocrine glands.

Gold C. Iridology: The origin. Available at: http://www.campbellmgold.com/archive_health/irid_origin.pdf Accessed July 11, 2017.

---

black. Each is thought to indicate pathology within the body, as shown in **BOX 10.2**.

The iridologist, besides observing the layers, colors, and markings on the iris, will assess the rings and spots on the iris that supposedly indicate certain body conditions. Spots that move across the iris are said to indicate deficiencies of a particular organ or system. Several types of rings may be found on the

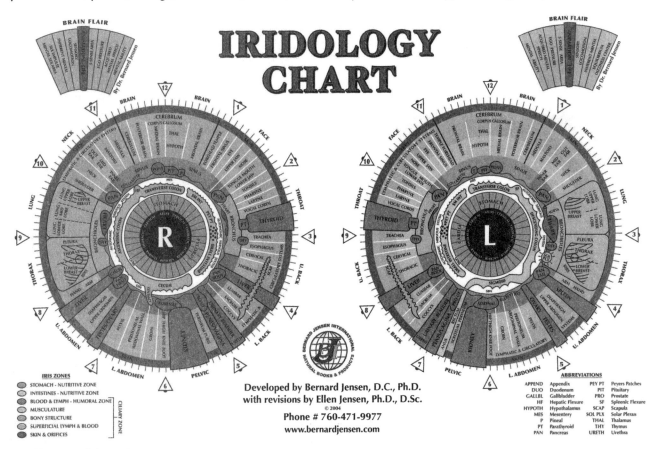

FIGURE 10.2 Iridology chart.

With permission from Bernard Jensen International.

BOX 10.2 Eye Markings and Their Relationship to Pathology

- White indicates an area of the body working hard to "maintain."
- Yellow-white indicates an area of the body losing a battle.
- Yellow indicates poor kidney function; yellow sclera (white part of the eye) suggests gallbladder disease.
- Orange indicates problems metabolizing carbohydrates and weakness in the liver and/or pancreas. Glucose levels should be checked.
- Red-brown indicates deterioration.
- Brown indicates poor liver function and "dirty blood."
- Black indicates dying tissue.

---

iris, each of which is said to indicate body deficiency. See **BOX 10.3** for a few examples of how iris rings relate to pathology.[19]

Practitioner qualifications vary. One can acquire a Diploma of Holistic Iridology in person or through distance education though the International Institute of Iridology and the DaVinci College of Holistic Medicine.[21] The International College of Iridology[22] is a professional society for the study and advancement of iridology. Its website states that it is dedicated to the education and unification of iridologists around the world. It provides continuing education forums, support research, and clinical practice of iridology.[22]

BOX 10.3 Iris Rings and Their Relationship to Pathology

- **Scurf Rim or Ring of Purpose** is a dark band around the iris. This may indicate that the skin is not functioning properly (perhaps does not easily sweat).
- **Stress Rings or Rings of Freedom** look like growth rings on a tree. They may indicate neuromuscular tension and stress.
- **Lipid Ring or Ring of Determination** is a heavy white ring partially or completely covering the outer edge of the iris. This ring is mostly found in older people, and it may be indicative of arteriosclerosis and other cardiovascular problems. It may also indicate problems with the liver and thyroid and an increased risk of Parkinson's disease.
- **Lymphatic Rosary or Ring of Harmony** looks like a tiny ring of clouds around the outer iris. People with this ring may have lymphatic congestion and swollen lymph nodes

---

Problems with Iridology

One of the problems associated with iridology is that this practice is not regulated or licensed by any government agency in the United States or Canada. What is more important, there seems to be no scientific evidence that iridology should be used for diagnostic purposes.[23] All double-blinded, rigorous tests of iridology have failed to find any statistical significance.[23] Usually, the studies were set up so that iridologists would view photographs or slides of individuals and then be asked to diagnose disease. For example, a kidney disease and iridology study was published in the *Journal of the American Medical Association* and a gallbladder disease and iridology study was published in the *British Medical Journal*.[24] Both showed no statistical significance for using iridology as a diagnostic tool for disease. Many more studies have been attempted. Even though there have been research studies that showed iridology was a valid diagnostic tool, they have been discounted because they did not use good scientific procedures such as control groups and unmasked studies. Studies like these are biased and should not be used to promote any benefit of the use of iridology for diagnostic purposes.[16,23,25]

Mineral Analysis

Naturopaths may analyze hair for trace mineral content. Testing is performed on hair that is cut one and half inches from the scalp, and the hair sample is then sent to a laboratory for analysis. Supposedly, the hair sample can reveal mineral status and toxic metal accumulation following long-term or even acute exposure. Diet, stress, medications, pollution, nutritional supplements, and inherited patterns are all factors that are believed to affect a mineral imbalance.[26] A study of six commercial U.S. laboratories, which analyze 90% of the hair samples in the United States, showed laboratory differences in highest and lowest reported mineral concentrations.[27] There were variations in laboratory sample preparation methods and **calibration** standards. The conclusion was that hair mineral analysis is unreliable and should not be used to assess individual nutritional status or exposure to environmental pollution.[27]

Bioresonance Diagnosis

Bioresonance is the practice of using an electronic device to measure the body's electromagnetic radiation and electric currents. The theory is that damaged organs and cancer cells emit electromagnetic oscillations that are different from healthy cells and that a Bioresonance device can detect this information.[28] Thus far, there is no scientific evidence that

Bioresonance works.[28] Bioresonance machinery was supposed to cure smoking addiction and cancer, but it was shown to be a fake gadgetry.[16,23] In March 2002, the Federal Trade Commission charged an Internet entrepreneur, David L. Walker, with making false claims about the efficacy of his supposed cancer cure, the CWAT-Treatments: BioResonance Therapy and Molecular Enhancer.[29] Walker had advertised his products, which also included herbal and mineral mixtures, as so effective in fighting cancer that people would not need surgery, chemotherapy, or other conventional cancer treatments. He also charged thousands of dollars for the treatment. The settlement with Walker and the FTC occurred in October 2002, with Walker having to pay $229,000 in fines and was permanently prohibited from making the same or similar claims.[29]

Kirlian Photography as Diagnosis

In **Kirlian photography**, colorful photographs of images surrounding the body and within the body are made after applying high-frequency electrical currents to a patient's body. An object is placed in contact with a photographic plate and connected to a source of high voltage, high frequency, but low current electricity. The electricity stimulates electrons so they ionize the surrounding air. Those promoting Kirlian photography say it is photography of the aura, or an electrical field, surrounding people. Those debunking Kirlian photography say it is due to natural phenomena such as pressure, electrical grounding, humidity, and temperature.[30] To date, there are no rigorous scientific studies showing the worth of Kirlian photography for use in diagnosing disease.

Thus far, several naturopathic diagnostic tests have been discussed, but either they have not been scientifically tested or they have been tested and shown not to be effective.

▶ What Are the Naturopathic Treatments?

Balancing Four Major Body Systems

Naturopaths employ a system of noninvasive health care and health assessment in which neither surgery nor drugs are the first treatment of choice, although they know that there are times and certain body conditions that require them.[30] Naturopaths believe that the key to successful treatment is in balancing four major body systems: the immune system, the elimination (or detoxification) system, the nervous system, and the hormonal system.[10] In order to achieve this balance, naturopaths encourage patients to use natural therapies such as fresh air, sunlight, water, rest, natural medicines and herbs, and exercise.[10,31]

Education and Counseling

Naturopaths rely on educating and counseling clients about lifestyle and diet. In fact, at Bastyr University in Seattle, a major hub for educating naturopaths, students take counseling courses so that they can better work with clients.[32]

Nutrition

Nutrition and its relationship to diseases is a primary focus of naturopathy. Naturopaths believe that diet alone or with the use of proper supplements may improve conditions. **Fasting** may be prescribed for a day or more (1-, 3-, 5-, and 7-day fasts). The purpose is to give the digestive system a rest and to detoxify the body. Juice may be drunk or grapes may be eaten during days of fasting.[5]

Botanicals and Traditional Medicines

Medicines prescribed usually come from nature rather than a laboratory. Naturopaths use botanical medicine (**phytotherapy**) for treating disease conditions. Vitamins and homeopathic substances (e.g., tissue cell salts) may also be prescribed. Different states have laws identifying the type of traditional medicines that naturopaths may prescribe. In the state of Washington, for example, naturopaths may prescribe antibiotics, thyroid medicine, progesterone, and other drugs.[10]

Energy Work, Massage, Physical Therapy, Traditional Chinese Medicine, and Bodywork

Naturopaths might use energy work, massage therapy, physical therapy, and traditional Chinese medicine **modalities** (such as acupuncture, herbal medicines). Naturopathic manipulation or bodywork comprises a variety of systematic movements to heal musculoskeletal and neurological conditions, very similar to **osteopathic** and **chiropractic** medicine.

Hydrotherapy

Hydrotherapy and colonic enemas (colon hydrotherapy) may be used, depending on the condition. Hydrotherapy is the treatment of physical disability, injury, or illness by immersion of all or part of the body in water to facilitate movement, promote wound healing, and relieve pain. It is usually done under the supervision of a trained therapist. Hydrotherapy may include the use of hot and cold water. Alternate hot and cold is used to stimulate the blood and lymph circulation and help to remove congestion and revive the body tissues.[5] Cold compresses may also be used to boost the elimination of toxins.

As described, naturopathic treatments are usually noninvasive and medicines are natural or herbal rather than prescription drugs. Naturopaths focus on the importance of nutrition and lifestyle not only as strategies for the prevention of disease, but also as treatment modalities.

You have now learned what naturopathy is, the diagnostic methods used, and an overview of treatment modalities. Next, we explain the training of the naturopathic physician.

▶ What Are the Naturopathic Classifications and the Training of Naturopathic Physicians?

There are three main categories of naturopathic practitioners[9]:

1. **Traditional naturopath**: The traditional naturopath does not have a university undergraduate or higher education degree. He or she can obtain training through distance learning (correspondence or Internet courses). The admission requirements are not rigorous, and naturopaths trained in this fashion are not eligible for certification. They may not prescribe drugs, X-rays, or surgery. The programs are not accredited by organizations recognized for accreditation purposes by the U.S. Department of Education and are not subject to licensing.
2. **Healthcare providers**: The second category is composed of medical doctors, osteopathic doctors, chiropractors, and nurses who pursued additional training in naturopathic treatment modalities.[9] Their training programs also vary.
3. **Naturopathic physician**: The third category is the naturopathic physician, whose training is similar to the training of the medical doctor.[9] Prerequisites include 3 years of premedical sciences at a university with a cumulative grade point average of 3.0 on a 4-point scale. The curriculum includes courses in the basic sciences (anatomy, physiology, histology, microbiology, biochemistry, immunology, pharmacology, and pathology), clinical disciplines (diagnostic medicine practices such as physical and clinical diagnosis, laboratory diagnosis, radiology, naturopathic assessment, and orthopedics), and naturopathic courses (clinical nutrition, botanical medicine, traditional Chinese therapeutic skills and treatments, homeopathic medicine, hydrotherapy, naturopathic manipulation, and lifestyle counseling). Clinical experience includes 1,500 hours of clinical requirements and proficiency in all aspects of naturopathic medicine. Students must also pass the board Naturopathic Physicians Licensing Examination (NPLEX) after the second and fourth years. Continuing medical education (CME) credits are required on an ongoing basis after becoming a Doctor of Naturopathy (ND).

Five universities in the United States and two Canadian universities offer a ND or Doctor of Naturopathic Medicine (NMD) degree.[33] According to the American Association of Naturopathic Physicians (AANP),[34] the 4-year, baccalaureate professional association, there are 3,000 licensed naturopathic physicians. See **BOX 10.4** for schools accredited by the Council on Naturopathic Medical Education.[33]

Currently, the following states and territories have licensing laws for naturopathic doctors[34]:

1. Alaska
2. Arizona
3. California
4. Colorado
5. Connecticut
6. District of Columbia
7. Hawaii
8. Kansas
9. Maine
10. Maryland
11. Massachusetts
12. Minnesota
13. Montana
14. New Hampshire
15. Oregon
16. Pennsylvania
17. Utah
18. Vermont
19. Washington
20. U.S. territories of Puerto Rico and Virgin Islands

What Is the Prevalence of Naturopathy Use?

According to the 2007 National Health Interview Survey (NHIS), an estimated 729,000 adults and 237,000 children in the United States had used a naturopathic treatment in the previous year. The 2012 NHIS shows a small but linear increase to 957,000 adults using a naturopathic treatment.[35] Some of the more common conditions that naturopaths treat are allergies, fatigue, colds, headaches, migraine headaches, shingles, genital warts (HPV), irritable bowel syndrome, gout, depression, urinary tract infections, kidney stones, constipation, arthritis, asthma, back problems, high blood pressure, menstrual problems, chronic pain, and stress.[1,10] Many individuals visit naturopathic practitioners not only for primary care, but also for prevention of disease and to support wellness.

What Are the Results of Research on Naturopathy?

Naturopaths have shown good success in treating some cancers because of the naturopathic treatments that focus on strengthening the body's immune system.[10] The National Center for Complementary and Integrative Health (NCCIH) is studying a naturopathic dietary approach for type 2 diabetes, naturopathic treatments for periodontal gum disease (**periodontitis**), and naturopathic herbal and dietary approaches to breast cancer prevention; currently, however, there are no study results. Another NCCIH study on naturopathic techniques to help a group of 70 warehouse workers who had lower back pain demonstrated positive results. Naturopathic care that included acupuncture, exercise, dietary advice, relaxation training, and a back care booklet was more cost effective than the employer's usual patient education program. Both workers and employers benefited from the naturopathic approach, which was associated with less absenteeism, lower costs for treatments, and better quality of life.[9]

The NCCIH[9] has reported that both naturopathy and traditional Chinese medicine were effective for

📄 *IN THE NEWS*

Article Presented at *The Health Site*, March 10, 2015

Naturopathic physicians believe in helping cancer patients cope with their illness in a more holistic and natural way. In an interview with Dr. Anjali Sharma, he explains some of those ways. Strict daily routine includes:

- Yoga
- Pranayama (breathing exercises)
- Relaxation
- Meditation
- Rehabilitative exercises
- Psychospiritual counseling
- Hydrotherapy
- Magnetotherapy
- Heliotherapy (light or sun therapy)
- Massage therapy
- Acupressure and acupuncture

What are your thoughts about these recommendations?

Source: Sampath S. How to cope with cancer the naturopathy way. *The Health Site.* March 10, 2015. Available at: http://www.thehealthsite.com/diseases-conditions/cancer-naturopathy-treatment-p214/. Accessed April 17, 2018.

treating **temporomandibular disorders (TMD)** in women. TMD is characterized by pain and tenderness when chewing and opening the mouth. Limitations of jaw opening are often accompanied by deviations in mandible path and clicking, popping, or grating sounds from the temporomandibular joint. Researchers evaluated two alternative healing approaches—traditional Chinese medicine (*n* = 50) and naturopathic medicine (*n* = 50)—to assess whether they were as effective as usual care (*n* = 50) provided by dental clinicians. Participants were females 25–55 years of age with multiple health problems.[9]

Two studies published in the 1990s showed positive results for naturopathic treatment of **rheumatoid arthritis** using a naturopathic-controlled diet.[36,37] Many other studies cited by Pelletier[10] were published in the 1970s, 1980s, and 1990s and showed fairly positive results for naturopathic treatment. One series of studies by Hudson showed the value of naturopathic botanicals and nutritional supplements that changed abnormal pap smears to normal. Also, a pilot study conducted at Bastyr University provided herbal and nutritional therapies to HIV-infected patients, which improved their immune function. Pelletier also presented studies showing the effects of naturopathic treatment on osteoarthritis, asthma, atherosclerosis, back pain, benign prostatic hypertrophy, depression, diabetes mellitus, eczema, HIV disease, irritable bowel syndrome, migraine headaches, middle ear infections, premenstrual syndrome, upper respiratory infection, and vaginitis. Refer to Pelletier's text,[10] *The Best Alternative Medicine: What Works? What Does Not?*, pages 184–194, for a closer examination of these results.

▶ What Is the Future of Naturopathy?

Naturopathy is cost-effective, and because of that is being integrated into conventional medicine practices. Naturopaths have lower overhead costs and charge patients less than do medical doctors or osteopaths. The treatments are less invasive and, therefore, cost much less. In many states, naturopathy is covered by insurance. Its practitioners are becoming well educated in the sciences, nutrition, and counseling practices. The future may comprise a new vision of health care that may include naturopathy. As more scientific studies are designed and implemented that demonstrate the effectiveness of naturopathy, the practice will likely increase.

The executive director of the AANP, Karen E. Howard, foresees that naturopathy will be a meaningful component in future health care. The AANP promotes naturopathy as a tool to change the health care system from disease management to health promotion by incorporating the principles of naturopathic medicine (presented earlier in this chapter).[38] The future of naturopathy appears to be bright.

▶ What Is the Homeopathy Healing System and How Did It Develop?

This chapter would not be complete without presenting information on homeopathy, one of the major tools of the naturopath. Homeopathy is a healing system developed in 1790 by a German physician and chemist named Christian Friedrich Samuel Hahnemann.[5,39] The word *homeo* refers to similar and *pathos or pathy* refers to suffering and disease. Homeopathy is a holistic and natural system of healing that aims to prevent illness as well as treat it. Homeopathy is based on the idea that like cures like. Substances that cause specific symptoms in a healthy person are thought to be able to cure individuals who are ill displaying the same type of symptoms.

History

Hahnemann became disenchanted with the unhygienic and often brutal medical techniques such as purging, emetics, bloodletting, and the use of large doses of chemical agents such as mercury and arsenic that were used in the late 1700s. He stopped his physician's practice and became a translator. While translating a text called *A Treatise on Materia Medica* by Scottish physician Dr. William Cullen, Hahnemann learned that quinine was supposed to cure malaria because of its **astringent** properties. Because he doubted that the astringent property of quinine was the reason for the cure, he began to experiment on himself. Each time he took a dose of quinine, he produced the symptoms of malaria in himself, supposedly a healthy individual.[5,39] His investigations continued as he began to experiment with small doses of substances thought to cure disease. Soon, Hahnemann began to dilute substances such as herbs, minerals, and animal extracts in an alcohol–water solution. Hahnemann found that the more he diluted substances, the less the side effects and the more he could boost the potency of the drug. As the solutions were diluted, shaking became a necessary action because this process released what Hahnemann called stores of vital energy.

Although Hahnemann popularized the idea of *like cures like*, Hippocrates, the Father of Medicine, and the Egyptians used the idea of similars in the 5th century BCE.[39] Over time, the more orthodox practice of curing with substances contrary to the symptoms took over. In folk medicine, however, the principle of similars persisted for hundreds of years until Hahnemann began his more scientific investigation of homeopathy.[1] The more that Hahnemann tested subjects, the more he found a "drug picture of substances," and then finally a "symptoms picture" of each patient that made his prescriptions more effective.[5] He developed three essential principles of homeopathy that remain today:

1. **The principle of similars**: Like cures like.
2. **The principle of infinitesimal dose**: The more diluted the dose, the more potent its curative effects.
3. **The principle of specificity of the individual**: If the remedy is to cure, it must match the symptom profile of the patient.[38]

Dr. Constantine Hering, a student of Hahnemann, introduced homeopathy into the United States. He opened a homeopathic medical school in 1835 in Allentown, Pennsylvania.[40] By 1900, there were 22 homeopathic medical schools, close to 100 homeopathic hospitals, and over 1,000 homeopathic pharmacies in the United States. About 15% of all U.S. physicians were homeopathic practitioners. During the 1930s, conventional pharmaceutical medications were being produced, and a powerful American Medical Association challenged homeopathy as a viable medical system. Consequently, the practice in the United States virtually died out.[40] Homeopathy did not, however, die out everywhere; it is still practiced worldwide. There are more than 6,000 German and 5,000 French practitioners. In Great Britain, homeopathy is a part of the medical and health care system. There are many homeopathic hospitals and outpatient clinics. The practice is also used in India, where there are over 100 homeopathic colleges.

▶ What Are Homeopathic Treatments?

Homeopathic treatments are minute (diluted) remedies made from animal, vegetable, and mineral substances.[1,39] Homeopaths believe that the energy or *vibrational* pattern from a homeopathic substance that is contained in the solution stimulates healing by activating the *vital force*, first identified by Hahnemann.

Remedies come in a variety of forms: tablets, powders, wafers, and liquids in an alcohol base. Like many traditional medicines, many homeopathic remedies are found as over-the-counter products.[1,39] This allows for self-treatment of minor conditions such as flu, sore throat, headache, and insomnia.

The process of dilution takes several weeks. Plant parts are dissolved in a mixture of alcohol and water and left to stand for 2–4 weeks. The mixture, called **mother of tincture**, is occasionally shaken and strained. That solution is then used to make different potencies by repeatedly diluting with water or alcohol and vigorously shaking it, a process called **succession**.[40] A dilution to a 4× remedy is done in the following way: The mother of tincture solution is diluted by a factor of 10 (1×), then again by a factor of 10 (2×), then again by a factor of 10 (3×), and again by a factor of 10 (4×). The dilution amount is calculated at 1:10,000. That seems very dilute, but many remedies are diluted even more. For instance, some solutions are diluted by 100 at each stage and use a C scale. A 4C solution (C = Roman numeral 100) is made in the following way: One part of the mother tincture is diluted with 99 parts of water. The dilution factor is then 100 or a 1C remedy. The solution is then repeatedly diluted by a factor of 100, leading to 2C, 3C, and 4C solutions. Many homeopathic remedies are diluted to 30C. The resulting solution is unlikely to contain even a molecule of the original solution.[23] There are even higher diluting scales used by some homeopaths: a millesimal (M) scale—1 part in 1,000 and a quintamillesimal (Q) scale—1 part to 50,000 parts. Homeopaths claim that the remedy has memory of the original solution and that is enough to influence body symptoms.

Currently, there are over 2,000 homeopathic remedies, often referred to by an abbreviated name. For instance, the abbreviation for *Argentum nitricum* is Arg-n; this is a homeopathic remedy made from silver nitrate and used for nervous complaints or anxiety. In addition, a homeopath might use tissue salts, made only from mineral sources. Tissue salts are also used in diluted solutions; in fact, they are so diluted that even if toxic substances such as snake's venom are used there are no possible side effects.[5]

Homeopathic practitioners consult repertories and materia medicas to determine the remedy to be used that matches the patient's symptoms or profile. The compendiums were written over a period of 200 years and include thousands of tests or "provings" on healthy individuals.[40] If given to a well person, the substances are supposed to cause illness, but given in diluted doses to a sick person, the substances are thought to cure illness. Rather than treating a person who has diarrhea with substances that could cause constipation, the homeopath would prescribe a minute dose of a substance that in a stronger preparation would cause diarrhea.

▶ How Safe Are Homeopathic Remedies?

According to the NCCIH, a review has found that homeopathic remedies are generally considered safe and unlikely to cause severe side effects. Even though the liquid homeopathic medicines contain alcohol, no adverse effects from alcohol levels have been found or reported to the FDA. Also, homeopathic remedies have not been found to interfere with conventional drugs, although people should let their doctors know if they are using them.

▶ What Types of Health Conditions Are Treated by Homeopathy?

A full range of health conditions are treated by homeopathic remedies. These include headache, sore throat, cough, earache, digestive disorders, colic, diarrhea, fever, sleep disturbances, mumps, measles, hemorrhoids, shingles, hives, allergies, joint pain, and more. See **TABLE 10.1** for homeopathic remedies for various health conditions.[1,38]

TABLE 10.1 Homeopathic Remedies and Health Conditions Treated

Homeopathic Remedy	Target Ailments	Where Found	Homeopathic Use
Aconite (Aconitum nacelles)	Angina, anxiety induced by shock, arthritis, asthma, colds, flu, fevers, headaches, sore throat, colic, diarrhea, cystitis, toothaches	Bluish violet flowers called monkshood. Found in the mountainous regions of Europe, Russia, and Central Asia. Juices traditionally used by hunters as an arrow poison	For symptoms similar to being poisoned; distress or fear, thirst, and unbearable aches and pains. Illnesses for which onset is sudden and acute
Alium cepa	Colds with sinus congestion; coughs that cause a ripping, tearing throat pain; inflamed eyes; hay fever; earaches	Red onion, a common garden vegetable. Applied to skin as a poultice. Used internally for intestinal worms	Used for same conditions as when exposed to onion: watering eyes and burning, runny nose
Aloe	Indigestion, diarrhea, hemorrhoids	Made from the juice of the flowering succulent plant native to Africa	Used to treat diarrhea, hemorrhoids, and indigestion
Antimonium tartaricum	Whooping cough, nausea, fever, chest colds	Substance found in metals, mostly sulfide stibnite	For gradual, progressive weakness; accumulation of mucus with rattling in the chest; cold sweat; and great sleepiness
Apis (apis mellifica)	Bites and stings with burning, itching, or swelling; conjunctivitis; general swelling from food allergies; hives; tonsillitis; mumps; red, swollen joints; cystitis; shingles; fever	Made from the body of the honeybee found all over the world	For ailments with symptoms similar to a bee sting: redness and swelling, restlessness, or irritability
Arg. N (Argentum nitricum)	Emotional problems, headaches, eye complaints, sore throat, digestive disorders, stomach ulcers, flatulence, diarrhea, constipation, trembling, weakness	Made from pure crystals of silver nitrate	Used for symptoms of mental exertion and anxiety. Good for exam nerves or stage fright

Homeopathic Remedy	Target Ailments	Where Found	Homeopathic Use
Arnica (*Arnica montana*)	Muscle aches and pain, bruises, sprains, strains	Mountain daisy found in higher elevations in Europe, Northern Asia, and the United States	Used for very active people (mountain climbers) and those who suffer some sort of accident
Arnica (*Leopard's Bane*)	For trauma, injury, and any case of major or minor physical stress, broken bones, bruises, swollen tissue, and inflammation	Known as leopard's bane. Grows in the mountains of Europe and in Siberia	Used as a first aid remedy, particularly to treat shock and trauma. As an application, used for bruises and swelling
Arsenicum album	Angina, anxiety disorders and panic attacks, Crohn's disease, influenza	Dilute form of arsenic made from separation from other metals such as iron, cobalt, and nickel by baking at high temperatures	Prescribed to treat patients with various digestive complaints accompanied by dehydration and burning pains
Belladonna	Common cold, flu, sore throat, earache, high fever with chills but no thirst, arthritis, colic, measles, mumps, sunstroke, toothaches, painful menstrual periods	Deadly nightshade plant that grows wild across Europe. Yellow flowers in July and dark red berries in late summer	For illnesses with symptoms of dry mouth and hot, flushed skin, nausea, convulsions, and delirium
Bryonia (*Bryonia alba*)	Irritability; vertigo, headache; dry, parched lips, mouth; excessive thirst; bitter taste; sensitive epigastric discomfort; constipation; dry cough; rheumatic pains and swellings	Flowered, vine-like plant that originated in England, often growing on hedgerows	Prescribed to patients to treat back pain, sciatica, neck pain, and other general aches and pains
Calcarea carbonica	Lower back pain, broken bones, sprains, muscle cramps, constipation, chronic ear infections, eye inflammations, headaches, insomnia, allergies, eczema, gastritis, gallstones, menstrual problems, asthma, arthritis	Comes from chalk, coral, and limestone	Used for conditions accompanied by symptoms of exhaustion, depression, and anxiety
Calendula	Promotes healing; used on cuts, tears, lacerations, burns, open wounds, and hemorrhages after tooth extraction; used as a mouthwash and an eyebath	Made from the fresh flowering tops and leaves of the marigold plant	Used for first aid; antiseptic; used to bathe and sterilize wounds and abrasions

(continues)

TABLE 10.1 *(continued)*

Homeopathic Remedy	Target Ailments	Where Found	Homeopathic Use
Cantharis	Bladder infections, sunburns, scalds	A beetle found in Southern France. The beetles are boiled and diluted before being used for treatment	Prescribed to patients whose ailments are coupled with symptoms like those of cantharis poisoning
Chamomilla	Irritability, toothaches, painful menstrual periods, earaches	The flowering German chamomile plant common in Europe	Prescribed to patients who are extremely sensitive to pain, irritable, and impatient. Most often given to children who work themselves into violent temper tantrums
Ferrum phosphoricum	Tickling, hacking coughs; headaches; fevers; rheumatic joints; early menstrual periods	Mineral compound of iron and phosphorus. Derived from mixing the solution with lactose to make it nontoxic	Prescribed to patients who suffer from conditions with low energy and anemia
Gelsemium (*Gelsemium sempervirens*)	Anxiety, flu with aches, exhaustion, headaches	A climbing vine with trumpetlike yellow flowers, commonly found in the United States	Prescribed in diluted forms for ailments accompanied by symptoms similar to those of gelsemium poisoning
Hepar sulphuris, Hepar sulphuris calcareum	Swollen and painful abscesses, colds, sore throat, earache, aching joints, coughing with chest pain, hoarseness, asthma, emphysema, croup, genital herpes, constipation	The flaky inner layer of oysters yields the calcium. Mixed with sulfur and heated in an airtight container. The powder is dissolved in hydrochloric acid and combined with lactose and diluted by trituration	For infections containing pus, mental and physical hypersensitivity, and intolerance to pain and cold
Hypericum (*Hypericum perforatum*)	Backaches, bites and stings, cuts and wounds	Also known as St. John's wort, it grows in Europe, Asia, and the United States from June to September	Prescribed to patients for bodily injuries because of the soothing effect it has on the nerves
Ignatia (*Ignatia amara*)	Anxiety, dry tickling cough, sore throat with feeling of a lump, tension headaches, indigestion, irritable bowel syndrome, painful hemorrhoids	Seeds (beans) from the fruit of a small tree native to China and the Philippines. Called St. Ignatius bean	Used for symptoms similar to poisoning symptoms: increased salivation, pounding headache, cramps, giddiness, twitching, and trembling
Ipecac, ipecacuanha	Nausea, vomiting, motion sickness, irritating cough, flu with nausea, gastroenteritis	The ipecacuanha shrub is native to Central and South America. The shrub is said to induce vomiting, but when diluted can help with these symptoms	Prescribed to patients for nausea and vomiting

Homeopathic Remedy	Target Ailments	Where Found	Homeopathic Use
Kali bichromicum	Acute bronchitis, mucus discharge, sinusitis	Also called potassium bichromate. Chemical compound acquired from chromium iron ore or by processing potassium chromate with a strong acid	Prescribed for conditions that are accompanied by pain in a specific spot
Lachesis	Choking coughs, croup, earaches, sore throats, indigestion, throbbing headaches, insomnia, hot flashes, heart arrhythmias, hemorrhoids, sciatica	South American bushmaster snake that grows to 7 feet. Venom is lachesis. Venom extracted and diluted in large quantities of lactose	Treats symptoms similar to venom poisoning: destruction of red blood cells and clotting impairment. Heart poisoning
Ledum (*Ledum palustre*)	Animal bites, insect sting, bruises that have discolored, deep cuts or puncture wounds, gout, aching joints	Ledum is a plant also called marsh tea. Found in bogs across Northern Europe, Canada, and the United States	Helpful for conditions accompanied by signs of infection or inflammation
Lycopodium (*Lycopodium clavatum*)	Backache with stiffness and soreness in lower back, bedwetting, colds with stuffy nose, cystitis, headache with throbbing pain, gout, indigestion with abdominal cramps, gas, heartburn, sciatica, eczema	Known as club moss, it grows in pastures and woodlands in Great Britain, Northern Europe, and North America	Used for complaints accompanied by symptoms of digestive upset, desire for sweets, and anxiety
Mercurius vivus	Abscesses (dental or glandular), backaches, chickenpox, earaches, eye inflammation	Made from the chemical element mercury by diluting the element with large quantities of milk sugar	Prescribed for conditions with symptoms of shaking, hot and cold sweats, and restlessness
Natrum muriaticum	Backaches; cold sores; colds with sneezing, watery eyes, and runny nose; constipation; fevers; genital herpes; eczema; anemia; hay fever; migraine headaches; indigestion; depression	Natrum is salt or sodium chloride	Given for conditions with symptoms of extreme thirst, emotional sensitivity, and a strong desire for salt
Nux vomica	Colic and stomach cramps from overeating, colds with sneezing and stuffy nose, constipation, cystitis, headache with dizziness, fevers with chills, gas and gas pains, hangovers, indigestion, insomnia, irritable bowel syndrome, stomach flu	Known as poison nut; it is made of seeds of an evergreen tree found in India, Thailand, China, and Australia. Seeds contain strychnine	For overindulgence of alcohol, food, or coffee

(continues)

TABLE 10.1 (continued)

Homeopathic Remedy	Target Ailments	Where Found	Homeopathic Use
Phosphorus	Bronchitis, pneumonia, coughs with congestion, visual problems resulting from eyestrain, gastritis, nosebleeds, indigestion, stomach ulcers, kidney infections, nasal polyps, hepatitis, anemia, hemorrhages, diarrhea	Found in inorganic phosphate rocks	For conditions accompanied by symptoms of fatigue and nervousness with a tendency to bleed easily and unquenchable thirst for cold water
Pulsatilla (Pulsatilla nigricans)	Bedwetting, breast infections, hay fever, aching joints, late menstrual periods, depression, urethritis in men	Plant found in the meadows of Northern and Central Europe	Prescribed to patients with conditions accompanied by yellow or white discharge
Rhus toxicodendron	Arthritis, backache with spine stiffness, bursitis, carpal tunnel syndrome, eye inflammation, itching, genital herpes, influenza, hives that itch, impetigo, poison ivy, sprains with stiffness, toothaches	Vine-like shrub known as poison ivy	Conditions accompanied by fever, restlessness, and swollen glands
Ruta (Ruta graveolens)	Carpal tunnel, eye strain, sciatica, groin strain, sprains, tennis elbow, tendon and cartilage injury	A plant native to Southern Europe	For conditions or injuries accompanied by symptoms of weakness or bruised sensation
Sepia	Backaches, violent coughing, cold sores and fever blisters, genital herpes, hair loss, gas, headaches, sinusitis, urinary incontinence, menstrual cramps, nausea from motion sickness or pregnancy	Cuttlefish, a soft-bodied mollusk related to a squid	For conditions with symptoms of apathy, moodiness, and weakness
Silica	Athlete's foot, constipation, hemorrhoids	Mineral present in the human body in trace amounts, but vital to the bones, cartilage, and skin	Minute doses prescribed to patients for excessive sweating, weakness, and sensitivity to cold
Sulfur	Asthma accompanied by rattling mucus, cough with chest pain, diarrhea, eye inflammation, bursitis, headaches, indigestion, joint pain, itching with redness, burning vaginal discharge, eczema with itching and burning	Also called brimstone	For conditions accompanied by irritability, intense itching, burning pains, and offensive odors

▸ What Steps Are Used When Prescribing Homeopathic Treatments?

Homeopaths use five essential steps to prescribe a remedy: note the symptoms; look up the symptoms; decide which remedy is appropriate; decide the dosage, and how often and when to repeat it; and evaluate the results. The dosage is dependent on the severity of symptoms, but the rule in homeopathy is that the minimum dosage required to initiate a healing response is first given. An important principle of homeopathy is that the whole person should be studied—their temperament, personality, and emotional and physical responses—before prescribing a homeopathic remedy. A person's genetic and personal health history and body type are also considerations when prescribing a homeopathic remedy.

▸ Where Is Homeopathy Used and How Many Are Using It?

Homeopathy is used in many countries: Australia, Canada, Czech Republic, France, Germany, Great Britain, Greece, Hungary, India, Israel, Latin America, Netherlands, New Zealand, and the United States.[38] According to the 2007 NHIS, approximately 3.9 million adults and approximately 900,000 children used homeopathy in the previous year in the United States.[9] The 2012 NHIS showed an increase to 5.04 million adults using homeopathy[35]; so, the evidence is clear that the use of homeopathy is rising.

▸ What Have Clinical Studies on Homeopathy Found?

According to the NCCIH, homeopathy is difficult to study using current research methods due to the problems in standardizing homeopathic remedies. They simply cannot be measured using current scientific methods, and therefore the NCCIH reports there is not enough evidence to support effectiveness as a medicinal treatment.[40] The following is an example of this.

Homeopaths take into account several considerations when prescribing the right homeopathic remedy for a headache, for example. Homeopathic clinicians have identified more than 200 symptom patterns for headaches. They would note where in the

brain the headache is occurring, and the individual's temperament, constitution, emotionality, and personality. They would next select a homeopathic remedy for headache that would meet these considerations. The problem is that there is not just one homeopathic remedy for headaches, but many that could be given depending on the patient's profile. It makes setting up clinical trials very difficult; consequently, the NCCIH believes that very little evidence has been demonstrated that supports homeopathy as an effective treatment for any specific condition.[40]

On the other hand, the following studies have reported effectiveness. Freeman and Lawlis described several randomized studies conducted in the 1980s and 1990s that were to assess whether homeopathy was significantly better than the placebo effect.[41] The first two described were conducted by David Reilly, a Scottish physician. Reilly and colleagues conducted a pilot study and then two randomized, double-blind, placebo-controlled trials on homeopathic treatment of allergies and treatment of asthmatics sensitive to house dust mites. A meta-analyis of the studies on allergies and house dust mites showed that homeopathic remedies were reported to be more effective than placebo. These studies were published in the international journal *Lancet*, a peer-reviewed publication that has editorial offices in London and New York. Cucherat and colleagues conducted a meta-analysis of homeopathy clinical trials.[42] They found some evidence that homeopathic treatments were more effective than placebo, but discounted it because of the poor quality of the trials. Townhill analyzed available homeopathic research and found evidence that homeopathy was effective in the treatment of some musculoskeletal disorders, but also reported that some studies had flaws in quality and design.[43]

Other earlier studies reported some positive effects of homeopathy when assessing whether homeopathic remedies were better than placebo. These involved treatment of fibromyalgia, influenza, carriers of hepatitis B virus, rheumatic arthritis, and childhood diarrhea.[41] Other studies involving homeopathic remedies, however, were not so positive and had methodological flaws. An outcome from previous research is that future studies will need to be high in quality and should be replicated for specific disease conditions.[41]

Cyril Smith, a researcher in England, purports that there is proof of evidence for homeopathy because of the phenomena of coherent frequencies.[44] His explanation holds that the frequency signature of the first dilution (mother tincture) causes a biological effect of coherent frequency pattern. It continues to

🔍 CASE STUDY

Lisa, a 22-year-old college student, has suffered every spring for as long as she can remember with sinus headaches, sore throat, cough, and congestion. Often, it would turn into a bad case of bronchitis, for which the doctor would order antibiotics. After several weeks, all of the symptoms would happen again. A friend has told Lisa about a naturopathic physician who uses homeopathic remedies, and is encouraging her to make an appointment. Lisa should take several steps before making the first appointment.

Question:

In what order should the following steps be taken?
1. Check credentials of the doctor.
2. Look up the definition of naturopathy and gain an understanding of the field.
3. Distinguish among the different types of naturopaths and select a doctor from the type most preferred.
4. Look up the definition of homeopathy and gain an understanding of the field.
5. Find a list of homeopathic remedies used for allergies and sinus congestion.
6. Notify family physician.

develop through dilution and succession. The physical and mathematical consequence of the mother tincture and the dilution and succession processes create the potency of the homeopathic substance.[44]

Homeopaths, however, are not perplexed about the inability of past research studies to demonstrate how homeopathic remedies actually work. They say that the mechanism of many allopathic drugs, such as aspirin and some antibiotics, also is not scientifically explained.[10]

▶ Are Homeopaths Licensed and Certified?

Currently, there are no uniform licensing or professional standards in the United States for homeopaths. What often occurs is that a homeopathic practitioner is licensed in one of the medical professions, such as an MD or osteopathic physician, which is the rule in Arizona, Connecticut, and Nevada. Naturopaths, chiropractors, dentists, physical therapists, nurses, and veterinary physicians are allowed to employ homeopathy within their practices in many states.

▶ Conclusion

It seems that naturopathy and homeopathy are an integral part of complementary and alternative medicine. Many traditional physicians are also embracing the ideas and practices of both naturopathy and homeopathy. Perhaps a fusion of the best of our traditional and alternative practices will offer hope of a better healthcare system in the United States.

Wrap-Up

Key Terms

Astringent A substance or preparation that constricts tissue. It can lessen discharges such as mucus or blood.

Bioresonance The practice of using an electronic device to measure the body's electromagnetic radiation and electric currents and to detect damaged body cells.

Biotypes Body types or body constitutions that naturopaths use to aid a diagnosis, because they believe each type has certain characteristics that are related to risk of particular diseases.

Calibration To adjust instrumentation so that it will be precise.

Chiropractic A discipline and profession that focuses on disorders of the musculoskeletal and nervous systems under the belief that the effects of these disorders negatively impact health.

Cholera An acute, infectious disease characterized by profuse diarrhea, vomiting, and cramps.

Degenerative arthritis Chronic breakdown of cartilage in the joints; the most common form of arthritis, occurring usually after middle age.

Ectomorph Body type in which the appearance of the body is thin.

Endomorph Body type in which the appearance of the body is round and soft. The physique presents the illusion that much of the mass has been concentrated in the abdominal area.

Epidemic Refers to an occurrence and rapid rise of an infectious disease in a community or region in a given time period.

Fasting To abstain from all food.

Homeopathy The use of extremely diluted substances given to cure disease using the law of similars: *like cures like.*

Hydrotherapy The treatment of physical disability, injury, or illness by immersion of all or part of the body in water to facilitate movement, promote wound healing, and relieve pain. It is usually done under the supervision of a trained therapist. May involve the use of hot, moist soaks or dry heat for pain relief and to promote healing.

Infrastructure The basic, underlying framework or features of a system or organization.

Iridology The examination of the iris or colored portion of the eye for markings that supposedly reveal changing conditions of every part and organ of the body.

Kirlian photography Colorful photographs of images surrounding the body and within the body that are made after applying high-frequency electrical currents to a patient's body.

Mesomorph Body type in which the appearance of the body is a natural, athletic physique.

Modalities The application of a therapeutic agent, usually a physical therapeutic agent.

Mother of tincture The homeopathic mixture first made from plants that is diluted in alcohol and left to sit for 2–4 weeks.

Naturopathic medicine A holistic, whole body health care system based on the belief that the body has the potential to heal itself and that the physician's role is to support the body's efforts. A system or method of treating disease that employs no surgery or synthetic drugs but uses special diets, herbs, vitamins, massage, and so on to assist the natural healing processes.

Osteopathic A therapeutic system originally based on the premise that manipulation of the muscles and bones to promote structural integrity could restore or preserve health. Current osteopathic physicians use the diagnostic and therapeutic techniques of conventional medicine as well as manipulative measures.

Pathogen A disease-producing agent such as a virus, bacterium, or other microorganism.

Periodontitis Gum disease that begins when permeability of the mouth tissue permits pathogenic bacterial components to invade deeper periodontal connective tissues and bone leading to tooth loss.

Phytotherapy Using botanical medicine to treat disease conditions.

Quinine A white, bitter, slightly water-soluble alkaloid, having needlelike crystals, obtained from cinchona bark. Used in medicine chiefly in the treatment of resistant forms of malaria.

Rheumatoid arthritis A chronic autoimmune disease characterized by inflammation of the joints, frequently accompanied by marked deformities, and ordinarily associated with manifestations of a general or systemic affliction.

Succession Act of shaking a homeopathic mother of tincture solution during the dilution process.

Temporomandibular disorder (TMD) A condition characterized by pain and tenderness of the jaw when chewing and opening the mouth.

Tuberculosis An infectious disease that may affect almost any tissue of the body, but especially the lungs. It is caused by the organism *Mycobacterium tuberculosis*, and is characterized by tubercles.

Suggestions for Class Activities

1. Invite a naturopathic physician to class. Ask about services rendered, fees for various stages of condition (from the first office visit on), academic background, philosophy of iridology, and any other questions students want to ask.

2. Visit a health food store and note the types of homeopathic remedies. Make a presentation to the class regarding your findings.

3. Demonstrate the homeopathic dilution process in class using a simple remedy. You can find these at various websites.

Review Questions

1. What is naturopathic medicine and how did it develop?
2. Name five major beliefs of naturopathy.
3. Explain what iridology is and how it is thought to aid in the diagnosis of body ailments.
4. Name and describe several main naturopathic treatments.
5. How do naturopaths use hydrotherapy?
6. What type of training does a naturopathic physician receive?

7. What are the three levels of training for a naturopathic physician?
8. What is the level of naturopathic use in the United States?
9. What does the research show about naturopathy?
10. What is homeopathy?
11. Who was the founder of homeopathy?
12. Define and differentiate among the three principles of homeopathy.
13. How did homeopathy evolve into a medical discipline?
14. What is mother of tincture?
15. What is the process of homeopathic dilution?
16. What types of health conditions are treated by homeopathy?
17. What do the clinical studies show regarding homeopathy?
18. How do homeopaths become licensed or certified?

References

1. Somerville R, ed. *The Alternate Advisor*. Alexandria, VA: Time Life Books; 1997.
2. Corinthian Naturopathic College. What is Naturopathy? Available at: http://www.corinthiannaturopathic-edu.org/what-is-naturopathy. Accessed April 16, 2018.
3. ND Health Facts. Benedict Lust. Available at: http://www.ndhealthfacts.org/wiki/Benedict_Lust. Accessed April 16, 2018.
4. Heartland Naturopathic Clinic. The History of Naturopathic Medicine. Available at: http://www.heartlandnaturopathic.com/history.htm. Accessed April 16, 2018.
5. Bradford N, ed. *The One Spirit Encyclopedia of Complementary Health*. Hong Kong: Hamlyn; 2000.
6. Snider P, Turner RN. Nature cure in Europe: The transatlantic journey from pragmatism to principles. *Naturopathic Doctor News & Review*. Oct 2, 2010. Available at: http://ndnr.com/education-web-articles/nature-cure-in-europe-the-transatlantic-journey-from-pragmatism-to-principles/ Accessed April 17, 2018.
7. The Natural Health Perspective. A History of Western Natural Healing Practices in Europe. Available at: http://naturalhealthperspective.com/tutorials/history.html. Accessed April 16, 2018.
8. Bastyr University. About Naturopathic Medicine. Available at: https://bastyr.edu/academics/naturopathic-medicine/about-naturopathic-medicine. Accessed April 16, 2018.
9. National Center for Complementary and Integrative Health. Naturopathy. Available at: https://nccih.nih.gov/health/naturopathy. Updated September 24, 2017, Accessed April 16, 2018.
10. Pelletier K. *The Best Alternative Medicine: What Works? What Does Not?* New York, NY: Simon & Schuster; 2000.
11. Vercillo K. 10 Underlying Beliefs of Naturopathy. *HubPages*. October 30, 2012. Available at: http://hubpages.com/hub/10-Underlying-Beliefs-of-Naturopathy. Accessed April 16, 2018.
12. Atwood KC 4th. Naturopathy: A critical appraisal. *MedGenMed*. 2003;5(4):39.
13. Micozzi M. *Fundamentals of Complementary and Alternative Medicine*. 3rd ed. New York, NY: Elsevier; 2006.
14. Natural Path Health Center. Core Beliefs of Naturopathy. Available at: http://naturalpathhealthcenter.com/core-beliefs-of-naturopathy/. Accessed April 16, 2018.
15. Ernst E, ed. *The Desktop Guide to Complementary and Alternative Medicine: An Evidence-Based Approach*. New York, NY: Mosby; 2001.
16. Ernst E, Pittler M, Wider B, eds. *The Desktop Guide to Complementary and Alternative Medicine: An Evidence-Based Approach*. 2nd ed. New York, NY: Mosby Elsevier; 2006.
17. Formerfatguy.com. A Solution for Hardgainers and Ectomorphs. May 16, 2009. Available at: http://www.formerfatguy.com/weblog/2009/05/solution-for-hardgainers-and-ectomorphs.asp. Accessed April 16, 2018.
18. Carter S. Iridology History. Available at: http://sandycarter.com/iridologynow/iridology-history.html. Accessed April 16, 2018.
19. Gold CM. Iridology: The Origin. 2008. Available at: http://www.campbellmgold.com/archive_health/irid_origin.pdf. Accessed April 16, 2018.
20. Iridology-What do your eyes say about you and your health? Available at: http://www.iridology.webs.com/. Accessed April 16, 2018.
21. Da Vinci College of Holistic Medicine. Available at: http://davincistudentlogin.com/. Accessed April 16, 2018.
22. International College of Iridology. Available at: http://www.iridologycollege.org. Accessed April 16, 2018.
23. Singh S, Ernst E. *Trick or Treatment: The Undeniable Facts About Alternative Medicine*. New York, NY: Norton; 2008.
24. Knipschild P. Looking for gall bladder disease in the patient's iris. *BMJ*. 1988;297(6663):1578-1581.
25. Simon A, Worthen DM, Mitas JA 2nd. An evaluation of iridology. *JAMA*. 1979;242(13):1385-1389.
26. Gero GB. Trace Mineral Analysis. Holistic Naturopathic Center. Available at: http://www.holisticnaturopath.com/hairmineral.htm. Accessed April 16, 2018.
27. Seidel S, Kreutzer R, Smith D, McNeel S, Gilliss D. Assessment of commercial laboratories performing hair mineral analysis. *JAMA*. 2001;285(1):67-72.
28. Memorial Sloan-Kettering Cancer Center. BioResonance Therapy. Available at: http://www.mskcc.org/mskcc/html/69136.cfm#References. Updated July 28, 2015. Accessed April 16, 2018.
29. Federal Trade Commission. Bogus cancer cure guru settles FTC charges. October 28, 2002. Available at: https://www.ftc.gov/news-events/press-releases/2002/10/bogus-cancer-cure-guru-settles-ftc-charges. Accessed April 16, 2018.
30. Towne R. What is Kirlian photography? The science and the myth revealed. *Light Stalking*. November 14, 2012. Available at: https://www.lightstalking.com/what-is-kirlian-photography-the-science-and-the-myth-revealed/. Accessed April 16, 2018.
31. Whole Health Wellness Center. About Naturopathic Medicine. Available at: http://www.wholehealthllc.com/jen-stagg/about-naturopathic-medicine/ Accessed April 16, 2018.
32. Bastyr University. Naturopathic Medicine. Available at: https://bastyr.edu/academics/naturopathic-medicine. Accessed April 16, 2018.
33. Council on Naturopathic Medical Education. Accredited Programs. Available at: http://www.cnme.org/programs.html. Updated November, 2017. Accessed April 16, 2018.

34. American Association of Naturopathic Physicians. Regulated States & Regulatory Authorities. Available at: https://www.naturopathic.org/regulated-states. Accessed April 16, 2018.

35. Clarke TC, Black LI, Stussman BJ, Bames PM, Nahin RL. *National Health Statistics Reports; No. 79. Trends in the use of Complementary Health Approaches Among Adults: United States, 2002-2012.* Hyattsville, MD: National Center for Health Statistics. 2015. Available at: https://www.cdc.gov/nchs/data/nhsr/nhsr079.pdf Accessed April 16, 2018.

36. Kjeldsen-Kragh J, Haugen M, Borchgrevinck CF, et al. Controlled trial of fasting and one-year vegetarian diet in rheumatoid arthritis. *Lancet.* 1991;338(8772):899-902.

37. Haugen M, Kjeldsen-Kragh J, Nordvåg BY, Førre O. Diet and disease symptoms in rheumatic diseases—results of a questionnaire based survey. *Clin Rheumatol.* 1991;10(4):401-407.

38. Restor Medicine. Naturopathic Medicine: The Medicine of the Future. Available at: https://restormedicine.com/naturopathic-medicine-the-medicine-of-the-future/. Accessed April 16, 2018.

39. Dannheisser I, Edwards P. *Homeopathy: An Illustrated Guide.* Boston, MA: Element; 1998.

40. National Center for Complementary and Integrative Health. Homeopathy. Available at: https://nccih.nih.gov/health/homeopathy. Updated April 2015. Accessed April 16, 2018.

41. Freeman L, Lawlis F. *Mosby's Complementary and Alternative Medicine: A Research-Based Approach.* St. Louis, MO: Mosby; 2001.

42. Cucherat M, Haugh MC, Gooch M, Boissel JP. Evidence of clinical efficacy of homeopathy. A meta-analysis of clinical trials. HMRAG. Homeopathic Medicines Research Advisory Group. *Eur J Clin Pharmacol.* 2000;56(1):27-33.

43. Townhill S. Homeopathy and musculoskeletal disorders—an overview and critique of available research. *Hpathy Ezine.* November, 2009. Available at: http://hpathy.com/scientific-research/homeopathy-and-musculoskeletal-disorders-%e2%80%93-an-overview-and-critique-of-available-research/. Accessed April 16, 2018.

44. Smith CW. Proof of evidence for homeopathy. *Altern Integr Med.* 2017;6:242.

CHAPTER 11

Botanicals: A Biologically Based Therapy

LEARNING OBJECTIVES

As a result of reading this chapter, students will be able to:

1. Explain what are biologically based therapies and botanicals.
2. Name and explain five different forms of herbs.
3. Distinguish among crude herbs, decoctions, and infusions.
4. Name five chemicals and properties of herbs.
5. Explain ways in which botanicals could be better standardized.
6. Discuss how the U.S. Government controls herbs.
7. Examine the impact of botanicals on the pharmaceutical industry.

▶ What Are Biologically Based Therapies?

Biologically based therapies use a variety of natural techniques to maintain health and/or treat diseases. A major biologically based therapy is the use of botanicals, which are fresh or dried plants, plant parts, or chemicals extracted from the plants. Some botanicals are classified as herbs and some as spices. Some botanicals are used in cosmetics, prescription drugs, and nonprescription drugs.

Biologically based therapies also make use of minerals, vitamins, fatty acids, proteins, and probiotics (live bacteria often found in whole grains, yogurt, and functional foods). Biologically based therapies may involve **orthomolecular medicine**

(which emphasizes supplementing diet with mega doses of vitamins, minerals, enzymes, hormones, and amino acids) and **chelation therapy** (use of a drug to bind with and remove excess or toxic amounts of metal or minerals from the blood). This chapter focuses mainly on the use of botanicals for therapeutic use.

▶ What Are Botanicals?

Botanical is a term for the use of plants or plant parts to create scents or to develop therapeutic medicinal treatments.[1] Several terms are also used synonymously: herbal medicine, **phytotherapy** (plant therapy), or medical herbalism. Botanicals may include using a mixture of different herbs or a single herb.[1] Herbal substances may come from all parts of plants such as roots, stalks, flowers, bark, and seeds, and may include chemicals extracted from the plants. Over 1,600 botanicals and their derivatives are sold in the United States as dietary supplements. The herbs are sold as dried materials of plant origin either in bulk whole form, cut and sifted, or powdered.[2,3] Herbal remedies are used to restore and maintain health by relying on the curative properties of certain herbs to stimulate our body's healing system.[4,5] Herbs are used to alleviate disease, prevent it from recurring, detoxify the body, and support the immune system.

Nutritional Supplementation, Spices, and Other Uses

Botanicals may be used to supplement a person's normal diet. This can be done by including **nutritional supplements** such as green tea, soy products, ginseng, Echinacea, garlic and red clover (not an exhaustive list). They also may be used to provide fragrance (aromatherapy). Botanicals classified as spices are used to flavor foods. Spices are said to be piquant (pungent or tart in taste; spicy). Aromatic plant materials, usually tropical in origin, such as cloves, cinnamon, nutmeg, and pepper are used in seasoning food.[3,4]

In addition, the cosmetics industry uses over 360 botanical additives to add fragrance and enhance the looks of their products. Moreover, botanicals are used in prescription and nonprescription drugs. They may be present in crude form (whole dried plants or plant parts) or as a chemical constituent.

▶ How Have Herbs Been Used Historically?

Herbs have been used by many cultures for centuries; in fact, before recorded history.[4,5,6] Herbs were used in Ayurvedic medicine as long ago as 1900 BCE and in traditional Chinese medicine (TCM) from around 2700 BCE. Chinese herbalism is based on the concepts of yin and yang and qi (chi) energy. Herbs used for cooling are yin herbs and those used for stimulating are yang herbs. For more information on the use of traditional Chinese herbal medicines, see Chapter 9; for more information on Ayurvedic herbal use, see Chapter 8.

The use of herbs has been traced back 5,000 years by the Sumerians, who wrote of well-established medicinal uses for such plants as laurel, caraway, and thyme. The ancient Egyptians (1000 BCE) relied heavily on garlic, opium, myrrh, cumin, caraway, fennel,

olive oil, and licorice. Native American Indians and early Americans used plants and the bark of certain trees. The native Indians of Peru used quinine to treat malaria and lime to prevent scurvy, a vitamin C deficiency. They also used a plant called foxglove to obtain a chemical, now known as digitalis, to treat certain heart conditions. In 1960, the body of a Neanderthal man living 60,000 years ago was uncovered and several herbs used to treat him were present. Eight different species of plants were found at the burial site, and seven of those are used for medicinal purposes today.[7]

▶ What Is an Herbalist?

An **herbalist** is a practitioner and contributor to the field of herbal medicine. Native healers, shamans, scientists, holistic medical doctors, nutritionists, pharmacists, naturopaths, TCM doctors, and traditional Ayurvedic medicine doctors may use and promote herbal medicines. Medical herbalists combine modern scientific concepts with their knowledge of herbs. They are academically trained in examination techniques and knowledge of the human body.[4,5]

▶ What Are the Different Forms of Herbs?

Herbs come in their natural state or are processed into many forms. The different forms are described as:

- **Crude herbs**: Herbs that are collected and dried, cut, and sifted. Stored in dark glass or closed containers made of plastic, the herbs may be stored for 6 months and still retain their properties.[4] Crude herbs may be cooked into teas.[5,7,8]
- **Concentrated herbal extracts**: These herbs may be in liquid or solid form and are anywhere from 2–100 times as concentrated as crude herbs.[6,7,8,9]
- **Powders**: Ground crude herbs. They may be ingested in natural form or cooked to make teas.
- **Teas**: Aqueous extractions of crude herbs or herbal powders.
- **Dried decoctions or concentrated granules**: Decoctions are concentrated brews made by simmering tougher forms or parts of herbs such as roots, barks, and woody stems.[4,5,6,7,8] Decoctions are cooked as teas and the solid residue is removed, after which the remaining liquids are dried until only the powders remain. The powders are about four times as potent as the original herbs.
- **Tinctures**: Herbal concentrates or extracts made by soaking herbs in solutions, usually alcohol,

glycerin, or a vinegar base.[4,6,7] These are designed to bring out the herbal properties.

- **Infusions**: Concentrates made by steeping 1 ounce of herb in 2 cups of water. The more delicate parts of the plant such as leaves, flowers, and light stems are used.
- **Bolus**: A suppository made from herbs that may be inserted into the rectum or vagina. Powdered herbs mixed with cocoa butter, water, or honey can be formed into a suppository. If made with cocoa butter or honey, the preparation needs to be refrigerated or it will lose its shape. If made with water, it needs to be heated on a cookie sheet at a low temperature of 120°F or so until hardened. At time of insertion, a lubricant should be applied to the bolus.[4,8]
- **Capsules**: Powdered herbs, dried decoctions, or concentrated extracts are placed in gelatin capsules.
- **Tablets**: Powdered herbs, dried decoctions, or concentrated herbal extracts are mixed with a binding substance and then pressed into tablets.
- **Gelcaps**: Sealed gelatin capsules that hold either tinctures or concentrated liquid herbal extracts.
- **Bath**: Two to four quarts of a decoction or infusion, strained and then added to a tub of bathwater.
- **Poultice**: A preparation of a fresh, dry, ground, or powdered herb or herbal mixture that is wrapped in thin cotton or wool cloth and applied to the skin. Sometimes, the poultice is applied directly to the skin.[6,8,9]
- **Fomentation**: A cloth is soaked in an infusion or decoction from which all the herb has been strained. The cloth is then applied to the skin.[6,8]
- **Liniment**: A liniment has a liquid base and is rubbed into sore muscles and joints. It is made by making a decoction or infusion and then adding one-fourth to half part olive oil and/or rubbing alcohol.[6,8]

▶ What Are the Chemicals and Properties of Herbs?

Various plants contain chemicals, many of which are used in today's prescription medications as well as herbal medicines. Some of the chemicals found in plants and herbs include:

- **Alkaloids**: Alkaloids are used in painkiller drugs, narcotics, hypotensives (to lower blood pressure), hypertensives (to increase blood pressure), bronchodilators, stimulants, antimicrobials, and anti-inflammatory herbs. Coffee bean

and the plant *Ephedra sinica* contain stimulating alkaloids.[9]
- **Cardiac glycosides**: These chemicals have a marked action on the heart, strengthening the force and speed of systolic contractions. The foxglove plant contains *Digitalis purpurea*, one of the glycosides.[9]
- **Carotenoid pigments**: These are pigments found in yellow and red plants such as carrots, sweet potatoes, red and yellow peppers, squash, and tomatoes. Two carotenoids are beta-carotene and lycopene (red pigment found in tomatoes). They help maintain healthy epithelial tissue and mucous membranes, aid growth and repair body tissue, and more. Carotenoid pigments transfer light energy to chlorophyll for use in photosynthesis and act as antioxidants for chlorophyll.[10]
- **Chlorophyll**: This is a pigment found in dark green leafy vegetables such as spinach, parsley, kale, green beans, and leeks. Chlorophyll absorbs energy from the sun to facilitate photosynthesis (synthesis of carbohydrates from carbon dioxide and water) in plants. According to Michael T. Simonich of the Linus Pauling Institute, chlorophyll has antioxidant properties and retards cancer cell growth.[11,12] Two types of chlorophyll are found in plants and green algae: chlorophyll a and chlorophyll b.
- **Fixed oils**: Fixed oils are referred to as vegetable, carrier, or base oils and contain nutrients such as minerals, antioxidants, and fat-soluble vitamins. They are not volatile and do not evaporate. Many fixed oils are used with essential oils for aromatherapy because they do not compete with the aroma. They may also be mixed with essential oils that are used for massage therapy.[13] Some examples of fixed oils are almond oil, avocado oil, aloe vera, castor oil, flaxseed oil, and evening primrose oil.[13,14]
- **Flavonoids**: Flavonoids are a set of chemicals that include brilliant plant pigments seen in fruits and vegetables. They are thought to be potent antioxidants, and have anti-inflammatory and metal-chelating properties.[15] There are six subclasses: anthocyanidins are found in red, blue, and purple berries; red and purple grapes; and red wine. Flavanols are found in teas, chocolate, grapes, berries, apples, and red wine. Flavanones are found in citrus fruits and juices. Flavonols are found in yellow onions, scallions, kale, broccoli, apples, berries, and teas. Flavones are found in parsley, thyme, celery, and hot peppers. Isoflavones are found in soybeans, soy foods, and legumes.

- **Lignans**: Lignans are phytoestrogens with weak estrogenic or antiestrogenic activity. Lignans may be found in nuts, seeds, breads, vegetables, fruit, and wine. Examples of nuts and seeds are milk thistle seed, flaxseed, sunflower seed, sesame seed, cashews, peanuts, and poppy seeds. Whole grain, multigrain, rye, and wheat bread also contain lignans. Vegetables such as broccoli, cauliflower, onions, and green beans contain lignans, as do fruits such as apricots, strawberries, peaches, and pears.[16] Research studies are conflicting about the health benefits of lignans. Although a diet rich in lignans lowers cardiovascular disease risk, research is unclear as to whether the effect is due to lignans alone or to other foods in the diet. Velentzis and colleagues[17] conducted a meta-analysis study of publications up to September 2008 and found there was little evidence to suggest that lignans with their mild estrogenic activity are associated with increased breast cancer risk. On the other hand, for postmenopausal women, the meta-analysis found that high lignan intake was associated with a 15% reduction in the risk for getting breast cancer.[17]

- **Phytoestrogens**: Phytoestrogens are estrogen-like chemicals that can act like the hormone estrogen. They come from three chemical classes: the lignans, the isoflavonoids, and the coumestans. More than 300 foods contain phytoestrogens.[17] Isoflavonoid phytoestrogens are found in the legume family (e.g., soybeans) and coumestan phytoestrogens are found not only in various beans such as pinto beans and lima beans, but also in alfalfa and clover sprouts. Research studies about the use of soy are conflicting. Some studies used soy isolates of soy protein and were shown to increase cancer growth, but isolates can only be made in a lab. Those studies, therefore, do not apply to soy foods that people consume, but may lead to discouraging the use of soy supplements. Studies that assessed breast cancer in people eating soy foods such as soybeans found no relationship to breast cancer and/or reduced risk of breast cancer. Women in Japan grow up eating soy foods in the amount of 25–50 mg per day, while women in the United States may intake less than 1–3 mg per day. No link was found between soy intake and breast cancer.[18]

- **Phytoprogesterones**: Phytoprogesterones are plant chemicals that bind to progesterone receptors. These are found in lignans, isoflavonoids, flavonoids, and coumestans. Examples of plant sources are flaxseed, soybeans, tofu, sesame seeds, blueberries, and almonds. The National Center for Complementary and Integrative Health (NCCIH) cites a 2008 study by Bloedon and colleagues that found flaxseed may reduce some risk factors related to heart disease by lowering LDL (bad) cholesterol levels.[19]

- **Plant coumarins**: Coumarin was first isolated from the tonka bean (*Dipteryx odorata*), which is in a classification known as coumarou; thus, similar plants were named plant coumarins. Coumarins are mainly synthesized in the leaves of plants, but occur at the highest levels in the fruits, next highest in the roots, and at the lowest levels in the stem. Coumarin has no anticoagulant activity, but once converted to dicoumarol by fungi it becomes anticoagulant in nature. Sweet clover disease in cattle is caused by cattle eating moldy, sweet clover silage, which results in death due to resultant hemorrhage.[20] Coumarin is also found in sweet woodruff, vanilla grass, sweet grass, Cassia cinnamon, and red clover blossoms. Prescription oral anticoagulants are derived from plant coumarins. For example, Warfarin was used as a rat killer (rodenticide) prior to its 1954 introduction into clinical medicine as an anticoagulant.[20]

- **Salicylates and salicins**: These are aspirin-like compounds that have pain-relieving and anti-inflammatory action. Salicin is a glycoside found in willow bark. It acts as antipyretic, antiseptic, and anti-inflammatory. It is a bitter tonic (gastric stimulant) and is useful for mild feverish colds, headaches, and rheumatic conditions.[21] Herman Kolbe synthesized salicylic acid from coal tar; it was found to be stronger than salicin.[21,22] Today, it is an active ingredient in many skin care products used to treat acne. Because salicin and salicylic acid use caused many side effects such as stomach irritation leading to nausea and vomiting and hearing problems (tinnitus), scientists synthesized acetylsalicylic acid, the main ingredient in today's aspirin products.

- **Saponins**: Saponins are glycosides or chemicals found in plants such as oats, vegetables, and beans that cause plants placed in water to "soap up" or froth to form lather. They are also found in several herbs: alfalfa, agave, fenugreek, and ginseng.[23] They get their names from the soapwort plant (*Saponaria*); the root of the plant was used for making soap.[24] Because of the detergent properties, saponins are used in shampoos, facial cleansers, and cosmetic creams.[25] They act on internal surfaces of membranes and blood vessels to lower surface tension. Saponins are thought to have several health benefits, including reducing blood cholesterol levels, boosting immunity, reducing cancer risk, reducing bone loss, and having antioxidant properties.[25]

- **Tannins**: Tannins are polyphenols obtained from various parts of plants. They are found in tree bark, wood, fruit, leaves, and roots. Tannins bind with proteins and form a protective layer on the skin and mucous membranes.[26] They are used in dyeing and photography, as an astringent in medicines, and for refining beer and wine.[27] They can reduce diarrhea or intestinal bleeding, and are used externally to inhibit infections of the eye, mouth, vagina, and rectum.[27] Coffee, black tea, green tea, and wine contain tannins.

- **Volatile oils**: Volatile oils come from plants and produce what is popularly known as essential oils. They are compounds of vegetable origin that evaporate at room temperature and allow us to enjoy the smell. Two of the many ways they are made are steam distillation and expression.[28] Steam distillation is done by immersing the plant in a still filled with water and then boiling it. The vapors are condensed on a cold surface and the essential oils then separate. During expression, the process calls for an abrasive action on the surface of fruit while being washed with water. The solid waste is eliminated and essential oil is separated by centrifugation. More information may be found in Chapter 12, "Aromatherapy and Bach® Original Flower Remedies." Volatile oils have many health benefits: antiseptic properties (oil of thyme); antispasmodic properties (ginger, lemon balm, rosemary, peppermint, chamomile, fennel, caraway); perfumes (oil of rose); and flavoring (oil of lemon). They may be used in medicine as stimulants, and some exhibit antifungal and insect-repellent actions. Eucalyptus, garlic, oregano, and tea tree also contain volatile oils.[28]

▶ How Are Herbs Used?

Shopping for Herbs

If you are considering obtaining herbs, you may buy them in bulk or buy standardized medicinal herbs.[29] Bulk herbs are those harvested from an herbalist who has grown them in an herb garden or those that you have grown. You may also purchase bulk herbs at a health food store or herbal shop where you may see bins of dried bulk herbs. One problem is that you cannot be sure of the level of constituents in the bulk herbs or plant material. But, buying bulk herbs allow you to learn how to process and store the herbs. You can also experiment by mixing some preparations.[29]

The advantage of buying standardized herbs is that they have been processed, so a known minimum level of one or more of the major active ingredients is present. They may be more expensive than bulk herbs, but are still quite a bit less expensive than pharmaceuticals that treat the same conditions.[29]

Care and Storage of Herbs

If you are considering obtaining herbs, you should gather them when they are as fresh as possible. You will need to be careful to obtain them from reputable sources and should buy them in a form allowing positive identification. You should check to be sure the herbs are free of insects, and you should store them in tightly closed glass containers in cool, dry places away from the sun. Empty 35 mm film containers are a good size for storing small amounts of herbs when traveling. They can be placed in glove compartments or backpacks and heat does not affect the 35 mm container.[4,8] Herbal brews can be kept in the refrigerator for a couple of days, but then begin to weaken in medicinal strength.

Utensils for Making Herbal Preparations

Pans that are aluminum or cast iron should not be used for brewing teas because the metals disintegrate into the herbal preparation. It is best to use stainless steel, glass, or ceramic pots and bowls. Even the stirring spoon should be stainless steel, but wooden spoons may be used. To avoid contaminating your herbs, you should keep a clean set of spoons that are used only for herbal preparation and nothing else.[4,8]

▶ How Does the Government Control Herbs?

Governmental Control of Herbs in Germany Compared with the United States

In 1976, the Federal Republic of Germany (then West Germany) developed a mechanism to assure herbal safety. The country commissioned an expert panel (German Commission E) composed of physicians, pharmacists, pharmacologists, toxicologists, and representatives of the pharmaceutical industry and laypersons. To determine with "reasonable certainty" the safety and efficacy of each herb being evaluated, the commission checks herbal data independently of other drugs. They assess data from clinical trials, field studies, case studies, and independent medical association members.[7] Approximately 600–700 different plant drugs are sold in pharmacies, health food stores, and markets. About 70% of German physicians prescribe registered herbal remedies, and government health insurance helps pay a significant proportion of the $1.7 billion in annual sales.

In the United States, the Food and Drug Administration (FDA) evaluates the safety and efficacy of new drugs based on data supplied by the drug manufacturer (pharmaceutical company). According to Tufts Center for the Study of Drug Development, the cost of getting a new drug to market is $2.56 billion. The drug developers' out of pocket expense is approximately $1.4 billion and $1.16 billion in time costs.[30] Even though the FDA was petitioned by phytomedicine manufacturers from Europe and the United States to allow well-researched European drugs the status of old drugs so they would not have to go through new drug applications (NDAs), the FDA has never responded to those petitions.[7]

In 1994, the U.S. Dietary Supplement Health and Education Act (DSHEA) allowed herbal products to be labeled with certain information such as side effects, potential safety problems, and contraindications.[31] Nutritional support information and how the product affects the body's physiology can be included, but the label cannot make a statement that the herb is therapeutic or can treat or cure a disease condition.

Herbals are defined by the DSHEA as dietary supplements.[31] They are described as a product that:

- is intended to supplement the diet.
- contains one or more dietary ingredients (including vitamins, minerals, herbs or other botanicals, amino acids, and certain other substances) or their constituents.
- is intended to be taken by mouth in forms such as tablet, capsule, powder, softgel, gelcap, or liquid.
- is labeled as being a dietary supplement.

▶ How the FDA Approves New Drugs and Medical Devices

The FDA's drug approval process, aimed at proving the safety and effectiveness of new drugs, is an important hurdle for new companies seeking a piece of the international market. If the FDA would accept herbal supplements for the approval process, the following steps would be taken:

1. **Investigational new drug application:** Researcher submits preliminary animal and lab testing data, a proposal for tests on humans, and expected findings. The FDA has 30 days to submit questions, which delays the process, or to allow the next step.[32]

2. **Clinical studies:** It involves the following three phases.
   a. *Phase 1*: Safety, dosage, and effects on the body are tested on 20–80 healthy volunteers (about 1 year).
   b. *Phase 2*: Effectiveness and side effects are tested on 100–300 people with the disease to be treated by the drug (about 2 years).
   c. *Phase 3*: The drug is tested on 1,000–3,000 people with the disease who are in clinics or hospitals. Benefits and long-term side effects are compared. Marketing information, including labels and warnings, are developed (about 3 years).

3. **New drug application:** An NDA is then submitted (usually about 100,000 pages). Researchers submit applications containing all scientific data, how the drug is processed, what it is made of, and how it would be packaged, along with samples and labeling. On receiving the NDA, the FDA starts a 180-day approval period that can be delayed at any time for questions and additional research. FDA chemists, pharmacologists, physicians, statisticians, microbiologists, and other specialists review the NDA. This approval process usually takes around 2½ years.

See **BOX 11.1** for the different types of applications required by the FDA.[33]

BOX 11.1 FDA New Drug Application Types

Following are the different FDA drug application types:

- Investigational New Drugs
- New Drug Applications
- Abbreviated New Drug Application (Generic Drugs)
- Over-the-Counter Drugs
- Biologic License Application

In addition, the FDA tests that following categories of products:

- Cosmetics
- Tobacco Products
- Foods
- Medical Devices
- Radiation-Emitting Products
- All Other Topics

Source: U.S. Food and Drug Administration. Types of applications. Available at: https://www.fda.gov/Drugs/DevelopmentApprovalProcess/HowDrugsareDevelopedandApproved/ApprovalApplications/default.htm Accessed August 3, 2017.

📄 *IN THE NEWS*

The FDA released a tips paper in January 2002 titled, *Tips for the Savvy Supplement User: Making Informed Decisions and Evaluating Information*, which has been updated regularly and can be found on the FDA website in the "Information for Consumers" section.[31]

- **Basic Points to Consider:** Think about total dietary needs. Check with your personal doctor before using supplements. Obtain information about prescription drug and over-the-counter medicine interactions. Check unwanted effects from supplements during pregnancy. Gain knowledge about adverse effects and who you should report it to. Learn who is responsible for ensuring safety and efficacy of dietary supplements.
- **Tips on Searching the Web for Information on Dietary Supplement:** Find out who operates the site, purpose of the site, source of the information, and references. Check to be sure information is current and if the Internet site is reliable.
- **More Tips and To-Do's:** Ask yourself if it sounds too good to be true. Think twice about chasing the latest headline. Check assumptions about safety of the herb such as equating the word, natural, and to mean healthful and safe or safe because there is no cautionary information on the label or safe because it has not been recalled. Contact the manufacturer if you cannot tell if the product meets the same standards as those in research studies you have read. Look for information about substantiating claims, tests conducted for safety or efficacy, what quality control systems are in place, and if the firm has received any adverse effects from people who have used the product.

Questions:

1. What are your thoughts about the FDA approval process?
2. How could the FDA speed up the approval process (or should it)?
3. What are your thoughts about the approval process for herbal products?
4. What main point did you learn from the FDA tips displayed in the "In the News" section?
5. Do you believe that the United States could learn from and adopt policies that have been developed in Germany?

Source: U.S. Food and Drug Administration. Tips for Dietary Supplement Users. Available at: https://www.fda.gov/food/dietarysupplements/usingdietarysupplements/ucm110567.htm. Updated February 23, 2018. Accessed July 15, 2018.

Sometimes, the FDA will move generic drugs or medical devices through a streamlined process.[33] An example of this process is exemplified by an article published in the *Healthcare Business News*.[34] Based on information presented, it could be that some herbals already approved by the German commission or other European commissions could be streamlined through the FDA process.

▶ How Safe Are Herbal Supplements?

Even though an herbal supplement is on the shelf of a store, the FDA is still supposed to monitor its safety. If the FDA finds a product unsafe, it could take action against the manufacturer and/or issue a warning. The product could also be removed from the market. Herbal supplements, however, do appear to have a better safety record than that of pharmaceutical drugs.[5] That does not mean that all herbals are safe or that they cannot be abused. Safety depends on many factors, including chemical makeup, how the herb works in the body, how it is prepared, dosage, and interaction with other herbs or pharmaceutical products.[35] We should be aware that many herbals contain ingredients that elicit strong effects in our bodies and could have potential side effects. Moreover, taking the products along with prescription drugs could be dangerous if the herb potentiates (adds to the effect) or negates the effect of the prescription drug. An example is the use of herbs such as ginkgo, garlic, ginseng, ginger, and St. John's Wort, which increase the effect of prescription drug blood thinners and blood thinning effects of over-the-counter medicines such as nonsteroidal anti-inflammatory drugs such as ibuprofen.[36] The FDA has issued a public health advisory concerning many of these interactions. Examples follow:

- Kava kava (an antianxiety herb) has been linked to liver toxicity. Kava has been taken off the market in several countries because of this toxicity.
- Valerian (taken as a sleep aid) may have the unexpected effect of overstimulating instead of sedating.
- Garlic, ginkgo, feverfew, and ginger, among other herbs, may increase the risk of bleeding.
- Evening primrose (*Oenothera biennis*) may increase the risk of seizures in people who have seizure disorders.
- St. John's Wort is taken to aid mild depression, but some people find it makes their skin more sensitive to the sun's ultraviolet rays which results in an allergic reaction.

- In 2007, the FDA put out a warning to consumers to avoid red yeast rice products promoted on the Internet as treatments for high cholesterol. Products put out by Swanson Healthcare Products Inc. and manufactured by Nature's Value Inc. and Kabco Inc. contained an unauthorized ingredient called lovastatin, which is found in a prescription drug called Mevacor. The ingredient does lower cholesterol, but has side effects of adverse muscle reaction and kidney complications.[36]

In addition, some herbal supplements, especially those imported from Asian countries, may contain high levels of heavy metals, including lead, mercury, and cadmium. Talk to your healthcare provider for more information. Certainly, you should talk to your doctor if you are thinking about buying and using herbal supplements.

What Are a Healthcare Professional's Knowledge of and Recommendations Regarding Herbal Supplements?

Research studies have been employed to ascertain healthcare professionals' knowledge and attitudes regarding herbal supplement use for various conditions. The first study discussed is a review of studies[37] through March 2006 of U.S. or Canadian pharmacists' attitudes, knowledge, or professional practice behaviors regarding herbal supplements. Results show inconsistency. A majority of respondents not only believed that herbal supplements could be beneficial, but they also believed that the majority of their colleagues do not accept herbal medicine. A majority believed that herbal medicine could increase the profit margin. Studies showed inconsistency about pharmacists' views regarding how selling herbal supplements affects the pharmacy's image. Some believed it affected the pharmacy negatively and some did not.[37]

Results of a survey study[38] of 184 board certified psychiatrists in New Jersey revealed that 62% did not recommend herbal products. Of the 38% responding who did recommend herbal remedies, 30% recommended St. John's Wort, 25% recommended gingko, 13% recommended valerian, and 8% recommended other herbal products.[38]

The last example presented is a survey administered to oncologists (cancer doctors). It was conducted by mail and e-mail and was administered to 1,000 members of the American Society for Clinical Oncology.[39] Approximately 66% (2 of 3) reported they did not know enough about herbal supplements to answer their patients' questions, and over 50% had not received any education regarding herbal supplements.[39] Clearly, physicians need to learn about herbal supplements in order to answer their patients' questions and to determine the safety of any that are taken by their patients and whether or not they negatively interact with their cancer therapies.

How Much Money Is Spent on Herbal Supplements Each Year?

According to the 2007 National Center for Health Statistics (NCHS) survey,[40] out-of-pocket spending for all complementary and alternative medicine (CAM) therapies was estimated at $33.9 billion. Of that amount, the cost of nonvitamin, nonmineral products was $14.8 billion and $2.9 billion was spent on homeopathic medicine.

Who Uses Herbals, and Which Herbals Are the Most Popular?

According to the same NCHS 2007 study,[40] 17.7% of U.S. adults had used natural products during the past 12 months. The 10 natural products most commonly used by U.S. adults during the last 30 days were fish oil omega 3 (37.4%), glucosamine (19.9%), echinacea (19.8%), flaxseed oil/pills (15.9%), ginseng (14.1%), combination herb pills (13%), ginkgo biloba (11.3%), chondroitin (11.2%), garlic supplements (11%), and coenzyme Q-10 (8.7%).

Certain precautions should be taken before buying an herb for medicinal use. The main one is to discuss your idea with your physician. If you are taking any prescription medications, talking with your physician is extremely important because of the possibility of drug interaction. A second precaution is to research the company that is producing the herbal. You might want to get a membership in Consumerlab.com, an Internet site that researches and tests herbals, minerals, and vitamins to ensure that the ingredients listed on the label are actually in the herbal preparation. There are hundreds of herbs—too many to include in one chapter of a textbook—but the following represents those more commonly used for certain disorders and disease conditions. Some have been studied scientifically, some are still being studied, and some have not been studied.

▶ What Are the Common Herbal and Nonplant-Based Dietary Supplements?

The following are some of the most commonly used herbal and nonmineral-based dietary supplements:

- **Alfalfa** (*Medicago sativa*): This versatile herb is a folk remedy for arthritis, diabetes, asthma, and hay fever. It is said to detoxify the body, especially the liver. It contains vitamin K, which helps the body form blood clots, and should not be taken in combination with warfarin (Coumadin), an anticoagulant drug. It is possibly effective for lowering cholesterol in people with high cholesterol levels. It may also lower blood sugar. Taking alfalfa seeds may cause extra sensitivity to the sun, and taking alfalfa pills along with estrogen birth control pills may lower their effectiveness. It may mimic lupus erythematosus symptoms and should not be taken by people with lupus.[41]

- **Aloe vera**: Aloe is known as burn plant, lily of the desert, and elephant's gall (**FIGURE 11.1**).[4] It is used topically for skin wounds and other skin conditions. Aloe supplements can be used for peptic ulcers and gastrointestinal health. Aloe latex (the green part of the leaf that surrounds the gel) contains a laxative compound. Aloe vera contains three anti-inflammatory fatty acids helpful for the stomach, small intestine, and colon. It alkalizes digestive juices to prevent overacidity and the leaves contain a clear gel that is used as a topical ointment.[4]

- **Arginine** (*L-arginine*): Arginine is an amino acid that can raise levels of nitric oxide in the blood and body tissues, which can increase blood flow necessary for arousal. Because of the vasodilation effect, conditions such as chest pain from clogged arteries and headaches due to blood vessel swelling may be helped. Arginine has also been studied for its wound healing properties, as an aid to sperm production, and for its bodybuilding properties. It is also being studied for wasting disease in people who have AIDS and similar conditions.[42]

- **Arnica** (*Arnica montana*): Arnica is an extract of a bright yellow, daisy-like flower. It is rubbed on the skin to soothe and heal bruises and sprains, and relieve irritations from trauma, arthritis, and muscle or cartilage pain. Applied as a salve, arnica is also good for chapped lips, irritated nostrils, and acne. It has also been used as a mouthwash for swollen gums and mouth ulcers.[43]

- **Astragalus** (*Astragalus membranaceus, Astragalus mongholicus*): The root of Astragalus is used in soups, teas, extracts, and capsules. Astragalus (**FIGURE 11.2**) is promoted as a tonic and immune-enhancing herb that is supposed to increase natural killer (NK) cell activity. This type of plant has been used in China for nearly 4,000 years for chronic hepatitis and as an adjunct in cancer therapy.[9,43] It is used by those with AIDS today. The herb is presently being studied by the NCCIH. Preliminary studies indicated some effectiveness for boosting the immune system, benefits for the heart and liver, and as a useful adjunct for cancer therapy.[44]

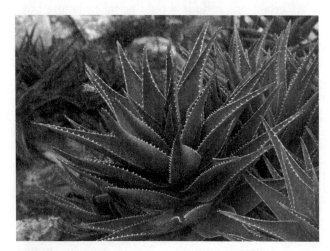

FIGURE 11.1 Aloe vera plant.
© Andrei Rybachuk/Shutterstock

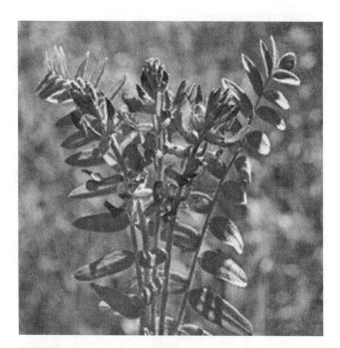

FIGURE 11.2 Astragalus.
© Starover Sibiriak/Shutterstock

- **Bee pollen:** Bee pollen is collected from flowers by honeybees and is their main food source. It is a popular energy booster, strengthens the immune system, and enhances vitality. It is said to slow the effect of premature aging of the skin as well as act as an aid for weight control. Animal studies on mice and rats showed benefits of bee pollen, and in a study of 60 men in Wales, researchers found that pollen extract was effective as a treatment for prostate enlargement and inflammation of the prostate.[9,45,46]

- **Bilberry:** Bilberry is a little blue berry related to cranberries and blueberries. It is said to be a powerful anti-inflammatory and antioxidant. It contains nutrients (e.g., flavonols, anthocyanosides) needed to protect eyes from eyestrain or fatigue and can improve circulation to the eyes. It may help with night vision and/or help the eyes to adjust to changes in light.[43,45] Clinical studies suggest that bilberry may prevent diabetic retinopathy and improve visual acuity and retinal function. Because of the coumarins present in bilberry, an additive effect with blood thinners could result.[47,48]

- **Black cohosh:** This is a plant native to North America that is a member of the buttercup family (**FIGURE 11.3**). It has been used as a treatment for arthritis and symptoms of menopause (hot flashes, night sweats, vaginal dryness). Scientific studies have not shown effectiveness for treating menopausal symptoms, but laboratory study of mice showed promotion of bone formation.[49]

- **Butterbur:** Butterbur is also known as butter dock, bog rhubarb, and exwort. It is an herb native to Europe, Asia, and North Africa. Both the leaf and roots may be used. Herbalists use an extract from its roots called petasins. Extracts have been used to treat allergies, bronchial asthma, headache, pain, and muscle and urinary tract spasms. Several clinical studies have demonstrated the effectiveness of butterbur for migraine headache.[50,51,52,53]

- **Calendula** (*Calendula officinalis*): Calendula is grown in the United States. The flower (**FIGURE 11.4**) is used medicinally to prevent muscle spasms, start menstrual periods, and reduce fever. The plant is said to be antibacterial, antifungal, anti-inflammatory, and antiviral. Calendula stimulates white blood cells to engulf harmful microbes and helps speed wound healing. It is also used in skin moisturizers, lotions, and salves. Commercial calendula flower ointments can be purchased and applied as needed.[54]

- **Cascara sagrada aged bark** (*Rhamnus purshiana*): Cascara is a species of buckthorn found predominantly in the Western United States. The aged bark has been used for centuries as a laxative herb because of the plant's glycosides. Only organic bark, aged at least a year, should be used; fresh bark induces vomiting and diarrhea. Cascara sagrada was a primary ingredient in many over-the-counter laxatives in the United States until the FDA banned its use along with aloe in 2002. The FDA banned cascara because of a controlled clinical study that found cascara sagrada could

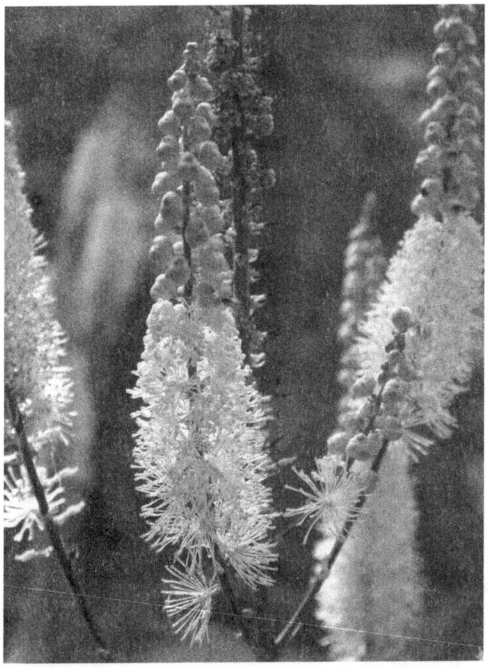

FIGURE 11.3 Black cohosh.
© pinkannjoh/age fotostock

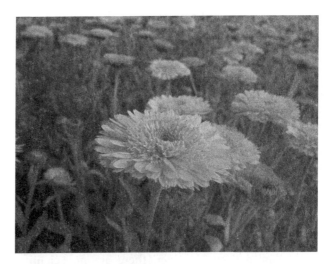
FIGURE 11.4 Calendula.
© iStockphoto/Thinkstock

potentially cause liver damage with long-term usage due to the glycosides present in the plant's chemical makeup.[55] Manufacturers were given the opportunity to submit studies showing safety, but they deemed the process too expensive to conduct. Currently, however, products containing aloe and cascara can still be sold as herbal supplements because the FDA does not test nor regulate herbal supplements.

- **Cat's claw** (*Uncaria tomentosa, Uncaria guianensis*): Cat's claw is most commonly used to support the immune system. Cat's claw is used to help treat viral infections, Alzheimer's disease, cancer, kidney disease, and arthritis.[43,45] The inner bark of cat's claw is used to make liquid extracts, capsules, and teas. Small studies in humans have shown a possible benefit of cat's claw in osteoarthritis and rheumatoid arthritis, but no large trials have been conducted. In fact, there is not enough scientific evidence to determine whether cat's claw works for any health condition. The National Institute on Aging has funded a study to look at how cat's claw may affect the brain. Findings may point to new avenues for research in Alzheimer's disease treatment.[45] Few side effects have been reported for cat's claw when taken at recommended dosages. Women who are pregnant or trying to become pregnant should avoid using cat's claw because of its past use for preventing and aborting pregnancy.[43]

- **Cayenne pepper** (*Capsicum anuum*): Also known as chili pepper, Cayenne is not cooked or used raw (undried) because of its irritant effect on the gastrointestinal system. Excessive ingestion also may cause gastroenteritis or liver or kidney damage. It is intended to be used in a dry, usually powdered, form to heal bleeding ulcers in the digestive system.[9] The chemical that causes the hotness is capsaicin which reportedly has antioxidant properties. Regular consumption of cayenne increases the resistance of blood lipids to oxidation and may slightly decrease insulin levels after a meal. Cayenne is reported to possibly interfere with MAO inhibitors and antihypertensive therapy, and may increase hepatic metabolism of drugs.[56]

- **Celery seed**: Celery seed is used primarily as a diuretic (increasing urine output to help the body get rid of excess water). It is also suggested for treating arthritis and gout, and to help reduce muscle spasms, calm the nerves, and reduce inflammation. However, there are no scientific studies in humans that show whether celery seed is effective for these conditions or any others. Studies do show that celery seeds act as a mosquito repellent. Pregnant women should not use celery seed because it may lead to uterine bleeding and muscle contractions in the uterus, which could cause miscarriage.[45]

- **Chaste tree extract** (*chasteberry*): Chasteberry is the fruit of the chaste tree, a small shrub-like tree native to Central Asia and the Mediterranean region (**FIGURE 11.5**). It is dried when ripe and used to prepare liquid or solid extracts that are put into capsules and tablets. It can cause gastrointestinal problems, rashes, and dizziness. Some studies show chasteberry improves premenstrual syndrome, breast pain, some types of infertility and even acne, but many of the studies were not well designed and/or not scientifically reliable enough to determine efficacy.[57]

- **Cranberry fruit** (*Vaccinium macrocarpon*): Historically, cranberry fruits and leaves were used for a variety of health conditions such as wounds, urinary disorders, diarrhea, diabetes, stomach ailments, and liver problems. Many people take cranberry juice or the fruit for preventing or treating urinary tract infections (UTIs). Research shows that components found in cranberry may prevent bacteria, such as *E. coli*, from clinging to the cells along the walls of the urinary tract and causing infection. Cranberry has been reported to have antioxidant and anticancer activity, but there is little scientific evidence that cranberry can treat urinary tract infections.[58] The NCCIH, however,

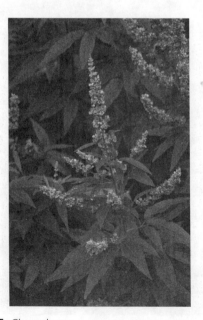

FIGURE 11.5 Chasteberry.
© FLPA/Keith Rushforth/age fotostock

reports there are scientific studies ongoing that are studying the effects of cranberry related to tumor cells and anemia found in cancer patients. Cranberry may be found in the form of fruit, fruit juice, extracts, capsules, or tablets.

- **Creatine**: Although not a plant herb, creatine is a dietary supplement used by athletes and we wanted to include information about it. Creatine is naturally synthesized in the human body, and during the 1800s was found to be an organic constituent present in meat. It began to be used by athletes as a "natural" way to enhance athletic performance and build lean body mass. Adolescent athletes have been found to take doses that are not consistent with scientific evidence and to frequently exceed recommended loading and maintenance doses. The National Collegiate Athletic Association has now banned the use of school funds to buy and supply creatine for athletes, although the athletes may buy creatine for themselves and consume it.[59]

- **Dong quai root** (*Angelica sinensis*): Dong quai is an herb in the celery family native to China, Japan, and Korea. The root (**FIGURE 11.6**) is medicinally active, and different parts of the dong quai root are believed to have different actions. The head of the root has anticoagulant activity; the main part of the root is a tonic; and the end of the root eliminates blood stagnation. It is considered the "female ginseng" because of its balancing effect on the female hormonal system. However, studies have not found dong quai

to have strong hormone-like effects.[60] Dong quai should not be used by people with bleeding disorders, excessive menstrual bleeding, diarrhea, or abdominal bloating, or during infections such as colds and flu. Dong quai may contain weak estrogen-like compounds and should not be taken by pregnant or nursing women, children, or people with breast cancer.[60]

- **Echinacea**: There are nine known species of echinacea, all native to the United States and Southern Canada. Echinacea is believed to stimulate the immune system to help fight infections and has been used to treat or prevent colds, flu, and other infections. The above-ground parts of the plant and its roots are used fresh or dried to make teas, squeezed (expressed) juice, extracts, or preparations for external use. Two NCCIH-funded studies did not find a benefit from echinacea, either as a fresh-pressed juice for treating colds in children or as an unrefined mixture of two strains of echinacea. However, other studies have shown that echinacea may be beneficial in treating upper respiratory infections. NCCIH is continuing to support the study of echinacea to identify the herb's active ingredients and to study the plant's bacteria (live within the plants) and their effects on the immune system.[61]

- **Ephedra or ephedrine**: Ephedra is an evergreen shrub-like plant native to Central Asia and Mongolia. The principal active ingredient, ephedrine, is a compound that can powerfully stimulate the nervous system and heart. Ephedra has been used for more than 5,000 years in China and India to treat conditions such as colds, fever, flu, headaches, asthma, wheezing, and nasal congestion. It has also been an ingredient in many dietary supplements used for weight loss, increased energy, and enhanced athletic performance. The dried stems and leaves of the plant are used to create capsules, tablets, extracts, tinctures, and teas. In 2004, the FDA banned the U.S. sale of dietary supplements containing ephedra after finding that the supplements had an adverse health risk (namely, cardiovascular complications). The ban does not apply to traditional Chinese herbal remedies or to products such as herbal teas regulated as conventional foods.[62]

- **Evening primrose** (*Oenothera biennis*): Evening primrose is a plant native to North America, but it grows in Europe and parts of the Southern hemisphere as well. It has yellow flowers that bloom in the evening. Evening primrose oil has

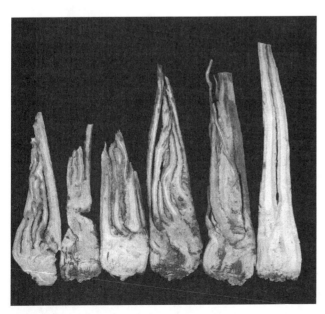

FIGURE 11.6 Dong quai root.

been used since the 1930s for skin disorders such as eczema (inflamed, itchy, or scaly skin) and for body inflammation such as experienced in rheumatoid arthritis. It is also used for breast pain associated with the menstrual cycle, for menopausal symptoms, and for premenstrual syndrome.[45]

- **Feverfew** (*Tanacetum parthenium*): Feverfew was originally found in the Balkan mountains of Eastern Europe. It now grows throughout Europe, North America, and South America. It is a short bush with daisy-like flowers (**FIGURE 11.7**) and has been used for centuries for many conditions such as fevers, headaches, stomachaches, toothaches, insect bites, infertility, problems with menstruation, and with labor during childbirth. Some research suggests that feverfew may be helpful in preventing migraine headaches; however, results have been mixed and more evidence is needed from well-designed studies. Feverfew may be helpful in treating mild rheumatoid arthritis symptoms.[45]

- **Flax** (*Linum usitatissimum*): The flax plant is believed to have originated in Egypt, but grows throughout Canada and the Northwestern United States. Flaxseed is used for many conditions: as a laxative, for hot flashes, and for breast pain. Studies of flaxseed preparations to lower cholesterol levels report mixed results, some positive and some not. There is not enough reliable information to determine whether flaxseed is effective for heart conditions.[45]

- **Garlic** (*Allium sativum*): Garlic is the edible bulb from a plant in the lily family. It is used to treat high cholesterol, heart disease, and high blood pressure. Garlic is also used to prevent certain types of cancer, including stomach and colon cancers. Some evidence indicates that taking garlic can slightly lower blood cholesterol levels; studies have shown positive effects for short-term use (1–3 months). However, an NCCIH-funded study on the safety and effectiveness of three garlic preparations (fresh garlic, dried powdered garlic tablets, and aged garlic extract tablets) for lowering blood cholesterol levels found little to no effect.[63] Preliminary research suggests that taking garlic may slow the development of atherosclerosis (hardening of the arteries), a condition that can lead to heart disease or stroke. Garlic may also slightly lower blood pressure and it may lower the risk of certain cancers. However, no clinical trials have examined this. A clinical trial on the long-term use of garlic supplements to prevent stomach cancer found no effect.[63]

- **Ginger root** (*Zingiber officinale*): Ginger is a tropical plant that has green-purple flowers and an aromatic underground stem (called a rhizome). The active ingredient in ginger is gingerol. Ginger can be consumed as a spice, in juice, or in oil.[64] Ginger has been used for centuries in Asian and Indian foods and medicines to treat gastrointestinal conditions such as stomachaches, nausea, diarrhea, and nausea from motion, chemotherapy, and pregnancy. It seems to not be effective in stopping vomiting episodes but does help with nausea. Ginger has been shown to be effective for reducing muscle pain and for conditions such as osteoarthritis of the knee.[64] In studies on rats, ginger intake increased insulin production and lowered blood sugar levels.[65] A study assessing ginger's effect on coronary heart disease showed that a single large dose (10 grams) showed significant platelet aggregation reductions while small doses of 4 grams per day had no effect.[65] More research on ginger is clearly indicated.

- **Ginkgo biloba**: Ginkgo comes from the leaves of the ginkgo biloba tree. Ginkgo leaf extract has been used to treat a variety of ailments and conditions, including asthma, bronchitis, fatigue, and tinnitus (ringing or roaring sounds in the ears). The NCCIH funded a study of the well-characterized ginkgo product EGb-761.[18] In a clinical trial known as the *Ginkgo Evaluation of Memory* study, researchers recruited more than 3,000 volunteers age 75 or older who took 240 milligrams of ginkgo daily. They were followed for an average of approximately 6 years. Results of the study found that EGb-761 was ineffective in lowering the overall incidence of

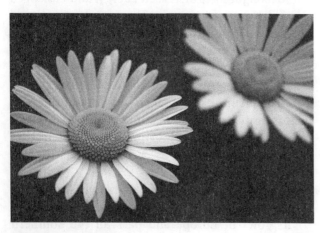

FIGURE 11.7 Feverfew.
© iStockphoto/Thinkstock

dementia and Alzheimer's disease in the elderly and ineffective in slowing cognitive decline, lowering blood pressure, or reducing the incidence of hypertension. Side effects of ginkgo may include headache, nausea, gastrointestinal upset, diarrhea, dizziness, or allergic skin reactions. More severe allergic reactions have occasionally been reported.[66]

■ **Ginseng** (*Panax ginseng*): Although Asian ginseng has been widely studied for a variety of uses, research results to date do not conclusively support health claims associated with the herb (**FIGURE 11.8**). Traditional and modern uses of ginseng include improving the health of people recovering from illness, increasing a sense of well-being and stamina, improving both mental and physical performance, and treating erectile dysfunction, hepatitis C, and symptoms related to menopause. Some studies have shown that Asian ginseng may lower blood glucose levels. Other studies indicate possible beneficial effects on immune function. Of all the studies, only a few large, high-quality clinical trials have been conducted.[67]

■ **Glucosamine and chondroitin**: Glucosamine and chondroitin are not plant herbs, but are dietary supplements used by many today. Glucosamine is a natural compound found in healthy cartilage. Available evidence from randomized controlled trials supports the use of glucosamine sulfate in the treatment of osteoarthritis, particularly of the knee. Glucosamine is commonly taken in combination with chondroitin, a glycosaminoglycan derived from articular cartilage.[68]

■ **Goldenseal** (*Hydrastis canadensis*): Goldenseal is a plant that grows wild in parts of the United States but has become endangered by overharvesting. Goldenseal is used for colds and other respiratory tract infections, infectious diarrhea, eye infections, and vaginitis (inflammation or infection of the vagina). It is also applied to wounds and canker sores, and is used as a mouthwash for sore gums, mouth, and throat. The NCCIH is funding research on goldenseal, including studies of antibacterial mechanisms and potential cholesterol-lowering effects. Few studies have been published on goldenseal's safety and effectiveness and there is little scientific evidence to support using it for any health problem. Goldenseal is considered safe for short-term use in adults at recommended dosages.[69]

■ **Gotu kola** (*Centella asiatic*): This is a perennial plant native to India, Japan, China, Indonesia, South Africa, Sri Lanka, and the South Pacific. Gotu kola has been used to treat leprosy, bronchitis, asthma, and syphilis. It also has been used in Ayurvedic medicine for wound healing. It is used most often to treat chronic venous insufficiency (a condition where blood pools in the legs). People with liver disease should not take gotu kola because it has been shown in clinical trials to adversely affect the liver.[70]

■ **Grape seed extract** (*Vitis vinifera*): Grape seed extract is used for heart and blood vessel conditions such as atherosclerosis (hardening of the arteries), high blood pressure, high cholesterol, and poor circulation. Grape seed extract has also been used for complications related to diabetes, such as nerve and eye damage; vision problems such as macular degeneration (which can cause blindness); and swelling after an injury or surgery. It has been used for cancer prevention and wound healing. Even though small randomized trials have found beneficial effects, larger clinical trials are needed to determine the efficacy of grape seed extract for diabetic retinopathy and for vascular fragility.[29]

■ **Green tea** (*Camellia sinensis*): Fresh leaves from the *Camellia sinensis* plant are steamed, producing green tea. Green tea and green tea extracts have been used to prevent and treat a variety of cancers, including breast, stomach, and skin cancers. Green tea and green tea extracts have also been used for improving mental alertness, aiding in weight loss, lowering cholesterol levels, and protecting skin from sun damage. Even though laboratory studies suggest that green tea may help protect against or slow the growth of certain cancers, studies in people have shown

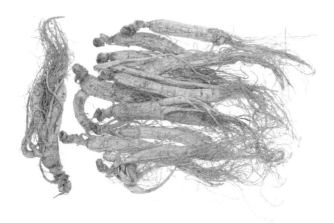

FIGURE 11.8 Ginseng.

mixed results. Green tea does contain some caffeine, giving a sense of mental alertness. There is not enough evidence to show whether green tea supports weight loss.[29]

- **Hawthorn** (*Crataegus laevigata*): Hawthorn is a spiny, flowering shrub or small tree of the rose family. Hawthorn is used for problems associated with heart disease, digestion, and kidney problems. The hawthorn leaf and flower are used to make liquid extracts, usually with water and alcohol. Dry extracts can be put into capsules and tablets. There is scientific evidence that hawthorn leaf and flower may be safe and effective for milder forms of heart failure, but study results are conflicting. There is not enough scientific evidence to determine whether hawthorn is effective for other heart problems.[29]

- **Hoodia** (*Hoodia gordonii*): Hoodia is a flowering, cactus-like plant native to the Kalahari Desert in Southern Africa (**FIGURE 11.9**). Hoodia currently is used as an appetite suppressant, although research does not support its use as a weight loss herb.[71] Dried extracts of hoodia stems and roots are used to make capsules, powders, and chewable tablets. Hoodia can also be used in liquid extracts and teas. The safety of hoodia is still unknown.[71]

- **Kava** (*Piper methysticum*): Kava is used primarily for anxiety, insomnia, and menopausal symptoms. A clinical trial conducted in Australia indicates that Kava may potentially be a choice for the treatment of chronic clinical anxiety.[72] The FDA, however, has issued a warning that using kava supplements has been linked to a risk of severe liver damage and has been associated with several cases of dystonia (abnormal muscle spasm or involuntary muscle movements). Kava can interact with drugs used for Parkinson's disease and cause scaly, yellowed skin when used over a long period of time.

- **Kudzu** (*Pueraria lobata*): Kudzu is a coiling, climbing, and trailing vine native to Southern Japan and Southeast China. It now grows in the Southeastern part of the United States. It has been used in China to treat alcoholism, diabetes, gastroenteritis, and deafness. A 2015 double-blind study found that an extract of the root reduces alcohol drinking in binge drinkers and that they drank more slowly than a placebo group.[73] The researchers concluded that Kudzu may be a safe alternative for alcohol abuse.

- **Lavender** (*Lavandula angustifolia*): The name "lavender" comes from the Latin root *lavare*, which means "to wash." Lavender is native to the mountainous zones of the Mediterranean region. It also flourishes in the Southern United States. Essential oil is extracted from the blue-violet flowers (**FIGURE 11.10**), and when diluted, may be applied to the skin. It is used for conditions such as anxiety, restlessness, insomnia, and depression. Lavender is also used for burns, headache, upset stomach, and hair loss. Dried lavender flowers can be used to make teas or liquid extracts that can be taken by mouth. There is little scientific evidence of lavender's effectiveness for most health uses. Small studies on lavender for anxiety showed mixed results.[74] Research on larger populations should be conducted in future studies.

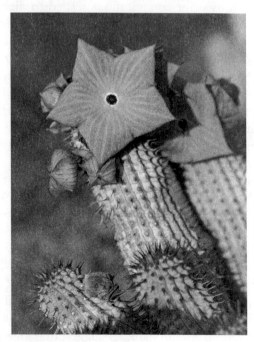

FIGURE 11.9 Hoodia.
© GFC Collection/age fotostock

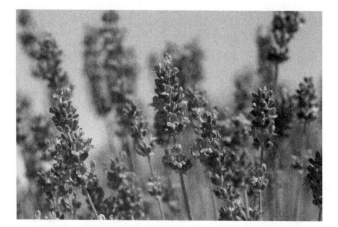

FIGURE 11.10 Lavender.
© iStockphoto/Thinkstock

- **Melatonin:** Melatonin may be found in animals, plants, and microbes. It is not considered a plant herb like most of the others in this section, but it is another dietary supplement used by many. Melatonin is a hormone normally secreted by the pineal gland and was first promoted as a cure for jet lag and then as a sleep aid. A review of studies showed weak evidence for jet lag, insomnia, and sleep,[75] although clinical research has found that melatonin may help elderly people with insomnia who are tapering off or stopping benzodiazepines. It may help with sleep problems associated with menopause. Positive studies have shown that melatonin can help with complications during chemotherapy for breast cancer, and it may also be an effective treatment for prostate cancer; however, more research is needed. Melatonin should not be taken if pregnant or nursing because not enough research has been conducted to demonstrate that it is safe for the developing fetus or the infant after birth.

- **Milk thistle seed** (*Silymarin, Silybum marianum*): The milk thistle seed plant is native to the Mediterranean and grows wild throughout Europe, North America, and Australia. It is a potent anti-inflammatory and antioxidant. The plant's small, hard fruits have been shown to protect the liver against a variety of toxins. It is purported to alter liver cell membrane structure, blocking the absorption of toxins into the cells. It is used to treat liver cirrhosis, chronic hepatitis (liver inflammation), and gallbladder disorders. However, in a 2012 clinical trial, silymarin given in higher than usual doses was no more effective than placebo in treating chronic hepatitis C.[76,77] Results from other studies of milk thistle for liver diseases have been mixed, and most studies have not been rigorously designed. The National Cancer Institute is studying the effectiveness of silymarin for patients with leukemia who experience chemotherapy-related liver damage.[78]

- **Nettle** (*Stinging nettle, Urtica dioica*): Nettle is a perennial flowering plant, native to North America and the Mediterranean region. Reports say that nettle can provide relief from painful muscles and joints, arthritic pain, and gout. Extracts also can be used to treat anemia, hay fever, kidney problems, and pain by inactivating inflammatory cytokines. It is used in Europe for benign prostatic hyperplasia. Stinging nettle may interact with several types of drugs such as blood thinners, high blood pressure drugs, diuretics, drugs for diabetes, and nonsteroidal anti-inflammatory drugs. Consumers should check with their doctors before using nettle. The potency and effectiveness of nettle are still being assessed.[79]

- **Peppermint** (*Mentha piperita*): Peppermint is a cross between two types of mint (water mint and spearmint), and it grows throughout Europe and North America. It is used for a variety of health conditions, including nausea, indigestion, and cold symptoms. Peppermint oil is also used for headaches and muscle and nerve pain. Although some studies have shown no effects, several suggest that peppermint oil may improve symptoms of irritable bowel syndrome.[80]

- **Pomegranate juice:** Pomegranate juice contains antioxidants at higher levels than do other fruit juices. Research has not yet proven that drinking pomegranate juice can help lower cholesterol or assist with any other health issue. If you choose to drink pomegranate juice, be sure that it is 100% pure pomegranate juice. Dr. Dean Ornish maintains that blood flow to the heart improved 17% in men and women with coronary heart disease who drank 8.5 ounces a day for 3 months. Research findings from Israeli studies showed that it can lower blood pressure and help shrink plaque buildup in the neck arteries. It also has been shown to help control dental plaque when taken as an extract in mouthwash.[81]

- **Probiotics:** Probiotics are not a plant herb but are live bacteria similar to beneficial microorganisms found in the human gut. They are also called "friendly bacteria" or "good bacteria." Probiotics are used by many as a dietary supplement, but they are not all alike. Some may be helpful while others are not. Probiotics are thought to prevent and treat certain illnesses and support general wellness. The largest group is lactic acid bacteria, the type found in yogurt (*Lactobacillus acidophilus*). Research suggests that probiotics are useful to treat diarrhea, irritable bowel syndrome, and urinary tract infection; shorten intestinal tract infections; reduce recurrence of bladder cancer; and prevent and manage atopic dermatitis.[82]

- **Red clover** (*Trifolium pratense*): Red clover is used for relieving coughing and skin problems and for preventing symptoms caused by menopause. Research studies, however, have not shown it to be effective for helping with the hot flashes known to women undergoing menopause. Some preliminary studies indicate there might be some benefit for people who have colon or prostate cancer, but more research is needed. The primary side effects reported were nausea and upset stomach.[83]

🔍 CASE STUDY

Robert is a 55-year-old man who has been experiencing urinary frequency during the night and sometimes during the day. He has been feeling fatigued at work because he has not been getting a good night's sleep. His wife, Sandy, has been urging him to see an urologist (genitourinary specialist). While playing golf, Robert revealed his problem to one of his friends. The friend told Robert that he had been having similar symptoms. He recommended an herb called saw palmetto because he was taking it and his urinary frequency problem had lessened.

Questions:
1. What steps should Robert follow before obtaining this herb?
2. How important is it that Robert consult with a physician?
3. If Robert did decide to purchase the herb, where should he get it?
4. What other precautions should Robert take?

- **Sage** (*Salvia officinalis, Salvia lavandulaefolia, Salvia lavandulifolia*): Sage is used for mouth and throat inflammation, indigestion, and excessive sweating. Sage is also used as an ingredient in some dietary supplements for mouth, throat, and gastrointestinal problems. Some people may use sage to improve mood or to boost memory or mental performance. Sage is available as dried leaves, liquid extracts and sprays, and essential oils. It may be gargled, applied topically, or drunk as a tea. Two small studies suggest that sage may improve mood and mental performance in healthy young people and memory and attention in older adults. Sage is the main herb used in the practice of smudging. Smudging is the burning of an herb to create smoke which is inhaled or breathed in (**FIGURE 11.11**). It is supposed to be beneficial due to decreasing the amount of bacteria in the air.[84]

- **Saw palmetto berry** (*Serenoa repens*): Saw palmetto is a small palm tree native to the Eastern United States. Its fruit was used medicinally by the Seminole tribe of Florida. It is mainly used for urinary symptoms associated with an enlarged prostate gland. It is also used for chronic pelvic pain, bladder disorders, decreased sex drive, hair loss, hormone imbalances, and prostate cancer. Older studies seemed to indicate some success in treating benign prostatic hyperplasia (BPH), but current research shows that taking saw palmetto has no or little benefit.[85]

- **St. John's Wort** (*Hypericum perforatum*): St. John's Wort is a plant with yellow flowers (**FIGURE 11.12**) whose medicinal uses were first recorded in ancient Greece. St. John's Wort has been used for centuries to treat mental disorders and nerve pain. It has also been used as a sedative and a

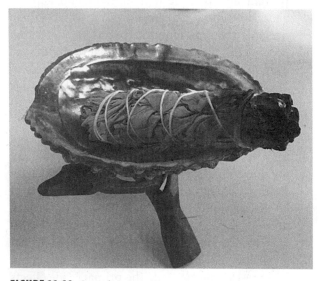

FIGURE 11.11 Smudging.

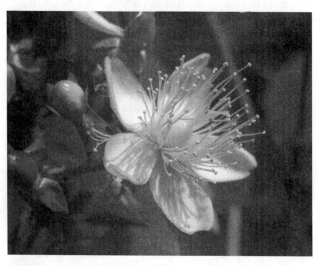

FIGURE 11.12 St. John's Wort.

treatment for malaria as well as a balm for wounds, burns, and insect bites. St. John's Wort is most commonly used today for depression, anxiety, and sleep disorders. There is scientific evidence that it may be useful for short-term treatment of mild to moderate depression.[45] Although some studies have reported benefits for more severe depression, others have not. St. John's Wort has significant interactions with some other medications.[45]

- **Valerian** (*Valeriana officinalis*): Valerian is a perennial plant native to Europe and Asia and is now grown in North America. The plant has an odor that is offensive. It was used by Hippocrates and Galen for insomnia, nervousness, headaches, and even heart palpitations. Valerian currently is used for sleep disorders and anxiety. Research suggests that valerian may be beneficial to sleep disorders; however, there is not enough evidence at this time to confirm this or any other uses of valerian.[86]

- **White willow bark**: White willow bark is used today for the treatment of pain, headache, and inflammatory conditions such as bursitis and tendinitis. Researchers believe that the chemical salicin, found in willow bark, is responsible for these effects. However, studies have identified several other components of willow bark that have antioxidant, fever-reducing, antiseptic, and immune-boosting properties. Some studies have shown white willow bark is as effective as aspirin for reducing pain and inflammation (but not fever), and at a much lower dose.[87]

- **Wild yam**: Wild yam is a plant that contains a chemical, diosgenin, which can be made into steroids such as estrogen and dehydroepiandrosterone (DHEA). It is used to treat menstrual cramps, nausea, and morning sickness associated with pregnancy; inflammation; osteoporosis; menopausal symptoms; and other health conditions. Several studies have found that wild yam has no effect at all on menopausal conditions, because by itself wild yam does not contain progesterone.[88]

- **Yarrow** (*Achillea millefolium*): Yarrow has been used for thousands of years for medicinal purposes. It is thought to have anti-inflammatory properties and has the ability to staunch blood flow from slow healing wounds. It is used by modern herbalists to treat wounds. Yarrow has also been used to make tea and to flavor beer, wine, and soft drinks. The leaves and flowers are used as

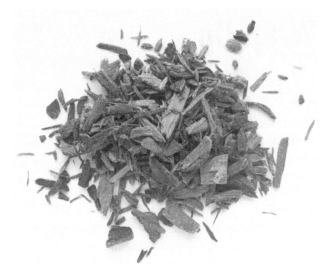

FIGURE 11.13 Bark from a yohimbe tree.
© TH Foto/age fotostock

seasoning and young leaves may be used in salads or boiled as greens. Yarrow has been found to have many properties. It has been used as an anti-inflammatory herb and gas relieving herb that may be helpful for those with ulcerative colitis. It has been used for sore throat and as a digestive stimulant. Used to make tea, it may be helpful for premenstrual syndrome.[89]

- **Yohimbe**: Yohimbe comes from the bark of the yohimbe tree that is found in Zaire, Cameroon, and Gabon in Africa (**FIGURE 11.13**). It is used to treat erectile dysfunction in males and also to increase weight loss. Studies are conflicting as to whether the herb is effective in increasing weight loss. An overdose can cause serious problems such as weakness and nervous stimulation, followed by paralysis, fatigue, stomach disorders, and ultimately death.[90,91]

▶ Conclusion

In summary, there are a myriad of herbs available, but you should become knowledgeable about the ones you use. Valid and reliable herbal information is available from the NCCIH, MedlinePlus, Mayo Clinic, University of Maryland Medical Center, and similar websites. The *Physician's Desk Reference for Herbal Medicines* also is a great resource. There are many herbals that can be safely used, but you need to take personal responsibility when selecting them for your bodily conditions or just as a preventive method for staying well.

Wrap-Up

Key Terms

Alkaloids A group of chemicals made by plants and are alkaloid in nature. Examples of alkaloids include cocaine, nicotine, and caffeine.

Biologically based therapies Use of natural techniques to maintain health and/or treat diseases.

Cardiac glycosides These chemicals have a marked action on the heart, strengthening the force and speed of systolic contractions.

Carotenoid pigments Pigments found in yellow and red plants such as carrots, sweet potatoes, red and yellow peppers, squash, and tomatoes.

Chelation therapy Use of a drug to bind with and remove excess or toxic amounts of metal or minerals from the blood.

Chlorophyll Pigment found in green plants and dark leafy green vegetables such as spinach, parsley, kale, green beans, and leeks.

Fixed oils Referred to as vegetable, carrier; or base oils; they contain nutrients such as minerals, antioxidants, and fat-soluble vitamins.

Flavonoids A set of chemicals that include brilliant plant pigments seen in fruits and vegetables.

Herbalist A practitioner of and contributor to the field of herbal medicine.

Lignans Phytoestrogens with weak estrogenic or antiestrogenic activity.

Nutritional supplements Also called dietary supplements. Nutritional supplements are preparations that provide additional nutrients and may include such things as green tea, soy preparations, ginseng, red clover, vitamins, and minerals (not an exhaustive list).

Orthomolecular medicine Emphasizes supplementing the diet with mega doses of vitamins, minerals, enzymes, hormones, and amino acids.

Phytoestrogen Estrogen-like chemicals that can act like the hormone estrogen.

Phytotherapy Plant therapy. Using botanical medicine to treat disease conditions.

Plant coumarins Oral anticoagulants. Coumarin was isolated from the tonka bean (*Dipteryx odorata*), which is in a classification known as coumarou; thus, similar plants were named plant coumarins.

Salicylates and salicins Aspirin-like compounds that have pain-relieving and anti-inflammatory action.

Saponins Glycosides or chemicals found in plants such as oats, vegetables, and beans that cause plants placed in water to "soap up" or froth to form a lather.

Tannins Polyphenols obtained from various parts of plants. Found in tree bark, wood, fruit, leaves, and roots.

Volatile oils Compounds of vegetable origin that evaporate at room temperature and allow us to enjoy the smell.

Suggestions for Class Activities

1. Invite an herbalist to class to discuss the properties of various herbs and how to grow them.
2. Visit an herbal garden and take photos. Bring the photos to class and let classmates guess the herbs. You can make a game of this by dividing the class into two teams.
3. Research the benefits and side effects of selected herbs. Present your findings to the class.
4. Start your own herbal garden using three common herbs. Report to the class the care required for the herbal garden.

Review Questions

1. What are biologically based therapies?
2. What are two examples of biologically based therapies?
3. What is the definition of phytotherapy?
4. Give two examples of nutritional supplements.
5. What is the definition of an herbalist?
6. What are the differences among crude herbs, decoctions, and herbal extracts?
7. What are four chemicals and properties of herbs?
8. What are phytoestrogens?
9. What is the difference between bulk and standardized herbs?
10. How should herbs be cared for and stored?
11. What is the difference between the United States and Germany regarding the assessment of the safety and efficacy of herbs?
12. What is the definition of herbals according to the DSHEA?
13. If an herb is found to be unsafe, what action can the FDA take?
14. How much money is spent on herbals each year and what percentage of U.S. adults use them?
15. Could you name five herbs and identify the conditions/diseases they are used for?

References

1. National Center for Complementary and Integrative Health. Herbs at a Glance. Available at: https://nccih.nih.gov/health/herbsataglance.htm. Updated September 24, 2017. Accessed April 23, 2018.

2. MedlinePlus. Herbal Medicine. Available at: http://www.nlm.nih.gov/medlineplus/herbalmedicine.html. Accessed April 23, 2018.

3. Answers.com. Botanical. Available at: http://www.answers.com/topic/botanical#ixzz1BsZLWhqI. Accessed April 23, 2018.

4. Tillotson A. *The One Earth Herbal Sourcebook: Everything You Need to Know About Chinese, Wester, and Ayurvedic Herbal Treatments*. New York. NY: Kensington Publishing Corp.; 2001.

5. Bradford N, ed. *The One Spirit Encyclopedia of Complementary Health*. London, UK: Hamlyn; 1996.

6. Raintree Tropical Plant Database. Methods of Preparing Herbal Remedies. Available at: http://www.rain-tree.com/prepmethod.htm#.WYN2jtPytBw. Updated January 2, 2013. Accessed April 23, 2018.

7. Freeman LW, Lawlis GF. *Mosby's Complementary and Alternative Medicine: A Research-Based Approach*. St. Louis, MO: Mosby; 2001.

8. Thomas L. *10 Essential Herbs*. Prescott, AZ: Hohm Press; 1996.

9. Boon H, Smith M. *The Complete Natural Medicine Guide to the 50 Most Common Medicinal Herbs*. 2nd ed. Toronto, Canada: Robert Rose Inc.; 2004.

10. Science Encyclopedia. Plant Pigment - Carotenoids. Available at: http://science.jrank.org/pages/5303/Plant-Pigment-Carotenoids.html. Accessed April 23, 2018.

11. Simonich MT. Cancer prevention by chlorophylls. *Linus Pauling Institute, Oregon State University Research Newsletter*. Fall/Winter 2006: 7-11. Available at: http://lpi.oregonstate.edu/sites/lpi.oregonstate.edu/files/pdf/newsletters/fw06.pdf. Accessed April 23, 2018.

12. Anderson E. Chlorophyll can help treat cancer. *Natural News*. June 12, 2008. Available at: http://www.naturalnews.com/023422_chlorophyll_cancer_carcinogen.html. Accessed April 23, 2018.

13. TheresaAnn LM. Essential oils versus fixed oils. *Hub Pages*. January 26, 2017. Available at: https://hubpages.com/health/essential-oils-versus-fixed-oils. Accessed April 23, 2018.

14. Henriette's Herbal Homepage. Olea Fixa. Fixed Oils. Available at: http://www.henriettes-herb.com/eclectic/usdisp/olea-fixa.html. Accessed April 23, 2018.

15. Linus Pauling Institute. Flavonoids. Available at: http://lpi.oregonstate.edu/sites/lpi.oregonstate.edu/files/pdf/newsletters/fw06.pdf. Accessed April 23, 2018.

16. Cholesterol and Fat Database. Lignans: Foods high in lignans. DietaryFiberFood.com. Available at: http://www.dietaryfiberfood.com/lignan.php. Updated October 28, 2012. Accessed April 23, 2018.

17. Velentzis LS, Cantwell MM, Cardwell C, Keshtgar MR, Leathem AJ, Woodside JV. Lignans and breast cancer risk in pre- and post-menopausal women: Meta-analyses of observational studies. *Br J Cancer*. 2009;100(9):1492-1498.

18. Susan G. Komen Cancer Center. Komen Perspectives – Answering Questions about Soy and Breast Cancer. Available at: http://ww5.komen.org/KomenPerspectives/Answeringquestionsaboutsoyandbreastcancer.html. Updated April 2015. Accessed April 23, 2018.

19. National Center for Complementary and Integrative Health. Flaxseed Reduces Some Risk Factors of Cardiovascular Disease. Available at: https://nccih.nih.gov/research/results/spotlight/062308.htm. Updated October 21, 2015. Accessed August 23, 2018.

20. Thangavelu A, Irizarry L. Coumarin Plant Poisoning. Medscape. Available at: http://emedicine.medscape.com/article/816897-overview. Updated March 31, 2014. Accessed April 23, 2018.

21. Schror K. *Acetylsalicylic Acid*. Weinheim, Germany: Wiley-Blackwell; 2009.

22. Singh AP. Salicin – A natural Analgesic. EthnoLeaflets.com. Available at: http://www.ethnoleaflets.com/leaflets/salicin.htm. Accessed April 23, 2018.

23. Sahelian R. Saponin in plants benefit and side effects, glycosides and extraction. February 10, 2016. Available at: http://www.raysahelian.com/saponin.html. Accessed April 23, 2018.

24. Cornell University College of Agriculture and Life Sciences. Department of Animal Science – Plants Poisonous to Livestock: Saponins. Available at: http://poisonousplants.ansci.cornell.edu/toxicagents/saponin.html. Accessed August 3, 2017.

25. Phytochemicals. What is saponins? Available at: http://www.phytochemicals.info/phytochemicals/saponins.php. Accessed April 23, 2018.

26. Goode J. Tannins. Wineanorak.com. Available at: http://www.wineanorak.com/tannins.htm. Accessed April 23, 2018.

27. Herbs 2000. Tannins. Available at: http://www.herbs2000.com/h_menu/tannins.htm. Accessed April 23, 2018.

28. Ahmad N. Volatile Oils (PowerPoint slides). SlideShare.net. June 5, 2016. Available at: https://www.slideshare.net/noumanahmad9085/volatile-oils. Accessed April 23, 2018.

29. Duke J. *The Green Pharmacy*. Emmaus, PA: Rodale Press; 1997.

30. Williams S. The cost of developing an FDA-approved drug is truly staggering, study shows. *Motley Fool*. April 30, 2016. Available at: https://www.fool.com/investing/general/2016/04/30/the-cost-of-developing-an-fda-approved-drug-is-tru.aspx. Accessed April 23, 2018.

31. U.S. Food and Drug Administration. Dietary Supplements. Available at: https://www.fda.gov/food/dietarysupplements/. Updated April 13, 2018. Accessed April 23, 2018.

32. U.S. Food and Drug Administration. The FDA's Drug Review Process: Ensuring Drugs Are Safe and Effective. Available at: https://www.fda.gov/drugs/resourcesforyou/consumers/ucm143534.htm. Updated November 24, 2018. Accessed April 23, 2018.

33. U.S. Food and Drug Administration. Drugs: Types of Applications. Available at: https://www.fda.gov/Drugs/DevelopmentApprovalProcess/HowDrugsareDevelopedandApproved/ApprovalApplications/default.htm. Updated October 23, 2018. Accessed April 23, 2018.

34. Daly R. FDA moves to speed device approval process. *Modern Healthcare*. January 19, 2011. Available at: http://www.modernhealthcare.com/article/20110119/NEWS/301199967/#. Accessed April 23, 2018.

35. National Institutes of Health Office of Dietary Supplements. Botanical Dietary Supplements. Available at: http://ods.od.nih.gov/factsheets/BotanicalBackground/#h5. Updated June 24, 2011. Accessed August 8, 2017.

36. Corwin A, Zahorik L, Hurlbutt M. Herbal supplements: Healthcare implications and considerations. *CDHA J*. 2009;24(2):7-14.

37. Kwan D, Hirschkorn K, Boon H. U.S. and Canadian pharmacists' attitudes, knowledge, and professional practice behaviors toward dietary supplements: A systematic review. *BMC Complement Altern Med.* 2006;6(31).

38. Scimone A, Scimone AA. Recommendation of herbal remedies by psychiatrists. College of Information Sciences and Technology - Penn State. Available at: http://citeseerx.ist.psu.edu/viewdoc /download?doi=10.1.1.628.3218&rep=rep1&type=pdf. Accessed April 8, 2018.

39. Lee RT, Barbo A, Lopez G, Melhem-Bertrandt A, et al. National survey of US oncologists' knowledge, attitudes, and practice patterns regarding herb and supplement use by patients with cancer. *J Clin Oncol.* 2014;32(36):4095-4101.

40. Barnes PM, Bloom B, Nahin RL. *National Health Statistics Reports No. 12. Complementary and Alternative Medicine Use Among Adults and Children: United States, 2007.* Hyattsville, MD: National Center for Health Statistics. 2008. Available at: http://www.cdc.gov/nchs/data/nhsr/nhsr012.pdf. Accessed April 23, 2018.

41. U.S. National Library of Medicine. MedlinePlus. Alfalfa. Available at: http://www.nlm.nih.gov/medlineplus/druginfo /natural/19.html. Updated November 30, 2017. Accessed April 23, 2018.

42. Mayo Clinic. L-arginine. Available at: http://www.mayoclinic .org/drugs-supplements/arginine/evidence/hrb-20058733. Updated October 24, 2017. Accessed April 23, 2018.

43. Duke J. *The Green Pharmacy.* Emmaus, PA: Rodale Press; 1997.

44. National Center for Complementary and Integrative Health. Astragalus. Available at: https://nccih.nih.gov/health /astragalus. Updated September 2016. Accessed April 23, 2018.

45. Quick Access, ed. *Professional Guide to Conditions, Herbs & Supplements.* Newton, MA: Integrative Medicine Communications; 2000.

46. Conrad R. Bee pollen: An overview. *Bee Culture.* January 23, 2017. Available at: http://www.beeculture.com/bee-pollen -overview-2/. Accessed April 23, 2018.

47. Gibb J. The health benefits of bilberry. *Ezine Articles.* December 14, 2006. Available at: http://ezinearticles.com/?The -Health-Benefits-of-Bilberry&id=386416. Accessed April 23, 2018.

48. Memorial Sloan-Kettering Cancer Center. Bilberry fruit. Available at: http://www.mskcc.org/mskcc/html/69134.cfm #Clinical Summary. Updated July 20, 2015. Accessed April 23, 2018.

49. Geller SE, Shulman LP, van Breemen RB, et al. Safety and efficacy of black cohosh and red clover for the management of vasomotor symptoms: A randomized controlled trial. *Menopause.* 2009;16(6):1156-1166.

50. Diener HC, Rahlfs VW, Danesch U. The first placebo-controlled trial of a special butterbur root extract for the prevention of migraine: Reanalysis of efficacy criteria. *Eur Neurol.* 2004;51(2):89–97.

51. Grossman W, Schmidramsl H. An extract of *Petasites hybridus* is effective in the prophylaxis of migraine. *Altern Med Rev.* 2001;6(3):303-310.

52. Lipton RB, Göbel H, Einhäupl KM, Wilks K, Mauskop A. *Petasites hybridus* root (butterbur) is an effective preventive treatment for migraine. *Neurology.* 2004;63(12):2240-2244.

53. Agosti R, Duke RK, Chrubasik JE, Chrubasik S. Effectiveness of *Petasites hybridus* preparations in the prophylaxis of migraine: a systematic review. *Phytomedicine.* 2006;13(9-10): 743-746.

54. Mercola. Here's why you can count on calendula oil. January 19, 2017. Available at: http://articles.mercola.com /herbal-oils/calendula-oil.aspx. Accessed April 23, 2018.

55. U.S. National Library of Medicine. MedlinePlus. Cascara. Available at: https://medlineplus.gov/druginfo/natural/773 .html. Updated March 5, 2015. Accessed April 23, 2018.

56. Sahelian R. Cayenne pepper supplement health benefit and use in medicine. July 15, 2016. Available at: http://www .raysahelian.com/cayenne.html. Accessed April 23, 2018.

57. National Center for Complementary and Integrative Health. Chasteberry. Available at: https://nccih.nih.gov/health /chasteberry. Updated September 2016. Accessed April 23, 2018.

58. National Center for Complementary and Integrative Health. Cranberry. Available at: https://nccih.nih.gov/health/cranberry. Updated November 2016. Accessed April 23, 2018.

59. WebMD. Creatine. Available at: http://www.webmd.com/vitamins -supplements/ingredientmono-873-CREATINE.aspx ?activeIngredientId=873&activeIngredientName=CREATINE. Accessed April 23, 2018.

60. U.S. National Library of Medicine. MedlinePlus. Dong Quai. Available at: https://medlineplus.gov/druginfo/natural/936.html. Updated November 30, 2017. Accessed April 23, 2018.

61. National Center for Complementary and Integrative Health. Ecchinacea. Available at: https://nccih.nih.gov /health/echinacea/ataglance.htm. Updated September 2016. Accessed April 23, 2018.

62. National Institutes of Health. Office of Dietary Supplements. Ephedra and Ephedrine Alkaloids for Weight Loss and Athletic Performance. Available at: https://ods.od.nih.gov /factsheets/EphedraandEphedrine-HealthProfessional/. Updated Updated July 1, 2004. Accessed April 23, 2018.

63. National Center for Complementary and Integrative Health. Garlic. Available at: https://nccih.nih.gov/health/garlic /ataglance.htm. Updated September 2016. Accessed April 23, 2018.

64. Ware M. Ginger: Health benefits, facts, research. *Medical News Today.* January 2016. Available at: http://www.medical newstoday.com/articles/265990.php. Updated September 11, 2017. Accessed April 23, 2018.

65. Pennington Nutrition Series. Ginger: A Potent Root. Pennington Biomedical Research Center, Louisiana State University. 2007 No. 6. Available at: https://www.pbrc.edu /training-and-education/pdf/pns/PNS_Ginger.pdf. Accessed April 23, 2018.

66. National Center for Complementary and Integrative Health. Ginkgo. Available at: https://nccih.nih.gov/health/ginkgo /ataglance.htm. Updated September 2016. Accessed April 23, 2018.

67. National Center for Complementary and Integrative Health. Asian Gingseng. Available at: https://nccih.nih.gov/health /asianginseng/ataglance.htm. Updated September 2016. Accessed April 23, 2018.

68. Mayo Clinic. Glucosamine. Available at: http://www.mayoclinic .org/drugs-supplements/glucosamine/evidence/hrb -20059572. Updated October 14, 2017. Accessed April 23, 2018.

69. National Center for Complementary and Integrative Health. Goldenseal. Available at: https://nccih.nih.gov

/health/goldenseal. Updated September 2016. Accessed April 23, 2018.

70. Healthline Newsletter. Everything You Need to Know About Gotu Kola. Available at: https://www.healthline.com/health/gotu-kola-benefits. Accessed April 23, 2018.

71. National Center for Complementary and Integrative Health. Hoodia. Available at: https://nccih.nih.gov/health/hoodia. Updated September 2016. Accessed April 23, 2018.

72. Sarris J, Stough C, Bousman CA, et al. Kava in the treatment of generalized anxiety disorder: a double-blind, randomized, placebo-controlled study. *J Clin Psychopharmacol.* 2013;33(5):643-648.

73. Penetar DM, Toto LH, Lee DY, Lukas SE. A single dose of kudzu extract reduces alcohol consumption in a binge drinking paradigm. *Drug Alcohol Depend.* 2015;153:194-200.

74. National Center for Complementary and Integrative Health. Lavender. Available at: https://nccih.nih.gov/health/lavender/ataglance.htm. Updated September 2016. Accessed April 23, 2018.

75. Costello RB, Lentino CV, Boyd CC, et al. The effectiveness of melatonin for promoting healthy sleep: A rapid evidence assessment of the literature. *Nutr J.* 2014;13:106.

76. Fried MW, Navarro VJ, Afdhal N, et al. Effect of silymarin (milk thistle) on liver disease in patients with chronic hepatitis C unsuccessfully treated with interferon therapy: A randomized, controlled trial. *JAMA.* 2012;308(3):274-282.

77. National Center for Complementary and Integrative Health. Milk Thistle. Available at: https://nccih.nih.gov/health/milkthistle/ataglance.htm. Updated September 2016. Accessed April 23, 2018.

78. National Cancer Institute. Milk Thistle (PDQ®)–Health Professional Version. Available at: https://www.cancer.gov/about-cancer/treatment/cam/hp/milk-thistle-pdq#section/_7. Updated June 19, 2017. Accessed August 10, 2017.

79. WebMD. Stinging Nettle. Available at: https://www.webmd.com/vitamins/ai/ingredientmono-664/stinging-nettle. Accessed April 23, 2018.

80. Alam MS, Roy PK, Miah AR, et al. Efficacy of peppermint oil in diarrhea predominant IBS - a double blind randomized placebo-controlled study. *Mymensingh Med J.* 2013;22(1):27-30.

81. National Center for Complementary and Integrative Health. Pomegranate. Available at: https://nccih.nih.gov/health/pomegranate/at-a-glance. Updated September 2016. Accessed April 23, 2018.

82. National Center for Complementary and Integrative Health. Probiotics. Available at: https://nccih.nih.gov/health/probiotics. Updated September 24, 2017. Accessed April 23, 2018.

83. Vadeboncoeur S. Red clover (Trifolium pratense). Complementary and Alternative Medicine for Cancer. Available at: http://www.cam-cancer.org/The-Summaries/Herbal-products/Red-clover-Trifolium-pratense. Updated February 8, 2017. Accessed April 23, 2018.

84. Mohagheghzadeh A, Faridi P, Shams-Ardakani M, Ghasemi Y. Medicinal smokes. *J Ethnopharmacol.* 2006;108(2):161-184.

85. National Center for Complementary and Integrative Health. Saw Palmetto. Available at: https://nccih.nih.gov/health/palmetto/ataglance.htm. Updated September 2016. Accessed April 23, 2018.

86. National Institutes of Health, Office of Dietary Supplements. Valerian. Available at: https://ods.od.nih.gov/factsheets/Valerian-HealthProfessional/. Updated March 15, 2013. Accessed April 23, 2018.

87. Goldman R, Watson K. Willow bark: Nature's Aspirin. *Healthline Newsletter.* January 9, 2017. Available at: http://www.healthline.com/health/willow-bark-natures-aspirin#overview1. Accessed April 23, 2018.

88. U.S. National Library of Medicine. MedlinePlus. Wild Yam. Available at: https://medlineplus.gov/druginfo/natural/970.html. Updated February 16, 2015. Accessed April 23, 2018.

89. Michigan Medicine, University of Michigan. Yarrow. Available at: http://www.uofmhealth.org/health-library/hn-2188008. Updated May 23, 2015. Accessed April 23, 2018.

90. WebMD. Yohimbe. Available at: http://www.webmd.com/vitamins-supplements/ingredientmono-759-YOHIMBE.aspx?activeIngredientId=759&act. Accessed April 23, 2018.

91. National Center for Complementary and Integrative Health. Yohimbine. Available at: https://nccih.nih.gov/health/yohimbe. Updated September 2016. Accessed April 23, 2018.

CHAPTER 12

Aromatherapy and Bach® Original Flower Remedies

LEARNING OBJECTIVES

As a result of reading this chapter, students will be able to:

1. Define aromatherapy and describe several historical examples of the use of aromatherapy.
2. Explain how aromatherapy has become a complement to traditional medical health care.
3. Examine ways in which nurses, health educators, and other health professionals could incorporate aromatherapy within their practices.
4. Analyze how Western medicine can learn from and build upon alternative methodologies such as aromatherapy to improve health and change behaviors.
5. Explain the history and philosophy of the Bach® Original Flower Remedies.
6. Name the three Bach® Original Flower Remedies groups.

▶ What Is Aromatherapy?

Aromatherapy is an ancient therapy that has gained in popularity in recent years. The word aromatherapy means "treatment using scents."[1] Aromatherapy is the use of concentrated plant oils, or **essential oils (EOs)**, to help improve general health and well-being.[2] It is a branch of herbal medicine, but unlike herbal medicines which are mostly taken internally, EOs are typically breathed in or inhaled and/or applied to the skin. Aromatherapy is a holistic practice that considers the mind, body, spirit, and emotions during the healing process. Many EOs have antiviral, antibacterial, and antifungal properties. Many help reduce stress, enhance relaxation, relieve anxiety, and alleviate some emotion-related disorders.[2,3]

▶ What Are the Most Common Ways to Use Aromatherapy?

Aromatherapy is most often used in one of three ways. The first is inhalation or breathing in the scent of EOs. A bottle of EO could be uncapped and the scent breathed in. Depending on the type of EO, a few drops can be placed in the palm of the hand, rubbed together, and then breathed in. Currently, breathing in EOs with the use of a diffuser seems to be a popular way to inhale them. Diffusers can be electrical, burners that use candles, or a simple ceramic ring that is warmed by a light bulb. Four to eight drops of EOs are placed in water within a diffuser so that molecules can be released into the air. Many people run diffusers in their homes, especially at night in the bedroom. Many run diffusers in their workplace. If you do not have a diffuser, drops of EOs may be placed nearby so that the scent is inhaled, or 1–2 drops may be placed in a handkerchief and inhaled.[4] Some individuals apply a few drops to their pillowcase at bedtime and breathe in the EO essence. Steaming with EOs is another way to use them, especially if you have a sinus or respiratory cold. Eucalyptus, peppermint, and several others are good choices. You could make your own inhalation tent by adding EO drops (ratio of 3–5 drops per 4 cups of water) to a large pan of steaming hot water, place a towel over your head, and then inhale.[4] **BOX 12.1** is Dr. Synovitz's personal story about the benefits for EOs.

The second way to use aromatherapy is to apply a diluted form of EO directly to the skin. Some EOs may be applied directly from the bottle to the skin, usually only a drop or two. The drops may be applied to any areas on the body, including the soles of the feet. To avoid skin irritation, many EOs are placed in a carrier oil such as sweet almond oil, olive oil, or coconut oil before rubbing onto the skin.[4] Massage therapist often use EOs in a light base carrier oil when giving massages. EOs can also be applied to the skin during a tub bath. Because some people experience adverse effects when the EOs are added before sitting in the water, it is important to fill the tub with water, sit down in it, and then add the EOs (usually 5–8 drops). EOs can also be mixed with bath salts and applied to tub water. (See **Appendix 12.A** for a bath salt recipe.) Some EOs are added to perfumes and lotions. Even hot/cold compresses can be made by soaking a cloth in a water solution of 1–2 drops of EO (e.g., lavender) in a bowl of water.[2,3]

A third method to use aromatherapy involves ingestion or internal retention (EO in a suppository). Ingestion is by pills, capsules, or drinking a liquid (e.g., orange juice) in which EOs have been placed. Most lay aromatherapy consumers use inhalation or skin application, but individuals certified in aromatherapy, naturopaths, and physicians who specialize in EOs use and prescribe some internal EO preparations. It is safer for individuals to consult a trained expert in aromatherapy before ingesting EOs.

BOX 12.1 Personal Story

Several years ago, when I was teaching at my university, the wing of my office building was renovated. Our building was old and had severe rain damage from topical storms and hurricanes. Our entire faculty was moved to another building while renovations were being carried out. After a couple months, we were all moved back. One day, I began to notice dark granules landing on my desk and floor that were coming from the overhead heating and cooling vent. At first, I did not think too much of it and thought it was residual dirt coming from the ventilation system. About this time, I began to develop a cough and made an appointment with a pulmonologist who diagnosed me with asthma and who subsequently prescribed medicine and an inhaler. I was hesitant, however, to use the medications because I doubted that I had asthma. About that same time, and because I was concerned about the dark granules in my office, I asked the university Environmental Health and Safety department personnel to test them. They found that the granules contained hyphal mold. The university responded by replacing the entire ventilation system in the building. At that time, I was buying and accumulating many EOs. I began to steam myself morning and night with several drops of eucalyptus, frankincense, and lavender. I had only used the inhaler a couple of times before starting my steaming method and discontinued its use. Within a couple of weeks, my cough was disappearing, and within a month, I went back to the pulmonologist who was amazed at my recovery. I am telling you this story to let you know I believe that steaming with EOs cleared my lungs of hyphal mold. Please keep in mind that my story is anecdotal, not sound research.

▶ What Are Some of the Terms Related to Aromatherapy?

The following are some common terms used in aromatherapy[4,5]:

- **Absolute**: Plant extraction obtained by using chemical solvents.
- **Carbon dioxide**: Plant oil extracted by the carbon dioxide (CO_2) method.
- **Hydrosol**: Floral water or distillate water that remains after distilling an EO.
- **Carrier oil**: Base or vegetable oil derived from the fatty portion of plants such as the seeds, kernels, or the nuts. They are used to dilute CO_2 and **absolutes** before applying them to the skin. Examples are olive oil, sweet almond oil, avocado oil, sesame oil, sunflower oil, and peanut oil.
- **Essential oil (EO)**: Distilled liquid from the leaves, stems, flowers, bark, roots, or other elements of a plant.
- **Infused oil**: A carrier oil that has been mixed with one or more herbs.
- **Resin**: A thick sticky substance produced by trees.

Although some sources differentiate plant extracts into EOs, absolutes, hydrosols, and CO_2, EOs are used as a blanket term to include all natural, aromatic, and volatile plant oils, including CO_2 and absolutes.[5]

What Is the Historical Record Regarding Aromatherapy Use?

Plant oils have been used as a therapeutic aid for thousands of years. Historical Chinese, Ayurvedic, and Arabic medical texts document the use of aromatic oils for spirituality and health. Roman soldiers bathed in water that contained scented oils and received massages with plant oils. In ancient Greece, Hippocrates recommended regular aromatherapy baths and scented massages.[2] One of the first aromatic practices was fumigation. Plant oils were burned, creating a great deal of smoke that engulfed sickrooms, supposedly combating evil spirits and getting rid of them from patients' bodies.[3] Hippocrates used aromatic oils as **fumigation** to rid Athens of plague.[1] A Greek perfumer, Megallus, created a perfume called Megaleion. Megaleion included myrrh in a fatty oil base that was used to produce a pleasing aroma, had anti-inflammatory properties toward the skin, and was used to heal wounds.

The Egyptians were the experts, however, in the use of EOs. Approximately 6,000 years ago, the Egyptian physician Imhotep recommended scented oils for massage and bathing.[2] In Egypt, the EOs were prepared by placing plants in a stone trough along with fatty oils. The plants would be crushed until the base oil was saturated with the EOs. Priests in Egypt administered scented ointments to worshipers during rituals. Incense was burned three times a day in the city of Heliopolis and was always burned at the opening of a shrine, at the coronation of a pharaoh, and at all national celebrations. One recipe that was supposedly a perfume for the gods was named Kyphi, a cocktail of EOs that contained peppermint, saffron, juniper, acacia, and henna.[2] These were combined with wine, honey, resin, myrrh, and raisins; made into a paste; and solidified. The solidified mixture was then burned as an offering to the gods. This passion for incense nearly wiped out the cedar forests of Lebanon because of the military campaigns that were mounted to ensure a large supply of the prized cedar.

Because the Egyptians believed in an afterlife, they went to great lengths to ensure a comfortable journey into the next world. Alabaster jars and ebony coffers

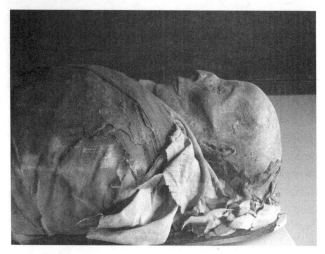

FIGURE 12.1 Mummification.
© James Wibberding/Shutterstock

contained ointments the Egyptians believed would make the skin of the deceased supple after he or she arrived in the new world.[2] During the embalming process, bodies were washed with salt and body cavities were filled with myrrh and oakmoss, imported from Greece. Oakmoss has an exquisite, sweet scent and contains usnic acid, an antibiotic that helped with the mummification process. Pine resin also had antimicrobial properties and was used for mummification[3] (**FIGURE 12.1**).

In daily lives, the Egyptians used heavy mascara on their eyelids and lashes to help protect their eyes from the sun. They also used many creams and lotions as antiaging remedies. They extracted oils from plants by a method of infusion for use as cosmetics. Their cosmetics contained scents from lily, bitter almond, mint, frankincense, and myrrh. Later, people from all around the world traveled to Egypt to learn the secrets of aromatherapy, because they finally understood that the Egyptians' aromatherapy practices were therapeutic for the skin and body.[1] At the time of the Crusades, the art of aromatherapy was carried to the West.

Avicenna (980–1037 CE), a Persia-born physician, developed the distillation method for oils that is still used today. Some argue that distillation had been used for many centuries and maintain that Avicenna merely refined the process. For example, within the 12th century, an abbess in Germany named Hildegard grew and distilled lavender for its medicinal properties. Avicenna, however, devised a coiled cooling pipe to condense steam and collect the evaporated essence.[1,2]

The methods of distilling oils were imported to northern Europe in the Middle Ages (14th century). Documents exist that show EOs were used to fight diseases such as the Black Death. At the end of the 15th century, Paracelsus, an army surgeon and alchemist, used aromatherapy to treat leprosy, and records also show that aromatherapy was used during the 16th and 17th centuries by European herbalists to treat several diseases.[1]

In the late 1930s, impressive research was conducted by Rene-Maurice Gattefosse, a French chemist who sparked interest in aromatherapy. In fact, it was Gattefosse who originated the term aromatherapy and defined the use of EOs as a healing discipline. His research began after he burned his hand in a laboratory experiment and quickly plunged it into a pot of the closest liquid, which happened to be lavender oil.[2] His hand healed with no infection or scarring. That event spurred him to do a great deal of research about aromatherapy's healing power. Dr. Jean Valnet, a French army surgeon, expanded the works of Gattefosse by using EOs as antiseptic during World War II. In 1977, Dr. Valnet wrote a book called *The Practice of Aromatherapy.*

Another key player in the establishment of modern aromatherapy was Marguerite Maury, an Austrian biochemist and two-time winner of an international prize for exceptional scientific contributions to cosmetic research. Maury introduced the concept of prescribing oils for people, but she developed a way to apply EOs in massage.[2] Micheline Arcier studied under Maury and opened clinics, now famous in Great Britain, using aromatherapy as a holistic health system.[3]

In the 1980s, California practitioners began to use EOs in treatment. Today, one can find a wide selection of books about aromatherapy and can find many EOs in local health food stores, although many are not considered pure EOs. Aromatherapy products are also easily accessible through the Internet. Most practicing **aromatherapists** in the United States are first trained as massage therapists, naturopaths, psychotherapists, chiropractors, sports medicine therapists, energy healers, Ayurvedic doctors/clinicians, and traditional Chinese medicine doctors, who then incorporate the use of EOs into their practices.

▶ Is Aromatherapy Safe?

Aromatherapy is safe from the young to the elderly, although some preparations are strong and instructions need to be followed very carefully. Adverse reactions are rare, but it is important to remember that EOs are powerful; taken in the wrong doses, they could be toxic to the body. Most undiluted EOs should not be applied directly to the skin or mucous membranes because they are too strong and could cause skin irritation or allergic reaction,[3,4] but some may be applied if only using a drop or two. For example, lavender and tea tree oil can usually be used undiluted; however, some individuals could be allergic. It is a good idea to perform a patch test to assess if you could be allergic to a particular oil. You could apply a couple of drops of the EO mixed in with some sort of carrier oil (e.g., olive oil or sweet almond oil) to the inside of your forearm. If there is no reaction, the EO should be safe to use.

Pregnant women should consult with their physician before using aromatherapy.[2,4] People with high blood pressure, asthma, epilepsy, or other health problems should also either avoid EOs or consult with their doctors before using them, because they may be taking medications that the aromatherapy oil may interact with.

Aromatherapy may be used on babies during massage. It is purported to speed the development of the nervous system and brain, help balance the baby's developing systems, and encourage growth.[3] Aromatherapy massage on babies should be done gently using a firm hand and special aromatic baby oils that contain no more than 2 drops of EO per 1¾ fluid ounces

🔍 CASE STUDY

Cathy has epilepsy and is taking medication for it. She also has insomnia many nights. She went to a spa and was impressed with an aromatherapy treatment she was given in conjunction with her massage. The aromatherapy scent made her remember smells associated with pleasant childhood memories, and now Cathy is very interested in obtaining her own EOs for home use. She found an online source and bought several, one of which was lavender, thought to be good for insomnia because of its sedative effect. That night, Cathy placed some drops of lavender EO in a diffuser, took her epilepsy medication (primidone [Mysoline]), and went to bed.

Questions:
1. What should Cathy have done before using lavender EO in her diffuser?
2. Research the potential interactive effects of lavender and medications for epilepsy. What did you find?

of carrier oil.[3] Generally accepted EOs for babies are lavender, rose, and chamomile.

To be very safe, if you are considering the purchase of EOs, you should check for an expiration date. Be sure to store your oils away from children. Always remember that less is more. If one drop will get the job done, do not use two drops. You should never take EOs internally based on your own judgment. Someone highly trained in aromatherapy such as a trained and certified aromatherapist, naturopathic doctor, or medical doctor could prescribe internal use, but you should not do this on your own. Finally, a very important safety tip is to keep EOs away from fire hazards because they are quite flammable.[3,4]

▶ Who Can Use Aromatherapy Essential Oils and for What Purposes?

An aromatherapist can use EOs because they are trained in their use, but the oils are available for anyone to use. That means you could buy your own supply of EOs for personal use.

The purposes for using aromatherapy vary. Some traditional physicians and naturopaths learn about the biochemistry of the oils and their action on our bodies, so their purpose is medicinal. They may use aromatherapy to treat the physical body or they may use it to treat emotional or psychological disorders.[3] Prescriptions may be for internal or external EO treatment.[3] Practitioners may use EOs as a part of beauty treatments or in cosmetics. Certainly, massage therapists use EOs in massage oil preparations. The main purpose of aromatherapy, however, is to maintain health by boosting the body's immune system via the senses of touch and smell.

▶ What Are the Various Processes for Making Essential Oils?

Just as with herbals (see Chapter 11), EOs are extracted from the bark, roots, leaves, stalks, flowers, berries, and sap of trees and plants, and they are very concentrated. For example, it takes about 220 pounds of lavender flowers to make about 1 pound of EO.

- **Steam distillation** is the most common method used to extract the oils. The plant parts are heated, and then the plant molecules evaporate and are carried in the steam along a pipe, where they are cooled and condensed into a liquid. Finally, the molecules separate, the water is drawn off the oil, and the result is a pure, natural EO.[3,5]

- **Macerating (or soaking)** is another method employed when the aromatic components of the plant could be ruined with high heat. Maceration involves soaking aromatic plants in animal fats or vegetable oils. Plates loaded with animal fat or vegetable oil are laid on wooden frames. Flower petals are then placed on the plates to soak. Every few days, new petals are placed on the plates so that the fat is soaked with scent. Later, the fat is washed with pure grain alcohol, which serves to dissolve the EO compounds while the fat is left behind. **Vacuum distillation** is used to remove the alcohol and what is left behind is the floral absolute. This method is costly and labor intensive, so it is rarely used anymore.[3]

- **Expression** is a method to extract EOs from the rinds of citrus fruit. Again, no heat source is used. First, the fruit is removed and the rinds and pith are soaked in water, then they are removed and turned upside down. The cells containing the oils break apart, and the oil drips out and soaks into nearby sponges. When the sponges become saturated, they are squeezed into containers.[2,3,6]

- **Cold-pressed extraction** is also used to extract EOs from citrus fruits as well as nuts and seeds. It is similar to expression, except this process involves high mechanical pressure to force the oils out. The oils contain water, which will eventually evaporate. Cold-pressed oils spoil more quickly than oils extracted from other processes, so you should purchase only small quantities at a time.[6,7]

- **Solvent extraction** is used for plants such as jasmine and linden blossom that cannot survive the distillation process. Blossoms are laid on perforated trays and washed with a solvent such as hexane. The solvent dissolves the nonaromatic waxes, pigments, and volatile aromatic molecules. The solution is filtered and the filtered material goes through a low pressure distillation process. A waxy mass called the **concrete** remains, which can contain as much as 55% of the volatile oil. The concentrated concrete is then processed to remove the waxy materials. The waxy concrete is warmed and stirred with alcohol, which breaks up the concrete into minute globules. The volatile oil separates, as does some of the wax. The solution is agitated and frozen to precipitate out the wax. The absolutes are left.[6,7]

- **CO$_2$ extraction** gives a richer, more intense scent because more of the aromatic chemicals are released. High pressure is placed on the CO$_2$, which turns it into a liquid and a solvent that can extract aromatic molecules in an extraction process similar to the solvent extraction process. The advantage to the CO$_2$ process is that no solvent residue remains because the CO$_2$ reverts back to gas and evaporates.[6,7]

- **Florasols/phytols extraction** is a process that uses other types of gaseous solvents. Dr. Peter Wilde used the solvent Florasol (R134a) in the late 1980s to extract aromatic oils and biologically active components from plant materials for use in the perfume industry as well as in food and aromatherapy. Because the extraction occurs at or below the outside (ambient) air temperature, there is no heat breakdown of the plant products used. A free-flowing clear oil free of waxes is obtained.[7]

How Do You Care for and Store Essential Oils?

Ultraviolet rays can decrease the storage life of EOs. They should be stored in dark amber, cobalt blue, or violet glass bottles. In addition, they should be kept in a cool, dark place away from direct sunlight, heater vents, and registers. Heat and water are major spoilers of EOs. They should never be left in the car, especially in the summer. If keeping EOs in the bathroom, the tops should be shut tightly to keep out moisture. The bottles should not be left in sun or in a window because the light will enter the bottle and warm up the oil. Heat will speed the oxidation process and make the oil prematurely age.[8]

The size of the bottle is also important. Smaller bottles expose the oil to less oxygen, which will keep the oil intact longer. With care, the shelf life can be greatly extended. The shelf life of most oils varies from 6 months to several years, although citrus oils have the shortest shelf life and should be stored carefully and/or kept in the refrigerator.[8]

What Are Carrier Oils?

Carrier oils are vegetable oils derived from the fatty part of a plant, usually from the seeds, kernels, or nuts,[9] and are used to dilute EOs prior to application. They "carry" the EO/s onto the skin. Some carrier oils are odorless, but many have a sweet, nutty aroma. If the scent is strong and bitter, the oil has probably become rancid. Several examples of vegetable oils that are used as a carrier in aromatherapy are sweet almond, coconut, apricot kernel, avocado, borage seed, camellia seed (tea oil), cranberry seed, evening primrose, grape seed, hazelnut, hemp seed, jojoba, macadamia nut, olive, peanut, pecan, pomegranate seed, rose hip, sesame, sunflower, and watermelon seed.[9]

Carrier oils are best if they have been cold pressed. The oil is pressed from the fatty portion of the botanical without the use of added heat. Cold expeller-pressed carrier oils are also acceptable. These oils have been processed under conditions that keep the heat to a minimum. If carrier oils are not processed with low heat, the nutrients in the oils are damaged.[9]

If you are attempting to select carrier oils for purchase, you should consider factors other than the processing methods. Some nutrients and essential fatty acids are contained within carrier oils. For example, some contain fat-soluble vitamins and minerals and act as antioxidants, helpful to the skin. Carrier oils that contain fatty acids are also nourishing to the skin, but may cause the oil to become rancid much faster.[9] You should select a carrier oil that has an aroma that will not conflict with the scent of the EO and a color that you will be satisfied with when mixed with your EO. Certainly, price is a consideration. For example, organic carrier oils are more costly than conventional oils. You should not purchase mineral oil or petroleum jelly for aromatherapy use because they clog pores and prevent the skin from breathing naturally.

To keep carrier oils for a longer period of time, they should be stored in dark glass bottles with tight fitting tops and in a cool, dark location. Carrier oils may, however, be stored in plastic, unlike EOs, which should always be stored in glassware. To prolong the lifespan of some fragile carrier oils, they should be stored in the refrigerator. Usually, the producer of the carrier oil will affix specific storage instructions on the carrier oil bottle. Some oils, such as avocado oil, should never be stored in the refrigerator; so, read the labels carefully.

What Do the Clinical Studies Show?

There are some completed aromatherapy studies, but very scant current research. Some of the previous studies have not been well designed and some are inconclusive. Cook and Ernst conducted a systematic review of the literature using Medline, Embase, British Nursing Index, CISCOM, and AMED to analyze randomized controlled trials of aromatherapy.[10]

The researchers found 12 trials: six had no replication and six found relaxing effects of aromatherapy combined with massage. The authors concluded that the effects of aromatherapy were not strong enough to be considered a treatment for anxiety, but that aromatherapy has a mild, transient anxiolytic (relaxing) effect.[9]

In a clinical study of the effects of lemon and lavender, the findings revealed that lemon appeared to enhance mood, but lavender had no effect on mood. Neither lemon (considered a stimulant) nor lavender affected participants' heart rate, blood pressure, wound healing, pain ratings, or levels of interleukin-6 or interleukin-10. The findings did show that blood levels of norepinephrine (stress hormone) remained elevated following participants' immersion in ice water after inhaling lemon scent. After smelling lavender, participants' levels of norepinephrine declined to pre-stressor levels.[11]

A controlled research pilot study to examine the effects of aromatherapy using clary sage and lavender showed positive results in decreasing stress and relieving anxiety in 14 ICU nurses over 42 nursing shifts.[12] The sample, however, was small and the authors concluded that the study should be replicated.

A 2010 review article on the antimicrobial and immune-modifying effects of eucalyptus EO revealed many positive effects on respiratory conditions such as bronchitis, asthma, and chronic obstructive pulmonary disease.[13] The authors point out that one can buy devices to inhale the vapor or by making a tent over steaming water.

Aromatherapy seems to promote relaxation in people with cancer and sleep disorders. Some of the oils or natural plants have been reported as useful when treating a wide variety of conditions such as burns, infections, depression, insomnia, agitation in Alzheimer's patients, and high blood pressure. The problem, however, is that there is very little clinical evidence to support claims that aromatherapy can prevent or cure diseases.[14] Some studies have shown that lavender and tea tree oils have been found to have some estrogenic (female hormone-like) effects. Lavender and tea tree oils may block or decrease the effect of androgens (male sex hormones). When lavender and tea tree oils were applied to the skin of prepubertal boys over a long period of time, there was a relationship to breast enlargement. If lavender and tea tree oil are indeed estrogenic, they may not be safe for women who have a high risk for estrogenic receptive breast cancer.[15] Another study of tea tree oil to assess if it is a possible antimicrobial affirmed that it was as effective as a standard type of antibacterial treatment for antibiotic-resistant bacteria.[15]

▶ What Are Some Common Aromatherapy Essential Oils?

The following are common aromatherapy EOs.[3,4,5,16] Even though they are presented as having benefits, keep in mind that most have not been scientifically tested here in the United States. (*Caution:* Before using any EOs, check for allergic reaction or sensitivity. Place a couple of drops in carrier oil such as sweet almond oil or coconut oil and place on forearm. If no reaction, you should be safe to use it.)

Bergamot Oil (*Citrus bergamia*)

Source: Comes from the pear-shaped yellow fruit of the bergamot tree that Christopher Columbus discovered in the Canary Islands, and then introduced to Italy and Spain. The rind of the fruit (**FIGURE 12.2**) is used. It takes peels from approximately 1,000 bergamot fruits to make 30 ounces of oil.

Action: Cooling and refreshing action to help nervous emotions and frustration. Benefits the gastrointestinal tract, aid for oily skin and acne, and used to soothe breathing difficulties.

Uses: Is a component in perfumes and is the main aromatic taste of Earl Grey tea. Used as a skin tonic and has a deodorizing action.

Cedarwood Oil (*Juniperus virginiana*)

Source: Flower from the cedarwood tree. It has the faint smell of sandalwood. Pale yellow to light orange in color.

Action: Helps calm and balance energy. Clears the respiratory system of excess phlegm. Aids urinary

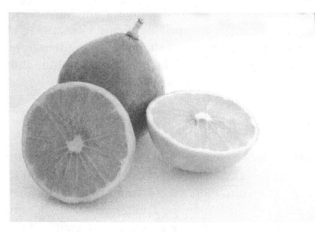

FIGURE 12.2 Bergamot.
© iStockphoto/Thinkstock

tract infections. Improves oily skin and dandruff. It should not be used on infants or women who are pregnant.

Uses: Egyptians used the oil in the mummification process, in cosmetics, and as an insect repellant.

Chamomile Oil (Roman chamomile, *Anthemis nobilis*, and German chamomile, *Matricaria chamomilla*)

Source: Flowers of the chamomile plant (**FIGURE 12.3**). The word chamomile comes from the Greek word meaning earth apple.

Action: The Roman chamomile is said to promote relaxation, whereas the German chamomile is reported to be a powerful anti-inflammatory. Benefits the gastrointestinal tract and relieves allergies, premenstrual syndrome, psychological problems, abdominal pain, gall bladder upsets, and ear and throat infections. Safe for use on children and pregnant women.

Uses: Used in teas, massage oils, as a poultice for wounds, in burners, and in steam baths.

Clary Sage Oil (*Salvia sclarea*)

Source: Clary sage plant. Gives a sweet, nutty, and floral aroma.

Action: Acts as anticonvulsant, antidepressant, antiseptic, antispasmodic, deodorant, sedative, and tonic. Helps with aging skin, diffuses hot flashes during menopause, relieves cramps, and reduces tension and stress.

Uses: Used in skin tonics, potpourri, poultice, massage oil, and baths.

Clove Oil (*Eugenia caryophyllata*)

Source: Evergreen tree native to Indonesia and the Malacca Islands. It has bright green leaves and nail-shaped rose-peach flower buds that turn deep red-brown when dried. Oil is extracted from the leaves, stems, and buds.

Action: Analgesic, antiseptic, antispasmodic, antineuralgic, carminative, antimicrobial, disinfectant, insecticide, and tonic.

Uses: Perfumes, mulled wines and liqueurs, dental products (toothache), pomade, insect repellant, lotions, creams, massage oil, burners and vaporizers, and as a mouthwash.

Eucalyptus Oil (*Eucalyptus radiata*)

Source: Eucalyptus plant native is to Australia. South Africa, Portugal, Spain, Brazil, and Chile also grow eucalyptus. The leaves (**FIGURE 12.4**) are steam distilled to obtain the oil.

Actions: Stimulant, decongestant, antimicrobial, anti-inflammatory, and breathing enhancer. Used to treat asthma, kidney infection, and sore muscles.

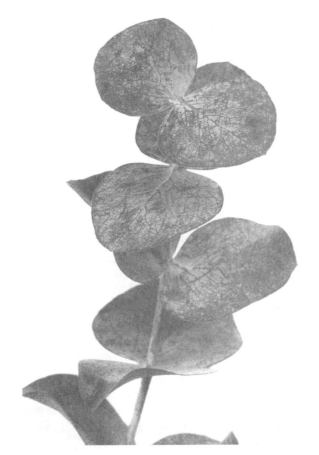

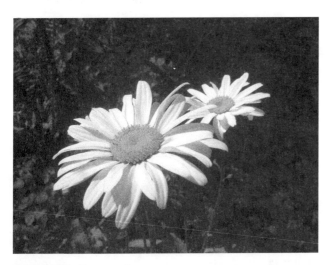

FIGURE 12.3 Chamomile.

FIGURE 12.4 Eucalyptus.

Uses: Steam inhalations, compresses, poultices, and massage.

Jasmine Oil (*Jasminum grandiflorum*)

Source: Evergreen, climbing shrub that can grow 33 feet high. Has dark green leaves and small white star-shaped flowers (**FIGURE 12.5**). Originally from China and Northern India, and then brought to Spain, France, Italy, Egypt, Morocco, Japan, and Turkey. Floral fragrance; rich sweet scent.

Action: Promotes feeling of optimism and well-being (antidepressant), helps muscular spasm, soothes irritating coughs and laryngitis, helps with labor and painful periods, and relieves anxiety and nervousness. Helps promote the flow of breast milk and reduces stretch marks.

Uses: Massage oils, baths, lotions, burners, and vaporizers.

Juniper Oil (*Juniperus communis*)

Source: Evergreen shrub. Oil is extracted by steam distillation from the berries, needles, and wood. Has a clear, slightly woody aroma and pale in color.

Action: Antiseptic, antirheumatic, antispasmodic, astringent, diuretic, stimulating, and tonic effect. Should not be used during pregnancy or by people with kidney problems. Helps with the digestive system and has a tonic effect on the liver. Effective for acne, eczema, oily skin, and dandruff.

Uses: Burners and vaporizers, massage oils, baths, lotions, creams, and compresses.

Lavender Oil (*Lavandula angustifolia*)

Source: Evergreen shrub with pale green leaves and violet flowers (**FIGURE 12.6**). Comes from the Latin word *lavare*, which means "to wash." Has a delicate floral fragrance. Oil is steam distilled from flowering tops.

Action: Disinfectant, pain relief (chronic muscle aches, back discomfort, menstrual pain, arthritic and rheumatic pain), and sedative. Helps to treat insomnia, anxiety, high blood pressure, burns, wounds, respiratory problems, and digestion disorders. Is used in skin care and hair care, stimulates urine production, and helps ease discomfort of insect bites. Should not be used by women who are pregnant or who are breastfeeding.

Uses: Cold compresses, massage oils, lotions, soaps, baths.

Lemon Oil (genus *Citrus* of the *Rutaceae* family of plants)

Source: Citrus lemon tree that grows to 15 feet high. Produces highly scented lemon fruit and white blossoms year-round. Early forms originated in China, and then were grown in Italy and the Mediterranean area. Columbus brought the

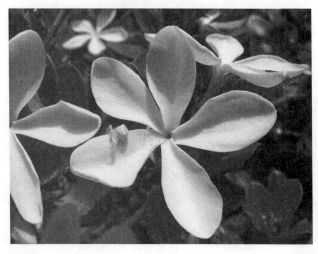

FIGURE 12.5 Jasmine.
© Yehuda Boltshauser/Shutterstock

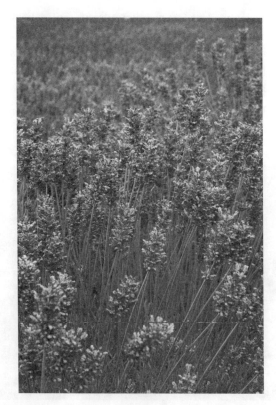

FIGURE 12.6 Lavender.
© iStockphoto/Thinkstock

lemon tree to the New World in 1493. Extraction by cold pressing the peel.

Action: Antiseptic, astringent, and detoxifying. Good for skin conditions, insomnia, fever, stomach disorders, weight loss, asthma, and hair care. Immune system booster.

Uses: Cleaner for cleansing the body and metal surfaces, perfumes, soaps, cosmetics, and drinks. Used in baths, massage, and inhalation.

Orange Oil (*Citrus sinensis*)

Source: Orange tree. Extraction is from peels of orange by expression or cold compression.

Action: Anti-inflammatory, antidepressant, antispasmodic, sedative, aphrodisiac, antiseptic, and carminative. Good for indigestion, dental care, respiratory problems, irritable bowel syndrome, urinary tract infections, hair care, and skin care. Can be used as a diuretic and tonic. Is a detoxifier.

Uses: Adds orange flavor to beverages and desserts. Used in soaps, lotions, creams, cosmetics, room fresheners, deodorants, and bakery items.

Peppermint Oil

Source: Cross between water mint and spearmint plants (**FIGURE 12.7**). Native to Europe. Known as the world's oldest medicine. Strong spicy mint flavor. May be safely ingested.

Action: Reduces pain of headache, digestive disorders, nausea, fever, stomach and bowel spasms,

sore throats, muscle aches, and toothaches. Can be used as a skin cleanser and breath sweetener.

Uses: Soap, shampoo, toothpaste, chewing gum, tea, perfume, and ice cream. Enemas, pills, cold rubs, tonics, massage, steam baths, and burners.

Rose Oil (*Rosa centifolia/Rosa damascena*)

Source: Flower. Deep floral, rich, sweet scent. It takes 30 roses to make a single drop of oil and 60,000 roses to produce just 1 ounce of rose oil. It is also known as rose otto (attar of roses) or rose absolute. Rose ottos are extracted by steam distillation while rose absolutes are made by solvent or CO_2 extraction.

Action: Antidepressant, antiseptic, antispasmodic, antiviral, aphrodisiac, astringent, laxative. Speeds up clotting for people suffering from hemorrhage. Good for liver health and as a tonic for the nerves. Soothes the stomach, helps the uterus function better, provides menstrual pain relief, and in mild concentrations is good for headaches.

Uses: Skin tonics, massage, baths, infused in the air.

Tea Tree Oil (*Melaleuca alternifolia*)

Source: Extracted by steam distillation of twigs and leaves of the tea tree (**FIGURE 12.8**).

Action: Antibacterial, antimicrobial, antiseptic, antiviral, expectorant, fungicidal, and insecticidal. Stimulates wound healing, circulation, and

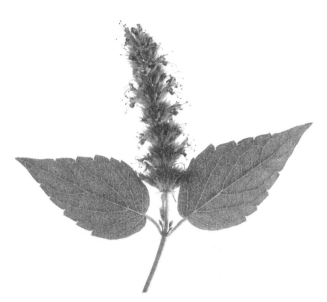

FIGURE 12.7 Peppermint.
© Madlen/Shutterstock

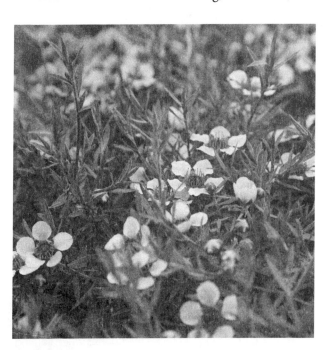

FIGURE 12.8 Tea tree leaves and flowers.
© Tamara Kulikova/Shutterstock

hormone secretions; boosts immunity; rids the body of toxins; and gives muscular pain relief.

Uses: Diluted doses for wounds, sores, or acne. A couple drops mixed with vodka can be given as a douche to treat yeast infections. Applied to toenails to treat fungus infections. Not recommended for baths because it can irritate sensitive areas.

Ylang Ylang Oil (*Cananga odorata*)

Source: Flowers of the ylang ylang tree, which is found in the rain forests of Asia-Pacific Islands such as Indonesia, Philippines, Java, Sumatra, Comoro, and Polynesia. Ylang ylang means "flower of flowers" (**FIGURE 12.9**). Extracted by steam distillation of fresh flowers of the tree.

Action: Antidepressant, antiseborrheic, antiseptic, aphrodisiac, lowers blood pressure, nerve booster, sedative, sleep enhancer, and anti-infective. Effective in maintaining moisture and oil balance of the skin.

Uses: Massage, baths, infused in the air.

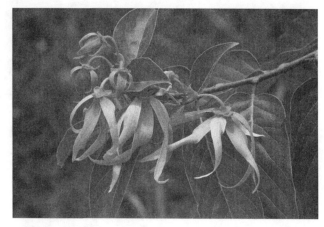

FIGURE 12.9 Ylang ylang flowers.
© Pierre-Yves Babelon/Shutterstock

Personal Note: Dr. Synovitz uses ylang ylang for this. (Be sure to test for allergic reaction.) Three to four drops of ylang ylang mixed in a ½ cup topical coconut oil is an effective measure to give moisture and bounce back to your hair. Rub the mixture onto the scalp and all over dry hair. Wrap a hot, wet towel around your head, let it sit for a half hour or so, then shampoo.

📄 *IN THE NEWS*

The following information is paraphrased and condensed from an online article from *eHow.com*.[17]

The first thing to do is gather your aromatherapy soy candle-making supplies (**BOX 12.2**). Lay the newspaper on a flat surface and place all your materials on it. Put the glue dots in the center of your jars so that you can secure the wicks, and then place the wicks on top of the glue dots. Next, heat water in the bottom pan of your double boiler. (If you do not have a double boiler, you can use two pans, placing two inches of water in the larger of the two.) Melt your wax in the top pan. Stir often to keep it from sticking to the bottom of the pan. Remove the top pan that contains the melted wax and add your dye (if using) in small increments. Stir so that the color is evenly distributed. Now, it is time to put in a few drops of EOs (5–10 per pound of wax). Mix them in quickly before the wax hardens. By this time, the wax should have begun to harden a little, and using your pouring container, you can pour the wax into your jars. You will need to hold the wicks so that they do not fall over in the jars. After the wax has been poured in and hardened, you will need to trim the wicks to about an inch from the top. If you want to make your jars attractive, tie ribbons around the mouth of the jars. Viola! You now have candles to keep or to give away as gifts. Caution: Remove the ribbons when lighting the candles so that the ribbons will not catch on fire.

BOX 12.2 Aromatherapy Soy Candle-Making Supplies

- Soy wax flakes, chips, or blocks (flakes and chips melt faster). There are approximately 20 ounces of volume per pound of wax. If your jars are 8 ounces and you want to make 8 jars, you will need 240 ounces in total. 240 divided by 20 equals 12 pounds of wax.
- EOs (5–10 drops per pound of wax)
- Wicks. Enough for one per jar. They should be trimmed to about 1 inch longer than the jar.
- Jars 8 or 16 ounces in size. Mason jars are good for soy candles. Number and size of jars will depend on the amount of wax you use.
- Newspapers
- Glue dots
- Double boiler pan
- Thermometer to measure the temperature of the wax (candy thermometer may be used)
- Pouring pot (aluminum)
- Candle dye is optional. May use liquid dyes or dye blocks.

Summarizing Essential Oils

The EOs listed and discussed earlier are the more common ones, but the list is certainly not exhaustive. If you are interested in learning about more EOs, check the reference list at the end of this chapter. In addition, see **Appendix 12.A** at the end of this chapter for several other simple aromatherapy recipes.

▶ What Are Bach® Original Flower Remedies and What Is Their History?

There are 38 bottles of tincture on the shelves of many health food stores and pharmacies that are known as the **Bach® Original Flower Remedies**. Dr. Edward Bach (pronounced Batch) was a renowned English physician and bacteriologist, who worked for years trying to find treatments that were less toxic than those he had available in the late 1920s and early 1930s. Dr. Bach (**FIGURE 12.10**) began to perceive that healing lay in nature rather than in the laboratory. In 1930, Dr. Bach gave up his practice and left London. He developed a holistic practice in which he talked to patients and comforted them.[2,18] Dr. Bach believed that disease was a manifestation of negative thoughts (fear, anxiety, jealousy, grief, frustration, despair), and the way to help and cure them was to address those negative thoughts. Dr. Bach had been trained in homeopathy, and while working at the London Homeopathic Hospital developed the seven Bach nosodes, still used

today. Nosodes are made from the discharges of diseases, but diluted so that only minute quantities or reminiscences of molecules are retained in the homeopathic solution.[2] Dr. Bach, however, wanted to develop medicines even less toxic than the nosodes.

Historical accounts relate how Dr. Bach began to use flowers as remedies for emotional disorders. One day, he strolled through the English countryside and stopped in front of several different flowers. As he was standing in front of a particular flower (such as a rose), he would feel a strong emotion, but after tasting the dew drop from the flower, the emotion would subside. He would move on to other flowers, experiencing different emotions that would subside after tasting the flower. Because of this, Dr. Bach conceived the idea that he could make liquid tinctures prepared from flowers. Over years of trial and error, Dr. Bach developed his 38 flower remedies to support every negative state of mind possibly conceived. Dr. Bach believed that if he could help rebalance his patients' emotions, then no matter what the disease condition, it would improve.

Dr. Edward Bach died in 1936 at the age of 50. He had been diagnosed with cancer some 20 years previously and finally succumbed to the disease. Before his death, Dr. Bach gave instruction that no more remedies should be formulated. Today, the Bach® Original Flower Remedies are used alone or as a supplement to homeopathy, herbalism, and aromatherapy, and the Bach Centre still thrives today in the house where he lived, Mount Vernon in Brightwell-cum-Sotwell, England.

The Remedies

The Bach® Original Flower Remedies are unique in that they are used to treat negative emotional states, not diseases, although the intent is to aid healing by treating the emotional disorder. The remedies were at one time classified into three groups: the *Twelve Healers*, the *Seven Helpers*, and the *Second Nineteen*. Currently, the remedies are classified into seven groups according to emotions (**TABLE 12.1**).

Following is a list of all the Bach® Original Flower Remedies; pictures of Remedies in the *Twelve Healers* and *Seven Helpers* classifications are featured. The use of each is paraphrased from the Bach Centre website,[18] wherein most of the explanations were developed by Dr. Bach.

- **Agrimony** (*Twelve Healers*): Used for people who keep their troubles and unhappiness hidden. They may use alcohol or other drugs to stay happy and like to be around friends, parties, and bright lights (**FIGURE 12.11**).

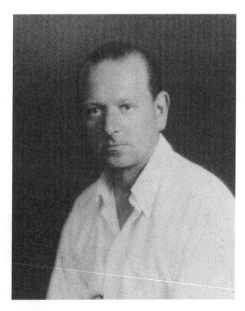

FIGURE 12.10 Dr. Edward Bach.

TABLE 12.1 The Bach® Original Flower Remedies Classified According to Emotions

Fear	Uncertainty	Insufficient Interest in Present Circumstances	Over-Care for Welfare of Others	Oversensitive to Influences and Ideas	Loneliness	Despondency or Despair
Aspen	Cerato	Chestnut Bud	Beech	Agrimony	Heather	Crab Apple
Cherry Plum	Gentian	Clematis	Chicory	Centaury	Impatiens	Elm
Mimulus	Gorse	Honeysuckle	Rock Water	Holly	Water Violet	Larch
Red Chestnut	Hornbeam	Mustard	Vervain	Walnut		Oak
Rock Rose	Scleranthus	Olive	Vine			Pine
	Wild Oat	White Chestnut				Star of Bethlehem
		Wild Rose				Sweet Chestnut
						Willow

Courtesy of The Bach Centre

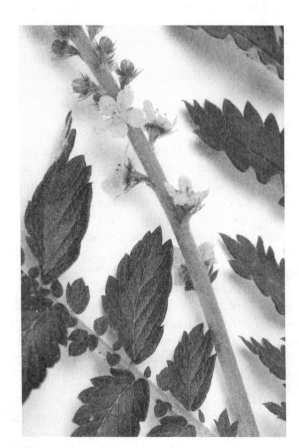

FIGURE 12.11 Agrimony.
© Kletr/Shutterstock

- **Aspen**: (*Second Nineteen*) Remedy for feeling of fear when one does not know what is causing the fear.
- **Beech**: (*Second Nineteen*) Flowers from the tree. In Dr. Bach's words, "Remedy for people who feel the need to see more good and beauty in all that surrounds them."
- **Centaury**: (*Twelve Healers*) For people who find it difficult to say no. They are usually kind, gentle people who are overanxious to serve others (**FIGURE 12.12**).

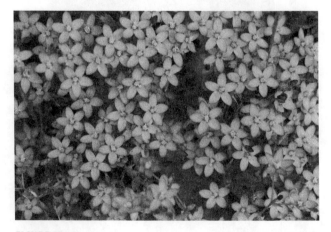

FIGURE 12.12 Centaury.
© Mauro Rodrigues/Shutterstock

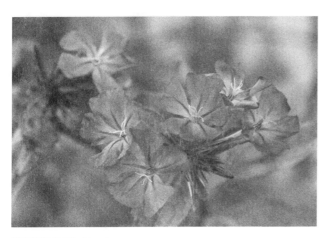

FIGURE 12.13 Cerato.
© Garden Picture Library/age fotostock

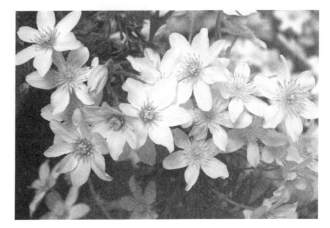

FIGURE 12.15 Clematis.
© iStockphoto/Thinkstock

- **Cerato**: (*Twelve Healers*) Remedy for people who make decisions, then question themselves or doubt if they have made the right decision (**FIGURE 12.13**).
- **Cherry plum**: (*Second Nineteen*) Flowers from the tree. Also a remedy for fear, but it is fear of losing control of oneself and doing something crazy. Cherry plum is an ingredient in Dr. Bach's **Rescue Remedy** or crisis formula.
- **Chestnut bud**: (*Second Nineteen*) Tree buds. For people who make the same mistake over and over because they have not learned the lessons of life.
- **Chicory**: (*Twelve Healers*) An aid to help someone love unconditionally rather than expecting to receive love and attention from someone after giving it. These people feel slighted and hurt if they do not get all they expect (**FIGURE 12.14**).
- **Clematis**: (*Twelve Healers*) Remedy for those who live in daydreams or whose minds drift away from reality into fantasies of the future (**FIGURE 12.15**).

- **Crab apple**: (*Second Nineteen*) Flowers from the tree. It is known as the cleansing remedy and is in the cream version of the Rescue Remedy. It is supposed to help people who have poor self-concept or self-esteem. They may not like their own personality or bodies.
- **Elm**: (*Second Nineteen*) Flowers from the tree. Remedy for people who have lost confidence in themselves or who have taken on a huge responsibility and do not feel they can handle it.
- **Gentian**: (*Twelve Healers*) Remedy for those times when people are feeling down. These people are easily discouraged, and small life delays cause doubts and the blues (**FIGURE 12.16**).
- **Gorse**: (*Seven Helpers*) Remedy for people who have given up belief and hope. Remedy for uncertainty; these people need to see things in a different light to move forward (**FIGURE 12.17**).
- **Heather**: (*Seven Helpers*) For people who do not like to be alone even though they are obsessed with themselves. Because of their need to talk about themselves, people avoid them and then

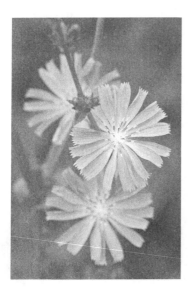

FIGURE 12.14 Chicory.
© Hemera/Thinkstock

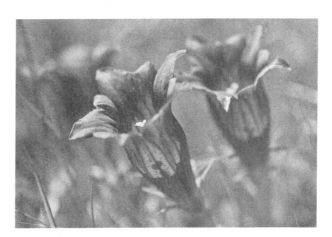

FIGURE 12.16 Gentian.
© zuender/Shutterstock

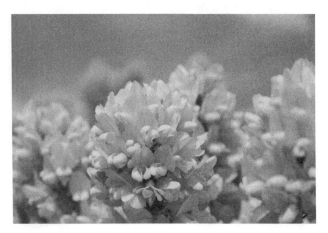

FIGURE 12.17 Gorse.
© iStockphoto/Thinkstock

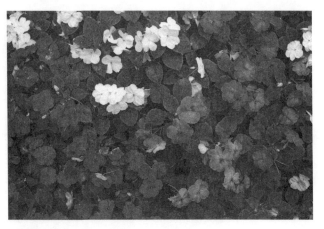

FIGURE 12.19 Impatiens.
© Jiri Sebesta/Shutterstock

they are alone, the one thing they do not like to be (**FIGURE 12.18**).

- **Holly**: (*Second Nineteen*) Remedy for negative, aggressive feelings toward others. They may feel hatred, suspicion, envy, and have an absence of love. The remedy is supposed to encourage openness and better feelings toward others.
- **Honeysuckle**: (*Second Nineteen*) Remedy for those who live in the past when they felt happy. These people believe their best days were those they lived in the past.
- **Hornbeam**: (*Second Nineteen*) Flowers from the tree. Remedy for those who feel they cannot take care of the burdens of life or daily affairs. Used to help those who feel exhausted and tired just thinking about what they have to do.
- **Impatiens**: (*Twelve Healers*) Remedy for those who are impatient and who feel frustrated and irritable. They may live life in a rush rather than in a methodical way, and they are impatient with people who are slow (**FIGURE 12.19**).

- **Larch**: (*Second Nineteen*) Cones from the tree. Remedy for people with a lack of confidence in themselves. They do not consider themselves as good as others around them, and they may expect failure.
- **Mimulus**: (*Twelve Healers*) Remedy for known fears such as fear of public speaking, getting sick, having an accident, being poor, being alone, and other misfortunes (**FIGURE 12.20**).
- **Mustard**: (*Second Nineteen*) Remedy for people who experience deep gloom or despair. They may

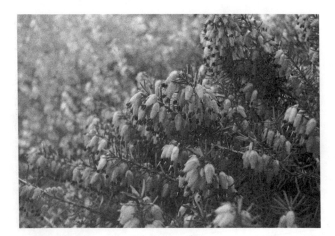

FIGURE 12.18 Heather.
© odze/Shutterstock

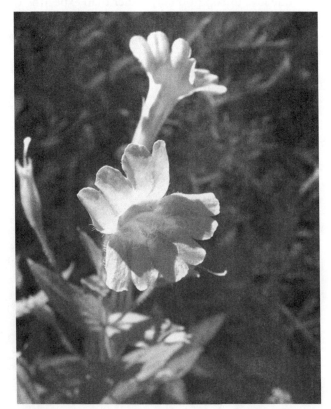

FIGURE 12.20 Mimulus.
© iStockphoto/Thinkstock

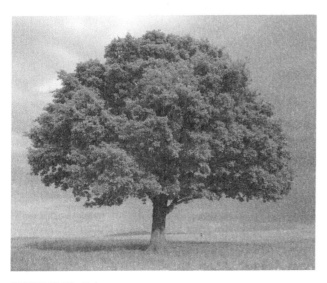

FIGURE 12.21 Oak tree.
© kosam/Shutterstock

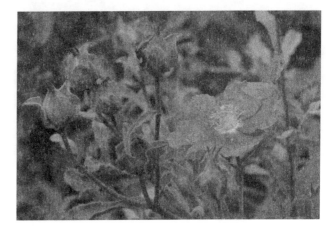

FIGURE 12.23 Rock rose.
© iStockphoto/Thinkstock

be able to state all the reasons they have to be happy, but still experience this gloom.

- **Oak**: (*Seven Helpers*) Remedy for people who are strong and steady and do not give up even when life hands them adversity. That seems very positive, but the negative side is that they do not rest or let others help them (**FIGURE 12.21**).
- **Olive**: (*Seven Helpers*) Remedy for those who have had severe mental or physical exhaustion after an illness or other tiring event. They may feel they have no strength left and no pleasure in their daily lives (**FIGURE 12.22**).
- **Pine**: (*Second Nineteen*) Remedy for people who blame themselves for an event or who may even blame themselves for mistakes made by others. They may be often asking for forgiveness even when they are not responsible.

- **Red chestnut**: (*Second Nineteen*) Remedy for those who experience fear because they are concerned or anxious about others. It can have a negative effect on the people who they are concerned about.
- **Rock rose**: (*Twelve Healers*) Remedy to help feelings of terror. It is an ingredient in the Rescue Remedy or crisis formula. This is a panicky and terror type of fear. The remedy is to help provide calm and courage (**FIGURE 12.23**).
- **Rock water**: (*Seven Helpers*) Remedy for those who deny themselves the joys and pleasures of life because it might interfere with their work. They take this self-denial to extremes and try to perfect themselves. The remedy is supposed to help people become kinder to themselves (**FIGURE 12.24**).
- **Scleranthus**: (*Twelve Healers*) Remedy for people who do not seem to be able to make up their minds or make a decision. They may end up with mood swings. The remedy is supposed to help people clarify what they want (**FIGURE 12.25**).

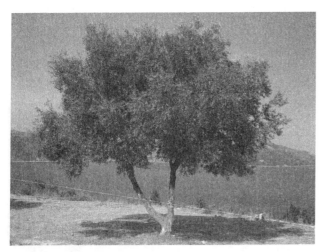

FIGURE 12.22 Olive tree.
© Irineos Maliaris/Shutterstock

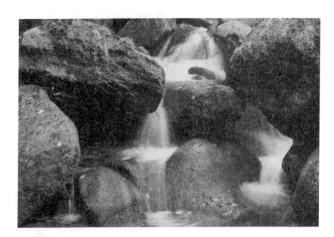

FIGURE 12.24 Rock water.
© Iafoto/Shutterstock

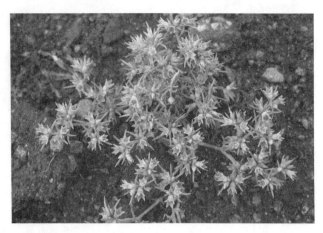

FIGURE 12.25 Scleranthus.

© Premaphotos/Alamy Images

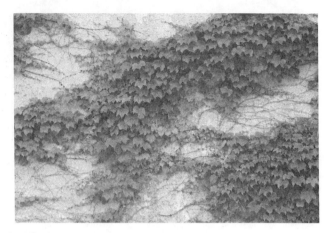

FIGURE 12.27 Vine.

© iStockphoto/Thinkstock

- **Star of Bethlehem**: (*Second Nineteen*) Included in the Rescue Remedy or crisis formula. Remedy for the aftereffects of shock that may have been caused by bad news (loss of family member or friend, car crash, etc.).
- **Sweet chestnut**: (*Second Nineteen*) Remedy for times of anguish so strong that people do not know if they can face it. This is final despair for them. The remedy is supposed to help people remain masters of their own lives and help them to renew hope and strength.
- **Vervain**: (*Twelve Healers*) Remedy for people who have rigid ideas and principles about life. They are perfectionists who try to persuade others to align their views with them. They are in danger, however, of becoming fanatics. The remedy encourages the wisdom to enjoy life, to calm themselves, and to listen to alternative views (**FIGURE 12.26**).

- **Vine**: (*Seven Helpers*) Remedy for people who know their own minds and who think they know best for others. They may try to dominate others, as tyrannical fathers or overbearing bosses. They may have a positive side from which they have the ability to make wise, gentle, and loving suggestions for others; the remedy encourages this disposition (**FIGURE 12.27**).
- **Walnut**: (*Second Nineteen*) Remedy to help protect against those times when others attempt to lead them away from their own ideas and convictions. The remedy helps protect them from outside influences.
- **Water violet**: Remedy for quiet and dignified people who are talented and capable but who seem proud and disdainful of others. The remedy is needed when a barrier appears between them and others and leaves them lonely (**FIGURE 12.28**).

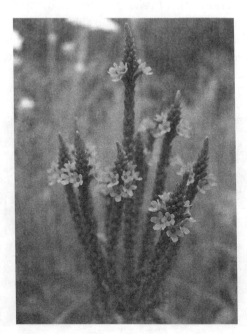

FIGURE 12.26 Vervain.

© Dale Wagler/Shutterstock

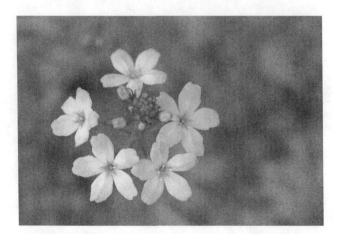

FIGURE 12.28 Water violet.

© Henk Verbiesen/age fotostock

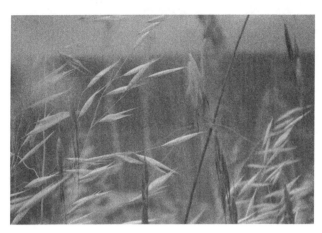

FIGURE 12.29 Wild oat.

© Hemera/Thinkstock

- **White chestnut**: Remedy for unwanted thoughts and mental arguments that cause a person to stop concentrating on other issues. The remedy helps them think more calmly and rationally.
- **Wild oat**: Remedy for people who have the ambition to do something worthwhile but do not know how to go about doing it. This remedy is supposed to help these people get in touch with their sense of purpose (**FIGURE 12.29**).
- **Wild rose**: Remedy for those who become resigned to life and do not make the effort to improve their lives or find joy. The remedy is supposed to help them reawaken their interest in life.
- **Willow**: Remedy for those who have suffered adversity and who feel resentful and bitter about their lives. They may begrudge others their success. The remedy encourages them to once again experience optimism and faith and to feel more generous about others.

Special Use of Bach® Original Flower Remedies

Rescue Remedy (also known as crisis formula) is a unique combination of five Bach® Original Flower Remedies.[3,18] The five flowers are rock rose for terror; impatiens for impatience; clematis for dreaminess or lack of interest in the present; star of Bethlehem for the aftereffects of shock; and cherry plum for fear of the mind giving way. Rescue Remedy is purported to help people cope with everyday situations such as taking an exam or driving test, the aftereffects of a bitter argument, wedding day nerves, going to the dentist, working toward a tight deadline, coping with bereavement, going for a job interview, speaking at an important meeting, fear of flying, receiving bad news, being stuck in a traffic jam, and coping with the kids. What do you think? Do you believe that one remedy can help all those emotions?

Another application of Bach Rescue Remedy is a cream called Bach Rescue Cream.[18] It is a general skin salve to soothe and restore and is supposed to help a wide range of skin conditions such as rough, flaking, or chapped skin. Bach Rescue Cream contains the same combination as Bach Rescue Remedy, but also contains crab apple, a cleansing remedy.

Choosing the Bach® Original Flower Remedies for Personal Use

Recognizing exactly how we are feeling is very important when it comes to choosing the most appropriate Bach® Original Flower Remedies for personal use. Certainly, we should carefully research all the remedies. Just as an exercise, let us talk about what you would

🔍 CASE STUDY

Michael is a college student who began feeling a lack of self-confidence that he could make it through nursing school. He has begun counseling and is learning a lot about himself. He learned that he is a worrier and is extremely fearful that he would make a nursing medical error. He also seems to need other people's permission to do and be what he wants. His mother was fine with his choice of profession, but his father wanted him to get a business degree. Michael has a quiet and sensitive nature. He has a part-time job, but his studies are getting more intense and soon he will need to do his clinical nursing practices. He could not make a decision about whether to keep his part-time job or to quit and take out more school loans. Michael's worries have led him to get irritable bowel syndrome and other stress-related conditions (e.g., his hair is thinning).

Questions:
1. List and describe all the emotions you identified when reading this case study.
2. For each emotion, which of the Bach Original® Flower Remedies might be appropriate to help Michael?

have to do to choose one of the Bach® Original Flower Remedies. First, you will have to pinpoint exactly how you are feeling at the moment or have been feeling during the past few weeks. Then, you would need to match the mood you are in with the appropriate remedy. It can be difficult to admit to ourselves some of our negative emotions—few of us want to be seen as jealous or overprotective. But, once we have admitted how we feel, we are halfway toward treating that emotion. If you find it too difficult to work out your feelings, why not ask someone who knows you well (your partner, a member of your family, or a work colleague) to describe you. With their help, you should be able to make an intelligent choice.

▶ Conclusion

This chapter has introduced you to aromatherapy and the Bach® Original Flower Remedies. If you are considering using them, please confer with your physician to be sure that the remedy or remedies will not interact with any prescription or over-the-counter drugs that you may be taking.

Wrap-Up

Key Terms

Absolutes Plant extractions that are obtained by using chemical solvents.
Aromatherapist A person trained in the use of essential oils.
Aromatherapy Means "treatment using scents"; the use of concentrated plant oils.
Bach® Original Flower Remedies Tinctures made from flowers to treat emotions rather than disease.
Carrier oils Base or vegetable oils used to dilute essential oils before applying them to skin.
CO_2 extraction High pressure is placed on the CO_2 turning it into a liquid and a solvent that can extract aromatic molecules. No solvent residue remains because the CO_2 reverts back to gas and evaporates.
Cold-pressed extraction Process involving mechanical pressure to force the oils out of citrus fruit, nuts, and seeds.
Concrete Waxy mass that remains after solvent extraction. The waxy concrete is then processed to remove the waxy materials.
Essential oils (EOs) Distilled liquid from the leaves, stems, flowers, bark, roots, or other elements of a plant.
Expression A method to extract EOs from the rinds of citrus fruit without using heat. Requires squeezing by hand and collecting oils with a sponge.
Florasols/phytols extraction A process that uses gaseous solvents to extract EOs.
Fumigation Burning of plant oils to create a great deal of smoke.
Hydrosol Floral water or distillate water that remains after distilling an EO.
Infused oil Carrier oil that has been mixed with one or more herbs.

Macerating (or soaking) Soaking aromatic plants in animal fats or vegetable oils for vacuum distillation.
Rescue remedy Five Bach® Original Flower Remedies flowers that make up a formula to treat a crisis.
Solvent extraction Process of washing blossoms with a solvent such as hexane to dissolve the non-aromatic waxes, pigments, and volatile aromatic molecules.
Steam distillation A process that involves heating the plant parts so that plant molecules evaporate, cool down, and then condense into a liquid. Water is drawn off the oil leaving a pure EO.
Vacuum distillation A process to remove alcohol and what is left behind to make the floral absolute.

Suggestions for Class Activities

1. Invite an aromatherapist to class to explain how he or she uses aromatherapy as a healing process.
2. Research the amount of money it would cost to acquire 10 aromatherapy EOs.
3. Make the aromatherapy candles in class or on your own at home. If you make them on your own, bring some samples in to show the class.
4. Make an aromatherapy treatment using a simple aromatherapy recipe found in the appendix at the end of this chapter.
5. Invite a Bach® Original Flower Remedies practitioner to discuss treatment procedures and costs.
6. If a Bach® Original Flower Remedies practitioner does not live in your area, research treatment procedures and costs and report back to class.

Review Questions

1. What does the term aromatherapy mean?
2. What are EOs?
3. What are three ways to use aromatherapy?
4. Who wrote the earliest written record of the therapeutic use of plant oils and in what year?
5. Why did early Greeks use aromatherapy for fumigation?
6. Which civilization was considered the experts in the use of EOs?
7. What aromatherapy plants were used in mummification?
8. Identify the French chemist who originated the term aromatherapy and defined the use of EOs as a discipline.
9. What are some side effects of the use of aromatherapy?
10. Name three EOs that may be safely used on babies.
11. Name and describe four of the seven ways to make EOs.
12. From which of the methods of making EOs are concretes formed?
13. What are four tips in the care and storage of EOs?
14. What are carrier oils? Give three examples.
15. Overall, what does the research show about the effects of aromatherapy?
16. What are four examples of aromatherapy oils? Please give a source, a benefit, and a use when answering.
17. How many Bach® Original Flower Remedies are there?
18. How many flowers are in the Bach® Original Flower Remedies Remedy formula?

References

1. Shealy C. N. *The Illustrated Encyclopedia of Natural Remedies.* Boston, MA: Element; 1998.
2. Bradford N. (ed.). *The One Spirit Encyclopedia of Complementary Health.* London, UK: Hamlyn; 1996.
3. Goldstein N. *Essential Energy: A Guide to Aromatherapy and Essential Oils.* New York, NY: Warner Treasures; 1997.
4. Wickell, D. Aromatherapy Foundations & Fundamentals. Class at: Prima Body LLC; June 11-12, 2011; Lake Park, FL. Accessed April 24, 2018.
5. Worwood V. *The Complete Book of Essential Oils and Aromatherapy.* San Rafael, CA: New World Library; 1991.
6. Shutes J. How Are Essential Oils Extracted? National Association for Holistic Aromatherapy. Available at: http://naha.org/explore-aromatherapy/about-aromatherapy/how-are-essential-oils-extracted/. Accessed April 24, 2018.
7. New Directions Aromatics Blog. How Essential Oils Are Made. March 20, 2017. Available at: https://www.newdirectionsaromatics.com/blog/articles/how-essential-oils-are-made.html. Accessed April 24, 2018.
8. Quinessence® Aromatherapy. Storing your Essential Oils. Available at: http://www.quinessence.com/essential-oil-storage-methods. Accessed April 24, 2018.
9. AromaWeb®. What are Carrier Oils? Available at: http://www.aromaweb.com/articles/whatcarr.asp. Accessed April 24, 2018.
10. Cook B, Ernst E. Aromatherapy: A systematic review. *Br J Gen Pract.* 2000;59(455):493–496.
11. Kiecolt-Glaser JK, Graham JE, Malarkey WB, Porter K, Lameshow S, Glaser R. Olfactory influences on mood and autonomic, endocrine, and immune function. *Psychoneuroendocrinology.* 2008;33(3):328-339.
12. Pemberton E, Turpin PG. The effect of essential oils on work-related stress in intensive care unit nurses. *Holist Nurs Pract.* 2008;22(2):97-102.
13. Sadlon AE, Lamson DW. Immune-modifying and antimicrobial effects of Eucalyptus oil and simple inhalation deices. *Altern Med Rev.* 2010;15(1):33-47.
14. WebMD. What Is Aromatherapy? Available at: http://www.webmd.com/balance/stress-management/tc/aromatherapy-essential-oils-therapy-topic-overview. Accessed April 24, 2018.
15. WebMD. Aromatherapy and Essential Oils (PDQ®): Complementary and alternative medicine - Patient Information [NCI] – Questions and Answers about Aromatherapy. Available at: http://www.webmd.com/cancer/tc/ncicdr0000458089-questions-and-answers-about-aromatherapy. Accessed April 24, 2018.
16. Organic Facts. 17 Surprising benefits of sage essential oil. Available at: https://www.organicfacts.net/health-benefits/essential-oils/sage-essential-oil.html. Accessed April 25, 2018.
17. Rogier, M. How to make a scented beeswax candle. *Our Pastimes.* September 15, 2017. Available at: https://ourpastimes.com/how-to-make-a-scented-beeswax-candle-12162933.html Accessed April 25, 2018.
18. The Bach Centre. Our founder, Dr Edward Bach. Available at: http://www.bachcentre.com/centre/drbach.htm. Accessed April 24, 2018.

Appendix 12.A

▶ Aromatherapy Recipes

Remember to do a patch test before placing any of the EOs on your body. Apply a few drops to the inside of your elbow and sole of your foot. If any irritation occurs, immediately clean it off and do not use. Some descriptions of oils in the following recipes were not described in this chapter and, therefore, are given.[1,2]

Digestive Aid Recipe

Makes 1 oz (30 ml) of abdominal massage oil.

> 7–8 drops sweet marjoram (steam distilled from an aromatic plant grown in the Mediterranean and Central European and North African countries)
>
> 22–25 drops tangerine
>
> 15 drops sweet fennel (steam distilled from crushed seeds of fennel plant)
>
> 7–8 drops peppermint
>
> 1 tablespoon (15 ml) olive oil
>
> 1 tablespoon (15 ml) grape seed oil
>
> 1 teaspoon (5 ml) sesame oil

Combine 30 drops of the EO mixture with 2 tablespoons (30 ml) of carrier oil in a 1 oz amber glass bottle.

Immune Support Foot Rub

Makes 1 oz (30 ml) of massage oil for feet after the morning shower.

> 7–8 drops geranium
>
> 15 drops Atlas cedar
>
> 22–25 drops hyssop decumbens (steam distilled from Hyssop herb)
>
> 1 tablespoon (15 ml) sesame oil

Musculoskeletal Injuries Massage Oil

Makes 1 oz (30 ml).

> 7–8 drops chamomile

¼ teaspoon plus 22 drops litsea (steam distilled from litsea cubeba fruit)

> 22–25 drops vetiver
>
> 1 tablespoon (15 ml) arnica
>
> 1 tablespoon (15 ml) St. John's Wort

Combine 30 drops of the EO mixture with 2 tablespoons (30 ml) carrier oil in a 1 oz amber bottle.

Moods and Emotions Recipe

Makes 1 oz (30 ml) of mood-balancing anointing oil.

> ¼ teaspoon plus 15–18 drops palmarosa (steam distilled from grass leaves of wild herbaceous plant)
>
> ¼ teaspoon plus 15–18 drops petitgrain (steam distilled from bitter orange plant)
>
> 2 drops rose

Put a drop on your finger and anoint the center of your chest and pulse points.

Respiration Recipe

This is an inhalation-diffusing blend recipe. Makes ½ oz. Do not use if you have asthma.

> 22–25 drops eucalyptus citriodora
>
> 22–25 drops pine
>
> 22–25 drops spruce
>
> ¼ teaspoon plus 8 drops ravensara (steam distilled from plant grown in Madagascar)
>
> (Could substitute frankincense or lavender for the pine and spruce)

Put 2-3 drops of the blend into a bowl of steaming hot water. Close eyes tightly, place towel over your head, and inhale the steam (good for colds and congestion).

> For sinus congestion, place a drop inside nostrils or on the center of your chest.
>
> You could also inhale any of the oils from their bottle or from a blend of the oils.

Skin Care Oil

Makes 2 oz of everyday body oil.

Combine 1½ teaspoons EO blend with 2 tablespoons Vitamin E and 7 oz hydrating carrier oil. Choose kukui nut, safflower, or sunflower oil.

¼ teaspoon plus 8 drops rosewood

7–8 drops sandalwood

2 drops lemon

1 tablespoon safflower, sunflower, or apricot kernel oil

½ teaspoon avocado oil

½ teaspoon vitamin E

Skin Care for the Face

Combine 20 drops of the EO blend with 2 tablespoons of a carrier blend. After washing your face, leave skin damp. Apply 2–3 drops to your fingers and rub them together.

To regenerate mature skin: Stroke skin in upward movement with Rose hip seed oil blend.

For oily skin: Jojoba. Pat on skin.

For dry skin: Avocado or olive oil. Use your fingers to spread the oil with upward strokes.

For hormone balancing and smoothing transitions of puberty or menopause: Massage lightly with evening primrose oil.

For sunburn: Rub gently with aloe vera gel.

Bath Salt Recipe (Lavender Mint Bath Salt)

Ingredients for bath salt recipe.[3]

2 cups epsom salts.

½ cup baking soda.

¼ cup sea salt (optional)

30 drops of lavender EOs.

10 drops of peppermint EO.

Mix all ingredients in a medium size bowl. Store in an airtight jar. Use 1/4th cup per bath.

References

1. Kroeger H. *Healing with Herbs A–Z.* Carlsbad, CA: Hay House; 1998.
2. Gillerman H, Arnold J. *The Essential Oils Deck: Simple Blends for Health and Beauty.* San Francisco, CA: Chronicle Books; 2009.
3. WellnessMama. How to Make Lavender Mint Bath Salts (Recipe). Available at: https://wellnessmama.com/24610/lavender-mint-bath-salts-recipe/. Updated January 28, 2018. Accessed April 24, 2018.

CHAPTER 13

Manipulative and Body-Based Therapies

As a result of reading this chapter, students will be able to:

1. Explain what chiropractic medicine is and trace the practice from its origins to its present-day place within the health care field.
2. Explain how internal philosophical conflicts within the various camps of chiropractors have impacted the entire chiropractic medicine field of study.
3. List and describe several reasons that bodywork therapies such as massage and reflexology benefit the physical, emotional, mental, and social domains of health.
4. Predict the future of chiropractic, massage, and reflexology as healing professions.

▶ What Is Chiropractic Medicine?

Chiropractic medicine is a method of treatment based on the belief that the nervous system (spinal column, nerves), skeletal system (bones, joints), and muscular system (muscles, ligaments, tendons) interact, and if that interaction is blocked, disease and/or pain will occur.[1] The chiropractic belief is that the body has an inherent ability to heal itself if nerve impulses can travel freely between the brain and the rest of the body. The chiropractic method of treatment is to relieve the blockage by using spinal manipulation or by manipulating joints throughout the body. Chiropractic doctors generally treat

people who present with neuromusculoskeletal disorders.[2] The word chiropractic is derived from the Greek words *cheir*, meaning hand, and *praktikos*, meaning done for.[3,4,5]

A major focus of chiropractic is to adjust the spinal vertebrae that surround the spinal cord to release pressure on the spine and spinal nerves that connect to and innervate the rest of the body. The term **subluxation** refers to one or more bones of the spine that have moved out of position and cause pressure on or irritate spinal nerves.[1] The chiropractic spinal manipulation or **adjustment** is a process of manipulating misaligned vertebrae or other joints in the body (e.g., wrist bones and joints) back into place.

The Origins of Chiropractic

Chiropractic care (spinal manipulation) can be traced back to 2700–1500 BCE in writings from China and Greece. Other ancient cultures, including Japan, Polynesia, India, Egypt, and Tibet, shared the concepts of basic manipulation. A variety of native North and South American cultures also practiced therapeutic manipulation, including the Aztec, Toltec, Tarascan, Inca, Maya, Sioux, and Winnebago. Even Hippocrates (460–379 BCE), the father of medicine, practiced manipulation and devoted two chapters of his text, *Corpus Hippocrateum*, to the use of manipulative procedures.[3] Later, the physician Galen (130–202 AD), who was influenced by the writings of Hippocrates, used manipulation within his practice. He was said to have used cervical manipulation to heal the paralysis of the right hand of a prominent Roman scholar, Eudemas.[3]

A form of chiropractic was practiced by people called **bonesetters**, who set the broken bones of people without conducting surgery. During the Middle Ages, bonesetting was practiced in Europe, North Africa, and Asia, where practitioners were apprenticed into the trade. Western folk medicine contains many references to "bonesetters," said to be early chiropractors, and those references contain many tales of bonesetters curing patients after doctors had failed.[4,6] Two English bonesetters, Sarah Mapp (an 18th-century bonesetter) and Sir Herbert Barker (1869–1950) became famous for their bonesetting skills.[3] Even today, in some countries such as England and Ireland, bonesetters still practice their bonesetting techniques.

Here, in the United States, Daniel David Palmer (1845–1913) founded the concept of chiropractic medicine in 1895 in Davenport, Iowa (**FIGURE 13.1**). Palmer had been a schoolteacher, a farmer, and a grocer before turning to magnetic healing, which he stayed with until chiropractic. He was a self-taught student of anatomy and physiology, at a time when many physicians had no formal medical education. One day, in a building where his office was located, he met a janitor who told Palmer he had been deaf for 17 years, ever since an occasion when he strained his back while in a small, cramped spot in a stooped position. After examining the man, Palmer found a prominent, painful, misaligned vertebra in the upper spine and convinced the man that he could help him. He used the spinous process of the vertebra as a lever and "racked" (gave a sharp thrust) the vertebra back into place.[3] The man could immediately hear again.

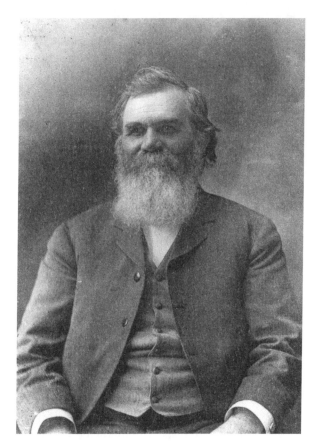

FIGURE 13.1 Daniel David Palmer.
Courtesy of Special Collections and Archives, Palmer College of Chiropractic.

Not only did Palmer have success on this one occasion, but some time later, he met a woman who had heart trouble that was not improving. After examining her spine, Palmer found a displaced vertebra that was pressing on the nerves that innervated the heart. After adjusting her vertebra, she had immediate relief from her heart symptoms. Palmer became confident that spinal manipulation could heal about 95% of all diseases.[7]

Many believe that Palmer learned manipulation from Dr. Andrew Taylor Still, the founder of osteopathy. Palmer had traveled from Davenport to observe Dr. Still's practice and had other things in common such as magnetic healing. Palmer, however, disputed that he was influenced by Dr. Still, and claimed that he learned his techniques from a person who lived in Davenport. In 1898, Palmer opened the Palmer School of Chiropractic in Davenport, Iowa; 4 years later, the school graduated four students, one of whom was his son, Bartlett Joshua (B.J.) Palmer.

Palmer had many problems as a founding chiropractor. In 1906, he was jailed for a short time (until he paid a fine) for treating people without a license. Soon after that, he sold his business to his son, B.J., who is credited with developing chiropractic medicine.

B.J. widely advertised the school, set up a correspondence program, and published two magazines. He also bought an X-ray machine and offered a course leading to a special diploma in X-ray technology. The school boasted 1,000 students by 1920.[3] During the ensuing years, chiropractic developed and changed.

Chiropractic Philosophy

Chiropractors believe that good health is determined by a healthy nervous system, particularly a healthy spinal column. The primary belief is in using natural and conservative methods of health care and to allow the body to heal itself without the use of surgery or medication.[2]

Tedd Koren, DC, wrote an article presenting a philosophical view of chiropractic and contrasted it with allopathic medicine.[8] His article stems from the philosophical roots of healing from the early writings of Hippocrates to the present. Even then, there were two conflicting views about healing. One camp was known as the Empiricists or Vitalists and the other camp was known as the Rationalists or Mechanists. Koren believes that chiropractic medicine is similar to the views of the Vitalists. The following quotes provide some of his philosophical comments. If you are interested in the full "debate," refer to the online article at www.chiro.org/links/abstracts/medical_philosophy .shtml.[8]

> "Living creatures are fundamentally different from non-living creatures," they say. "The laws of physics, chemistry, mechanics, and mathematics cannot give us a complete knowledge or understanding of biological systems because the whole body is greater than the sum of its parts." Vitalists learn how the body works by studying the living body, not isolated chemicals in a test tube or by making up theories.
>
> "The body is intelligent and reacts to the environment. Symptoms are its response to environmental stress, a sign that the body is fighting to return to its homeostatic balance. Symptoms must be permitted to express themselves so the body may cleanse and heal and return to normal balance."[8]
>
> "More important than diagnosing and treating disease, the individual's innate power of resistance needs to be strengthened so it may heal. People are chemically, emotionally, and structurally unique. When caring for a sick person, we should try to learn why that

one person is sick in his or her own unique way, and we should not generalize to other people. 100 people with cancer are, if you look closely enough, really expressing 100 unique conditions that have some things in common but many things unique to their situation. The more their care is tailored to their unique needs, the more successful the results."[8]

> "The body is essentially unknowable. It has billions of parts, each doing its own thing at a fantastic rate. The body is constantly reacting to its environment and changing moment by moment. How can anyone know what is happening at any one time to all those parts? And doesn't the very act of observing alter our results?"[8]

Chiropractic philosophy differs depending on views about chiropractic treatment. It is rooted in mystical concepts, leading to internal conflict between two camps called straights and mixers, which continues to this day. Even though there are two distinct camps of chiropractic, both believe in subluxations and the use of spinal manipulation,[9] and each of those two camps have offshoots.

Philosophy of Chiropractic Straights

There are two straight camps: **objective straights** and **traditional straights**. Objective straights focus solely on the correction of chiropractic vertebral subluxations, whereas traditional straights claim that chiropractic adjustments are a plausible treatment for a wide range of diseases.[10] Traditional straights believe in the concept of innate intelligence, which has been called a faith-based, unscientific belief, and which has led to criticism for chiropractors.[5,10,11] The traditional straights strictly adhere to chiropractic origins, limiting the scope of their practice to manual manipulations of the spine. They follow Palmer's doctrine that vertebral subluxations can either cause or contribute to most diseases and disorders. Traditional straights do not claim to be able to diagnose diseases but only that they can detect and cure subluxations. They recognize the Palmer School of Chiropractic in Davenport, Iowa, and two other schools having similar views about the use of chiropractic for treatment of disorders and also diseases. Rather than using treatment adjuncts such as heat and electricity, traditional straights use only spinal manipulation or joint manipulation to treat every sort of disease. Members see pinched nerves as the cause of dizziness, eye and ear problems, high or low blood pressure, skin disorders, hay fever, congestion, asthma, and other diseases. About 15% of all chiropractors are identified as straights.[11] The International Chiropractic Association, based in Davenport, Iowa, supports the views of the straights.

Philosophy of Chiropractic Mixers

Chiropractic mixers believe that disease can be caused by pathogens such as bacteria, viruses, fungi, and the like.[5,11] However, they believe that subluxations can lower resistance to disease or cause a neurological imbalance within the body, thus lowering resistance to disease. They use adjustments to treat back pain, neck pain, and other musculoskeletal disorders. Mixers comprise the majority of practitioners,[11] and are supported by the American Chiropractic Association (ACA) based in Arlington, Virginia. Members offer consultation, education, and various treatment modalities. Besides spinal manipulation and adjustments, mixers may use heat, light, water, electricity, vitamins, colonic irrigation, and other physical and mechanical adjuncts.

Philosophy of Reform Chiropractic

For several years, there was an offshoot of the mixers called the **reform chiropractors**. They rejected traditional Palmer philosophy and tended not to use alternative medicine methods. Reform chiropractors promoted scientific studies and practices and were considered the most biomedical of the groups.[12] They recommended chiropractic care only for musculoskeletal disorders and did not believe that spinal joint dysfunction is the cause of disease; therefore, they did not focus on subluxations only.[12,13] The association they developed was the National Association for Chiropractic Medicine (NACM), an association of chiropractors working for reform.[14] Their aim was to create a new profession called the orthopractic group.[14] However, the group was unable to influence the number of chiropractors needed to maintain their existence. At present, there is no longer a website for the NACM, and the group is now defunct.

Chiropractic Philosophy Regarding Vaccination and Fluoridation

Chiropractors have historically been opposed to vaccination and water fluoridation, based on their belief that all diseases were traceable to causes in the spine, and therefore could not be affected by vaccines.[15] They believe that the body is conditioned to fight off disease and that vaccines may be lulling people into a "false

sense of security."[16] Some chiropractors continue to be opposed to vaccination, but others are beginning to accept the practice. Many chiropractors do not promote the use or nonuse of vaccinations with their patients. If asked their view, they tell them to check with their children's pediatricians and to research vaccination information on their own.[16] Fluoridation, however, remains perhaps more controversial. Many countries in Europe are rejecting water fluoridation because they believe drinking water is not the appropriate vehicle for delivering medication. Many believe that ingesting fluoride is much less effective than topical application, and therefore, there is no need to swallow it. Another major reason against drinking fluoridated water is that there are known toxic effects.[17] Children are developing dental fluorosis or discolored teeth, and before dialysis units filtered out fluoride, people on dialysis were developing bone disease. Research is ongoing to assess any relationship to arthritis, thyroid function, and possibly osteosarcoma in adolescent males.[17]

Now that chiropractic philosophy has been presented, it is important to gain an understanding of the techniques employed by chiropractors. How do chiropractors adjust or align spinal vertebrae? Are there side effects from adjustments? Do people die from having adjustments? What does the research show? Answers to these questions follow.

The Process of Chiropractic

Occasionally, vertebrae become misaligned and place pressure on the nerves exiting the spinal cord. The misalignment of a vertebra is called subluxation. When subluxations occur, chiropractors use specific techniques to return the vertebrae into their proper positions or mobilize them so they can move freely. These techniques are called spinal manipulations or adjustments. During an adjustment, the vertebra is freed from the misaligned position and returned to the proper position in the spinal column. Once performed, chiropractors believe the adjustment allows the body to heal and maintain homeostasis.

Chiropractic Diagnosis

X-ray studies are a major diagnostic tool for chiropractors and are often used during the initial evaluation. In addition, a physical examination of the injured area is completed and a history is taken. Based upon the diagnosis, the chiropractor will formulate a treatment plan.

Chiropractic Techniques

There are a variety of chiropractic techniques. The most common technique is the chiropractic adjustment, which includes a wide variety of manual and mechanical procedures usually directed at specific joints. The adjustment may be delivered in many ways using the basic techniques: high or low velocity speed, short or long lever (direct application of force to spinous processes), high or low force, and with or without recoil.[3] The combination most used is high velocity, short lever, and low force.[3]

A direct or indirect thrust technique may be used. Different parts of the hand may be used to direct the thrust. If the neck is to be adjusted, the middle or base of the index finger may be used. If the lumbar spine is adjusted, the chiropractor may use the wrist bone to direct the thrust. If a direct thrust would be too painful, the chiropractor could use an indirect thrust by gently stretching the joint over a pad or wedge-shaped block.

The Thompson chiropractic technique involves analyzing the length of the legs and uses a drop table for adjustment. A gentle thrust is applied to the joints, which sets the drop table into motion. After the leg check analysis, the chiropractor adjusts the legs using a combination of multiple thrusts.[18]

The Cox Flexion/Distraction chiropractic technique is thought to restore range of motion in joints and muscles. It is performed on a special table that flexes and bends various muscles and joints to restore herniated discs, reduce headaches, and improve posture.[18]

One mechanical aid to chiropractic adjustment is the **activator**, a small tool that delivers a light and measured force to correct a misalignment. It gently and painlessly moves the vertebrae.[18]

The Gonstead chiropractic technique is the application of different levels of pressure to address specific misaligned joints (subluxations). It is used to increase muscle and joint mobility.[19] It is "short lever, high velocity and low amplitude" used with the chiropractor stabilizing the region above or below the area being adjusted. Several different types of chairs and tables are utilized for the Gonstead technique.[19] Many chiropractors use a drop table that drops down when an adjustment is made that allows for a lighter adjustment. Gonstead technique chiropractors might use this type of table.

Often, before the adjustment is done, soft tissue techniques may be used to relax joints or muscle tension. This could include **massage** therapy, which also serves to increase blood circulation, reduce swelling, and aid in recovery and range of motion. One type of massage therapy is a technique called **active release technique (ART)**, developed by P. Michael Leahy, a certified chiropractic sports physician.[20] It is designed to treat scar tissue adhesions that can cause symptoms such as pain, weakness, and restricted range of motion. It is also used to treat overused muscles that may have small tears or that are not getting enough oxygen. ART uses motion and hands-on muscle manipulation of the affected part. Exercises and stretches would be taught to the patients as an adjunct to this therapy.[20]

Another adjunct employed by chiropractors (and physical therapists) is dry needling. This procedure involves inserting an acupuncture needle into the affected area (trigger point area, muscle knot, or a tendon).[21] This technique seems to break up the muscle tension and tone and to promote scar tissue changes. It also serves to increase blood flow and helps the body's natural healing system.[21] Chiropractors have to become certified in acupuncture before dry needling certification. It involves over 100 hours of clinical training and passing a national board examination.[21]

More adjuncts that many chiropractors use include the following:

- **Hydrotherapy and heat therapy**: Use of hot, moist soaks or dry heat for pain relief and to promote healing. Many chiropractors use heat to loosen back muscles before giving adjustments.[1]
- **Cold therapy**: Use of ice packs to decrease swelling and relieve pain.[1]
- **Immobilization therapies**: Use of splints, casts, wraps, and traction to immobilize body parts so that the injured part may heal.[1]
- **Electrotherapy**: Use of several techniques to provide deep tissue stimulation and improve circulation.[22]
- **Galvanic stimulation**: High-voltage pulsed galvanic stimulation using direct current to stimulate deep tissue without producing tissue damage.
- **Radiofrequency rhizotomy**: Application of heated radio frequency waves to the joints' nerves.
- **Transcutaneous electrical nerve stimulation (TENS)**: Delivery of alternate current electrical stimulation through small electrodes placed inside an elastic-type belt. Usually applied to tissue by the spine before spinal adjustments by chiropractors.
- **Interferential current (IFC)**: A kind of TENS therapy in which high-frequency alternate current electrical impulses are introduced into the tissue near the pain center.
- **Ultrasound**: Use of deep heat by sound waves. Used to treat muscle pain and spasms and to reduce swelling and inflammation.[1]
- **Diet and nutrition counseling**: Chiropractors may educate people about their nutrition and lifestyle. They may give modification counseling

regarding exercise, smoking, mental stress, poor posture, improper lifting, and more.[18]

Contraindications and Adverse Effects of Chiropractic

Contraindications to having chiropractic adjustment include advanced osteoporosis, bleeding abnormalities or being on anticoagulants, or having spinal malignancy or other spinal inflammatory disease. Chiropractic side effects could include temporary headaches, tiredness, or local discomfort.[23] Serious adverse effects are reportedly rare. A 2007 study by Thiel and colleagues[24] covering 19,722 patients in the United Kingdom concluded that minor side effects such as local tenderness or soreness were fairly common, but serious adverse events were low to very low immediately or even up to 7 days post treatment.

Although rare, some serious side effects have occurred. Upper spinal manipulation could cause arterial dissection and stroke; lower spinal manipulation could cause cauda equina syndrome. The cauda equina are a bundle of spinal nerve roots that arise from the lower end of the spinal cord. The syndrome is characterized by dull pain in the lower back and upper buttocks and lack of feeling in the buttocks, genitalia, and thigh, together with disturbances of bowel and bladder function.

A study by Cassidy and colleagues[25] reinforced findings that stroke is not associated with chiropractic manipulation. The authors concluded that the increased risks of vertebral artery (VBA) stroke associated with chiropractic and primary care physicians was likely due to patients with headache and neck pain from VBA dissection seeking care before their stroke. The researchers found no evidence of excess risk of VBA stroke associated with chiropractic care as compared to primary care.

A 2015 study was conducted to assess risk of stroke in 1.1 million Medicare recipients, ages 66–99, who were treated for neck pain by chiropractors versus standard care given by primary care physicians.[26] After noting the first incidence of stroke after treatment, they found that the incidence of stroke among the entire group was very low. At 7 days, the risk of stroke was lower for those visiting a chiropractor (1.2 per 1,000), but at 30 days it was slightly elevated (5.1 per 1,000). Researchers doubted any significant difference.[26]

Training of the Doctors of Chiropractic (DC)

According to the ACA, the proper title for doctors of chiropractic (DC) is "doctor" because they are considered physicians under Medicare in an overwhelming majority of states. They are often also referred to as chiropractic physicians.

The formal training of a chiropractic physician is: Students must complete at least 3 years (90 hours) of undergraduate courses with a major emphasis on science courses. Chiropractic training then involves 4–5 years at a chiropractic college accredited by the Council on Chiropractic Education (CCE) and is certified by the U.S. Department of Education. The curriculum includes a minimum of 4,200–4,485 hours of classroom, laboratory, and clinical experience and 555 hours devoted to learning about adjustive techniques and spinal analysis. A major focus is on the structure and function of the human body in health and disease. The educational program includes training in the basic medical sciences, including anatomy with human dissection, physiology, and biochemistry. The curriculum also includes differential diagnosis, radiology, and therapeutic techniques. If interested, you can view National University of Health Sciences Doctor of Chiropractic Medicine Program curriculum online.[26] Total program credits in their curriculum totals 248.[27]

After their course of study, candidates must pass the national board exam and any exams required by the state in which they want to practice. In addition, they must meet all individual state licensing requirements. Doctors of chiropractic can both diagnose and treat patients, which separate them from nonphysician status providers. Specializations require an additional 3 years of study. Some of the postgraduate programs available include family practice, clinical neurology, orthopedics, sports injuries, pediatrics, and nutrition.

Critics' Thoughts on Chiropractic

There are those who remain critical of chiropractic. Ernst[6] conducted a narrative review of selected articles from chiropractic literature and came to the conclusion that the core concepts of subluxation and spinal manipulation are not based on sound science. He says chiropractic therapeutic value has not been demonstrated beyond reasonable doubt. During the 1960s, the American Medical Association (AMA) began a campaign to discredit the chiropractic profession, but in 1976 their efforts backfired. A source called "Sore Throat" leaked materials that revealed the AMA's tactics, prompting a Chicago chiropractor to file an antitrust lawsuit against the AMA. After a decade, the lawsuit ended. The judge on the case agreed that the AMA had acted unfairly against chiropractors. The AMA then took the case to the Supreme Court, but the appeal failed in 1990.[7] Thereafter, the AMA could not make the same claims nor discourage patients from seeing chiropractors.

Research on Chiropractic

Freeman and Lawless[3] reviewed and presented in their text several published studies from the 1980s and 1990s comparing chiropractic adjustments for treating various conditions to therapies that included heat, bed rest, soft tissue massage, hospital outpatient treatment, and physical therapy. Please refer to the Freeman and Lawless text for more details (*Mosby's Complementary and Alternative Medicine: A Research-Based Approach*).[3]

In two studies assessed in 1987 and 1999, chiropractic was found to be more effective during the first 2 weeks.[27,28] In two other studies during that time period, there was no difference between chiropractic and physical therapy results in the treatment of neck pain[29] or lower back and neck pain.[30] In 2010, Bronfort and colleagues[31] published a study that indicated positive results for some conditions and inconclusive or negative results for others. The study consisted of systematic reviews of randomized clinical trials using U.K. and U.S. evidence-based guidelines. The authors concluded that spinal manipulation/mobilization is effective in adults for acute, subacute, and chronic lower back pain; for migraine and cervicogenic dizziness; and for several extremity joint conditions. They also concluded that thoracic manipulation/mobilization is effective for acute/subacute neck pain and that massage is effective in adults for chronic lower back pain and chronic neck pain. On the other hand, they found that the evidence was inconclusive that chiropractic adjustment alone was effective for neck pain and mid-back pain for any duration, tension headaches, sciatica, temporomandibular joint disorders, fibromyalgia, and other conditions such as asthma and dysmenorrhea. They found the evidence was inconclusive regarding the effects of chiropractic care to help children who had middle ear infections (otitis media) and bedwetting (enuresis).[31]

A 2014 study involving 241 senior citizens was funded by the U.S. Department of Health and Human Services to assess the effect of spinal manipulative therapy and exercise on chronic neck pain. Results showed a 10% decrease in pain in those receiving spinal manipulation compared to those receiving home exercise only.[32] A 2015 study assessing the manual thrust spinal manipulation showed positive results. A total of 107 adults with low back pain onset during the previous 12 weeks were randomly assigned into one of the three following groups: group receiving manual thrust spinal manipulation, group receiving mechanical-assisted manipulation, and group receiving usual medical care. Results showed a statistically significant reduction in pain scores and self-reported disability in those receiving manual thrust spinal manipulation compared to both mechanical-assisted manipulation and usual medical care.[33] Although several studies have been cited, obviously there is a need to conduct future studies of the effects of chiropractic adjunct treatment combined with spinal manipulation.

The Pros and Cons of Chiropractic

The pros of chiropractic care are that it has been shown to be effective for back and neck pain, can help decrease frequency of headaches,[1] and provides benefits for several other conditions. Chiropractic does not require drugs and is considered a natural treatment. Because of the nature of chiropractic, many doctors develop close relationships with patients, and they stress educating patients about their backs and healthy lifestyles.

The cons of chiropractic care stem from those chiropractors who adhere to a philosophy that spinal manipulation can cure diseases. That has not been scientifically proven and could deter people from seeking medical advice. Chiropractors seem to have a rigorous course of study and have learned much about the neuromusculoskeletal system and body pathology, but future scientific studies need to confirm or not confirm spinal manipulation as a treatment for diseases.

In conclusion, we feel that chiropractic definitely has its place in the healing professions. It is a relatively safe and effective practice for many conditions and offers a complement or an alternative to traditional medicine or physical therapy.

One of the adjuncts to chiropractic is massage, and we present that topic next.

▶ What Is Massage?

Massage therapy is a system of manipulating soft tissue and muscles using a variety of physical methods, including applying fixed or moveable pressure, holding, vibrating, rocking, applying friction, kneading and compressing, and/or causing movement to the body. Therapists mainly use their hands, but some use their feet, forearms, and elbows. Even though craniosacral, Feldenkrais and Traeger therapies are sometimes identified as massage, manipulation of soft tissue is not their main focus, and therefore, are not included in the pure definition of massage therapy.[34] The definition of massage also excludes energy therapies such as healing touch (Therapeutic Touch), Reiki, acupressure, and **reflexology**.

Massage uses touch, a sense that most of us are especially responsive to. As an infant, a time when we are most dependent on safe handling, we rely on touch. Perhaps, as adults, when we are touched as in massage therapy, the experience may cause a memory or feeling about the touch we experienced as infants.[35]

The Origins of Massage

Massage is a therapy that has been used since ancient times in Eastern and European cultures. The word *massage* may come from the Arabic verb *mass*, meaning to touch, or from the Greek word *massein*, meaning to knead.[36] In the Far East, performers in dance and music used massage as an aid to their artistic development. In the Chinese book, *The Yellow Emperor's Classic of Internal Medicine*, written in 2700 BCE, massage of the skin and flesh was recommended. In the traditional Indian system of medicine, Ayurveda, great emphasis was placed on the therapeutic benefits of massage.[37] Egyptian tomb paintings depict people being massaged.[37] Evidence of writing about massage in India was noted during 1500–500 BCE, and even currently, massage is an important component of Ayurveda healing methods.[38]

In Europe, massage was an important practice of the Roman Empire and Greece. Hippocrates believed that all physicians should be familiar with the practice. He reported that the act of rubbing up (**anatripsis**) during massage was more effective than rubbing down, and outlined four guidelines concerning how massage should be conducted.[39] Massage schools were incorporated into Greek centers for health, called gymnasiums. In the 16th century, doctors in France praised massage as a treatment for many ailments. Massage was seen as an important part of movement therapy and gymnastics long before the practice was adopted by the medical community. In the 19th century, Swedish massage was developed by Per Henrik Ling (1776–1839), a Swedish doctor, poet, and educator. Dr. Ling was a gymnast and educator who developed the "Swedish Movement System" based on the techniques of China, Egypt, Greece, and Rome. Massage was used for the treatment of fatigue, illness, and injury. In fact, physiotherapy (physical therapy) was originally based on Ling's manual methods.[38]

Beginning in the 1970s to the present, there has been a movement to establish massage as a treatment for stress and a way to maintain health outside the medical practice; however, it has yet to receive a uniform definition by the various U.S. states. Massage therapists are licensed in 43 states and those states specify what a massage therapist may do or not do. Massage therapists are not allowed to diagnose conditions, prescribe drugs, or conduct spinal or joint manipulation.

Types of Massage

There are two main categories of massage: Western and Eastern.[40] Western massage methods tend to focus on stretching and are more soothing and calming, whereas Eastern massage methods use direct and focused pressure and are more stimulating. Eastern methods incorporate the concept of chi (qi) energy; massage is used to help chi flow through the body better.[40] Most types of massage therapy use massage lotions, soothing music, and aromatherapy. Various essential oils may be added to the massage lotion.

Western Massage

Western massage methods include Swedish massage, Esalen, and holistic massage.

- **Swedish massage** uses firm but gentle pressure to promote relaxation, ease muscle tension, and create other types of health benefits (e.g., stress relief, improvement of blood circulation).[41] Swedish massage may include deeper pressure on specific areas of muscle tension. This is called deep tissue massage.
- **Esalen massage** was developed in California at the Esalen Institute. Its staff has trained massage practitioners in the Esalen techniques, and they practice all over the world. The Esalen Institute is located at Big Sur and massage is conducted with the view and sound of waves breaking. Massages are done near the cliffside natural geothermal (hot) springs.[42] If not at the Institute, Esalen massage incorporates the sound of waves in the background, and if not close to water, uses recordings of waves breaking onto a beach or rocks. The rationale is that the ocean provides a slow-moving rhythm said to be similar to the internal rhythm of our bodies. Long, slow strokes are given to awaken awareness, and then the contact deepens and muscles are kneaded. It is said to be a wellness/stress management type of massage.[43]
- **Holistic massage** therapy claims to deal with the person as a whole. The massage therapist does not just focus on symptoms, but will attempt to address the underlying cause of the symptoms. At first consultation, the client completes a detailed health history, including what they have eaten and what they have eliminated. The massage combines kneading strokes on tight muscles with strokes to aid lymphatic drainage.[35,44]

Eastern Massage

Eastern massage includes Ayurvedic (India), tuina (China), lomi lomi (Hawaii), and shiatsu (Japan).

- **Ayurvedic massage** does not use a massage table, but rather a massage mat, usually made of reeds, placed on an Indian-style futon or cotton mattress. Massage chairs may also be used. These massages are said to provide relaxation, help circulation, and rid the body of toxins. Ayurvedic traditional Indian massage techniques are based on the Ayurvedic doshas and **marmas** (pressure points). They may also include Muslim massage techniques with pressure points called **muqame makhssos**. Massages are always given using Ayurvedic massage oils. Specific Ayurvedic massage techniques are practiced for certain disease conditions under the supervision of an Ayurvedic doctor.[45]

- **Tuina** is a bodywork therapy that has been used in China for over 2,000 years and uses the theory of the flow of chi through the meridians. Through the application of massage, chi flow is increased and allows the body to heal itself. The therapist uses hand techniques that massage soft tissues, muscles, and tendons, and uses acupressure to directly move the flow of chi. External herbal poultices, compresses, liniments, and salves may also be used.[46]

- **Lomi lomi** Hawaiian massage therapy also uses massage to increase energy flow in the body. The words *lomi lomi* mean massage. It is a unique healing massage derived from ancient Polynesians and master healers of Hawaii. The Hawaiian healing philosophy is called *Huna*, and it holds the assumption that everything seeks harmony and love. Massage is related to that philosophy through gently, yet deeply, working the muscles with loving hands. It uses continuous, long flowing strokes and relaxes the entire being. The therapist may use the forearms as well as the hands so that people who experience it say it feels like gentle waves moving over the body. The massage therapist may work on more than one part at a time (e.g., massaging a shoulder with one hand while massaging a hip with the other).[47]

- **Shiatsu** massage is a holistic type of body work and is a method to gain relaxation. In earlier days, it was mainly used within families. In this century, Japanese therapists like Namikoshi and Masunaga developed shiatsu into a professional therapy and introduced it in Europe. Shiatsu uses acupressure techniques applied with hands, thumbs, elbows, and knees. Acupressure is used to unblock meridian points where chi energy is blocked so that health and energy will be restored. The basic acupressure techniques focus on specific acupuncture points called Tsubo, which are located on the 12 meridians. Pressure is applied slowly and softly, but deeply, and it may feel uncomfortable. The client has to change positions during the massage, lying on the back, the stomach, and both sides.[48] Watsu is a form of shiatsu massage given in a therapeutic pool of water. It involves focusing on deep breathing while the massage therapist moves the client through the warm water. The therapist maneuvers the client into gentle stretches and will rock their client's body into cradle position. The therapist will then apply acupressure to the upper and lower body while continually supporting the spine.[49]

Massage Techniques

Massage is given in a flowing sequence so that one stroke blends into the next one. The first four described in the following list are used in Swedish massage, although they also may be used in other massage forms. Just enough massage oil is used to decrease friction on the skin, but not so much that the massage cannot be given deeply.

- **Effleurage** is a stroke that can blend all strokes (**FIGURE 13.2**). In effleurage, the hands are placed across the body with fingers together and thumbs slightly stretched. The stroke should be smooth, initially without pressure. The contours of the body should be followed and the skin should be smoothed toward the heart.[50]

- **Petrissage** is the act of kneading using the whole hand, with fingers together and thumbs outstretched so that the rounder contours of the body are squeezed (**FIGURE 13.3**).

- **Percussion** is lightly striking the body using different parts of the hands, keeping the wrists loose.

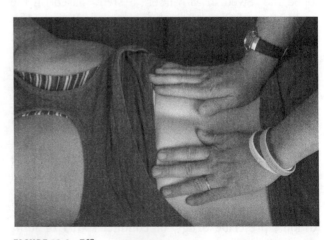

FIGURE 13.2 Effleurage.

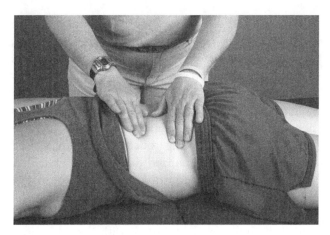

FIGURE 13.3 Petrissage.

This stroke should begin slowly and increase to moderate speed, then build to a crescendo and stop abruptly.

- **Tapotement** is a superficial form of percussion that can be carried out with great speed. It is given by tapping the body or face. It may be done by cupping, hacking, and pinching (**FIGURE 13.4**). It makes a great end to a facial massage.
- **Deep sustained pressure** up the full length of the sausage-shaped muscles on either side of the spine may be given during massage. The pressure is eased, however, at the cervical neck area.
- **Fan stroking** is done by placing hands palm side down and smoothly sliding upwards by leaning into it with a straight back. The fingers are then fanned out on both sides, slowly releasing pressure.

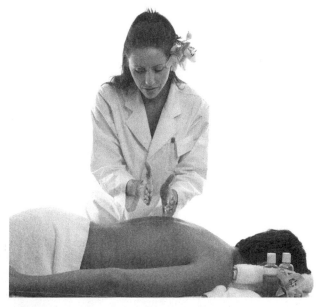

FIGURE 13.4 Tapotement.
© Hemera/Thinkstock

- **Circular stroking** is a variation of fan stroking. Both hands work on the same side at once. One hand completes a full circle motion, while the other applies a half circle. It is good for large areas like the back.
- **Thumb stroking** is used by stroking firmly upward and out using the left thumb. The stroke should be repeated higher using the right thumb.
- **Basic kneading** is done flat and smooth, just as in kneading dough. It is good for fleshy areas and for the front of the thighs.
- **Circular pressure** is applying light pressure with the thumbs in a circular motion while gradually increasing the pressure.
- **Static pressure** is good for releasing tension in the neck, shoulders, back, and feet. The thumbs are placed on the skin and the therapist leans into them, increasing the pressure. It is to be held for 10 seconds and then moved to another pressure point.
- **Cat stroking** is simply placing hands at the top of the area that is being massaged and, with very light pressure, gliding the hands down the body (like petting a cat).
- **Knuckling** is using the knuckles of the hand against the skin. The knuckles should rotate in a rippling movement in small circles on the shoulders, chest, palms, and feet.

Some therapists rock, jostle, vibrate, and/or shake their clients. Some roll, rake, and pummel the skin. Some use passive stretching. Some use aromatherapy oils or light aromatherapy candles. Some use hot stones along the muscles of the spine and some use hot or cold compresses. As you can see, massage therapists are taught many techniques, which are selectively used depending on their clients and their clients' conditions.

Training of the Massage Therapist

We have discussed many types of massage, but there are many more that we have not presented. Massage therapists can specialize in more than 80 different types of massage. Education programs vary by state, but can require 500 hours or more of study to complete. A high school degree or equivalent is a prerequisite to massage therapy school. The course of study includes anatomy and physiology, kinesiology (study of movement), and clinical massage techniques. Many states regulate massage therapy programs, and students in those states need to attend state-approved programs that may be accredited by independent agencies. After graduating, workers in states with massage therapy regulations must obtain a license prior to practicing massage therapy. They may be required to take only a state exam or one of two nationally recognized tests: the National Certification Examination for Therapeutic Massage and Bodywork (NCETMB) and the Massage and Bodywork Licensing Examination (MBLEx). A fee and periodic renewal of licensure also may be required.[51]

Benefits of Massage

Massage has physiological and psychological benefits.[52] Massage may eliminate waste products such as lactic acid from overworked muscles. Symptoms of overworked muscles are soreness, stiffness, and muscle spasms. Massage can improve circulation, bringing fresh oxygen to body tissues. It can stimulate the lymph system to rid the body of toxins. It can enhance a sense of well-being and reduce stress, and it can improve mood and sleep patterns.[52] Massage has been shown to decrease the level of lower back pain[52,53] and increase range of motion.[54]

Research on Massage

Much research has taken place to show the effects of massage therapy as a healing technique, but many studies have methodological limitations that included small sample size, inadequate control groups, lack of follow-up studies, and samples that included special patient populations. Massage is thought to be beneficial for chronic lower back pain,[52,53,54,55] as a treatment for anxiety and stress,[56,57] premenstrual symptoms,[58] and for pregnant women.[59]

Massage has been found to be beneficial in lowering blood glucose levels in children with diabetes mellitus.[60,61] A study of 598 infants by a team of researchers at the University of Warwick Medical School and Institute of Education found that massage may help infants age 6 months or younger sleep better, cry less, and be less stressed.[62] A review of 34 studies did not, however, find any significant benefits regarding several physical attributes of infants (weight/height, etc.) or mental/social development.[63] Others believe that infant massage helps in the bonding process by giving the caring touch.[64] Techniques used on infants are individualized depending on whether the infant muscles need to be relaxed or stimulated. A vegetable or plant oil such as grape seed or sweet almond oil is used because these are readily absorbed, and if the infant sucks a thumb with the oil on it, it will not be harmful. On the other hand, mineral oils are not used because they are not readily absorbed and may even be harmful. A study by Livingston and colleagues.[65] demonstrated the feasibility and safety of massage for infants with complex medical conditions. Massage was also found to create satisfaction among the caregivers, the massage instructors, and the nurses in neonatal intensive care units.

Massage has been found to be beneficial during pregnancy, but has to be conducted by someone trained in pregnancy massage to avoid pressure points that could cause uterine contractions. Massage is beneficial for relaxing anxiety during pregnancy, relieving back pain associated with muscle tension, relieving edema by stimulating circulation throughout the body, and helping promote sleep.[66] Aromatherapy oils may be used in massage lotions, but some are contraindicated during pregnancy, including arnica, clary sage, fennel, cinnamon, clove, and juniper.[67] Some of those that are beneficial are lavender, tangerine, lemon, grapefruit, eucalyptus, bergamot, Roman chamomile, geranium, tea tree, ylang ylang, and mandarin.[67]

🔍 CASE STUDY

Amy is a 54-year-old woman who has been experiencing a great deal of shoulder and neck tension. She is a computer analyst whose job requires sitting in front of a computer for long periods of time. In addition, Amy is worried about losing her job. A friend recommended that Amy should see a massage therapist, but Amy was skeptical that it could help. She felt that her problem was a pinched nerve in her neck. Eventually, Amy decided to try massage therapy.

The massage therapist took a careful history and then examined Amy's neck and shoulder. The therapist found many knots along the shoulder line and tightness in the back muscles. Simple Swedish massage and static pressure on shoulder knots was given on this first visit. Amy was instructed to do some neck and back exercises every 2 hours while sitting at the computer. Amy did feel some relief. On her next visit, the therapist began to more aggressively work out the shoulder knots. This caused Amy some discomfort but in a "good pain" way. During the third visit, the massage therapist continued to work on the shoulder knots and back muscles. Amy was feeling much better. She was trying to help herself by continuing to do her neck and back exercises and scheduled herself for regular massage therapy treatments.

Question:

1. Have you ever received a massage? If yes, why did you go? If no, why not?

📰 *IN THE NEWS*

Results of two surveys funded by the American Massage Therapy Association (AMTA)[74] found that 19% of consumers answering the survey reported they had a massage during the past year by a professional massage therapist. Respondents were 1,005 adults (504 men and 501 women) living in the United States. Top reasons for getting a massage were as follows:

- 50% for medical reasons (injury, soreness, pain relief, keeping fit, and prenatal).
- 28% for relaxation.
- 14% for pampering.
- 7% Other reasons.

Of those interviewed, 71% reported that massage therapy should be regarded as a viable healthcare procedure.

Question:

1. Have you had a massage? If yes, what could you tell your classmates about it? If not, what may be a potential barrier or reason for not getting a massage?

American Massage Therapy Association. AMTA consumer survey shows men neglecting massage therapy in past year. Available at: http://www.amtamassage.org/articles/2/PressRelease/detail/2219. Accessed September 3, 2017.

Older people also benefit from massage therapy. Many who have age-related illnesses such as Parkinson's disease, arthritis, diabetes, and heart disease gain benefits due to improved circulation of lymphatic fluid and blood.[68] In addition, the psychological impact of loving touch may help with feelings of isolation, depression, and loneliness.[68] Usually, geriatric massage is given in 30-minute sessions, and passive stretching of shoulders, legs, and feet is given along with massage. Geriatric massage improves mobility and reduces age-related stiffness.

Massage is recommended for some medically fragile individuals to improve relaxation and circulation. Techniques need to be suited to the individual so that the medically fragile person will not feel worse after the massage. The massage time may need to be shortened and the pressure may need to be light.[69] The hallmark thought is "less is better." Providing comfort for the patient is the ultimate goal. To do this, the hands of the massage therapist must be gentle, soothing, nurturing, comforting, calming, restful, simple, slow, nonjudgmental, and spacious.[69]

A review by the Agency for Healthcare Research and Quality on CAM practices for back and neck pain showed that massage significantly reduced the intensity of acute or subacute lower back pain compared with a placebo, but did not show a difference for chronic (long term) back pain.[70] A study of a single session of Swedish massage on hypothalamic–pituitary–adrenal and immune function produced measurable biologic effects and may have implications for managing inflammatory and autoimmune conditions.[71]

A randomized study to assess therapeutic massage benefits for chronic neck pain found that subjects receiving massage had a reduction in neck pain compared with a control group receiving a self-care book.[72] Massage therapy compared with simple touch

therapy was more effective in reducing pain and improving mood in patients with advanced cancer.[73]

It seems that several studies have shown efficacy of massage for select conditions, but most of the research scientists recommend continuing research.

The next section describes a practice known as reflexology, which physical therapists as well as massage therapists use. The most skilled practitioner, however, is known as a reflexologist.

▶ What Is Reflexology?

Reflexology is a form of massage that involves applying pressure to points on the feet, hands, and ears. The theory of reflexology is that the body is divided into 10 energy loops that start at and then return to the hands and feet. By stimulating the origins of these loops in the feet or hands, reflexologists believe that the pressure will cause a response in any of the organs or systems found within that particular loop. It is a holistic and relaxing therapy that is thought to balance homeostasis within the body and to boost the immune system.

The body is believed to be mirrored in the shape of the feet, so if you are lying down with your feet together, heels resting on the floor and toes pointed toward the ceiling, the shape of your feet would match the outline of your body. Pressure on certain points of the feet, hands, and ears are thought to heal parts of the body that correspond to the pressure points.

The Origins of Reflexology

Reflexology techniques can be traced back 5,000 years to ancient Egypt, India, and China. During the time of the Egyptian Sixth Dynasty (2323–2150 BCE), a high-ranking official, Ankhmahor, was buried in the ancient burial ground at Saqqara.[75,76] Pictographs (hieroglyphs) display multiple scenes of people undergoing medical treatment and work on hands and feet. Another Egyptian pictograph was found in the temple of Amon at Karnak, which was built during Ramses II's reign (1279–1213 BCE), and depicts a "healer tending to the feet of foot soldiers at the battle of Qadesh."[75,76] From observations of pictographs in the Americas (Latin America), the Incas practiced what is thought to be reflexology and the practice is believed have been passed down to North American Indian tribes (Cherokee) sometime in the 17th century. Tribes practiced zone therapy or reflexology to cure themselves of various diseases.[75,76,77]

In 1900, William Fitzgerald, a medical physician, introduced zone therapy to the United States. He researched zone therapy practiced by individuals in the United Kingdom and the Cherokee tribes and based the practice on those studies.[78,79] In zone therapy, the body is divided into 10 vertical zones, running from the tips of the toes to the top of the head. He wrote and published a book called *Zone Therapy*. Fitzgerald shared his knowledge with Dr. Joe Riley, a chiropractor, who began to apply pressure to his patients' feet and hands to relieve pain in other parts of their bodies. Through Riley, Eunice Ingham, a physiotherapist, began to use zone therapy on her patients (**FIGURE 13.5**). Ingham noticed her patients' healing time improved and developed the theories into a manual therapy.[79]

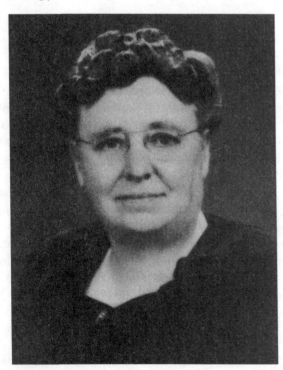

FIGURE 13.5 Eunice Ingham.

Courtesy of International Institute of Reflexology, www.reflexology-usa.net

Ingham renamed zone therapy as "reflexology," and mapped out the feet's reflex zones into charts that are still used today (**FIGURE 13.6**). Ingham also discovered that applying pressure to reflex points could have a much wider effect on the body than just pain relief.[78,79] In 1938, Ingham published her findings in her first book, *Stories the Feet Can Tell*, and in 1951, she wrote *Stories the Feet Have Told*.

Reflexology Techniques

Reflexology is a gentle, noninvasive technique with no known side effects and is complementary to other medical therapies such as chiropractic, acupuncture, and massage. It can be an avenue to increasing human touch, which is a basic human need. No special equipment is needed and it can be performed anywhere.

The practitioner applies pressure to the hands or feet, moving them back and forth and stretching them (**FIGURE 13.7**). A typical session will last about 30–60 minutes. If practicing on the feet, only the shoes and socks need to be removed. Using foot reflexology as an example, the basic technique uses the following steps[80]:

1. The client sits down with feet resting on a support.
2. The feet are bathed before the treatment. Rose water is often used because it helps to soothe the feet, and clients feel they are being pampered when their feet are bathed.
3. The reflexologist positions the feet close to each other and imagines looking at a map of the body.
4. Various points on the feet are pressed to stimulate the circulation.
5. Pressure is applied from the big toe down the foot, moving from side to side.

The reflexologist will hold the foot firmly and steadily. Sometimes, clients feel uncomfortable or they may feel ticklish.

Oil is not used for reflexology because the fingers may slip and cause extra pressure or pain. Instead, a light dusting of talcum powder is used on the foot. Sometimes, the reflexologist may feel tiny crystals under the skin and will record those on a piece of paper. To the reflexologist, it means that a particular area of the body may need special attention.

Training of the Reflexologist

Massage therapists receive some reflexology training, and many use it in their practices. Physical therapists also use reflexology. There are no licensing laws requiring special reflexology training, but it may allow a

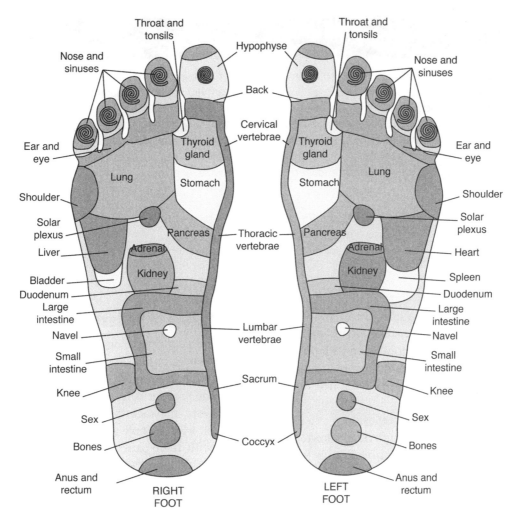

FIGURE 13.6 Foot reflexology chart.

© Peter Gardiner/Photo Researchers, Inc.

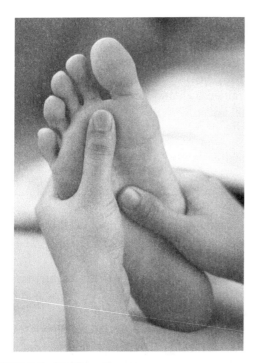

FIGURE 13.7 Reflexology therapy.

© Hywit Dimyadi/Shutterstock

practitioner to be more effective. A national education standard has been set by the American Reflexology Certification Board (ARCB).[81] The ARCB provides a written and practical examination for certification in both hands and feet. The training course consists of 110 hours of hands-on training: 40 hours in reflexology history and theory, 55 hours of anatomy and physiology, 5 hours of business ethics and standards, and 10 hours of supervised practicum. Upon graduating from such a course, an additional 90 hours of postgraduate sessions are required, bringing the total number of hours to 200 for national certification.[81]

Research on Reflexology

Reflexology has been shown to be effective on anxiety and pain in 23 patients with breast and lung cancer.[82] The majority of the sample were female, white, and age 65 or older. Following foot reflexology, those with breast and lung cancer experienced a significant decrease in anxiety, and patients with breast cancer showed a decrease in pain levels. Ear, hand, and foot

🔍 CASE STUDY

Susan is 45 years old, divorced, has two children, and works two part time jobs to make it financially. During the last year, Susan has been suffering with migraine headaches. A friend said that her migraine headaches had been helped after she started getting reflexology treatments. Since Susan had been trying conventional medical treatments that had not helped, she made an appointment to see a reflexologist. At the initial consultation, Susan revealed that she had a history of migraine headaches. They had stopped during pregnancy with her second child 10 years ago, but had returned approximately a year ago. During the past few months, she was getting them more often. After 3 months of a series of reflexology treatments on both her hands and feet, Susan was no longer experiencing migraine headaches.

Questions:

1. What do you think might be some reasons for the return of Susan's migraine headaches?
2. How could reflexology help Susan's migraine headaches?
3. What other reasons could explain her apparent recovery?

reflexology were shown to be effective in a randomized controlled study of 35 women with premenstrual symptoms.[83] Compared to women with placebo treatment, there was a significantly greater decrease in premenstrual symptoms for women given true reflexology treatment.

Two studies did not support reflexology as a treatment for either lower back pain or irritable bowel syndrome (IBS). In a randomized controlled study for the management of chronic lower back pain, 243 patients were assigned to one of three groups: reflexology, relaxation, or usual care. No significant differences were found among the groups on pre- and post-test lower back pain measures.[84] In the second study, reflexology was not shown effective in a single blind trial for 34 patients diagnosed with IBS.[85] Some patients were assigned to a reflexology massage and some were assigned to a nonreflexology massage. Abdominal pain, constipation/diarrhea, and abdominal distention were monitored. There was no significant difference between the reflexology group and the control group.[85]

The Future of Reflexology

The effects of reflexology in some of the clinical studies are encouraging. Some medical staff have taken up reflexology training to use as a complementary therapy. The practice is favorably received among physical therapists, massage therapists, and the nursing profession. More people are seeking out reflexologists to help with their pain conditions and body disorders. Because of these reasons, it seems that the future of reflexology is promising.

▶ Conclusion

We hope this chapter has given you a better understanding of the manipulative-based therapies of chiropractic, massage, and reflexology. If you are considering a treatment using one or more of these modalities, be sure to select a practitioner who has been trained well and who is licensed or certified for their field of study.

Wrap-Up

Key Terms

Activator A small tool that delivers a light and measured force to correct a misalignment.

Active release technique (ART) Technique designed to treat scar tissue adhesions, which can cause symptoms such as pain, weakness, and restricted range of motion. It is also used to treat overused muscles that may have small tears or are not getting enough oxygen.

Adjustment A process of manipulating misaligned vertebrae or other joints in the body (e.g., wrist bones and joints) back into place.

Anatripsis The act of rubbing up during massage.

Bonesetters People who set the broken bones of people without conducting surgery.

Chiropractic medicine A method of treatment based on the belief that the nervous system, skeletal system, and muscular system interact, and if that interaction is blocked, disease and/or pain will occur.

Chiropractic mixers Believe that subluxations can lower resistance to disease or cause a neurological imbalance within the body, thus lowering resistance to disease. They would use adjustments to treat back pain, neck pain, and other musculoskeletal disorders.

Reform chiropractic Reform chiropractors promote scientific studies and practices and are considered the most biomedical of the groups. Recommend chiropractic care only for musculoskeletal disorders. The group no longer functions.

Effleurage Massage using contours of the body; uses a smooth stroke.

Galvanic stimulation High-voltage pulsed galvanic stimulation using direct current to stimulate deep tissue without producing tissue damage.

Hydrotherapy and heat therapy Use of hot, moist soaks or dry heat for pain relief and to promote healing.

Immobilization therapies Use of splints, casts, wraps, and traction to immobilize body parts so that the injured part may heal.

Interferential current (IFC) A kind of TENS therapy in which high-frequency alternate current electrical impulses are introduced into the tissue near the pain center.

Marmas Ayurvedic massage pressure points.

Massage May come from the Arabic verb *mass*, meaning to touch, or from the Greek word *massein*, meaning to knead. It is manipulating soft tissue and muscles using a variety of physical methods, including applying fixed or moveable pressure, holding, vibrating, rocking, applying friction, kneading and compressing, and/or causing movement to the body.

Muqame makhssos Muslim massage pressure points.

Objective straights Focus only on the correction of chiropractic vertebral subluxations.

Petrissage The act of kneading using the whole hand, with fingers together and thumbs outstretched so that the rounder contours of the body are squeezed.

Radiofrequency rhizotomy Application of heated radio frequency waves to the joints' nerves.

Reflexology A form of massage that involves applying pressure to points on the feet, hands, and ears.

Subluxation Refers to one or more bones of the spine that have moved out of position and are causing pressure on or irritating spinal nerves.

Tapotement Massage that is given by tapping the body or face. It may be done by cupping, hacking, and pinching.

Traditional straights Claim that chiropractic adjustments are a plausible treatment for a wide range of diseases.

Transcutaneous electrical nerve stimulation (TENS) Delivery of electrical stimulation through small electrodes placed inside an elastic-type belt. Usually applied to the tissue by the spine before spinal adjustments by chiropractors.

Ultrasound Use of deep heat by sound waves to treat muscle pain and spasms and to reduce swelling and inflammation.

Suggestions for Class Activities

1. Invite a chiropractor to class. Ask questions of the chiropractor about his or her philosophical beliefs and what chiropractic "camp" they belong to. Also ask about their educational background, the cost of treatments, and whether they use any adjuncts to chiropractic.
2. Invite a massage therapist to class. Ask the therapist to show class participants some simple massage techniques. Practice on each other.
3. Invite a reflexologist to class. Ask the therapist to show class participants some reflexology movements. Practice on each other.

Review Questions

1. What was the origin of chiropractic medicine?
2. Define the terms "subluxation" and "adjustment."
3. Who was the founder of chiropractic in the United States?
4. What is the difference between chiropractic and osteopathic medicine?
5. What is the overall chiropractic philosophy?
6. What is the difference in chiropractic philosophy among the straights, the mixers, and the reform group?
7. What are the Thompson, Gonstead, and Cox Flexion/Distraction chiropractic techniques?
8. What is the active release technique (ART)?
9. Name three contraindications to chiropractic adjustment.
10. What is the training of a chiropractic doctor?
11. What do the critics say about chiropractic?
12. For which conditions does research show that chiropractic is effective and for which has research shown it to be ineffective?
13. What does the word massaged mean?
14. Name several physical methods used during massage.
15. What are the two major categories of massage and what are their philosophical differences?
16. Describe Swedish, Esalen, and holistic massage.
17. Name the four Eastern massage therapies and their countries of origin.

18. Describe tuina and lomi lomi massage therapy.
19. How does a practitioner perform shiatsu?
20. What is effleurage, petrissage, and tapotement?
21. What is the origin of reflexology and what individuals are responsible for its development as a therapy today?
22. What professions use reflexology?

References

1. Pelletier K. *The Best Alternative Medicine: What Works? What Does Not?* New York, NY: Simon & Schuster; 2000.

2. American Chiropractic Association. What is Chiropractic? Available at: https://www.acatoday.org/Patients/Why-Choose-Chiropractic/What-is-Chiropractic. Accessed April 24, 2018.

3. Freeman LW, Lawlis GF. *Mosby's Complementary and Alternative Medicine: A Research-Based Approach.* St. Louis, MO: Mosby; 2001.

4. Bradford N (ed.). *The One Spirit Encyclopedia of Complementary Health.* London, UK: Hamlyn; 1996.

5. Somerville R (ed.). *The Alternative Advisor.* Alexandria, VA: Time Life Books; 1997.

6. Ernst E. *The Desktop Guide to Complementary and Alternative Medicine: An Evidence-Based Approach.* New York, NY: Mosby; 2001.

7. Singh S, Ernst E. *Trick or Treatment: The Undeniable Facts About Alternative Medicine.* New York, NY: Norton; 2008.

8. Koren T. Medical Philosophy vs. Chiropractic Philosophy. Available at: http://www.chiro.org/LINKS/ABSTRACTS/Medical_Philosophy.shtml. Published March 14, 2003. Accessed April 24, 2018.

9. Ernst E. Chiropractic: A critical evaluation. *J Pain Symptom Manage.* 2008;35(5):544-562.

10. Strauss J. Position Paper #1-Objective Straight Chiropractic (OSC). Chiropractic Outside the Box. June 11, 2014. Available at: http://chiropracticoutsidethebox.com/2014/06/11/position-paper-1-objective-straight-chiropractic-osc/. Accessed April 24, 2018.

11. Holisticonline.com. Chiropractic: Two Schools of Chiropractors. Available at: http://www.holistic-online.com/Chiropractic/chiro_straight-and-mixers.htm. Accessed August 24, 2018.

12. Wikipedia. National Association for Chiropractic medicine. Available at: https://en.wikipedia.org/wiki/National_Association_for_Chiropractic_Medicine. Accessed April 26,2018.

13. Bellamy JJ. White paper: Chiropractic. Institute for Science in Medicine. Available at: https://www.chirobase.org/01General/ism.pdf. Published August 2012. Accessed April 26, 2018.

14. Editorial Staff. No more NACM. *Dynamic Chiropractic.* 2010; 28(8). Available at: http://www.dynamicchiropractic.com/mpacms/dc/article.php?id=54548. Published April 9, 2010. Accessed April 24, 2018.

15. Campbell JB, Busse JW, Injeyan HS. Chiropractors and vaccination: A historical perspective. *Pediatrics.* 2000;105(4).

16. Lombroso L. Some chiropractors turn their backs on vaccines. *USA Today.* February 17, 2015. Available at: https://www.usatoday.com/story/news/nation/2015/02/17/some-chiropractors-turn-their-backs-on-vaccines/23582549/. Accessed April 24, 2018.

17. Total Health. Water Fluoridation – Outdated, Unnecessary and Dangerous. September 14, 2013. Available at: http://www.totalhealthchiropractic.com.sg/water-fluoridation-outdated-unnecessary-and-dangerous/. Accessed April 24, 2018.

18. ChiropractorGuide.com. Understanding Chiropractic Technique. Available at: http://www.chiropractorguide.com/alternatives/understanding-chiropractic-techniques.html. Accessed April 24, 2018.

19. ChiroAccess. Technique Summary: Gonstead Technique. February 8, 2010. Available at: http://www.chiroaccess.com/Articles/Technique-Summary-Gonstead-Technique.aspx?id=0000128. Accessed April 24, 2018.

20. Dr. Axe Food is Medicine. 5 Active Release Technique Benefits, Including Lowered Pain & Increased Performance. Available at: https://draxe.com/active-release-technique/. Accessed April 24, 2018.

21. Premier Sports and Spine Center. Dry Needling Therapy and Acupuncture. Available at: https://premiersportsandspine.com/dry-needle-therapy/. Accessed April 24, 2018.

22. ChiroFind. Chiropractic Tools and Techniques. Available at: http://www.chirofind.com/resources/chirotools.php. Accessed April 24, 2018.

23. National Center for Complementary and Integrative Health. Chiropractic: In Depth. Available at: https://nccih.nih.gov/health/chiropractic/introduction.htm#hed6. Updated February 2012. Accessed April 24, 2018.

24. Thiel HW, Bolton JE, Docherty S, Portlock JC. Safety of chiropractic manipulation of the cervical spine: A prospective national survey. *Spine.* 2007;32(21):2375-2378.

25. Cassidy JD, Boyle E, Côté P, et al. Risk of vertebrobasilar stroke and chiropractic care: Results of a population-based case-control and case-crossover study. *J Manipulative Physiol Ther.* 2009;32(2 Suppl):S201-S208.

26. Whedon JM, Song Y, Mackenzie TA, Phillips RB, Lukovits TG, Lurie JD. Risk of stroke after chiropractic spinal manipulation in medicare B beneficiaries aged 66 to 99 years with neck pain. *J Manipulative Physiol Ther.* 2015;38(2):93-101.

27. National University of Health Sciences. Doctor of Chiropractic Medicine Program. Available online at: http://www.nuhs.edu/academics/college-of-professional-studies/chiropractic-medicine/curriculum/trimester-by-trimester/. Accessed April 24, 2018.

28. Mathews JA, Mills SB, Jenkins VM, et al. Back pain and sciatica: Controlled trials of manipulation, traction, sclerosant and epidural injections. *Br J Rheumatol.* 1987; 26(6):416-423.

29. Andersson GB, Lucente T, Davis AM, Kappler RE, Lipton JA, Leurgans S. A comparison of osteopathic spinal manipulation with standard care for patients with low back pain. *N Engl J Med* 1999;341(19):1426-1431.

30. Jordan A, Bendix T, Nielsen H, Hansen FR, Høst D, Winkel A. Intensive training, physiotherapy, or manipulation for patients with chronic neck pain: A prospective, single-blinded, randomized clinical trial. *Spine.* 1998;23(3): 311-318.

31. Bronfort G, Haas M, Evans R, Leininger B, Triano J. Effectiveness of manual therapies: The UK evidence report. *Chiropr Osteopat.* 2010;18:3.

32. Maiers M, Bronfort G, Evans R, et al. Spinal manipulative therapy and exercise for seniors with chronic neck pain. *Spine J.* 2014;14(9):1879-1889.

33. Schneider M, Haas M, Glick R, Stevans J, Landsittel D. Comparison of spinal manipulation methods and usual medical care for acute and subacute low back pain: A randomized clinical trial. *Spine.* 2015;40(4):209-217.

34. University of Minnesota. Massage therapy. Available at: http://www.takingcharge.csh.umn.edu/explore-healing-practices/massage-therapy. Accessed April 24, 2018.

35. Mitchell S. *The Complete Illustrated Guide to Massage: A Step-by-Step Approach to the Healing Art of Touch*. Boston, MA: Element; 1997.

36. Calvert R. *The History of Massage: An Illustrated Survey from Around the World*. Rochester, VT: Healing Arts Press; 2002.

37. All Allied Health Schools. The history of Massage Therapy. Available at: http://www.allalliedhealthschools.com/massage-therapist/massage-therapy-history/. Accessed April 24, 2018.

38. WorldwideHealth.com. What is Holistic Massage Therapy? Available at: http://www.worldwidehealth.com/health-article-What-is-Holistic-Massage-Therapy.html. Accessed April 24, 2018.

39. Greek Medicine. Massage and Bodywork. Available at: http://www.greekmedicine.net/therapies/Massage_and_Bodywork.html. Accessed April 24, 2018.

40. Alternative Healthcare Solutions. The differences between Eastern and Western massage techniques. Available at: http://www.thermocaresolutions.com/the-differences-between-eastern-and-western-massage-techniques/. Published July 6, 2015. Accessed April 24, 2018.

41. Brown A. The Swedish massage: Full body therapy. *Trip Savvy*. Available at: http://spas.about.com/od/swedishmassage/a/Swedish.htm. Updated February 5, 2018. Accessed April 24, 2018.

42. Esalen. Available at: https://www.esalen.org/. Accessed April 24, 2018.

43. The Healing Art of Deep Bodywork®. Esalen® Massage. Available at: http://www.deepbodywork.com/about/esalen-massage/. Accessed April 24, 2018.

44. MassageTherapy.com. Dimensions of holistic massage. Available at: http://www.massagetherapy.com/articles/index.php/article_id/1830/Dimensions-of-Holistic-Massage. Accessed April 24, 2018.

45. Sanatan Society. Ayurvedic massage. Available at: http://www.sanatansociety.org/ayurvedic_massage.htm#.Wa8DmHeGNBw. Accessed April 24, 2018.

46. Pacific College of Oriental Medicine. Tui Na Massage. Available at: https://www.pacificcollege.edu/news/blog/2014/10/26/tui-na-massage. Accessed April 24, 2018.

47. Lakainapali T. Hawaiian Lomi Lomi Massage. Available at: http://www.huna.org/html/lomilomi.html. Accessed April 24, 2018.

48. Dharmananda S. Zen Shiatsu: The Legacy of Shizuto Masunaga. Available at: http://www.itmonline.org/arts/shiatsu.htm. Published September 2002. Accessed April 24, 2018.

49. Massage Therapy 101©. Watsu. Available at: http://www.massagetherapy101.com/massage-techniques/watsu.aspx. Accessed April 24, 2018.

50. Healthepic.com Basic Technique. Available at: http://www.healthepic.com/massage/static/massabasic.htm. Accessed April 24, 2018.

51. Bureau of Labor Statistics, Occupational Outlook Handbook. Massage Therapists. Available at: https://www.bls.gov/ooh/healthcare/massage-therapists.htm. Updated April 13, 2018. Accessed April 24, 2018.

52. Cherkin DC, Sherman KJ, Deyo RA, Shekelle PG. A review of the evidence for the effectiveness, safety, and cost of acupuncture, massage therapy, and spinal manipulation for back pain. *Ann Intern Med*. 2003;138(11):898-906.

53. Furlan AD, Brosseau L, Imamura M, Irvin E. Massage for low back pain. *Cochrane Database Syst Rev*. 2002;(2):CD001929.

54. Hernandez-Reif M, Field T, Krasnegor J, Theakston H. Lower back pain is reduced and range of motion increased after massage therapy. *Int J Neurosci*. 2001;106(3-4):131-145.

55. Preyde M. Effectiveness of massage therapy for subacute low-back pain: A randomized controlled trial. *CMAJ*. 2000;162(13):1815-1820.

56. Ferrell-Torry AT, Glick OJ. The use of therapeutic massage as a nursing intervention to modify anxiety and the perception of cancer pain. *Cancer Nurs*. 1993;16(2):93-101.

57. Sherman KJ, Ludman EJ, Cook AJ, et al. Effectiveness of therapeutic massage for generalized anxiety disorder: A randomized controlled trial. *Depress Anxiety*. 2010;27(5):441-450.

58. Hernandez-Reif M, Martinez A, Field T, Quintero O, Hart S, Burman I. Premenstrual symptoms are relieved by massage therapy. *J Psychosom Obstet Gynaecol*. 2000;21(1):9-15.

59. Field T, Hernandez-Reif M, Hart S, Theakston H, Schanberg S, Kuhn C. Pregnant women benefit from massage therapy. *J Psychosom Obstet Gynaecol*. 1999;20(1):31-38.

60. Field T, Hernandez-Reif M, LaGreca A, Shaw K, Schanberg S, Kuhn C. Massage therapy lowers blood glucose levels in children with diabetes mellitus. *Diabetes Spectrum*. 1997;10:237-239.

61. Sajedi F, Kashaninia Z, Hoseinzadeh S, Abedinipoor A. How effective is Swedish massage on blood glucose level in children with diabetes mellitus? *Acta Med Iran*. 2011;49(9):592-597.

62. Warwick News & Events. Research says massage may help infants sleep more, cry less and be less stressed. Available at: http://www2.warwick.ac.uk/newsandevents/pressreleases/ne1000000231138/. Published November 8, 2006. Accessed April 24, 2018.

63. Bennett C, Underdown A, Barlow J. Massage for promoting mental and physical health in typically developing infants under the age of six months. Cochrane Database of Systematic Reviews. Available at: http://onlinelibrary.wiley.com/doi/10.1002/14651858.CD005038.pub3/abstract;jsessionid=BAEEF9FA7BFAE7EA69F68CB6A4E34AB9.f03t02. Published April 30, 2013. Accessed April 24, 2018.

64. Sinclair A. Infant Massage. Childbirth Solutions. Available at: http://childbirthsolutions.com/postpartum/infant-massage/. Accessed April 24, 2018.

65. Livingston K, Beider S, Kant AJ, Gallardo CC, Joseph MH, Gold JI. Touch and massage for medically fragile infants. *Evid Based Complement Alternat Med*. 2009;6(4):473-482.

66. American Pregnancy Association. Massage and Pregnancy – Prenatal Massage. Available at: http://americanpregnancy.org/pregnancy-health/prenatal-massage/. Accessed April 24, 2018.

67. Fit Pregnancy. Essential Oils: Essential oils that are safe during pregnancy and which ones to avoid. Available at: https://www.fitpregnancy.com/gear/maternity-fashion/essential-oils. Accessed April 24, 2018.

68. Massage Envy. Geriatric Massage. Available at: https://www.massageenvy.com/massage/massage-types/geriatric-massage/. Accessed April 24, 2018.

69. MacDonald G. *Massage for the Hospital Patient and Medically Frail Client*. Philadelphia, PA: Lippincott Williams & Wilkins; 2004.

70. Furlan A, Yazdi F, Tsertsvadze A, et al. *Complementary and Alternative Therapies for Back Pain II*. Rockville, MD: Agency for Healthcare Research and Quality; 2010. Available at: http://www.ncbi.nlm.nih.gov/books/NBK56295/. Accessed April 24, 2018.

71. Rapaport MH, Schettler P, Bresee C. A preliminary study of the effects of a single session of Swedish massage on

hypothalamic-pituitary-adrenal and immune function in normal individuals. *J Altern Complement Med.* 2010; 16(10):1079-1088.

72. Sherman KJ, Cherkin DC, Hawkes RJ, Miglioretti DL, Deyo RA. Randomized trial of therapeutic massage for chronic neck pain. *Clin J Pain.* 2009;25(3):233-238.

73. Kutner JS, Smith MC, Corbin L, et al. Massage therapy versus simple touch to improve pain and mood in patients with advanced cancer: A randomized trial. *Ann Intern Med.* 2008;149(6):369-379.

74. Newswise. AMTA consumer survey shows men neglecting massage therapy in past year. *Massage Magazine.* September 23, 2010. Available at: http://www.amtamassage.org/articles/2 /PressRelease/detail/2219. Accessed April 24, 2018.

75. International Institute of Reflexology. The History of Reflexology. Available at: http://www.reflexology-uk.net /site/about-reflexology/reflexology-history. Accessed April 24, 2018.

76. Egyptian Reflexology. Egyptian Footwork: Therapy, Beauty, Foot Rub or All Three. Foot-Reflexologist.com. Available at: http://www.foot-reflexologist.com/EGYPT_1.HTM. Accessed April 24, 2018.

77. Medindia Content Team. Reflexology—History. Available at: http://www.medindia.net/alternativemedicine/reflexology /reflexology2.htm. Updated December 21, 2016. Accessed April 24, 2018.

78. Contemporary Reflexology College. About Reflexology. Available at: https://www.contemporaryreflexologycollege. com/about/about-reflexology. Accessed April 24, 2018.

79. The History of Reflexology. Foot Reflexology: A Brief History. Available at: http://reflexologyhistory.com/History. html. Accessed April 24, 2018.

80. Wright J. *Reflexology and Acupressure: Pressure Points for Healing.* Summertown,TN: Hamlyn and Healthy Living Publications; 2001, and London, UK: Octopus Publishing Group; 2003.

81. American Reflexology Certification Board®. Reflexology Certification. Available at: https://arcb.net/take-the-arcb-exam/. Accessed April 24, 2018.

82. Stephenson NL, Weinrich SP, Tavakoli AS. The effects of foot reflexology on anxiety and pain in patients with breast and lung cancer. *Oncol Nurs Forum.* 2000;27(1):67-72.

83. Oleson T, Flocco W. Randomized controlled study of premenstrual symptoms treated with ear, hand, and foot reflexology. *Obstet Gynecol.* 1993;82(6):906-911.

84. Poole H, Glenn S, Murphy P. A randomised controlled study of reflexology for the management of chronic low back pain. *Eur J Pain.* 2007;11(8):878-887.

85. Tovey P. A single-blind trial of reflexology for irritable bowel syndrome. *Br J Gen Pract.* 2002;52(474):19-23.

CHAPTER 14

Mind–Body Intervention

LEARNING OBJECTIVES

As a result of reading this chapter, students will be able to:

1. Assess the impact of mind–body interventions on health care in the United States.
2. Distinguish among six types of meditation and describe each one's intended effect.
3. Analyze several positive or negative effects of the use of mind–body interventions and the reason for each.
4. Explain why yoga and the Alexander Technique are considered mind–body interventions.
5. Identify the function and several benefits of yoga.
6. Explain how hypnosis is used as a therapeutic technique.
7. Explain how biofeedback works.
8. Analyze whether prayer and faith healing are beneficial as healing techniques.

▶ What Are Mind–Body Interventions?

Mind–body interventions focus on a communication system between the mind and body, in an attempt to affect the mind's ability to improve health status.[1] This includes the mental, emotional, spiritual, social, sexual, and physical domains of health. Both Western and Eastern medical practitioners and physicians have come to the realization that this communication system is powerful, and many believe it promotes self-healing and overall health. Mind–body medicine encompasses the idea that healing does not always mean the cessation of physical symptoms, but it indicates the power to "make whole."[2]

Mind–body interventions are considered to be complementary medicine therapies, with many of the practices originating out of Chinese or Ayurvedic medicine. Some examples of mind–body interventions include **meditation**, **hypnosis**, **biofeedback**, **Alexander Technique**, **yoga**, faith healing, aromatherapy, autogenic and visual imagery training, progressive muscle relaxation, and tai chi. Dance movement, art therapy, and music therapy may also be included as mind–body interventions.

A variety of mind–body interventions have been shown to have measurable physiological responses such as lowered heart rate, blood pressure, and respirations. Stress hormones such as norepinephrine, epinephrine, and **cortisol** are kept in check, and blood glucose levels are decreased. One explanation for the relaxation state is that mind–body interventions may cause a placebo effect that tends to modify cognitive and body responses in a positive way by changing physiology. These positive responses are thought to boost the body's immune system.[3]

According to Pelletier,[2] there are six basic principles of mind–body interventions:

1. The mind, body, and spirit are connected with one another and environmental influences.

2. Stress and depression contribute to the development of and hinder recovery from chronic diseases because they create measurable hormonal imbalances.

3. Psychoneuroimmunology explains how mental functioning provokes physical and biochemical changes that weaken immunity, lowering resistance to disease.

4. Overall health improves when people are optimistic and have a positive outlook on life. Health and wellness are harmed by anger, depression, and chronic stress.

5. The placebo effect—improved health and favorable physical changes in response to inactive medication such as a sugar pill—confirms the importance of mind–body medicine and is a valuable intervention.

6. Social support from family, friends, coworkers, classmates, or organized self-help groups boosts the effectiveness of traditional and CAM therapies.

This chapter is intended to introduce you to a few of the previously identified mind–body interventions. These are meditation, hypnosis, Alexander Technique, biofeedback, yoga, and faith healing.

▶ What Is Meditation and How Does It Work?

Most people think of the person who meditates as someone sitting on a cushion, legs folded in lotus position, eyes closed, and in a deep meditative trance. People, however, can meditate sitting on chairs, walking, and even dancing.

Meditation has been practiced by many cultures throughout the world. Most forms of meditation practiced today come from ancient Eastern or other religious traditions, including **Buddhism** and Christianity. Sakyong Mipham says that learning how to meditate is like learning how to ride a horse while staying balanced, and that we can learn how to balance our lives through meditation.[4] This introduction to meditation will explain what meditation is and how it works as a healing and "balancing" methodology.

According to Jon Kabat-Zinn,[5] a well-known mindfulness awareness meditation instructor, researcher, and author of meditation books, meditation is not a collection of techniques but is *a* way of being, a way of seeing and even a way of loving. Kabat-Zinn is the founder of the Mindfulness-Based Stress Reduction program at the University of Massachusetts Medical Center. He says that even though there are hundreds of meditation techniques and methods, those who are learning to meditate can get so caught up in learning specific techniques that it may impede their understanding of the full richness of meditation practice and what it has to offer.[5] Meditation may be considered a state in which the body is consciously relaxed, the mind is allowed to become calm and focused, and deep feelings of well-being are experienced. Meditation also may stimulate people to become aware of many feelings such as mental anguish, boredom, impatience, frustration, or body tension. Even experiencing those feelings is thought to result in a healing effect because they allow an opportunity for insight and learning.[4]

Sogyal Rinpoche,[6] renowned Buddhist teacher from Tibet, says that meditation brings our mind home. It is "abiding by the recognition of our true nature." It is not "out there" but "here within." Additionally, the meditator is not required to stop thinking. Further, Rinpoche explains that meditation is a spiritual journey and that we need to persevere along the path. We may find one day good and the next day, not so good.[6]

Rinpoche's teachings are supported by Allan Wallace,[7] a renowned writer and translator of Tibetan Buddhism in the West. In his book *Tibetan Buddhism: From the Ground Up*, he writes:

> The point of Buddhist meditation is not to stop thinking, for … cultivation of insight clearly requires intelligent use of thought and discrimination. What needs to be stopped is conceptualization that is compulsive, mechanical and unintelligent, that is, activity that is always fatiguing, usually pointless, and at times seriously harmful.

Meditation is intended to facilitate growth in three main areas.[8] The first is "getting to know the mind" so that a person can carefully study his or her feelings, thoughts, emotions, and various mental states. The second is "training the mind." This is the process of developing awareness, concentration, and serenity, all necessary for mental well-being. The third involves "freeing the mind," a process that is not easy but is necessary to diminish negative tendencies that decrease a sense of inner peace and harmony within oneself and the world.

Forms of Meditation

Even though there are many forms of meditation, several are acknowledged worldwide, including **Vipassana** meditation, Transcendental Meditation®, Zen meditation, Taoist meditation, Buddhist meditation, and **mindfulness meditation**.

Vipassana meditation is one of India's most ancient techniques and was later rediscovered by Gautama Buddha more than 2,500 years ago.[9] The word *Vipassana* may be defined in several ways: "to see things clearly," "deep insight," "to come and see," or "to come inward and see." That is why Vipassana meditation is also known as insight meditation. The Buddha believed that the cause of suffering could be erased if people could see their true nature.[10] This form of meditation is said to be a rational method for purifying the mind of all those thoughts that cause stress and pain. To exercise the technique and benefit at a maximum level, we are encouraged to take instruction from a person who is highly trained and competent to teach. During Vipassana meditation, mindfulness is employed. Mindfulness is meditating by being in the present moment. For example, we would be instructed to practice nonbiased attention, awareness, and acceptance of whatever is occurring in the present moment. Further, we would be asked to observe our own body and our mind in a nonjudgmental and unbiased way.[10] During Vipassana meditation, the most important aspect is to be watchful of our breath as it comes and goes.[11] We are not supposed to attempt to control the breath. If the breath is deep, we are supposed to let it be, and if it is shallow, the same is true. Vipassana is said to be a simple, gentle technique that is suitable for men and women of any age or race and is said to be the easiest meditation technique of all time.

Transcendental Meditation® (TM) was founded and introduced to the Western world in 1958 by a **guru** (one regarded as having great knowledge) named Maharishi Mahesh Yogi.[12] TM helps people to see or transcend beyond their thoughts and to experience the source of their thoughts. This process is identified as transcendental consciousness of our most inner self, a supposedly very peaceful place and state of mind. If this state of "restful alertness" is achieved, our brain is supposed to function with significantly greater coherence and our body would gain deep rest.[13] Contrary to many other forms of meditation, TM does not require a person to concentrate (focus on something) or contemplate (think about something).[12] TM is a practical form of meditation that may be used by everyone, particularly those who lead especially hectic lives. Many forms of meditation may call for an hour or more to practice, whereas to practice TM, you just need 15–20 minutes twice daily, sitting comfortably with the eyes closed. You could do this on the bus or train, during lunch hour, or anyplace that is safe and comfortable where you could sit with eyes closed for those 15–20 minutes.

Zen Buddhist meditation, also called **zazen**, is practiced by way of sitting in preparation for calming the body and mind. Zazen means the "study of self." Zen Buddhism is a way to see clearly who we are, and the meditation process is supposed to help us discover insight into the nature of our being. The technique of Zen meditation gradually takes us to the state of absolute stillness and emptiness. When we think of the mind, the body, and the breath, we see them separately, but in Zen meditation, they come together as one.[14] The position used to practice Zen meditation is the pyramid structure, similar to the seated Buddha.[14] This meditation technique requires that we sit to close our mind to thought and images. Following a period of fixed concentration, our heart rate will begin to slow down and breathing will become shallow. We would then let go of past and future thoughts, and focus and react to what is being experienced in the now.[15] See **Appendix 14.A** at the end of this chapter for a basic Zen Buddhist exercise.

Taoist meditation is said to be much more practical than those forms requiring deeper contemplation. The fundamental principle in this form of meditation is to generate and circulate internal energy. When this particular flow of energy or force is achieved, it is known as "deh-chee," which then may be used to promote better health and longevity.[16] The first primary guideline in Taoist meditation is that we should be quiet, still, and calm. The second guideline is that we should concentrate and focus. The purpose of stillness, both mental and physical, is so that we can turn our attention inwards and cut off external sensory stimuli.[16] Within that silent stillness, we should focus attention on our breath so that we can develop intuitive insights. Taoist meditation involves breathing with the nostrils and expanding and contracting the abdomen. This form of meditation is a method that enhances self-awareness and insight.

Buddhist meditation is intended to bring our mind, body, and soul to a natural and tranquil balance. It is a method for transforming our view of reality or for getting in touch with ourselves. In Buddhist meditation, we are to become detached and objective about our thoughts, which aid us to think more clearly. Buddhist meditation is supposed to help us focus our minds and attention on a single point (*ekaggata*, or one-pointedness). As stated by Francis Story, author of *Buddhist Meditation*, "The mind is hard to tame; it roams here and there restlessly as the wind, or like an untamed horse, but when it is fully under control, it is the most powerful instrument in the whole universe."[17] Buddhist meditation is a disciplined practice and must become habit to benefit our minds, bodies, and souls effectively. Through consistent practice, we should become aware of many noticeable changes such as becoming free from fear and anxiety.

Mindfulness meditation involves our focusing on the present, to be aware of our present thoughts and actions in a nonjudgmental way. There is universal agreement that at the heart of most forms of meditation lies the concept of mindfulness, or as Kabat-Zinn describes it, "Mindfulness is none other than the capacity we all already have to know what is actually happening as it is happening."[5] Kabat-Zinn has further defined mindfulness in the following way[5]:

> Mindfulness can be thought of as moment to moment, nonjudgmental awareness cultivated by paying attention in a specific way, that is, in the present moment, and as nonreactively, as nonjudgmentally, and as openheartedly as possible. It means paying attention in a particular way; on purpose, in the present moment, and nonjudgmentally.

Mindfulness meditation means that we need to become aware of our physical, emotional, and mental activities in the present, meaning the here and now. This is ultimately the goal of all meditation—to awaken us to the present. Kabat-Zinn explains that the concept of mindfulness involves purposely paying attention to our experience during meditation, whether it is our breathing or our emotions. This includes deliberately noticing sensations and our response to those sensations.[5] When meditating, it is not about trying to get anywhere else, but allowing ourselves to be in the moment. Once we have learned to stay with the experience, we can then purposefully direct awareness toward some anchor to decrease the effect on our lives. In so doing, meditation can help us shape our minds.

Kabat-Zinn further points out that any state of mind can be a meditative state (anger, sadness, enthusiasm, delight) and is much more valuable than a blank mind or one that is out of touch.[5] Being aware of these emotions is an opportunity to learn more about ourselves. If we practiced this form of meditation, we would focus on what is happening in and around us at that very moment and become aware of all our thoughts and feelings that might be taking our energy from moment to moment. We would start by watching our breath, and then move our attention to the thoughts going through our minds, to the feelings in our bodies, and even to the sounds and sights around us. Most importantly, we would not judge or analyze ourselves. If you are considering starting meditation, you should select a form that seems to be in keeping with your philosophy and life values. The next section describes some meditation positions that allow for individual preference and comfort.

A Few Notes on Mindfulness

Have you ever had a moment where you said to someone or told yourself, "I completely missed that part of the discussion...." Odds are you were thinking about your own feelings about the conversation, or your response, or the Netflix show on your computer, or a text message that came in on your phone. We are busy, constantly bombarded with stimuli and information. So much so that we miss what is happening right in front of us. Mindfulness or being mindful goes well beyond the meditative practice described in the last section. It is a conscious choice on how to live your life. And the choice is to be present in the moment. In THAT moment ... and the next one ... and the next. We all want to experience joy.

So, you might be wondering how you can get it. What steps do you need to take to become more aware of what is happening around you and experience greater joy? The Vietnamese Buddhist Thich Nhat Hanh states that being mindful is what allows us to see the happiness in our lives that is already here; that we do not have to wait for. Here are some suggestions to get you started:

- Practice the mindfulness meditation breathing and focus activities described earlier.
- Find joy in what you are doing right now. Consider that others may not have the same opportunity for the experience you are having.
- Release your expectations of the situation. Take the moment for what it is and move with the moment. When you are focused on expectations, you miss what is happening right now.
- Practice kindness, especially to yourself. Disappointment and frustration, especially with self, are outcomes of being focused on future expectations and not what the moment can bring you.

The key to it all is to remember that what is happening right now is what is most important. It is, for almost all of us, a very different way to think and a very different way to behave. You might be thinking, "So what happens if I can accomplish those things?" The short answer is: lots of things. First, there will be greater joy in your life. When you live in this moment and this moment is the most important, you get the most out of it. Are all moments wonderful? No. And that brings us to the next benefit: resiliency. When we release expectations and practice kindness, we develop understanding and empathy. Those qualities help us manage the challenging times more successfully. Conflicts become less severe when you can empathize with another person. Disappointments become less traumatic when you can appreciate where you are right now and not fear the future. Less expectation means less conflict. Less conflict can lead to less anxiety and depression. Less anxiety leads to less fear and less fear to greater joy. And we are back to where we started—we all want greater joy.

Meditation Positions

Even though meditation may be practiced while walking, moving, or even dancing, we will explain the seated positions first.

Seated Positions

The point of the seated positions is to allow us to be still and quiet while meditating.

The first seated position, the **Burmese position**, is likened to the pyramid structure of the seated Buddha, as reflected in **FIGURE 14.1**. You would sit on the floor and use a zafu (small pillow) to raise your hips just a little, so that your knees could touch the ground. Sitting on the pillow with two knees touching the ground forms a tripod base that gives 360-degree stability. There are other versions of Burmese. In one, the legs may be crossed and both feet placed flat on the floor or one leg may be crossed and the other extended.

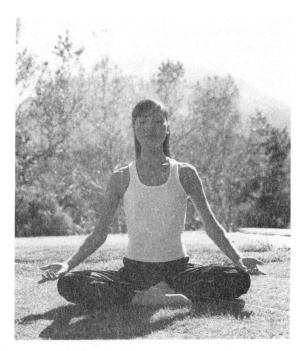

FIGURE 14.1 Burmese position.
© Motoyuki Kobayashi/Digital Vision/Thinkstock

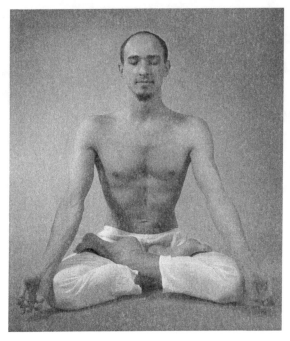

FIGURE 14.2 Full lotus position.
© Lakhesis/Shutterstock

The **half lotus position** is also used when meditating. In this position, the left foot is placed up onto the right thigh and the right leg is tucked under. The position is somewhat asymmetrical, and the upper body may need support to stay straight. The **full lotus position** is very stable and symmetrical.[14] In this position, both legs are placed on the opposite thigh, as reflected in **FIGURE 14.2**. An alternative to the seated floor positions is to sit on a chair or kneel on the floor.

Movement Positions

The movement meditation positions are quite interesting. Some people and cultures like to meditate while walking, doing **martial arts**, or even dancing.[16] Walking while meditating has been formalized as a Zen meditation practice called *Kinhin*. **Walking meditation** focuses on awareness of self, the process of walking, and the environment. It may be practiced inside or outside. The point of walking meditation is to be in the present moment. While walking, you would first pay attention to the movement of your legs, your breathing, and your body. You would then feel your feet contacting the ground. If your mind wanders, you would refocus on the process of walking and breathing. Meditating outside can be difficult because of the distractions, but if you choose to do this outside, find a quiet place with level ground.

Some martial arts practices include Zen archery (kyudo[18]; **FIGURE 14.3**), tai chi, and qigong. All encompass understanding the relationship of the power of

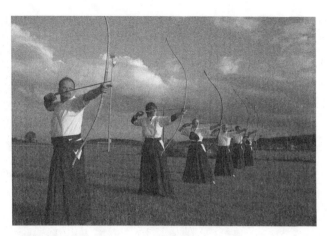

FIGURE 14.3 Zen archers.
© Paul Prescott/Shutterstock

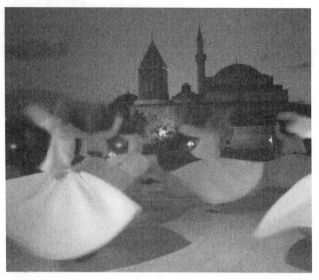

FIGURE 14.4 Sufi dancing.
© Hemera/Thinkstock

breath, the life force (qi energy), the mind, and the concept of oneness.

Dance is said to be a great method to build awareness, get rid of negative feelings, and get into the present moment. Many examples of dance meditation follow. **Sufi dancing** is said to be the dance of universal peace. It originated in the Islamic world and has been practiced for centuries, but not by all orders of Sufi. Sufi dancing is a part of **Sama**, a ritual practice developed in the mid-9th century that uses music, poetry recital, singing, and dance. The dances were first performed by religious men. All practices are intended to bring participants to a mystical experience.[19] The individual responsible for making the Sama dance a focus of Sufi doctrine is Jala-luddin Rumi, a spiritual master and a genius at poetry making who was also known as Mevlana. He was born in Iran, but eventually settled in Konya, Turkey. Rumi established his Sufi order. He taught his followers how to use the Sama dance to guide followers to a spiritual uplifting to the Immortal one.[19]

Sufi whirling is a version of Sufi dance. In this movement, dancers whirl by themselves with arms in various positions, such as reaching out and reaching to the heavens. Sufi whirling may also be danced with a partner and is known in the West as the dance of the "whirling dervishes." It is choreographed, performed under strict and controlled conditions, and is led by a Sufi master as a means to "commune with the devine."[20] The steps and motions symbolically depict the "cosmos in motion." The dance is supposed to cultivate inner peace and harmony with the Earth. The dances are simple circle dances wherein dancers move around a dance floor from partner to partner (**FIGURE 14.4**).[20] They are to let their thoughts fall away and connect on a spiritual level with other dancers. As they dance, they are to focus on the chants and songs while they connect with one another.

Another form of Sufi dance is Dervish dancing by Turkish dancers, who dress in a particular style. The **Dervish dancers** can be said to dance to the rhythm of the cosmos or the universe as they seem to represent the solar system and the planets that revolve around the sun. During the dance, they seem to yield the body to the earth's movement. They let their bodies sway to the changing tempos of the music. As they are doing this, their consciousness also changes. They seem to be in a trance-like state as they begin to understand the possibility of the eternity of the soul. They are said to have given away the body to the earth and that the mind and soul can now concentrate on the fully transcendental.[21]

A very different dance meditation is that of Master George Ivanovich Gurdjieff. The **Gurdjieff sacred dances** use well-defined movements in which different parts of the body seem not to be related with each other.[22] The dancer is expected to coordinate different rhythms at the same time. The movements and the dance are very energetic, sometimes strange, and sometimes depict ancient rituals. The purpose of the dance is to train the dancers to be in the present moment with no thoughts of the past or future. They are to accept themselves and to be playful and relaxed (**FIGURE 14.5**).

Again, if you are considering meditation, find the meditation form that fits your lifestyle and find the position (sitting, walking, dancing, etc.) in which you will feel most comfortable. Next is a discussion of meditation techniques.

Meditation Techniques

There are numerous types of meditation techniques. The following presents several meditation techniques

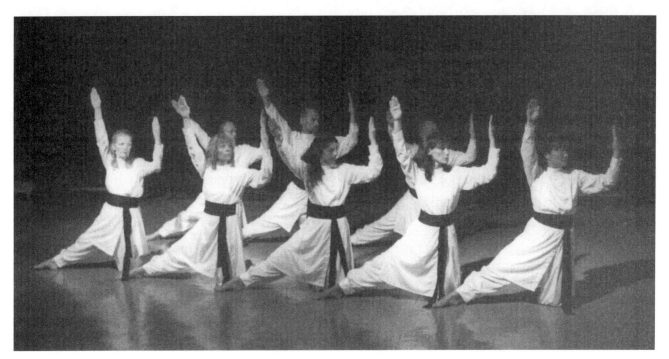

FIGURE 14.5 Gurdjieff dancers.
© OSHO International Foundation, www.osho.com

that are common to most forms of meditation, whether it is Vipassana, Transcendental, Taoist, Zen, Buddhist, mindfulness, or others.

Concentration and Visualization Techniques

To achieve concentration and visualization, you need to learn to be aware of your breath; this may occur using Zen breathing (zazen) or Vipassana breathing methods.[23] Both methods involve awareness and concentration during the breathing process to help build or shape your mind and to feel the mind and body as one. You would practice watching your breath and relax in whatever position works best. Close your eyes and start to pay attention to your breathing. Take in air through your nose and take a deep, slow breath. If your mind wanders from your breath, refocus attention to the air going in and out of your nose. As this is practiced, it is supposed to become easier to do.

Vipassana breathing entails extending awareness from the breath to the body and the sensations that rise and fall within it, and it requires being watchful of our breath as it comes and goes. Self-observation is intended to give insight into the workings of the mind.[11] Vipassana may be practiced anytime and anywhere, although when people are first practicing this form of meditation, they are encouraged to set aside a time and quiet place to meditate in a comfortable position. More experienced practitioners

practice Vipassana breathing while reading, playing, swimming, and the like.

Concentration techniques may involve focusing on an external object.[23] You could focus on anything from a point on the ceiling, to a flower, to a candle flame, to external sounds in the environment. Concentration meditations are thought to help develop focus, concentration, self-knowledge, and calmness, and to become aware of our consciousness. It allows for greater awareness and clarity to emerge.[23] After you become skilled at concentrating, you can stop concentrating on the focus point (ceiling, flower, etc.) and begin to concentrate on your mind and body as one.

Visualization techniques can range from simply moving awareness to various areas of the body, to visualizing internal flows of light, to imagining places. You could visualize images of God or places of power or peace. You could imagine that you are in a place that you love to visit and experience (**BOX 14.1**).

BOX 14.1 Imagery as a Visualization Technique

Take a moment to feel the warm sand between your toes. Look at the gentle, crystal blue water. Listen to the gentle sounds of the waves as they come in while smelling the fresh, clean air. Taste the freshness of this air. Try to totally submerge yourself into the picture you have created within your mind to ultimately create a place of total relaxation.

Insight Techniques

Techniques to acquire insight about ourselves are the **WHO AM I**, Koan, contemplation, silent mind, and empty mind techniques.

The WHO AM I technique was popularized by Shri Ramana Maharishi (**FIGURE 14.6**).[24] It focuses on negating our false self so that we can realize our true nature or enlightenment. In the Maharishi's words:

> The moment you start looking for the self and go deeper and deeper, the real Self is waiting there to take you in. Then whatever is done is done by something else and you have no hand in it. In this process, all doubts and discussions are automatically given up just as one who sleeps forgets, for the time being, all his cares.[24]

The **Koan meditation technique** comes from the Zen School of Buddhism and is designed to break down an ordinary pattern of thinking. It often includes a story, question, or statement that cannot be understood by rational thinking but can be solved through intuition. For example, "Two hands clap and there is a sound; what is the sound of one hand?"

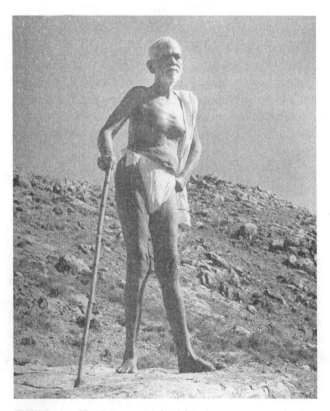

FIGURE 14.6 Shri Ramana Maharishi.
© Eliot Elisofon/Time Life Pictures/Getty Images

Contemplation meditative techniques use introspection, self-study, and reflection. Contemplative meditation is supposed to help us gain a deeper understanding of some aspect of reality. The Buddhists have a technique called "meditation on the corpse," which involves imagining our own death, the burial of our body, and then our body's decomposition. It also includes instructing us to see worms feeding on our flesh and finally watching our body return to the earth.[25] Meditation on the corpse is an example of an exercise in helping us to face reality. These meditations have their roots in many Western religions and are also a part of Eastern philosophies.

The **silent mind meditation** technique involves directly perceiving and feeling the world around us by focusing on how we are thinking. These meditations are an extension of the teachings of Jiddu Krishnamurti (1895–1986), who was born in India and died in California.[26] Krishnamurti was a writer and speaker on philosophical and spiritual issues. The silent mind technique is described as being sensitive of the senses, the movement of the mind, the emotions, and to others. Further, it involves being sensitive to the present. A part of the task is to develop moment to moment sensitivity of our physical, mental, and emotional dimensions.

The **empty mind meditation** technique is one that creates a kind of "awareness without object," an emptying of all thoughts from your mind.[26] The techniques for doing this involve sitting still, often in a full lotus or cross-legged position, and letting our mind go silent on its own. It is said to be difficult, because any effort seems to just cause more business in the mind.

Sound, Thought, Feeling, and Emotion Techniques

Sound (**mantra**) and thought meditation techniques are thought to enlighten people and to improve their health, wealth, happiness, and so forth.[27] Sound and thought vibrations as well as music are used to purify the heart and mind. While meditating, many of us find it difficult to keep our mind from wandering, and it seems to help if we concentrate on something specific. A mantra can help. This is a word or phrase that is repeated during meditation. It may be chosen by us or by an experienced master in some traditions. The mantra may be either repeated aloud or silently as meditation progresses. Mantras supposedly help people tune into their energy field. See **Appendix 14.B** at the end of this chapter for an example of a sound meditation exercise.

Rhythm and song methods of meditation are a combination of rhythm, chanting, music, and breath, and are sometimes used during meditation to achieve a desired state of calmness. Many religious denominations achieve the meditative state through song. Some meditations use positive thinking, self-hypnosis, power of intention (strong thought), and even laughter to achieve the meditative state.[23]

Often, **feeling and emotion meditation techniques** are used independently, but they also can be combined with other types of meditations. Bhagwan Shree Rajneesh used laughter, crying, and silence as meditative techniques.[28] He was known as Osho and was born in 1931 in Central India (**FIGURE 14.7**). Osho obtained a master's degree in philosophy, and later founded his own spiritual movement based on an eclectic mixture of religion and philosophy.[29] Osho, like the Maharishi, was also considered a guru (one regarded as having great knowledge). Osho developed a new type of meditation that advocated letting go of all attachments to the past, future, and ego. To achieve this, Osho recommended laughter and tears, the human emotions. In letting go of attachments, Osho believed that people would become enlightened[28]:

> You will see it yourself; if you can laugh without any reason, you will see something repressed within you … From your very childhood you have been told not to laugh— "Be serious!" You have to come out of that repressive conditioning.
>
> The second step is tears. Tears have been repressed even more deeply. It has been told to us that tears are a symptom of weakness—they are not. Tears can cleanse not only your eyes, but your heart too. They soften you; it is a biological strategy to keep you clean, to keep you unburdened. It is now a well-known fact that less women go mad than men. And the reason has been found to be that women can cry and weep more easily than men. Even to the small child it is said, "Be a man, don't cry like a woman!"
>
> But if you look at the physiology of your body, you have the same glands full of tears whether you are man or woman. It has been found that fewer women commit suicide than men. And of course, no woman in history has been the cause of founding violent religions, wars, massacres. If the whole world can learn to cry and weep again it will be a tremendous transformation, a metamorphosis.
>
> The third step is silence. I have called it "The Watcher on the Hills." Become as silent as if you are alone on the top of a Himalayan peak, utterly silent and alone, just watching, listening … sensitive, but still.

The Use of Mandalas as an Aid for Meditation

The word **mandala** comes from the classical Indian language of **Sanskrit** and means completion or circle. In both Hindu and Buddhist religious traditions, mandalas have a spiritual and ritual significance. The circle is a symbol found in many cultures.[30,31] They are seen in halos, prayer wheels, and other religious symbols.

Mandalas are complex designs with a circular pattern or motif. They might be incorporated into a square or rectangle, but the design retains a circular focal point and symmetry.[30,31] Sometimes, line drawings of mandalas can be filled in with color (**FIGURE 14.8**). There are several ways to color or make mandalas, including by using paint, pencils, crayons, pastels, and even colored sand. One can also buy pictures of mandalas (**FIGURE 14.9**).

Mandalas are said to appear in all aspects of life, such as the earth, sun, and moon. They could also represent circles of friends, family, and community.

Their use in meditation is to aid us to focus attention and to progressively move into deeper levels of the unconscious. Ultimately, mandalas are used to help us experience a mystical sense of oneness with the cosmos. We would eventually extract some sort of meaning from the mandala as we practiced

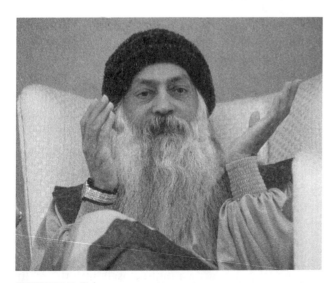

FIGURE 14.7 Osho.
© Matthew Naythons/Liaison/Getty Images

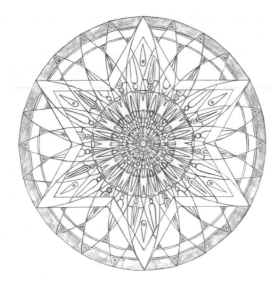

FIGURE 14.8 Mandala 1.
© MedusArt/Shutterstock

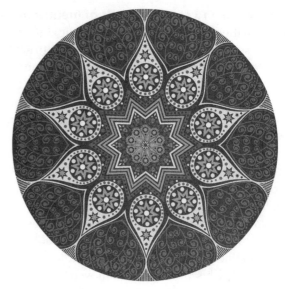

FIGURE 14.9 Mandala 2.
© Markovka/Shutterstock

meditation. The main purpose is to help us enter into the mandala and receive a sense of being blessed.[30,31]

Thus far, we have defined what meditation is and discussed various forms and techniques, but what does the research say about the benefits of meditation?

Benefits of Meditation

There seem to be many benefits for people who practice meditation. Some of the physiological benefits include the following[32,33]:

- Deep rest, as measured by decreased **metabolic rate**, lower heart rate, and reduced workload of the heart
- Lower levels of **blood lactates** and thus reduced anxiety
- Lower levels of cortisol and lactate, two chemicals associated with stress
- Reduction of **free radicals**—unstable oxygen molecules that can cause tissue damage
- Increased **serotonin**, which influences moods and behavior. Low levels of serotonin are associated with depression, headaches, and insomnia
- Improved blood pressure
- Higher skin resistance to wrinkles from stress-related conditions. Low skin resistance (more wrinkles) is correlated with higher stress and anxiety levels
- Drop in cholesterol levels. High cholesterol is associated with cardiovascular disease
- Improved flow of air to the lungs resulting in easier breathing. This has been very helpful to asthma patients

- Slowed aging process (through increased blood flow)
- Maintenance of normal blood pressure
- Reduced symptoms of premenstrual tension (PMT)
- Reduction of heart disease
- Increased weight loss

Some of the psychological benefits of meditation include the following[32,33]:

- Increased brain wave coherence
- Greater creativity
- Decreased anxiety
- Decreased depression
- Decreased irritability and moodiness
- Improved learning ability and memory
- Increased self-actualization
- Increased feelings of vitality and rejuvenation
- Increased happiness
- Increased emotional stability
- Increased self-confidence
- Enhanced energy, strength, and vigor
- A state of deep relaxation and general feeling of well-being

Besides the physiological and psychological benefits, there are spiritual benefits. The longer an individual practices meditation, the greater the likelihood that his or her goals and efforts will shift toward personal and spiritual growth. Many individuals who initially learn meditation for its self-regulatory aspects find that as their practice deepens they are drawn more closely into the realm of the "spiritual." In her work with many cancer and AIDS patients, Borysenko observed that people who meditated became more attuned to the spiritual dimension of life. Borysenko reported that many die "healed," in a state of compassionate self-awareness and self-acceptance.[34]

Meditation Research

A 2012 nationwide U.S. survey conducted by the National Center for Health Statistics regarding CAM use found that 8%, or nearly 18 million, U.S. adults had used meditation in the past 12 months. Reasons for using meditation were to help with anxiety, pain, depression, stress, insomnia, and physical or emotional symptoms associated with chronic illnesses such as HIV/AIDS, heart disease, and cancer.[35]

Research has shown that meditation does induce changes in the body. The **sympathetic nervous system** is responsible for the "fight-or-flight" response produced during times of stress. Symptoms of stress include an increased heart rate, increased respirations, and a narrowing of blood vessels causing blood flow to be restricted.[36] Meditation reduces activity of the sympathetic nervous system and increases activity of the **parasympathetic nervous system**, which is responsible for causing heart rate and breathing to slow down, blood vessels to dilate, and digestive juices to increase.[36] Research also is focusing on meditation's effects on psychological feelings of anxiety, depression, and coping.

A 2009 study by Nidich and colleagues,[37] funded in part by the National Center for Complementary and Integrative Health (NCCIH), found that TM showed positive effects by helping young adults cope with stress. The researchers studied 298 students from the American University and other schools in the Washington, D.C. and randomly assigned students to a TM group or a control group. The TM group had significant improvement in feelings of psychological distress, anxiety, depression, anger/hostility, and coping ability.

A 2013 NCCIH review of literature on mind–body techniques[38] revealed that meditation has a positive impact on smoking cessation. The study, published in Drug and Alcohol Dependence, reviewed 14 studies, 8 of which involved meditation as a method for cessation. The summary reports positive outcomes for those using meditative practice in the areas of abstinence, reduction in cravings, desire to smoke, and in daily usage of cigarettes. Other NCCIH-supported studies[39] showing positive or potential benefit include investigating meditation benefits for relieving stress, lower back pain, musculoskeletal pain, insomnia, suicidal ideation,

ulcerative colitis, HIV-related stress, and in improving empathy.

The NCCIH also funded a review of the scientific literature and found evidence that meditation has potential beneficial effects.[39] Some of the research studies reviewed were on the following topics: impact on chronic illness, alterations in brain and immune function produced by mindfulness meditation, meditation and relaxation, meditation and attention, meditation and cancer therapy, and the neural basis of the complex mental task of meditation. The researchers, however, concluded that future research needs to be more vigorous before confirming that meditation results in health benefits.

Davidson, Kabat-Zinn, and others[40] recorded the brain waves of stressed-out employees of a high-tech firm in Madison, Wisconsin. The subjects were split randomly into two groups—25 people were asked to learn meditation over 8 weeks and the remaining 16 were left alone as a control group. All participants had their brain waves scanned three times during the study: at the beginning of the experiment, when meditation lessons were completed 8 weeks later, and 4 months after that. The researchers found that participants who had meditated showed a pronounced shift in activity to the left frontal lobe, a pattern previously associated with positive effect (calmer and less stressed).[40]

Meditation is considered a safe practice, although there have been rare reports of worsening symptoms in people with certain psychiatric problems such as depression or anxiety.[39] Advice on the NCCIH website to people who are thinking about using meditation practices includes:

- Do not use meditation as a replacement for conventional care or as a reason to postpone seeing a doctor about a medical problem.
- Ask about the training and experience of the meditation instructor you are considering.
- Look for published research studies on meditation for the health condition in which you are interested.
- Tell all your healthcare providers about any complementary and alternative practices you use. Give them a full picture of what you do to manage your health. This will help ensure coordinated and safe care.

Meditation is practiced by many and is one of the most important mind–body interventions of all. It is safe, and has been proven to alter body physiology in a positive way.

▶ What Is Yoga?

The yoga of today stems from a wide variety of people, practices, and time periods. The word *yoga* comes from the Sanskrit word meaning *union*.[42] Yoga dates back thousands of years in the Indian tradition. Because yoga supposedly began before the written word (prehistoric period), people learned the concepts and practices of yoga from a guru or teacher in an intimate, one-on-one, personal manner. The major purpose was to attain the highest spiritual goals: self-realization, enlightenment, and the liberation of the soul. From 7000 BCE to 1500 AD, the teachings were written down in several pieces of classical literature related to yoga and in the Vedas, four volumes written in Sanskrit: *Rigveda, Yajurveda, Samaveda,* and *Atharvaveda*.[42,43]

In those years, yoga was a way of life, a culture, and a lifestyle that was more than specific yoga techniques. It included eating and bathing habits, prayer, work, and social interaction. From 1500 AD onward, yoga teachers began to focus more on the practices of Hatha Yoga, which include **asanas** (postures), pranayama (breath control), and dhyana (meditation).[44] The higher spiritual aims began to be overlooked.

In 1893, Swami Vivekananda (1863–1902) from Calcutta, India, made a historic address to the World Parliament of Religions in Chicago, where he introduced the religious practice of Hinduism. Because yoga is a major part of Hinduism, this event has often been said to be the beginning of the modern era of yoga.

In the century since then, yoga has increased in popularity and has moved a long way away from its historical foundations. Physical fitness, enhanced sexuality, and personal achievement have become the primary goals. People who practice yoga say it helps them relax and stay centered. Yoga is believed to increase the body's store of prana or vital energy and, due to better posture, facilitate energy flow.[42] Today, the practice of yoga has become a multi-billion dollar industry. Various types of yoga wear are a part of fashionable clothing lines, prepackaged snacks and supplements are sold as yoga food, yoga mats are sold, and yoga images of athletic people are on the covers of glossy magazines.

Function and Benefits of Yoga

Kabat-Zinn calls yoga a profound meditation practice, especially when mindfulness is incorporated.

📄 *IN THE NEWS*

Meditation a Hit for Pain Management by Allison Aubrey—Audio version played by National Public Radio on August 19, 2011

Previously in this chapter, under Buddhist Meditation, I wrote much about the philosophy of Jon Kabat-Zinn who uses mindfulness meditation, which Kabat-Zinn says is the heart of Buddhist meditation. In an article published in 2007, Allison Aubrey interviewed Jon Kabat-Zinn and a man with shoulder and neck pain. On August 19, 2011, National Public Radio played the entire audio of this interview.[41] A summary[39] is as follows:

Back in 1979, Jon Kabat-Zinn was a biologist at the University of Massachusetts. Because he was trained in Vipassana tradition of Buddhist mediation, he believed that the technique could help patients at the university's medical center. His clinic was in an underground office in a medical building and had no windows. Physicians and pain specialists at the university referred patients to Kabat-Zinn and he began teaching people his mindfulness technique. Subsequently, mindfulness classes were set up in other areas of the country and they were modeled on Kabat-Zinn's teachings. Bill Mies, a man with shoulder and neck pain, learned mindfulness meditation to help him cope with his discomfort. He had received injections by doctors and had learned some exercises from physical therapists but nothing had helped until he began to learn mindfulness techniques. Mies also participated in one of the class techniques called the body scan. The instructor walked him and others in the class through a sort of mental tour of the body so that they could bring awareness into specific areas of their bodies. The techniques did not cure the pain but he and the others reported they felt better. Mies says it is a struggle because his mind would wander as he attempted to focus on body parts. He admits that it is difficult to stay "in the moment" and that it takes a lot of practice.

Questions:

1. Before you read this summary, did you ever consider that meditation could be an aid to coping with pain?
2. Please discuss with classmates how meditation may have aided Bill Mies and others.

Source: Aubrey A. Meditation a hit for pain management. NPR September 4, 2011. Available at: http://www.npr.org/templates/story/story.php?storyId=7654964 Accessed September 6, 2011.

He believes that yoga develops strength, balance, and flexibility of the mind.[5] Kabat-Zinn explains that his patients in the Stress Reduction Clinic have found yoga to be a powerful form of mindfulness practice.

Yoga is believed to be helpful for a myriad of health disorders and diseases,[9,45] ranging from back pain to pain management, respiratory problems, arthritis, weight management, stress, depression, mental performance, heart disorders, and hypertension. Studies have shown that yoga lowers blood pressure, heart rate, and body temperature, and that people who practice yoga are more resistant to stress and have reduced anxiety, lower blood pressure, better respiratory function, and improved physical and sexual fitness.[9] There are claims that yoga even has antiaging properties.

Benefits of yoga include increasing flexibility, strength, and posture. The yoga poses are called asanas, and they work by safely stretching muscles. The stretches are thought to release lactic acid from the muscles, resulting in decreased feelings of stiffness, tension, pain, and fatigue. Yoga is thought to increase joint range of motion and lubrication. Muscle tone is improved in most forms of yoga, especially the ashtanga and power yogas. Even less vigorous forms of yoga, however, are thought to increase muscle tone. Upper body strength is increased after mastering poses such as Downward Dog, Upward Dog, and Plank. Poses that strengthen the lower back include Upward Dog and Chair pose.[46] The Halasana position is known as the Plough position (**FIGURE 14.10**) because Hala refers to plough. This position is good for stretching the neck and lower back muscles. The Shirshasana position is a headstand position (**FIGURE 14.11**). It is supposed to be the king of the asanas because it has many benefits. It increases circulation to the brain and aids nervousness, tension, and fatigue. The Shirshasana position is also thought to aid correct spinal alignment.

Posture is improved when strength and flexibility are increased. A stronger core allows a person to sit and stand "tall."[47] Full awareness of posture and movements

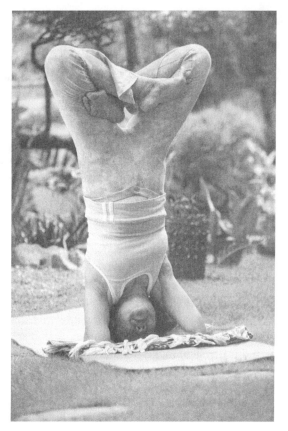

FIGURE 14.11 Shirshasana pose.
© OtnaYdur/Shutterstock

are common in all types of physical yoga. Moreover, attention is focused on the breath during all movements, which is supposed to help open up the energy channels.

Even though yoga has been deemed safe for all ages, critics of yoga are concerned that beginners will injure themselves by trying to do the more advanced yoga positions. For example, the upside-down headstands could be dangerous for people with hypertension.[9] Critics are also concerned that people will use yoga as an alternative rather than a complementary therapy to their prescribed, traditional course of treatment for some specific disease or disorder.[44] Yoga experts are aware of these problems and encourage people to talk with their doctors before beginning yoga and to start with easier poses until their bodies are conditioned for the more advanced ones.[9] The secret of yoga is to be gentle to reduce the likelihood of overstretching or straining muscles.[5]

How Yoga Works

Yoga works by promoting harmony of body, mind, and spirit, which requires correct breathing, posture, and meditation. The first thing you need to learn in doing yoga is to breathe correctly so that you make full use of your lungs, increase your circulation, and improve your energy and vitality.[44]

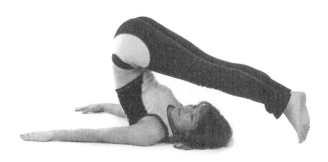

FIGURE 14.10 Halasana, or plough pose.
© grafvision/Shutterstock

Power of the Breath

Breathing during meditation (or yoga) is not just the process of taking air into the lungs and breathing it out. Those are only the first and last stages of breathing (prana).[48] After air is taken in, the second form of energy occurs. This is known as samana, wherein the oxygen is transported to your cells. Samana is supposed to be the balancing energy, the digestive breath. The third form of prana is called vyana, an energy that governs the circulatory system and makes sure that oxygen reaches all cells in our bodies. This energy is supposed to awaken us emotionally. A cleansing breath is called apana. It eliminates stale air from our lungs each time we breathe out. The energies we have taken in are returned to the external environment.[48] The last form is called udana, which means "air that flies upward." This is energy that starts in our solar plexus and gains strength as it rises upwards toward the throat and mouth. Udana is energy that is said to govern our physical make-up, our ability to stand and move, our enthusiasm, and our voice.[48]

Asana Poses

After mastering the breath, you would learn yoga poses (asanas) appropriate for a beginner so that you could exercise your body muscles to improve strength and tone. The asanas are performed in a particular sequence so that all the muscle groups are exercised and toxins are flushed out. As you improve, you can move to more advanced positions. During the process of becoming more skilled with breathing and poses, you become more relaxed and gain the ability to meditate.

Yoga should be performed no less than 2 hours after eating so that food has been digested. The lessons may take from 1 to 2 hours, and you should wear loose fitting clothing that allows movement (such as a leotard or sweat suit). Usually, people go barefoot or wear a light slipper and exercise on a mat. The first 10 minutes of the class usually focus on breathing control followed by 15–20 minutes of warm up. You would then be asked to perform the first position while concentrating on your breathing. All positions should be obtained slowly and smoothly and should be held only for as long as you are comfortable. After approximately 25 minutes of performing asanas, you would engage in about 20 minutes of relaxation exercises.

Clinical Studies

The NCCIH helped to support a study by Kiecolt-Glasser and colleagues[49] and featured the study results on its website. Long-term female yoga practitioners had lower blood levels of a stress-related compound thought to play a role in cardiovascular disease and type II diabetes. In addition, the long-term practitioners had five times lower levels of C-reactive protein, which serves as a marker for inflammation.[49]

Many other studies support yoga as an adjunct for various conditions. A 2017 study of 55 adults with mild to moderate depression were randomized in a controlled trial using yoga twice weekly for 8 weeks. Results indicated those in the yoga group experienced both statistically and clinically significant reduction in depression symptoms.[50] A 2014 study of 120 college girls indicated that yoga gave anxiety relief.[51] Another study found that yoga provided significant improvements, equal to structured breathing exercise, for bronchial asthma in children 7–12 years old.[52] A review of literature by Raub[53] found that Hatha yoga had significant psychophysiologic effects on healthy people and those compromised by musculoskeletal and cardiopulmonary disease.

Thus far, we have explained how meditation and yoga function as mind–body interventions. The next intervention discussed is hypnosis, a seemingly mysterious practice, and one people seem to fear because they feel that they will lose control over their minds and bodies. Do we?

▶ What Is Hypnosis?

Hypnosis is a mind–body technique that focuses on awareness and attention to internal stimuli, much like what is learned during meditation. The word hypnosis comes from the Greek word *hypnos*, meaning sleep. Hypnosis often, but not always, produces a trancelike state wherein the participant is highly responsive to suggestion.[2] When under hypnosis, people feel calm and relaxed, which allows them to concentrate more closely on a specific thought, memory, feeling, or sensation.[54]

Therapeutic hypnosis is used to promote health and is different from entertainment-type stage hypnosis. Free will remains intact, and people do not lose control over their behaviors.[54] Instead, hypnosis can help people learn to master their own states of awareness. A myth is that hypnosis causes people to lose consciousness and to lose memory of what happened during the hypnotic state (amnesia). A very small percentage might fit this description, but most people remember everything that occurs during the experience.[55]

History

Hypnosis has been used for centuries, even before the written language.[36] Trance states were used as a part of mystical and shamanic traditions since the beginning of humankind. Shamanic customs teach that the true shaman travels between many states of consciousness. In so doing, the shaman can heal people, prophesize the future, retrieve lost souls, and gain the ability to use any energies encountered.[36] However, it was not until the 18th century that it was used clinically by a German physician, Dr. Franz Anton Mesmer, who created and defined a discipline using hypnotism that he called "animal magnetism."[2,36] The term **mesmerize** comes from Mesmer's hypnotism practice. During the 20th century, Milton Erickson, a psychiatrist, began to scientifically study hypnotism as a part of his treatment process. Erickson focused his research on the process, the state, and the effects of hypnosis.[36]

Philosophies Regarding How Hypnosis Functions

Two main philosophies are used to explain hypnotic effects. The first is the **neodissociation model**, which suggests that hypnosis activates a subsystem of both psychological and physiologic parts. This activation results in an altered state of consciousness. The second is the **social psychological model**, which suggests that an altered state of consciousness does not occur during hypnosis; instead, hypnosis is explained by suggestibility, positive attitudes, and expectations.[36]

Researchers are at odds as to whether hypnosis affects the brain from the posterior part to the anterior or whether it affects the left and right hemispheres of the brain. Also, undetermined are the types of brain waves affected—beta, alpha, theta, and delta—although most research seems to point to theta waves.[36] Theta waves are thought to be associated with mental imagery, meditation, rapid eye movement during sleep, problem solving, focused attention, and cessation of a pleasurable activity. Theta waves are also most related to hypnotic susceptibility during hypnotic states.

There are several stages of hypnosis. As a participant is being hypnotized, he or she will become very relaxed. At this stage, the participant will gain the capacity to deeply contemplate a selected theme or focal point (absorption). Absorption helps the person to become deeply engaged in the words or images that the hypnotherapist presents. The next stage is dissociation, in which the participant can let go of critical thoughts and gain the capacity to compartmentalize his or her experience. The stage of responding to or complying with a hypnotherapist's suggestion occurs next. The last stage is when the participant returns to usual awareness and reflects on the experience.

Hypnosis as Therapeutic Treatment

Hypnosis (**hypnotherapy**) is currently used to gain access to the deeper levels of the mind so that a change in thinking and behavior will occur. During a first visit, the therapist will ask about your medical history, the reason for coming in, and what you want to address. The hypnotherapist then will explain what hypnosis is and how it works. He or she may teach several relaxation techniques and ask you to practice them at home. The sessions last about an hour, and usually you would begin to see results within 4–10 sessions.[56]

Hypnotherapy is used to modify feelings of pain, fear, and anxiety, and may be used as an adjunct to other conventional treatments such as analgesia in surgery, to help reduce stress, and to control allergies.[2] Research has demonstrated the effectiveness of hypnosis in treating cancer and cancer pain,[57,58,59] burn pain,[60,61] fibromyalgia pain,[62] and gastrointestinal disorders such as duodenal ulcers and irritable bowel syndrome.[63] Hypnosis has been helpful in treating nausea and vomiting during cancer chemotherapy,[64] pregnancy-induced nausea, and asthma, and has been used to help people who are obese lose weight. The power of suggestion from hypnosis has been used to cure warts, a condition caused by a virus. There are many published studies[65,66] of the use of hypnosis to cure warts, with a cure rate between 27% and 55%. Interestingly, once cured by hypnosis, the warts reportedly do not return, as they often do after traditional medical therapy.

Risks of Hypnosis

Hypnosis is considered safe when conducted under the care of a trained therapist. Adverse reactions might occur but they are rare; they could include headache, dizziness, nausea, anxiety, panic, and even the creation of false memories.[54]

How to Find a Hypnotherapist

Most hypnotherapists are physicians, registered nurses, social workers, family counselors, psychiatrists, or psychologists who have received additional training in hypnotism.[56] The National Board for Certified Clinical Hypnotherapists and the American Association of Professional Hypnotherapists[67] maintain websites where people can access a list of board-certified hypnotherapists in their state or area of the state.

The U.S. Department of Health and Human Services' Healthfinder.gov website offers a link to find a licensed (not certified) hypnotherapist. The sponsoring agency is the American Society of Clinical Hypnosis.

Hypnosis is a valid complementary and alternative therapy and is used by traditional and alternative healthcare professionals. It is a safe mind–body intervention that allows for introspection and reflection.

The next mind–body intervention to be explored is the Alexander Technique, an intervention that allows people to use their brains (mind power) to control their body posture and function.

▶ What Is the Alexander Technique?

The Alexander Technique is a process in which people can learn to release muscular tension. Over time, our muscles become habitually overtightened, which causes our bodies to become distorted, unbalanced, and compressed.[68] Some say that we have learned walking and postural habits that cause us bodily problems and that we can learn to retrain ourselves. Proponents of the Alexander Technique say that the technique will help us learn how to monitor the way we coordinate ourselves in activities so that the activities can be carried out with a minimum of strain. Performers who sing, act, or dance often acquire this type of muscle imbalance and turn to the Alexander Technique for aid. The area in which people feel this strain is in the muscles of the back and neck, causing a stiffening of the head on the neck. Alexander Technique helps people reeducate the mind and body. It is supposed to help people discover a new balance in the body by releasing unnecessary tension.[68]

History

Frederick Matthias Alexander (1869–1955), an Australian actor, began to experience chronic laryngitis while performing, and doctors were not able to help him.[68] After he realized that his personal stress and resultant tension in his neck and body were causing his physical problems, he began to find ways to speak and move more easily. Alexander learned how to change his breathing technique.[69] Eventually, Alexander began to teach others his technique. As people came to him for vocal training, many who had respiratory difficulties began to improve. As a result of this, medical doctors began referring their patients with respiratory ailments to Alexander (**FIGURE 14.12**).

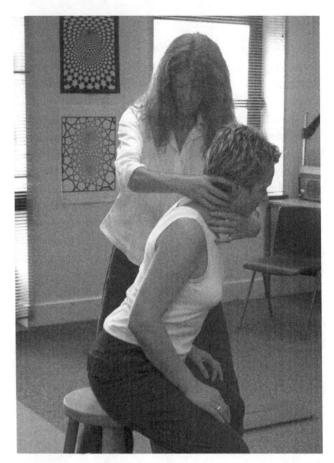

FIGURE 14.12 Alexander Technique.
© Sally and Richard Greenhill/Alamy Images

The Technique

The Alexander Technique can be applied when a person is sitting, lying down, standing, walking, lifting, and/or conducting other daily activities. The technique does not involve exercises, medical therapy or treatment, psychotherapy, or spiritual healing techniques.[69] It is a technique that helps people achieve core stability without specific muscle strengthening exercises. A lesson in Alexander Technique may last 30–45 minutes, and learning it appropriately will probably take a few lessons. A lot depends on how fast the participant learns new skills.[68] Many people come for several months, taking 20–40 lessons, and later come back for refresher lessons.

During the lesson, you would not need to remove your clothes or wear special clothing, although women feel more comfortable wearing pants or jeans rather than a skirt. You would be asked to walk and move around while the teacher observes your posture and movement patterns. The teacher might gently place his or her hands on your neck, shoulders, back, and hips while you are moving or sitting in a chair. This helps the teacher get more information about your patterns of breathing and moving.[70] At the same time, you would learn to think about your own movement and breathing techniques and, hopefully, be motivated to effectively change habits.

From *The F.M. Alexander Technique* by Marian Goldberg[69]:

> *Try this technique*: Try to breathe from high up in your chest or from low down in your abdomen; try walking or moving your arms while you breathe in one of these ways. Do you walk or move your arms differently when you change your breathing? Or make a conscious effort to change the way you walk or the way you hold your neck, or try clenching your arms: Do these efforts affect your breathing or your voice? What if these were habitual efforts—efforts which you made all the time but you were unaware that you were making them? We do make habitual excessive efforts most of the time, but we are generally unaware of making them. Excessive stress in one part of the body is usually part of a larger pattern of habitual malcoordination.

The Benefits

The benefits of the Alexander Technique are many.[69] The technique supposedly results in freer and more comfortable movement, relief from muscle strain and chronic tension, better posture, easier and healthier breathing, increased strength, and increased vitality.

Training of the Teachers

The training period to become a teacher of the Alexander Technique is quite long. Instructors in the Alexander Technique are members of a professional teaching society in the country in which they reside, and the society requires successful completion of a 3-year full-time study program at an accredited teacher training site. Student trainees are required to take 1,500–1,600 hours of instruction and attend classes four to five times each week during that time.[69] Alexander teachers may move from a focus on the postural aspects of the physical body to a focus on healing. This is commonly called "direction," in which the intent of the teacher is to allow his or her life force to be available to the life force within the student. To practice direction, the teacher will be quite still and allow his or her hands to sense what might come. The teacher might let the hands rest lightly on the student's body at whatever locations they are guided to intuitively, but does not physically manipulate the student, although the teacher might use some sort of guided movement. During lessons the hands of the teacher may become very hot or vibrate, and students often experience a release of emotions.[71]

Research Studies

Several recent studies have shown benefits of the Alexander Technique. One was a randomized study in which 579 participants with chronic or recurrent lower back pain were divided into treatment groups: 147 to massage, 144 to 6 Alexander Technique lessons, and 144 to 24 Alexander Technique lessons. In addition, half of each of these groups was randomized to exercise prescription. The exercise and Alexander Technique groups remained effective in lowering lower back pain level after 1 year, but the massage groups did not.[72] Another study by Austin and Ausubel[73] found enhanced ease of breathing in participants who learned Alexander Technique compared to a control group. A 2010 study[74] conducted at the Cincinnati Children's Hospital found that Alexander Technique training resulted in significant improvement in posture and trunk and shoulder endurance from pre- to post-Alexander training in four pediatric urology fellows and three urology residents. The study involved assessing endurance and posture discomfort when performing basic laparoscopic skills. Another investigation was a case study of a 49-year-old woman with a 25-year history of left-sided, idiopathic (unknown cause), lumbar-sacral back pain. The Alexander Technique improved her postural coordination, and after the treatment period, she had decreased lower back pain.[75]

It seems that there are many benefits of the Alexander Technique that involve using one's own mind power to control posture and body function, including pain. It is a noninvasive and gentle technique that results in long-lasting bodily changes.

Next is a discussion of biofeedback, a mind–body intervention used by a wide variety of health and medical professionals.

▶ What Is Biofeedback?

Biofeedback is a mind–body intervention used by many professions to train people to improve their health by using their own body's electrical signals from the muscles or brain. Physical therapists use it to help stroke victims regain movement in paralyzed muscles. Health educators use biofeedback when teaching stress management. Psychologists use it to help tense and anxious clients learn to relax. Many health and medical specialists use biofeedback to help their patients cope with pain.

Origins of Biofeedback

In the 1960s, scientists were hopeful that they could train research subjects to alter brain activity, blood pressure, heart rate, and other bodily functions. They thought that biofeedback could make it possible to decrease the amount of or could stop the need for medications in patients with high blood pressure or other serious conditions. The research showed that we do have more control over involuntary body functions than we thought possible, but it also showed the limitations of mind over body functions.[76]

How It Works

When something frightens us or when we get angry, the stressful event produces a body response that is controlled by our sympathetic nervous system, a network of nerve tissues that help our bodies prepare to meet emergencies as in the "fight-or-flight" response. Hormones (epinephrine, norepinephrine, and cortisol) are secreted from the adrenal gland. Our pupils dilate to let in more light and we begin to sweat. Our blood vessels contract near the skin and our gastrointestinal tract slows down. Our heart beats faster and our blood pressure rises. When the event is over, we begin to relax again and our body responses return to normal. Scientists have used this knowledge to teach people how to relax.

The biofeedback practitioner will initiate a visual or auditory signal to stimulate stress responses. Several kinds of devices are used to monitor a variety of responses. The most regularly used are brain wave activity (electroencephalography, or EEG), skin temperature (thermal feedback), muscle tension (electromyography, or EMG). Used to a lesser degree are galvanic skin resistance (GSR), electrodermal resistance (EDR), blood pressure, respiratory rate, and blood flow.[77] Some of these are handheld portable devices, whereas others are connected to computers. Sensors attached to the skin send information to a monitoring box or a computer that translates the measurements into an audio tone and/ or a visual meter that varies in brightness. Patients see the displayed responses and are then taught to consciously control their own body responses (e.g., respirations and heart rate). The aim is for the patient to control the stress response when not connected to the machine. The exact mechanism for how this is possible is unknown, but scientists believe that the mind–body interaction acts on the limbic system and affects the hypothalamus–pituitary axis and autonomic control.[45]

Effectiveness of Biofeedback

Biofeedback seems to be effective for a range of health and medical problems. For example, biofeedback helps treat urinary incontinence[77] and may also help people with fecal incontinence.[78,79] Thermal biofeedback has been found to ease the symptoms of Raynaud's disease (a condition that causes reduced blood flow to fingers, toes, nose, or ears) and EMG biofeedback has been shown to help people with fibromyalgia.[66] Biofeedback has also been used effectively in children. For example, EEG biofeedback revealed significant reduction in cortical stimulation in children with attention deficit disorder.[80] Thermal biofeedback helped relieve migraine and chronic tension headaches among children and teens as well.[77]

Finding a Qualified Practitioner

Psychiatrists, psychologists, nurses, dentists, physicians, physical therapists, exercise scientists, and health educators may provide biofeedback training. The Association for Applied Psychology and Biofeedback is a good resource for finding qualified biofeedback practitioners,[77] and the U.S. Department of Health and Human Services website, Healthfinder.gov,[81] contains a link to a site that explains how to find a biofeedback practitioner. The sponsoring agency is the Biofeedback Certification Institute of America.

The next two mind–body interventions explored in this chapter are prayer and faith healing. Can prayer work? Can people really heal others through touch? If so, how? Is healing based on faith? These are questions that perhaps will not be answered definitively, but many people offer possible explanations.

▶ Are Prayer and Faith or Spiritual Healing Powerful Mind–Body Interventions?

Prayer for Healing

All religions believe in prayer for healing, although people of different faiths may pray in different styles and ways.[9] In times of illness especially, religious people look toward their God or their figure of authority to help them get well.

Even people who may not believe in a particular religion hold spiritual beliefs that help them get through times of sickness, and those spiritual beliefs are said to be powerful enough to help them regain a sense of well-being.[9] Spirituality is a term that could be synonymous with religiosity, but often it is not. It may be considered an inner sense of believing that something is greater than oneself or some sense that there is a meaning to existence that is higher than oneself. As an example, Alcoholics Anonymous and other similar groups use the concept of a "higher power" to help people overcome addictions.

Questions remain about whether religion, spirituality, or prayer can be effective to help people in the healing process. To answer these questions, scientists have been inspired to use modern scientific tools and methods to test the power of prayer to cure others. Formally, studies of the mind and health healing are considered **noetic science**. "Noetic" means the power of inner knowing, and is a branch of metaphysics.[82] Skeptics believe it is a waste of money to validate the supernatural. On the other hand, proponents say the research is valuable because so many people believe in the power of faith and prayer to heal themselves or others.

Distant healing is perhaps the most controversial healing method. It involves people praying for and healing others great distances away (sometimes without the ill person knowing it). It is also known as **intercessory prayer**. In a 1988 study, a San Francisco cardiologist, Randolph Byrd, asked born-again Christians to pray for 192 people who had heart disease and who were hospitalized. He compared those individuals with 201 people not targeted for prayer and who had heart disease. No one was told which group they were in, but those who were prayed for seemed to need fewer drugs and needed less help breathing. In a landmark 1998 publication, Sicher and colleagues[83] published a study reporting the results of a double-blind randomized trial of distant healing in 40 patients with AIDS. Treatment subjects acquired significantly fewer new AIDS-related illnesses, had lower illness severity, required significantly fewer doctor visits, had fewer hospitalizations, and had a more positive mood compared with controls who did not receive distant healing. A randomized, controlled, double-blind study published in 1999 by William Harris and colleagues[84] involved almost a thousand heart patients, and about half of them were prayed for without their knowledge. The prayer group had lower coronary care unit scores that were derived from a chart review (scored from 1 to 6 on specific coronary needs).[84] Critics, however, say the Sicher and Harris studies were flawed because they were analyzed in the most positive ways and were due to chance, not real science.[85] Further, a behavioral scientist at Columbia University says there is nothing that could account for how the prayers of someone in Washington, D.C., could influence the health of a group of people in Iowa.

The study of intercessory prayer and healing continues. A study led by Dr. Mitch Krucoff[86] in 2001 at Duke University Medical Center studied the effects of intercessory prayer on cardiac patients. Those who received intercessory prayer in addition to having stents placed in their diseased coronary arteries had better clinical outcomes than those not receiving prayer. Another study published in 2004 looked at how a belief in intercessory prayer affected patients.[87] Even though patients did not know they were being prayed for, those who were prayed for did better. A study published in *Research on Social Work Practice* in 2007 found that a meta-analysis of intercessory prayer among social workers indicated a small but significant healing effect.[88]

Does this research mean that intercessory prayer is the main reason the people who participated in these studies gained better health? The answer is no. Even most of the authors agree that there are problems in their research: short time periods of study, other uncontrolled and unknown confounding reasons, small samples, statistical methodology, and so forth. Most, however, are promoting the value of and need for future studies.

Faith or Spiritual Energy Healing

In Chapter 7, we wrote about the practices of shamans—healers among Native American people—and provided a review of healers from other cultures around the world. **Faith or spiritual energy healing** has occurred since earliest times among all cultures, religions, and medicinal practices. Healers have used various healing techniques such as chants and prayer, touching, or hands placed close to the body within the energy fields that surround the body. Popular current methods used for energy healing include Reiki therapy, Therapeutic Touch, qigong healing, and crystal healing. These are discussed in Chapter 15.

Examples of Faith Healing Throughout History

Many examples of faith healing have been recorded throughout history. By 1000 BCE, the Egyptian, Imhotep, had become a famous healer; so much so that on his death, he was deified as the Egyptian god of healing. A symbol of medicine and healing showing snakes entwined around a staff originated from the temples of Imhotep,[89,90] and reoccurred in the Greek and Roman Rod of Asclepius (**FIGURE 14.13**).

Many references to healing can be found in the Bible in both the Old and New Testaments. In the New Testament, Jesus was recorded as having cured both physical and spiritual illnesses after touching people

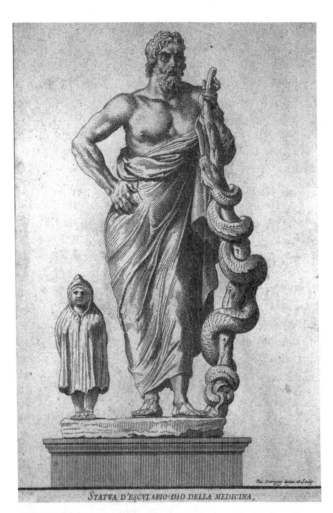

FIGURE 14.13 Asclepius with his serpent entwined staff.
Courtesy of National Library of Medicine

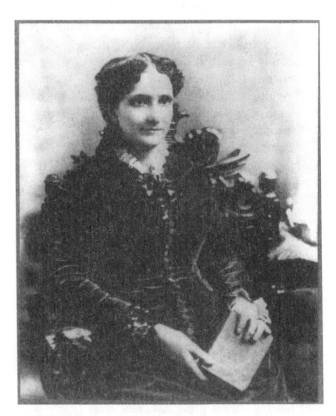

FIGURE 14.14 Mary Baker Eddy.
Courtesy of Library of Congress, Prints & Photographs Division [reproduction number LC-USZ62-53514]

with diseases and disorders such as blindness, lameness, deafness, and insanity.

In 1858, a 14-year-old peasant girl visited a grotto on the edge of Lourdes, a town in France. The girl was Bernadette Soubirous, who was said to have seen visions of the Blessed Mother on 18 different occasions. During one of those incidents, Bernadette was told to dig in the grotto soil and drink the water that would be released. A natural spring was found below the grotto, and the water was thought to have curative powers. This event led to thousands of sick and injured people coming to the spring in hopes of getting cured. They prayed at the spot and bathed in the waters. The healing Grotto of Bernadette was constructed on the site, and visited by people from all around the world. Claims of being cured of cancer, blindness, and other conditions through the ensuing years has led to Lourdes being one of the busiest tourist spots in France.[91]

Mary Baker Eddy (**FIGURE 14.14**) established the first Christian Science church in 1879. She was a notable faith healer who believed she was the recipient of cures after professing to the "truth in Christ." Mary Baker Eddy believed that the basis of all disease was psychosomatic. She wrote that disease was an illusion and could be erased by mind control. Her philosophy became imbedded in the philosophy of the Christian Science church, which holds that the real person is spiritual and reflects God, whereas the material body is unreal. Christian Scientists, therefore, believe that the proper treatment for illness is prayer.[92]

Agnes Sanford (1891–1982), an Episcopalian, is viewed as an important 20th-century healer. In her first book, *The Healing Light*, she outlined her experiences with the healing power of God. In it, she described healing a child's knee. After having touched the knee, the child called to Agnes to take away her hand because "it's hot." Sanford told the child that it was God's electricity and power working in her knee.[93]

Edgar Cayce (1877–1945) is said to be one of the most famous, if not the most famous, healer of the modern era. He was a psychic healer and psychic trance channeller who claimed that he was a devout Christian, though others say he was the founder of the New Age movement. Cayce was most famous for channeling answers to questions concerning the

🔍 CASE STUDY

The following is a synopsis of a case study published on the Spiritual Science Research Foundation (SSRF) website.[96] A man who had been addicted to alcohol for 17 years attended a meeting in March 1999 held by two seekers of the SSRF. They explained the science of Spirituality in brief and explained its influence on various aspects of people's daily lives. They talked about how to begin spiritual practices and explained scientifically how specific spiritual remedies helped in overcoming many of the otherwise insurmountable difficulties in life. One of the examples they gave was an explanation about addictions and their belief that they were caused by spiritual factors such as negative energies. The man attended a second meeting that was led by another spiritual advisor. He began to feel optimistic that by applying the science of Spirituality he could overcome his drinking habit. The advice the spiritual advisors offered was that he should begin chanting the name of God as per his religion of birth and that he should chant the Name of Lord Datta, which is a specific remedy to overcome difficulties due to ancestral problems. He was also instructed to pray to God. The following response is in his own words:

> I started chanting the name of my family deity on the spot. Over the next few days, I slowly started experiencing a change within me. My restlessness and anxiety decreased. I could attend to my job better and I actually started enjoying it. Previously, I would find it stressful to complete obligations at work but now I found that I could meet all the deadlines and still find enough time, energy and enthusiasm to participate in the preparations for the public discourse. I found myself looking forward to the evenings, when I would meet with the seekers of SSRF and work till late into the night with the preparations. The need for alcohol that ordinarily would have been at the top of my mind took a backseat without my knowledge or conscious effort. Soon I found that I did not need it to sustain my day. In one and a half months, my drinking habit of 15 years was gone. Since then for the last 6 years, I have been totally abstinent.

Questions:

1. After reading the case study, what explanations could you give for the man's apparent recovery from alcohol addiction?
2. Why does he believe that chanting aided his recovery?
3. Do you think it is possible that prayer and chanting could be a healing methodology?

Source: Spiritual Science Research Foundation. Overcoming addiction to alcohol. Available at: https://www.spiritualresearchfoundation.org/addiction/overcoming-addictions. Accessed September 7, 2017.

health problems of distant patients. He was known as the Sleeping Prophet because he would lie down, enter a trance state, and then give his readings. It is reported that he gave about 20,000 readings in his lifetime.[94]

Barbara Brennan is a famous healer who runs the Barbara Brennan Healing School. Brennan teaches her students about the human energy field or aura and how to heal it. She is a scientist, healer, author, and trainer. One of her most popular healing books is *Hands of Light: A Guide to Healing Through the Human Energy Field*.[95] In her book, she cites medically verified case studies of a variety of people with diverse illnesses being healed by healers.

Historical and present-day spiritual healers hold some common beliefs. Healers believe that the mind, body, and spirit are one interdependent unit and that all three must work in harmony.[44] They believe that all of us have an energy force around our physical bodies, our minds, and our spirits. Healers believe that the energy force gets disrupted from adverse factors such as stress, negative attitudes, poor dietary habits, and

lack of exercise, and when that occurs, our own power to heal gets blocked. They believe that illness begins in the mind or the spirit and affects the body. When healers lay their hands on people, they believe they can channel or direct energy from some unknown spiritual source via themselves into their patients or clients. Healers also believe that they can help people die more peacefully.

▶ Conclusion

You have now been introduced to many mind–body interventions, some of which have valid scientific studies that indicate they are effective. Some need much more study before reaching that conclusion. Our hope is that the contents of this chapter will motivate you to explore and experience some of these practices so that you can assess for yourself whether they are healing techniques that you could use when needed.

Wrap-Up

Key Terms

Alexander Technique A process in which people can learn to release muscular tension and habitually overtightened muscles that cause our bodies to become distorted, unbalanced, and compressed.

Asanas Another name for yoga poses.

Biofeedback A mind–body intervention that helps train people to improve their health by using their own body's electrical signals from the muscles or brain.

Blood lactate A chemical associated with stress.

Buddhism A religion that originated in India by Buddha (Gautama) and later spread to China, Burma, Japan, Tibet, and parts of Southeast Asia. It holds that life is full of suffering caused by desire, and the way to end this suffering is through enlightenment that enables one to halt the endless sequence of births and deaths to which one is otherwise subject to.

Burmese position Sitting on the floor and using a zafu—a small pillow—to raise the hips just a little so the knees can touch the ground. Sitting on the pillow with two knees touching the ground forms a tripod base that gives 360-degree stability.

Concentration technique Involves concentrating on an external object as a focus point for the mind.

Contemplation meditative techniques Use introspection, self study, and reflection. Contemplative meditation is supposed to help people gain a deeper understanding of some aspect of reality.

Cortisol A chemical associated with stress.

Dervish dancers Turkish dancers who dress in a particular style and seem to dance to the rhythm of the cosmos or the universe.

Distant healing Involves people praying for and healing others at great distances away (sometimes without the ill person knowing it). Also known as intercessory prayer.

Empty mind meditation Involves sitting still, often in a full lotus or cross-legged position, and letting the mind go silent on its own.

Faith or spiritual energy healing Spiritual energy healing has occurred since earliest times among all cultures, religions, and medicinal practices. Various healing techniques are used (including chants and prayer, touching, or placing the hands close to the body within the energy fields that surround the body). Popular current methods used for energy healing include Reiki therapy, Therapeutic Touch, qigong healing, and crystal healing.

Feeling and emotion meditation techniques These may be used independently, but also may be combined with other types of meditation practices.

Free radicals Unstable oxygen molecules that can cause tissue damage.

Full lotus position A seated position in which each leg is placed on the opposite thigh.

Gurdjieff sacred dances A technique wherein the movements are very defined and different parts of the body seem not to be related to each other.

Guru One who is regarded as having great knowledge, wisdom, and authority in a certain area and who uses it to guide others.

Half lotus position A seated position in which the left foot is placed onto the right thigh and the right leg is tucked under the left thigh.

Hypnosis A mind–body technique that focuses on awareness and attention to internal stimuli, much like what is learned while doing meditation. The word "hypnosis" comes from the Greek word *hypnos*, meaning sleep. It was first termed "animal magnetism."

Hypnotherapy Therapy using hypnosis to gain access to the deeper levels of the mind so that a change in thinking and behavior will occur.

Intercessory prayer Involves people praying for and healing others at great distances away (sometimes without the ill person knowing it). Also known as distant healing.

Koan meditation technique Meditations from the Zen School of Buddhism that are designed to break down an ordinary pattern of thinking.

Mandala Means completion or circle. A word coming from one of the languages of India called Sanskrit.

Mantra A word or phrase repeated during meditation.

Martial arts Encompass understanding the relationship of the power of breath, the life force (qi energy), the mind, and the concept of oneness.

Meditation A way of being, a way of seeing, and even a way of loving; a state in which the body is consciously relaxed, the mind is allowed to become calm and focused, and deep feelings of well-being are experienced.

Mesmerize Term stemming from Dr. Franz Anton Mesmer, who defined the discipline of hypnotism.

Metabolic rate The amount of energy liberated or expended in a given unit of time.

Mindfulness meditation To become aware of your physical, emotional, and mental activities in the here and now.

Neodissociation model A model that suggests hypnosis activates a subsystem of both psychological and physiologic parts.

Noetic science The study of the mind and health healing. Noetic means the power of inner knowing, and is a branch of metaphysics.

Parasympathetic nervous system Responsible for causing heart rate and breathing to slow down, blood vessels to dilate, and digestive juices to increase.

Rhythm and song methods of meditation A combination of rhythm, chanting, music, and breath used during meditation to achieve a desired state of calmness.

Sama A ritual practice developed in the mid-9th century that uses music, poetry recital, singing, and dance.

Sanskrit Is one of 22 languages spoken in India and is the liturgical (church language) of Hinduism and Buddhism. The language originated about 1500 BCE.

Serotonin Levels of this chemical influence moods and behavior; low levels are associated with depression, headaches, and insomnia.

Silent mind meditation Technique involving directly perceiving and feeling the world around us by focusing on how we are thinking.

Social psychological model A model that suggests that during hypnosis, an altered state of consciousness does not occur; instead, hypnosis is explained by suggestibility, positive attitudes, and expectations

Sufi dancing Said to be the dance of universal peace and is supposed to bring participants to a mystical experience and cultivate inner peace and harmony. The dance involves whirling by oneself or with partners. Dancers whirl with arms in various positions, such as reaching out and reaching to the heavens.

Sympathetic nervous system Responsible for the "fight-or-flight" response produced during times of stress.

Vipassana Is known as insight meditation. Mindfulness is employed during meditation. Requires being watchful of your breath during inhalation and exhalation.

Visualization techniques Used to achieve a meditative state.

Walking meditation Focuses on awareness of self, the process of walking, and the environment.

WHO AM I Focuses on negating the false self in order to realize one's true nature or enlightenment.

Yoga Requires full awareness of posture and movements. Attention is focused on the breath during all movements and helps open up the energy channels. Thought to be a powerful meditation technique.

Zazen The breathing technique of Zen meditation, also known as the meditation of the Buddha. This involves awareness and concentration during the breathing process to help build or shape the mind and to free oneself from dualistic thinking (separation of mind and body).

Suggestions for Class Activities

1. Invite a person skilled in meditation to class and practice a simple meditation technique. Write a reflection paragraph about how you felt practicing meditation. If a meditation instructor is not available, practice a walking meditation routine.
2. Invite a yoga instructor to class. Be sure that you can obtain a room in your building suitable for practicing some simple yoga techniques. Write a reflection paragraph about how you felt practicing yoga.
3. Invite a hypnotist into class to talk about their techniques when using hypnotism for healing.
4. Obtain a biofeedback machine or computerized biofeedback DVD. Practice biofeedback in class.

Review Questions

1. What are mind–body interventions?
2. Define meditation and discuss three overall benefits.
3. Name five forms of meditation.
4. Who was the founder of TM and how is it used?
5. What is Vipassana meditation and how is it practiced?
6. What is zazen meditation and how is it practiced?
7. Which of the forms of meditation focus on generating and circulating internal body energy?
8. How would you describe mindfulness meditation?
9. Name four meditation positions.
10. Name and explain four meditation techniques.
11. What are five physiological and five psychological benefits of meditation?
12. How can meditation aid spiritual growth?
13. What does the research on the effects of meditation indicate?
14. What is the history and origin of yoga?
15. What are six health benefits of yoga?
16. Why is posture important when practicing yoga?
17. What does "the power of breath" mean?
18. Name three asanas.
19. What does the research indicate about the benefits of yoga?
20. How would you define hypnosis?
21. What is the history of hypnosis?
22. Name and discuss two philosophies explaining hypnotic effects.

23. What are the four stages of hypnosis and what occurs at each stage?
24. How is hypnosis used as a therapeutic treatment?
25. How could you find a qualified hypnotist?
26. What is the Alexander Technique process?
27. What are three benefits of the Alexander Technique?
28. What is the history of the Alexander Technique?
29. Describe a typical Alexander Technique session.
30. How are Alexander Technique teachers trained?
31. What does the research indicate regarding the benefits of the Alexander Technique?
32. What is biofeedback and what are its origins?
33. How does biofeedback work as a mind–body intervention?
34. Explain the biofeedback process.
35. What does the research indicate regarding the benefits of biofeedback?
36. How could you find a qualified biofeedback practitioner?
37. What does the research indicate about the effects of prayer and faith or spiritual healing?
38. What is noetic science?
39. What is intercessory prayer?
40. Name and explain three examples of faith or spiritual healing through the ages.
41. Who was Mary Baker Eddy and what was her contribution to faith healing?

References

1. Complementary and Alternative Medicine for Cancer. Mind-body medicine. Available at: http://cam-cancer.org/The-Summaries/Mind-body-interventions. Accessed April 26, 2018.
2. Pelletier K. *The Best Alternative Medicine: What Works? What Does Not?* New York, NY: Simon & Schuster; 2000.
3. Begley S. Placebo effect may reveal some of its secrets in a new study. *Stat News.* July 4, 2016. Available at: https://www.statnews.com/2016/07/04/placebo-effect-brain-immune-system/. Accessed April 26, 2018.
4. Mipham S. *Turning the Mind Into an Ally.* New York, NY: Riverhead Books; 2003.
5. Kabat-Zinn J. *Coming to Our Senses: Healing Ourselves and the World Through Mindfulness.* New York, NY: Hyperion; 2005.
6. Rinpoche S. Essential Advice on Mediation. Available at: http://www.sacred-texts.com/bud/tib/essmed.htm. Accessed April 26, 2018.
7. Wallace A. *Tibetan Buddhism: From the Ground Up: A Practical Approach for Modern Life.* Somerville, MA: Wisdom; 1993.
8. Cianciosi J. *The Meditative Path: A Gentle Way to Awareness, Concentration, and Serenity.* Wheaton, IL: Quest; 2001.
9. Somerville R, ed. *The Alternative Advisor.* Alexandria, VA: Time Life Books; 1997.
10. Vipassana Dhura Meditation Society. What is Vipassana? Available at: http://www.vipassanadhura.com/whatis.htm. Accessed April 26, 2018.
11. Meditation is Easy. Vipassana: The meditation technique of Gautama Buddha. Available at: http://www.meditationiseasy.com/meditation-techniques/vipassana-the-meditation-technique-of-gautama-buddha/. Accessed April 26, 2017.
12. Maharishi University of Management. Transcendental Meditation Technique. Available at: https://www.mum.edu/about-mum/transcendental-meditation-technique. Accessed April 26, 2018.
13. Transcendental Meditation®. What are the evidence-based benefits? Available at: http://www.tm.org/#benefits. Accessed April 26, 2018.
14. Zen Mountain Monastery. Zazen Instructions. Available at: https://zmm.mro.org/teachings/meditation-instructions/. Published December 30, 2012. Accessed April 26, 2018.
15. A View on Buddhism. What is Meditation? Available at: http://viewonbuddhism.org/meditation_theory.html. Updated December 29, 2016. Accessed April 26, 2018.
16. Holistic Online. Meditation Techniques: Taoist Meditation Methods. Available at: http://1stholistic.com/Meditation/hol_meditation_taoist_meditation.htm. Accessed April 26, 2018.
17. Story F. *Buddhist Meditation.* Sri Lanka: Buddhist Publication Society; 1986. Available at: http://www.freemeditations.com/buddhist_meditation.html. Accessed April 26, 2018.
18. Zen Mountain Monastery. Beginner's Kyudo: Zen Archery Intensive. Available at: https://zmm.mro.org/program/begkyudo-aug-2016/. Accessed April 26, 2018.
19. Kiann N. Persian Dance and its forgotten history. Iran Chamber Society. Available at: http://www.iranchamber.com/cinema/articles/persian_dance_history02.php. Updated November 10, 2014. Accessed April 26, 2018.
20. Gorgani R. 10 things about Sufi dance. Available at: http://www.ranagorgani.com/10-things-about-sufi-dance/. Accessed April 26, 2018.
21. Erzen J. The Dervishes Dance – The Sacred Ritual of Love. Available at: http://www.contempaesthetics.org/newvolume/pages/article.php?articleID=514. Published October 2008. Accessed April 26, 2018.
22. Gurdjieff Dances. Introduction. Available at: http://gurdjieff-dances.com/eng/. Accessed April 26, 2018.
23. Mehta A. Best Meditation Techniques, Types & Practice: Guide to Meditation Practice & Types of Meditation. Available at: http://anmolmehta.com/meditation-techniques-types-and-practice-a-comprehensive-guide/. Accessed April 26, 2018.
24. Maharshi R. Practical Eastern Philosophy—It is Intention that is Action. Available at: http://hello.feilhauer.net/index.php?entry=entry110107-105533. Accessed April 26, 2018.
25. Rosenberg L. Shining the Light of Death on Life: Maranasati Meditation (Part I). Barre Center for Buddhist Studies, *Insight Journal.* Spring 1994. Available at: https://www.bcbsdharma.org/article/shining-the-light-of-death-on-life-maranasati-meditation-part-i/. Accessed April 26, 2018.
26. J. Krishnamuti Online. An Overview of Krishnamurti's Life and Work. Available at: http://www.jkrishnamurti.org/about-krishnamurti/biography.php. Accessed April 26, 2018.
27. Mehta A. Sound Awareness Meditation Technique. Available at: http://www.anmolmehta.com/blog/2007/04/18/free-online-guided-meditation-book-sound-awareness-meditation-technique-ch-2/. Accessed April 26, 2018.
28. Osho. The Osho Mystic Rose Meditation. Available at: http://www.osho.com/highlights-of-oshos-world/mysticrose. Accessed April 26, 2018.
29. Biography Online. Osho Biography. Available at: http://www.biographyonline.net/spiritual/osho.html. Accessed April 26, 2018.

30. Hurley T. Mandalas for Meditation and Coloring. Available at: http://stress.lovetoknow.com/Mandalas_for_Meditation_and_Coloring. Accessed April 26, 2018.

31. Wong C. Coloring mandalas as a meditation technique. *Very Well Mind.* August 23, 2016. Available at: https://www.verywell.com/coloring-mandalas-as-a-meditation-technique-89818. Accessed April 26, 2018.

32. Project Meditation®. Benefits of Meditation. LifeFlow® Audio Technology. December 16, 2015. Available at: https://www.project-meditation.org/benefits-of-meditation/. Accessed April 26, 2018.

33. Giovanni D. Scientific benefits of meditation: 76 things you might be missing out on. Live and Dare. Available at: http://liveanddare.com/benefits-of-meditation/. Accessed April 26, 2018.

34. Borysenko J. *The Beginner's Guide to Meditation* [CDs]. Hay House; 2006.

35. Clarke TC, Black LI, Stussman BJ, et al. *National Health Statistics Reports; No 79. Trends in the use of complementary health approaches among adults: United States, 2002–2012.* Hyattsville, MD: National Center for Health Statistics. 2015.

36. Lawlis F. *Mosby's Complementary and Alternative medicine: A Research-Based Approach.* St. Louis, MO: Mosby; 2001.

37. Nidich SI, Rainforth MV, Haaga DA, et al. A randomized controlled trial on effects of the transcendental meditation program on blood pressure, psychological distress, and coping in young adults. *Am J Hypertens.* 2009;22(12):1326-1331.

38. Carim-Todd L, Mitchell SH, Oken BS. Mind-body practices: An alternative, drug-free treatment for smoking cessation? A systematic review of the literature. *Drug Alcohol Depend.* 2013;132(3):399–410.

39. National Center for Complementary and Integrative Health. Spotlighted Research Results—Meditation. Available at: https://nccih.nih.gov/health/223/research. Accessed September 26, 2018.

40. Davidson RJ, Kabat-Zinn J, Schumacher J, et al. Alterations in brain and immune function produced by mindfulness meditation. *Psychosom Med.* 2003;65(4):564-570.

41. Aubrey A. Meditation a hit for pain management. *National Public Radio.* March 1, 2011. Available at: http://www.npr.org/templates/story/story.php?storyId=7654964. Accessed April 26, 2018.

42. Weil R. Yoga. Medicine Net. Available at: http://www.medicinenet.com/yoga/article.htm. Accessed April 26, 2018.

43. Yoga Basics. The Vedas. Available at: http://www.yogabasics.com/learn/the-vedas/. Accessed April 25, 2018.

44. Bradford N, ed. *The One Spirit Encyclopedia of Complementary Health.* London, UK: Hamlyn; 1996.

45. Ernst E. *The Desktop Guide to Complementary and Alternative Medicine: An Evidence-Based Approach.* New York, NY: Mosby; 2001.

46. Google. Yoga images. Available at: https://www.google.com/search?q=yoga+images&tbm=isch&tbo=u&source=univ&sa=X&ved=0ahUKEwibmufu7NfaAhVEM48KHfdhCDsQsAQIJQ&biw=1366&bih=662. Accessed April 26, 2018.

47. Watson S. The health benefits of yoga. WebMD. Available at: http://www.webmd.com/fitness-exercise/a-z/yoga-workouts. Accessed April 26, 2018.

48. Saradananda S. *The Power of Breath: The Art of Breathing Well for Harmony, Happiness, and Health.* London, UK: Duncan Baird; 2009.

49. Kiecolt-Glaser JK, Christian L, Preston H, et al. Stress, inflammation, and yoga practice. *Psychosom Med.* 2010;72(2):113–121.

50. Prathikanti S, Rivera R, Cochran A, Tungol JG, Fayazmanesh N, Weinmann E. Treating major depression with yoga: A prospective, randomized, controlled pilot trial. *PLoS One.* 2017;12(3):1-36.

51. Chettiar C. Yoga as an intervention method in the reduction of anxiety in college girls. *Res Horizons.* 2014;4:184-187.

52. Ramadan Azab AS, Moawd SA, Abdul-Rahman RS. Effect of Buteyko breathing exercises versus yoga training on pulmonary functions and functional capacity in children with bronchial asthma: A randomized controlled trial. *Int J Therap Rehabil Res.* 2017;6(1):148-153.

53. Raub J. Psychophysiologic effects of hatha yoga on musculoskeletal and cardiopulmonary function: A literature review. *J Altern Complement Med.* 2002;8(6):797-812.

54. Mayo Clinic. Hypnosis. Available at: http://www.mayoclinic.org/tests-procedures/hypnosis/basics/definition/prc-20019177/. Accessed April 26, 2018.

55. American Society of Clinical Hypnosis. General Info on Hypnosis. Available at: http://www.asch.net/Public/GeneralInfoonHypnosis/GeneralInfoTemplate.aspx. Accessed April 26, 2018.

56. Howard, P. Just what does a hypnotherapy session involve? Available at: https://www.sich.co.uk/7410/just-hypnotherapy-session-involve/ Accessed April 25, 2018.

57. Goudas L, Carr DB, Bloch R, et al. *Management of Cancer Pain. AHRQ Pub No. 02-E002.* Rockville, MD: Agency for Healthcare Review; 2001.

58. Potié A, Roelants F, Pospiech A, Momeni M, Watremez C. Hypnosis in the perioperative management of breast cancer surgery: Clinical benefits and potential implications. *Anesthesiol Res Pract.* 2016; 2016:2942416.

59. Schnur JB, David D, Kangas M, Green S, Bovbjerg DH, Montgomery GH. A randomized trial of a cognitive-behavioral therapy and hypnosis intervention on positive and negative affect during breast cancer radiotherapy. *J Clin Psychol.* 2009;65(4):443-455.

60. Berger MM, Davadant M, Marin C, et al. Impact of a pain protocol including hypnosis in major burns. *Burns.* 2010;36(5):639-646.

61. Askay SW, Patterson DR, Jensen MP, Sharar SR. A randomized controlled trial of hypnosis for burn wound care. *Rehab Psychol.* 2007;52(3):247-253.

62. Thieme K, Gracely RH. Are psychological treatments effective for fibromyalgia pain? *Curr Rheumatol Rep.* 2009;11(6):443-450.

63. Moser G, Trägner S, Gajowniczek EE, et al. Long-term success of GUT-directed group hypnosis for patients with refractory irritable bowel syndrome: A randomized controlled trial. *Am J Gastroenterol.* 2013;108(4):602-609.

64. Richardson J, Smith JE, McCall G, Richardson A, Pilkington K, Kirsch I. Hypnosis for nausea and vomiting in cancer chemotherapy: A systematic review of the research evidence. *Eur J Cancer Care (Engl).* 2007;16(5):402-412.

65. Shenefelt PD. Use of hypnosis, meditation, and biofeedback in dermatology. *Clin Dermatol.* 2017;35(3):285-291.

66. Shenefelt P. Biofeedback, cognitive-behavioral methods, and hypnosis in dermatology: Is it all in your mind? *Dermatol Ther.* 2003;16(2):114-122.

67. National Board for Certified Clinical Hypnotherapists. Find a Hypnotherapist. Available at: http://www.natboard.com/index_files/Page548.htm. Accessed April 26, 2018.

68. The Complete Guide to the Alexander Technique. What happens during an Alexander Technique lesson or class? Available at: http://www.alexandertechnique.com/lesson.htm. Accessed April 26, 2018.

69. Goldberg M. The F.M. Alexander Technique. Alexander Technique Center of Washington. Available at: http://www.alexandercenter.com. Accessed April 26, 2018.

70. Rickover RM. The Alexander lesson. In: *Fitness Without Stress*. Portland, OR: Metamorphous Press; 1988: Chapter 4.

71. Benor DJ. Spiritual healing: A unifying influence in complementary therapies. *Compl Ther Med*. 1995;3(4):234-238.

72. Little P, Lewith G, Webley F, et al. Randomised controlled trial of Alexander Technique lessons, exercise, and massage (ATEAM) for chronic and recurrent back pain. *Br J Sports Med*. 2008;42(12):965-988.

73. Austin JH, Ausubel P. Enhanced respiratory muscular function in normal adults after lessons in proprioceptive musculoskeletal education without exercises. *Chest*. 1992;102(2):486-490.

74. Reddy PP, Reddy TP, Roig-Francoli J, et al. The impact of the Alexander technique on improving posture and surgical ergonomics during minimally invasive surgery: Pilot study. *J Urol*. 2011;186(4 Suppl):1658-1662.

75. Cacciatore TW, Horak FB, Henry SM. Improvement in automatic postural coordination following Alexander Technique lessons in a person with low back pain. *Phys Ther*. 2005;85(6):565-578.

76. Runcke B. What is Biofeedback? Psychotherapy.com. Available at: http://psychotherapy.com/bio.html. Accessed April 26, 2018.

77. Mayo Clinic. Biofeedback. Available at: https://www.mayoclinic.org/tests-procedures/biofeedback/about/pac-20384664 Accessed April 26, 2018.

78. Collins J, Mazor Y, Jones M, Kellow J, Malcolm A. Efficacy of anorectal biofeedback in scleroderma patients with fecal incontinence: A case-control study. *Scand J Gastroenterol*. 2016;51(12):1433-1438.

79. Vonthein R, Heimerl T, Schwandner T, Ziegler A. Electrical stimulation and biofeedback for the treatment of fecal incontinence: A systematic review. *Int J Colorectal Dis*. 2013;28(11):1567-1577.

80. Flisiak-Antonijczuk H, Adamowska S, Chładzińska-Kiejna S, Kalinowski R, Adamowski T. Treatment of ADHD: Comparison of EEG-biofeedback and methylphenidate. *Archives Psychiatr Psychother*. 2015;17(4):31-38.

81. Association for Applied Psychophysiology and Biofeedback. Finding a Practitioner for Biofeedback and Applied Psychophysiological Interventions. Available at: https://www.aapb.org/i4a/pages/index.cfm?pageid=3281. Accessed April 26, 2018.

82. Mamun S. Noetic sciences definition & experiments—science of subconscious mind power & thoughts. *Hub Pages*. April 8, 2017. Available at: https://hubpages.com/education/noetic-sciences-experiments-definition-science-of-subconscious-mind-power. Accessed April 26, 2018.

83. Sicher F, Targ E, Moore D 2nd, Smith HS. A randomized double-blind study of the effect of distant healing in a population with advanced AIDS—report of a small-scale study. *West J Med*. 1998;169(6):356-363.

84. Harris WS, Gowda M, Kolb JW, et al. A randomized, controlled trial of the effects of remote, intercessory prayer on outcomes in patients admitted to the coronary care unit. *Arch Intern Med*. 1999; 159(19):2273-2278.

85. Carroll RT. Healing Prayer (HP) & Distant Healing (DH). Skeptic's Dictionary. Available at: http://skepdic.com/essays/healingprayer1.html. Published March 6, 2008. Accessed April 26, 2018.

86. Krucoff MW, Crater SW, Green CL, et al. Integrative noetic therapies as adjuncts to percutaneous intervention during unstable coronary syndromes: Monitoring and actualization of noetic training (MANTRA) feasibility pilot. *Am Heart J*. 2001;142(5):760-769.

87. Palmer RF, Katerndahl D, Morgan-Kidd J. A randomized trial of the effects of remote intercessory prayer: Interactions with personal beliefs on problem-specific outcomes and functional status. *J Altern Complement Med*. 2004;10(3):438-448.

88. Hodge DR. A systematic review of the empirical literature on intercessory prayer. *Res Soc Work Pract*. 2007;17(2):174-187.

89. Google. Image of Caduceus. Available at: http://www.google.com/images?hl=en&rlz=1G1GGLQ_ENUS368&q=image+of+Caduceus.&um=1&ie=UTF-8&source=univ&ei=OoXoTNaRHoI.6lwf-uYJpCw&sa=X&oi=image_result_group&ct=title&resnum=1&ved=0CC0QsAQwAA&biw=1194&bih=1136. Accessed April 26, 2018.

90. Castro J. Religion: A shrine to faith and healing. *Time*. August 29, 1983. Available at: http://www.time.com/time/magazine/article/0,9171,949777,00.html. Accessed April 26, 2018.

91. Kime R. *The Informed Health Consumer*. Guilford, CT: Dushkin; 1992.

92. Christian Science. Mary Baker Eddy. Available at: http://www.christianscience.com/what-is-christian-science/mary-baker-eddy/. Accessed April 26, 2018.

93. Way of Life Literature. Agnes Sanford. Available at: https://www.wayoflife.org/reports/agnes_sanford.html. Published July 22, 2008. Accessed April 26, 2018.

94. Do famous spiritual energy healers manifest miracles? October 6, 2008. Available at: https://www.slideshare.net/marcwiliam/do-famous-spiritual-energy-healers-manifest-miracles. Accessed April 26, 2018.

95. Brennan B. *Hands of Light: A Guide to Healing Through the Human Energy Field*. New York, NY: Bantam; 1987.

96. Spiritual Science Research Foundation. Overcoming addiction to smoking, drinking and marijuana with spiritual practice. Available at: https://www.spiritualresearchfoundation.org/addiction/overcoming-addictions. Accessed April 26, 2018.

Appendix 14.A

▶ Guided Basic Zen Meditation Technique

It is important to meditate in a quiet and still environment. This might be in a bedroom or den in your house. The lighting should be low or, if daytime, sit without the sun directly on you. You can set a timer, but it is not necessary.

1. Sit in a comfortable position. You can sit on a zafu in a lotus or cross-legged position.[27] People who use a zafu sit on the forward part of the cushion so that the hips are higher than the knees. Sometimes it may require sitting on more than one zafu to raise the hips higher than the knees. You may also sit on a chair. If so, keep both your feet planted on the floor.

2. Lengthen your spine. It should be upright, but allowing for the spine's natural curve.

3. Rest your hands on your thighs.

4. Try to relax your shoulders and your arms.

5. Tuck in your chin a little.

6. Shut your eyes until they are half open. You may focus your gaze on the floor in front of you or on some other point in the room.

You also may close your eyes completely if you wish.

7. Relax your face and jaw. It helps to relax the jaw by placing your tongue on the roof of your mouth. Stillness of the body is important at this time. It is the time to calm the mind as well as the body.

8. Concentrate on your breathing. You may take a few deep, slow breaths through the nose and breathe out through the mouth. Try not to manipulate your breathing after those first few breaths. Just pay attention to it and become aware of when the breath is relaxed.

9. Some people are taught to count their inhalations and exhalations up to a certain number and then to start again. You may try that for the first week of meditating. Inhale deeply and count one. Exhale deeply and count two. Inhale again and count three. Exhale again and count four.[27] The next week, try counting only the inhalations but not the exhalations. The 3rd or 4th week that you meditate, try not counting at all. Just sit in stillness and be aware of the moment, the state of stillness.

Appendix 14.B

▶ Guided Sound Awareness Meditation Technique

Guided sound awareness meditation is another variation on meditation. The first steps are the same as guided Zen meditation. The last steps are a little different.

1. Sit in a comfortable position. You can sit on a zafu in a lotus or cross-legged position. People who use a zafu sit on the forward part of the cushion so that the hips are higher than the knees. Sometimes it may require sitting on more than one zafu to raise the hips higher than the knees. You may also sit on a chair. If so, keep both your feet planted on the floor.

2. Lengthen your spine. It should be upright, but allowing for the spine's natural curve.

3. Rest your hands on your thighs or your lap.

4. Try to relax your shoulders and your arms.

5. Tuck in your chin a little.

6. Close your eyes or shut your eyes until they are half open. You may focus your gaze on the floor in front of you or on some other point in the room.

7. Relax your face and jaw. It helps to relax the jaw by placing your tongue on the roof of your mouth.

8. Take a few deep, slow breaths through the nose and breathe out through the mouth. Do not try to control your breathing, but pay attention to it.[27]

9. When your breathing becomes relaxed, begin to pay attention to sounds in your immediate environment.

    Then, begin to pay attention to sounds that are more distant. Try to just listen and attend to those sounds. Note if the sound is loud or soft, high or low, or it changes beat. Try not to get involved with the sounds, but become a detached observer who is listening to the music of life.[27] You may find yourself thinking about personal issues. If so, observe those thoughts, but then return to attending to the sounds in your environment.

10. After a period of time, turn your attention from distant sounds to sounds closer to you.

11. Finally, turn your attention to only the sounds closest to you and to your breath.

12. Open your eyes and slowly become aware of all your surroundings. Stand and breathe deeply.

CHAPTER 15

Energy Therapies

LEARNING OBJECTIVES

As a result of reading this chapter, students will be able to:

1. Identify typical practices considered to be energy therapies.
2. Characterize chi and its role in energy therapies.
3. Contrast the practices of Reiki and Therapeutic Touch.
4. Examine the challenges related to "mainstreaming" energy therapies.
5. Identify whether research exists to support the use of energy therapies.

▶ What Are Energy Therapies?

Energy therapies, or energy health therapies, are defined by the National Center for Complementary and Integrative Health (NCCIH) as "A technique that involves **channeling** healing energy through the hands of a practitioner into the client's body to restore a normal energy balance and, therefore, health."[1] They are a group of methods that attempt to harness, manipulate, or direct energy in and around the body. In Eastern cultures and alternative medicine practice, as discussed in earlier chapters, believe **qi (chi)** is a therapeutic force. The central concept is that life force energy qi is embodied in all things living and nonliving, and as such that energy can play a role in one's well-being. Energy therapies are sometimes broken down into two categories: **biofield** and bioelectrical therapies. Biofield practices are said to affect the energy in and around the body. There is no effective and efficient mode of measuring biofield energy; thus, these forms of treatment are quite controversial. Bioelectrical energy is measurable, with energy forms using a specific frequency or wavelength, and is most often a magnetic force, light energy, or a type of radiation.

▶ What Is the Human Biofield?

Energy healers believe that the body possesses and emits "**subtle energy**," and it is the disruption in the flow of this energy that causes disease and illness. The human biofield is a multidimensional, vibrational reflection of the emotional and mental energy of the physical form[2] and links our cellular activity to the meridians of the body. It is comprised of measurable electromagnetic energy and qi, and is more generally referred to as the human energy field or an aura.[3] Thus, therapy and healing involve the restoration of a positive and efficient flow of human energy. As you might imagine, not all medical professionals believe in this form of healing. Most practitioners of Western medicine acknowledge that the human body emits a low level of energy, but see it as a by-product of cell activity, nothing of significance, and most certainly not something that can be manipulated for personal well-being.

This chapter will introduce readers to **putative** (yet to be measured successfully) energy therapies such as **qigong**, **Reiki**, and **Therapeutic Touch**, and **veritable** (measurable) therapies such as bioelectromagnetic, light, and sound therapies.

▶ What Is Qigong?

Qigong (also spelled qi gong) is an ancient method of Chinese health care utilizing physical forms, focused breathing, and deliberate movement. According to the Qigong Association of America, qigong comes from the combination of two Chinese words: *qi*, meaning energy, and *gong* (pronounced "kung") referring to action or more specifically, skill.[4] There are many **forms** of qigong, but all involve posture, breathing, and mental focus. As mentioned earlier, qi is described as an energy force found in all things living and nonliving. Therefore, energy is all around us. Practitioners of qigong believe energy can be manipulated, gathered, utilized, and influenced through meditation and movement designed to increase and focus the flow of that energy. In this sense, it has both a physical component and an intellectual one, where the mind is used as much as the body in gathering and directing energy. Qigong, therefore, is a reference to the skill or practice of cultivating energy. Not everyone believes this is a legitimate form of healing and explain potential effects and benefits in other ways. See **BOX 15.1** for an example of the placebo effect.

As in all Chinese medical practices, practitioners of qigong believe disease or illness takes hold when there is a blockage or disruption in the flow of qi. Qigong is designed to activate the meridian system (discussed in Chapter 9) and improve or redirect the flow of energy, and as a result, improve well-being.

When used strictly as a form of exercise, proponents of qigong point to the multidimensional nature of the art form as "better" than traditional exercise. Benefits are expanded because you must integrate mind with body.[4]

History of Qigong

Summarizing 3,500 years of history is no easy task, and we can provide only minimal information here. In short, qigong history falls into four predominant time frames. The first starts when art was introduced

---

BOX 15.1 Placebo Effects

People get better because they believe they will get better. That is the explanation many physicians and researchers give to explain the "benefit" of most energy therapies (and many other complementary medicine therapies). It is called the placebo effect. A placebo effect is a situation in which people believe a particular medicine or treatment is curing their illness, but they are experiencing a pill or treatment known to have no medicinal benefit (e.g., sugar pill). In short, studies have shown a percentage of people who are told they are taking real medicine, even though it is fake medicine (commonly referred to as a sham), will perceive that their health has improved. They get better because they have the *expectation* that they will get better. The more a person believes they will improve, the better they may become.

When it comes to energy medicine, and the practitioners and patients are working with a form of energy that has yet to be accurately measured like chi (through Therapeutic Touch or Reiki), physicians tend to believe that the placebo effect is occurring.

---

around 1000 BCE, and continues for approximately 800 years. It is during this time that shamans performed traditional animal dances as a form of spiritual cleansing at New Year's.[5] In addition, the *Chinese Book of Changes* introduced the concept of qi and the relationship among man, heaven, and Earth. Qi was first recorded as a source of energy in ancient carvings. In 300 BCE, Zhuang Zi, a Daoist philosopher, described the connection between breathing and personal health.

The second phase occurred during the Han Dynasty (206 BCE to 220 AD). Meditation and Buddhism were introduced in China from India, where qigong had been used for thousands of years. Because of the new Buddhist influence, this time is often referred to as the religious era of qigong. In this phase, qigong focused only on health and well-being, and the introduction of faith practice to the art significantly broadened its emphases. Unfortunately, the masses were not allowed to practice, because the religious leaders kept most of the information secret. If the practice had not been secretly passed on through the Buddhist monasteries, we may not have ever seen qigong in the general population.

The third phase (500 AD to 1911) began during the Liang dynasty, when qigong started being used as a martial art, and ran through the end of the Qing dynasty. Many, many martial art forms were created using the principles of qigong. It was deemed to increase physical strength in addition to simply improving general health and well-being. It is also during this phase when the animal forms came to being: the tiger, leopard, dragon, snake, and crane. Each form represents a different style and sequence of movement representing the most cherished and revered animals of the time.

The final phase runs from 1911 to the present time. Qigong today is a mix of practices from a multitude of countries. The secrecy of the religious elders has been broken and qigong has become an activity of the masses. It is during this current phase that research began to take place, a more pronounced emphasis on wellness and qigong was seen, and its worldwide visibility increased.[6]

Forms of Qigong

According to the Wudang Taoist Traditional Kung Fu Academy, qigong can be categorized as internal or external.[7] **Internal qigong** is similar to meditation, using mind, breath, and visualization to guide bodily energy and energy immediately surrounding an individual. Internal qigong is designed to increase qi, open meridians, to open the lungs and improve respiration, and strengthen organs. **External qigong** involves greater movement. This movement is said to hold many health benefits, from reduction of blood pressure to increased flexibility. External qigong is used in conjunction with internal qigong to strengthen mind and body connection.

Activities and movements included in qigong are done either as a singular movement, in combination, or in sequence. These movements or sequences are referred to as forms. Forms are generally designed to address a specific health issue such as heart health or lung health. Some forms are designed for general well-being or lifelong fitness. They go by names such as Everyday Stretching Qigong and Eight Brocade Exercises.[8] See **BOX 15.2** for an example of Remedy Routines.[9] There are countless forms available to learn and practice, with a growing number of videos and community-based exercise programs available to teach qigong, as well. Most forms involve a significant emphasis on flexibility. All forms incorporate an emphasis on the flow of qi, the opening of the body's meridians, and breathing. Because of the physical nature of the external form, as with any form of activity, it is recommended you discuss a new program with your physician before initiating practice.

What Does Research Say About Qigong?

A challenging component to interpreting the research on qigong is that most is completed in Chinese culture, where the concept of qi as a universal life force found in all things is a given, not something to be proven. Qigong is famous in China for curing chronic disease and promoting health. Western practitioners do not appear to have a clear consensus on the effect of practicing qigong, because there is still the challenge of measuring qi itself.

In a 2016 article published in the *International Journal of Behavioral Medicine*,[10] researchers examined the effect of one month of qigong practice on the immune system of 43 randomly assigned participants. Analysis indicated a significant improvement in the experimental groups' immune system to both recognize disease and mobilize to attack disease. In 2015, 87 postmenopausal breast cancer survivors were enrolled in a double-blind controlled study[11] to determine if qigong practice (compared to a sham technique) would improve survivors' fatigue, depression, and sleep issues. After three months of participation and subsequent follow-up, the researchers determined that qigong can improve posttreatment fatigue in survivors.

Clinical research on qigong is more extensive, with many studies having a primary focus on cancer patients. Klien and colleagues[12] conducted a systematic review of randomized-controlled studies encompassing a total of 831 patients from multiple countries. They found a consistent pattern of significant positive effects of qigong on cancer patient quality of life, levels of fatigue, immune function, and cortisol levels. Mayer conducted a review of 33 studies, the vast majority again published in Chinese literature, to gain a sense of the overall success of qigong as a method of controlling hypertension.[13] The analysis revealed a results pattern supporting the notion that qigong can reduce or stabilize blood pressure for those who use the technique. In many of the studies, participants were able to reduce or eliminate their medication. Along with blood pressure adaptations, results included increases in blood flow, reductions in vascular tension, reduced viscosity (thickness) of the blood, and increased volume of blood flow to the limbs. Mixed results exist on the effectiveness of qigong in addressing fibromyalgia,[14] mental illness, heart disease, and lower back pain.[15]

As with lab studies, these results are not without controversy, particularly in research methodology. Lack of random assignment of subjects, lack of specific measurement of treatment effects (was it the

BOX 15.2 The Remedy Routine: Qigong

Remedy Routine: Discharging Turbid Substances from the Liver

Part 1. Preparation

Stand with your feet as wide apart as your shoulders and pointing straight ahead, knees slightly bent. Let your shoulders relax. Allow your hands to fall at your sides naturally. Place the tip of your tongue on your upper palate, just behind your teeth. Relax the root of your tongue. Smile slightly. Keep your eyes level and open, thinking of nothing.

Use your mind to relax your head, your neck, your shoulders, your elbows, your wrists, your fingers, your chest, your stomach, your back, your waist, your hips, your knees, your ankles, your feet, and your toes. Gather qi into your lower dantian (belly button level). Concentrate your mind on your lower dantian for a little while.

Direct qi from your lower dantian down to hui yin (groin area) and back up and along du mai (channel through the center middle of the body) to da zhui (neck level). At this point, split the qi into two streams and direct it through the middle of the shoulders, down through the arms to lao gong (middle of palm). Shift your body weight onto your left leg and place your right foot a half step forward with the heel on the ground and toes up pointing to a tree, some wood, or wooden furniture.

Part 2. Taking Back the Qi

Turn your palms forward and using your shoulders as pivot, raise your arms while holding a ball of outer qi, and then beam it into bai hui (point at top of skull). Open your chest by spreading out your elbows. With palms down and fingertips pointing at each other, let your hands descend in front of your body guiding qi through your middle channel into shan zhong or heart area. See Forms 1–4 in **FIGURE 15.1**.

Part 3. Discharging Turbid Substance from the Liver

Move your hands parallel to your right chest and then descend along your right side thinking that you are guiding the turbid substance (spent qi) from your liver through the inner side of your right leg. Discharge it out of your body from da dun (the inner side of your right big toe) to the tree, wood, or wooden furniture. When your hands have descended and become straight, turn your palms facing the tree, wood, or wooden furniture thinking the spent qi has been pushed into it. Then, allow your arms to fall naturally at your sides. See Forms 5–8 in Figure 15.1.

If you do it continuously, you should separate your two hands instead of allowing them down, and then push your hands out a bit to draw an arc and raise your hands along your hips, and then turn your palms forward and start to do it again. You may do it continuously from 9–30 times until you feel your liver area is comfortable. It all depends on the need of the individual, but you cannot do it too many times.

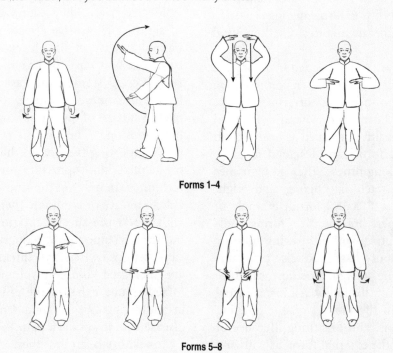

Forms 1–4

Forms 5–8

FIGURE 15.1 Remedy routine associated with cleansing of the liver.

Courtesy of Qigong Association of America (www.qi.org).

qigong, or was it just being active, or did the ailment just run its natural course), and expectancy bias all were common issues with the studies included in the review.

What does this mean for the practice of qigong and its health benefit? By Eastern standards and measures, qigong is rooted in 7,000 years of historical success, and the documentation of that success is clear and evident. Identifying, measuring, and studying qi are not necessary in Eastern culture—it is readily accepted that life force energy exists and can be accessed at the individual level. Through the eyes of a Western medical practitioner, however, there has not been enough controlled experimentation, accounting for all potential bias, to determine clinical significance of the practice. That being said, there appears to be a positive health effect to the practice of qigong, and at a time when two out of three U.S. adults are overweight or obese, movement such as qigong for healthy purposes is a positive alternative.

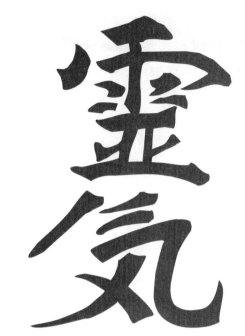

FIGURE 15.2 Japanese Reiki character.
© Daniela Illing/Shutterstock.

▶ What Is Reiki?

Combining two Japanese words, *Rei* and *Ki*, gives the word Reiki. Literal translation is always challenging when trying to describe something unseen, but Rei has been defined as the wisdom of God, a higher power (in general), or a reference to a cosmic, universal energy. Ki (essentially the same as qi) is the unseen energy that gives or causes life.[16] When placed together, Reiki becomes a reference to an energy force guided by a greater power. However, practitioners are quick to point out that the general public should not associate a "greater power" reference to religion or specific dogmatic practice. Reiki is considered to be a universal practice that, once trained, any individual can use to help themselves or others. The symbol for Reiki is two Japanese kanji, one over the other: the top representing Rei and the bottom, Ki (**FIGURE 15.2**). A person undergoing Reiki healing is shown in **FIGURE 15.3**.

The International Center for Reiki Training (ICRT) describes the practice of Reiki as a Japanese technique for stress reduction and relaxation that also promotes healing.[17] Like other Eastern philosophy techniques, Reiki focuses on qi, the life force energy. It is this energy that causes us to be alive. ICRT summarizes the notion by stating, "If one's life force energy is low, then we are more likely to get sick or feel stress, and if it is high, we are more capable of being happy and healthy."

The exact history of Reiki involves some uncertainty. According to Tanmaya Honervogt, in her book *The Power of Reiki*, the development of Reiki is attributed to a Japanese professor, Dr. Mikao Usui, who left a faculty position to search for the secrets behind the healing and miracles of Jesus Christ.[16] On his journey, which included an extended stay at a Buddhist monastery, Usui was meditating upon a mountain. During that meditation, he was given the power of healing. Although he was able to assist others in their physical healing, he did not feel as though he was helping people change their lives, and from this notion he created the Reiki rules for life or the Reiki Principles (**BOX 15.3**). He also discovered that the desire to be healthy was not by itself enough for

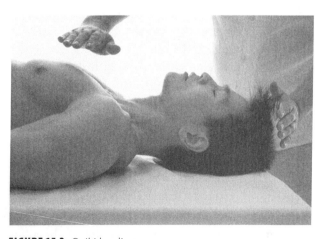

FIGURE 15.3 Reiki healing.
© Jupiterimages/Goodshoot/Thinkstock.

According to Muller and Gunther in their book, *A Complete Book of Reiki Healing*, the principles of Reiki are:

- Just for today, be free and happy.
- Just for today, have joy.
- Just for today, you are taken care of.
- Live consciously in the moment.
- Count your blessings with gratitude.
- Honor your parents, teachers, and elders.
- Earn your living honestly.
- Love your neighbor as yourself.
- Show gratitude to all living things.

Muller B, Gunther H. *A complete book of Reiki healing.* Mendocino, CA: LifeRhythm USA; 1995.

healing to occur. A person must *ask* for healing and one must *give* something in return. The history presents a challenge in that all records of the "lineage" of Reiki were destroyed in World War II, and it has now become more like folklore than fact.

The principles were written to help people understand that you must make a conscious decision to improve oneself, and accept responsibility for your healing, for the process to have lasting results.

Reiki came to the United States after World War II through a Reiki master named Hawayo Takata. She carried on the practice of Reiki in the United States, and began training new masters in 1975. Before her death in 1980, she had trained 22 new masters. Reiki healers are not trained in a school, but rather have the art passed on to them from another master. Today, one can find Reiki practitioners all over the world.

The Reiki practitioner is said to serve as a channel for life force energy. A relatively simple concept, the practitioners use their hands to transmit life force energy to the ill. The ICRT website describes the treatment experience as "a wonderful glowing radiance that flows through and around you ... including body, emotions, mind and spirit, creating many beneficial effects that include relaxation and feelings of peace, security and wellbeing."[17]

Reiki Symbols

Reiki symbols (**TABLE 15.1**) are used through movement of the center of the palm or the fingers, through a visualization of the symbol, or by spelling the symbol name three times. Whichever method of activation is used, it is done over an energy center or the ailing component of the recipient of services. Symbols and mantras (words spoken internally that represent the symbols) are used during the healing process to create vibration. Vibration creates and accesses energy. The first symbol increases power from the surrounding area. The second symbol promotes harmony for mental/emotional healing. The third symbol sends Reiki over distance. The fourth symbol balances energy. The fifth symbol is the most powerful and is only used by masters as it is purported to heal the soul.[16]

The Concept of Attunement

The process of using Reiki as a healing modality, or of using Reiki on another person, begins with **attunement**. Attunement is the ceremony of initiation to the force of energy and is the precursor to an individual becoming a practitioner. The student receives this energy or attunement from a master, opening up the chakras and channels to allow the energy to flow through the body. Energy is released through the hands, and once "attuned," a student can then use the energy on another person. The energy never leaves you once your channels are opened.[18]

Reiki Degrees

Reiki practitioners can progress through three levels of training or **Reiki degrees**.[19] The first degree, and most basic, contains the initial attunements, opening up the energy channels for transmission of energy to another person (or animal; **BOX 15.4**).[20,21] The energy will go where it is needed, so there need not be any specific placement of the hands.[19] The Reiki practitioner could rest his or her hands on the patient's hands, and the energy flow would make its way from the practitioner, through the patient's hands, and continue through the patient's body until it reaches the area of need. All hand placements for healing physical ailments are trained at level one. A second degree Reiki practitioner integrates symbolism into the healing process. At this level, the practitioner has been further trained in the placement of hands for the purpose of healing the nonphysical realm, and can send energy over distance to a person or event.[19] The third degree, or Master Healer/Teacher/Grandmaster, is studied when one is ready to lead a life of healing. The Reiki master training is much more personalized, with mastery of the Reiki symbols the focus. The Reiki master is expected to then train new practitioners, passing along skills and attunements.[18,19]

TABLE 15.1 The Reiki Symbols

Symbol Name	Alias	Symbol	Use
Cho Ku Ray (choh-koo-ray)	The Power Symbol		Increases power by drawing energy from the surrounding area
Sei Hei Ki (say-hay-key)	The Harmony Symbol		Mental, emotional healing; calming the mind; balance
Hon Sha Ze Sho Nen (hanh-shah-zay-show-nen)	The Distance Symbol		Sends Reiki over distance and time (past, present, future) to anyone and anything
Tam A Ra Sha (tam-a-ra-sha)	The Balancing Factor		Grounds and balances energy; unblocks chakra centers
Dai Ko Myo (dye-ko-me-o)	The Master Symbol		Most powerful symbol; used only by Reiki masters; heals the soul

Modified from reiki-for-holistic-health.com.

BOX 15.4 It's Not Just for Humans

One of the fastest growing areas for the use of Reiki is in the animal kingdom. Reiki masters are using their training to heal pets and farm animals.[20] The International Association of Reiki Professionals indicates that the number of specialists utilizing Reiki on animals is growing and that animals respond very well to the practice.[20] One area of specialty is equine Reiki, practiced on horses. This specialty claims to help horses heal from abuse or neglect and become more calm, making it easier for owners to manage the animal's behavior.[21] In New Mexico, a local Reiki healer works with family pets to ease anxiety and fear in the animals, helping them to be more pleasant and cope with being in a home with more success.[22]

Most of the pet owners, and even some of the practitioners, cannot fully describe what is at work. Skeptics will say it is simply the one-on-one attention the pet receives—something the owner should be doing anyway. Believers in Reiki will reinforce the tenets of healing and the ability of energy to be focused for the good of the animal. Most pet owners simply know that their animal is calmer, less noisy in many cases, and overall better behaved.

Ellis S. Healing for your horse: find out the best therapy yourself. *Farmer's Weekly.* 140:21, 2004.; Farida M. Much cheaper way to heal pets. *New Strait Times.* June 21, 2008:7.

What Is Therapeutic Touch?

Therapeutic Touch, in practice, is much like Reiki. An individual unfamiliar with either practice would not be able to distinguish them, with the notable exception that does *not* involve touch (in most instances).[23,24] Reiki, in most cases, involves actual placement of the hands on the recipient. Other distinctions between the two are found primarily in philosophy, history, and training. The actual art of laying on of hands and healing through touch is almost as old as mankind. It is described in virtually every historical or spiritual practice available. Therapeutic Touch's specific form, description, and function of healing was designed and introduced in the 1970s by a New York University nursing professor, Dolores Krieger, PhD, RN.[25] Dr. Krieger took the ancient philosophies and designed a form of healing to be used by nurses in practice, although her vision was that anyone and everyone could be a healer (**FIGURE 15.4**).

Therapeutic Touch is performed in five stages.[25,26] The first stage, centering, is a form of meditation that allows the Therapeutic Touch practitioner to focus on their own energy field in preparation for transmission to the patient. McCormack describes the necessity of the process, stating the importance of the healer working without judging the patient, and that doing so

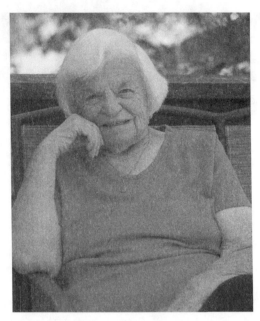

FIGURE 15.4 Dolores Krieger, PhD, RN, designer of Therapeutic Touch.

Courtesy of Therapeutic Touch Dialogues, Inc.

requires a clear mind.[25] Once the practitioner is centered, an **assessment** of the energy surrounding and emanating from the patient is performed. This stage is a clear distinction from Reiki practice. Assessment involves the passing of the healer's hands 2–6 inches away from the patient's body in an attempt to detect disruptions in energy flow or in the patient's energy field. The practitioners will move their hands in a sweeping motion, palms facing the patients, attempting to sense a distinction in energy in moving systematically from one area of the body to the next.

The third stage of the process **rebalances** the energy of the patient, clearing excess energy into the environment. Hands are moved in long sweeping strokes, much like one would use to smooth out a bed sheet while making a bed. This effort is designed to rebalance the energy field; allow for energy to flow in a positive, undisturbed fashion; and allow the patient to then heal more efficiently. The fourth stage is the treatment phase, sometimes referred to as modulation. In this phase, the practitioner uses stationary hand positions to direct energy to a specific location. This is said to transfer energy from the practitioner to the patient, correcting any further imbalance in the patient's energy field.[25] The fifth stage is the evaluation stage. During this stage, the practitioner completes a final assessment of the patient's human energy field to compare changes in the field with original assessment and to formally end the session. Following completion of the Therapeutic Touch session, the practitioner recommends that the patient rest to integrate the changes in his or her energy field.

Recipients of Therapeutic Touch report a variety of outcomes, some positive, some not. In her 2004 article in *Nursing Standard*, Annie Hallett reported on seven cancer patients and their experience with Therapeutic Touch.[26] Reactions varied with some patients mentioning relaxation, peace, focus, or understanding. In the rare occasion a patient has a negative experience, it is usually associated with the release of strong emotions.

▶ What Does Research Say About Reiki and Therapeutic Touch?

As you might imagine, therapy and healing based on the presence of a biofield surrounding the human body is likely to be criticized. Significant debate is present as to whether a field of energy surrounding the body even exists. The manipulation of that energy, then, would seem even more debatable. Although proponents of energy therapies say there is proof of the human energy field, demonstrated for instance with Kirlian photography, others believe such techniques are not measuring a "manipulatable" field of energy. Nonetheless, significant published research exists. In general, research on these two practices seem to carry a similar challenge—scientific methodology. Evidence presented demonstrating positive effect ranges from purely anecdotal to research with rigor. While often criticized for a weak scientific approach, the vast majority of research shows some positive influence on a broad spectrum of ailments; however, there are also articles containing significant criticism of both practices. What follows is a brief summary.

Supporting Research

In 2015, Gronowicz and colleagues[27] studied the effect of Therapeutic Touch on the development of cancer in mice, compared to a control and a sham treatment. While the animals receiving treatment did not experience chances in the development of the tumor itself any differently than the comparison groups, the mice receiving Therapeutic Touch did have significantly lower levels of cancer metastasis and significantly higher immune functions. A study with one of the largest samples of recipients of Therapeutic Touch was published in 2003 in the journal *Holistic Nursing Practice*.[28] As part of a quality improvement process at a New York hospital, more than 600 recipients of Therapeutic Touch were surveyed and monitored. The results indicated patient satisfaction with the process and improvements in pain reduction, calmness, and overall well-being.

Two recent studies measured perceptions in the treatment group after exposure to Reiki sessions. In a randomized trial, Rosada[29] and colleagues studied the effect of a 30-minute Reiki session on burnout symptoms in mental health professionals. Analysis from patient Maslach Burnout Inventory-Human Services Surveys and Measure Your Medical Outcome Profiles showed significant reductions in burnout, depersonalization, and fatigue in the experimental group versus the sham Reiki participants. Rosenbaum and Van de Velde (2016)[30] measured cancer center users' perceptions pre- and post-participation in Reiki. Patrons expressed significantly lower levels of stress and anxiety as well as increases in mood and perceived quality of life.

A 2003 Kumar and Kurup[31] study reviewed the impact of Reiki and meditation practices on individuals with seizure disorders proving untreatable by other means. The 15 people in the study participated in Reiki sessions over a 3-month period. In the end, participants showed significant positive changes to the imbalances in magnesium, tryptophan, tyrosine, dopamine, and norepinephrine, all of which were related to an increase in seizure frequency. All participants experienced a reduction in seizure frequency of at least 50%, with most experiencing a decrease of 75% (e.g., a drop from 12 seizures per month to two seizures per month).

A short-term 2006 study of 24 seniors with mild levels of Alzheimer's disease, half of whom received four weekly Reiki treatments and half of whom did not, revealed small but nonstatistically significant improvements in the mental function of those involved in the study.[32] Participants, between 60 and 80 years of age, most commonly reported improvements on scales related to memory and depression. Short-term memory of recent events, recall of location of items, and concentration ability showed improvement. Emotional state improvements in degree of sadness, degree of worry, and measures of self-esteem were seen as well.

Stress reduction is often a desired impact in the practice of energy therapies. According to an article published in the *Journal of Alternative and Complementary Medicine* in 2014,[33] the perceptions of well-being among oncology patients was studied over a 4-year period. Significant improvements were found for those participating in Reiki in reducing stress and pain as well as increasing levels of happiness. A 2004 study measured the influence of Reiki on several mechanisms in the autonomic nervous system, the component of the central nervous system responsible for initiating and disengaging the stress response.[34] The study found significant positive influences for the reduction of mean blood pressure, diastolic blood pressure (a reflection of the relaxation response), heart rate, frequency of respirations, and vagal tone (pre- and post-Reiki measurement). Vagal tone is the difference in the pace of the heartbeat when breathing in versus when breathing out. Heart rate normally increases during an inhalation and slows during an exhalation. A small difference in heart rate during inhalation and exhalation would indicate a weak or poor vagal tone and a reflection of increased stress levels. Participating in an activity that increases the vagal tone would suggest the reduction of stress. It should be noted that differences were also significant when compared to a control group receiving no treatment. Interestingly, a placebo group (subjects believed they were receiving Reiki, but were not) also showed a pretest/posttest improvement in several of the measured areas. Environmental stress has also been positively affected by Reiki. Baldwin and Schwartz compared the Reiki practice to a sham practice (people simply sitting next to the subject with their hands up and facing) and a control group, and found Reiki to be an effective tool in reducing the impact of white noise on systematic stress in laboratory animals.[35]

Some Examples Against Therapeutic Touch

One of the historical and most compelling pieces pointing to Therapeutic Touch as fraudulent is a 1998 article published in the *Journal of the American Medical Association*, featuring a study conducted by a sixth grade student in Colorado.[36] The study asked 21 practitioners of Therapeutic Touch to show they could detect a human energy field. Practitioners sat at a table with their hands on the table, palms up. The researcher placed one of her own hands 3–4 inches above one of the practitioners' hands. The practitioner, with vision of the hands blocked, was to indicate which hand was covered. The practitioners were only able to correctly identify to researcher's hand placement 42% of the time, less than what would be expected by random guessing.

A 2014 Best Practices in Mental Health study[37] reviewed the impact of Reiki treatments on the development of secondary traumatic stress in 67 social workers and social work graduate students. Reiki tenets also have been challenged in the literature. It is believed the Reiki practitioner is independent of the energy transmission process and functions merely as a "go-between" in the healing process. One 2006 study found the practitioner's own energy field did have an impact on the healing and growth of *E. coli* cultures in a laboratory setting.[38]

A 2002 study again placed doubt on the legitimacy of a Reiki practitioner to accurately identify energy fields, or to have a significant effect on the health

process for, in this case, stroke victims.[39] A Reiki master trained several hospital employees in Reiki, with only half going through full initiation, the process giving them the ability to be a healer. Results did not indicate a difference in treatment responses between fully initiated and fake Reiki healers nor a difference in the new healers' ability to determine whether they had been fully initiated.

▶ What Is Bioelectromagnetic Therapy?

As stated earlier, veritable (measurable) energy therapies use a predetermined wavelength and/or frequency to emit energy on a patient as a healing force.[40] Although light and sound therapies are included in this subcategory of energy therapies, magnet or magnetic therapies are the most commonly seen and most controversial of the group. The use of magnets for healing has occurred for centuries. The relationship between human energy and magnets became more popularized in the late 1700s when Franz Mesmer "demonstrated" his ability to use magnets to alter the human energy field.[41]

Magnets, Polarity, and Healing

If one accepts the concept that we each possess a human energy field, or biofield, as discussed throughout the chapter, then what is acknowledged is the existence of **universal polarity**. Consider a time in your childhood when you played with magnets. Magnets, you were told, had a north pole and a south pole. One end of the magnet attracted and one end repelled, and most kids figured out how to make one magnet spin by turning another magnet above it. The strength of the magnetic pull is called **gauss rating** (**BOX 15.5**).[41] Also see **FIGURE 5.5** for an image of a healing magnet bracelet.

The energy found in and around the human body, chi, is said to move because of the tension between polarities.[40] Anderson explains the tension between opposing polarity "pulls" energy through the body, and keeps it in constant motion.[40] If illness is a disruption or blockage in the flow of energy, then the manipulation of polarity can return flow to normal. This is the basis of **magnet therapy**.

Research Related to Bioelectromagnetic Therapies

The majority of research on the use of magnets for health purposes is in the area of pain control. Ratterman and colleagues report the literature claims

BOX 15.5 Gauss Ratings

The claim reads, "We have the most powerful magnets on the market today! 12,500 gauss! There is nothing better for your health, so buy yours now. Supplies are limited on this incredibly powerful magnet!" The key to the advertisement is the term "gauss."

Gauss is used to describe magnetic strength or power. In general, the term is used to answer the question, "How magnetic is it?" A typical consumer often believes that bigger is better. If 300 gauss is a good magnet, then 12,500 gauss must be awesome! When it comes to products for magnetic therapy, however, consumers should know that gauss ratings are only part of the story. You must also consider the size, weight, and material used for the magnet.[43]

An example of this is the Earth's magnetic field, which possesses a gauss rating of 0.5, compared to a refrigerator magnet, which has a gauss rating of about 8–10. Is the refrigerator magnet 50 times more powerful than the Earth? Well, no, of course not. Because it is not *just* about the gauss rating; it has to do with the size and mass of the Earth compared to the size and mass of the refrigerator magnet. A round iron magnet with a quarter-inch diameter has the same gauss rating as a 12-inch by 12-inch iron plate. The gauss rating is based on the material, iron. The plate would be more powerful overall, because of its greater size, and would have a magnetic pull from a greater distance, as opposed to just right next to the magnet.

If you are interested in utilizing magnet therapy, do not be manipulated by claims like the one above. Most therapy-related magnets range from 300–3,000 gauss. When looking for products, be certain to investigate. Check the company's reputation, any business claims made by consumers, and cost. Use the gauss rating, but also review the size and mass of the magnet, its cost, and return policies if you experience no benefit from the therapy.

Source: Richmond SJ, Gunadasa S, Bland M, MacPherson H. Copper bracelets and magnetic wrist straps for rheumatoid arthritis—analgesic and anti-inflammatory effects: A randomised double-blind placebo controlled crossover trial. *PLoS One.* 2013;8(9):e71529.

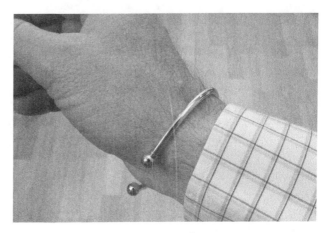

FIGURE 15.5 Healing magnet bracelet.

related to magnetic therapy's impact on fibromyalgia and chronic and soft tissue pain.[42] The group points out that research supporting the claims is sparse and what exists is predominantly anecdotal. Of the seven pieces of research summarized in the article, six show a positive improvement on pain and/or fatigue, but all show deficiencies in study design.

Like the other energy therapies, some magnet therapy research also shows little to no benefit from the method. A typical article of this nature is a 2013 study on the use of magnetic wristbands on 70 individuals with rheumatoid arthritis compared to demagnetized bracelet with no polarity.[43] Changes in health status were not significant in the areas of pain management, inflammation, or functionality. This is a common finding throughout the literature. Authors generally mention the lack of rigor and scientific merit in energy therapy research.

The NCCIH essentially states[44] that there is no scientific support for the medical use of magnets as a therapeutic device. In fact, magnets may be dangerous for those who were on an insulin pump or have a pacemaker. The magnet can interfere with the function of these devices. There are some studies that show evidence for the use of magnets for pain, but in general, they are small studies, were conducted for too short a time frame, or were not controlled to Western medical standards.

▶ How Should I Choose an Energy Therapy?

A quick search of the Internet will identify thousands of people identifying themselves as therapists using energy-based techniques, and about 350,000 hits for a search on "healing magnet dealers." Like all alternative therapy practices, follow the basic guidelines from the NCCIH to protect yourself.[45]

- Keep your primary healthcare provider informed. Seek their recommendation for a practitioner in the type of healing you seek.
- List CAM practitioners and gather information about each before making your first visit. Check on their education, training, and licensure. Read the research for use of a practice for your ailment.

⌕ CASE STUDY

Janine is a 47-year-old woman who recently has been struggling with her health. In the last 12 months, Janine has been feeling extremely fatigued. Continuous aching throughout her body compounds this sense of "tired." She has been to see her family practice doctor on several occasions, who first treated her for flu, then arthritis, but has now determined that the symptoms are too random and are therefore untreatable. She feels like she has been on every medication in the book. The pain for Janine has become almost unbearable. She has lost her job because she cannot make it through the day without taking breaks due to her tiredness and her pain. Money is getting tight in her family, and her husband is working extra to try and support Janine and their two children. She is starting to think that no one believes her, and that this is all in her head. She has even contemplated suicide, although she has no real desire to die, she just has had enough of the pain.

Questions:

1. What might Janine's issue be?
2. Which energy therapies discussed in this chapter, if any, have been shown, at some level, to assist with Janine's issue?
3. How might Janine go about determining whether an energy therapy, or a specific energy therapist, is right for her?

- Determine if the alternative practitioner will work with your primary care provider.
- Ask the practitioner some basic questions: What are your credentials? How long have you been in practice? Where did you receive your training? What licenses or certifications do you have? What is your success rate? Can I talk to other clients of yours?
- Ask how much the treatment will cost. How many sessions of treatment would you need? Do not assume your insurance will cover the cost.
- Make a list of questions for the first visit, and come prepared to answer questions about your personal health history. Decide after the first visit if the practitioner is right for you. Did you feel comfortable with the practitioner? Could the practitioner answer your questions? Did he or she respond to you in a way that satisfied you? Does

the treatment plan seem reasonable and acceptable to you?

▶ Conclusion

Energy therapies are often considered some of the most controversial of alternative medical practices. The emphasis on the mental and spiritual aspects of healing leaves room for much debate over the actual physiological influences and what might be attributed to mere suggestion, and the research, generally, does not conclude that energy healing can be used for any and all disorders. Those who claim to have benefitted from these practices, as well as the growing number of practitioners in the realm of energy therapies, will continue to tout the advantages of taking part in mind–body–spirit modalities.

Wrap-Up

Key Terms

Assessment A process in Therapeutic Touch wherein the practitioner determines where and how the energy of the patient is moving.

Attunement A Reiki rite of passage where the ability to heal is passed on to a new Reiki practitioner from a Reiki master.

Biofield The energy emitted from the human body.

Channeling In Reiki, the role of practitioner. Energy sent to the patient simply flows through the Reiki healer, who is the channel.

Reiki degrees Levels of advancement in the art of Reiki.

External qigong Bodily movement related to the practice of qigong.

Form A series of predetermined and/or scripted movements designed to increase, unblock, or promote healing through the acquisition of energy (qi).

Gauss rating The degree of magnetic strength based solely on materials used to construct the magnet.

Internal qigong A form of qigong emphasizing breathing, meditation, and visualization.

Magnet therapy The use of magnets on or around the human body to restructure the flow of energy in the human body for purposes of healing and well-being.

Putative A type of energy that has yet to be effectively measured by science.

Qi (chi) According to TCM, qi is a bodily energy that flows through unseen channels in the body called meridians. Illness is believed to occur when qi is blocked.

Qigong A type of energy therapy that uses gentle movement to access and redistribute energy surrounding and within the human body.

Rebalance A process in Therapeutic Touch to clear or release excess energy from the human energy field into the environmental field.

Reiki An energy therapy characterized by laying hands on an individual at specific locations, and the transfer of energy from the practitioner to the patient.

Subtle energy Generic term used to describe all energy not easily or readily categorized by modern science.

Therapeutic Touch An energy therapy characterized by holding the hands several inches away from the patient, sending energy to the patient via the hands, in an effort to heal.

Universal polarity Concept of all energy being influenced and moved by opposing polar magnetism.

Veritable A form of energy that can be measured scientifically.

Suggestions for Classroom Activities

1. Conduct a search for an energy therapy practitioner in your area. Conduct an interview using the guidelines for selecting a practitioner and report back to class.
2. Conduct an experiment with the use of a magnetic bracelet or device designed to balance your electrical aura. Report your results.

Review Questions

1. What is a veritable energy therapy?
2. What is a putative energy therapy?
3. For what ailments is qigong potentially an appropriate therapy?
4. How do Reiki and Therapeutic Touch differ? Explain each difference.
5. Why might the mystic/spiritual component of touch therapies present a problem for researchers?
6. What is the theory behind the use of magnet therapy as an approach to healing?
7. What steps should a person take before committing to an alternative medical practitioner?

References

1. National Center for Complementary and Integrative Health. Terms Related to Complementary and Integrative Health. Available at: https://nccih.nih.gov/health/providers/camterms.htm. Updated September 24, 2017. Accessed April 30, 2018.
2. Red Spirit Energy Healing. The Human Biofield. Available at: http://www.red-spirit-energy-healing.com/human-biofield.html. Accessed April 30, 2018.
3. Biofield Tuning. The Biofield Anatomy. Available at: https://biofieldtuning.com/biofield-tuning-institute/the-biofield-anatomy/. Accessed April 30, 2018.
4. National Qigong Association. What is Qigong? Available at: http://www.nqa.org/what-is-qigong-. Accessed April 30, 2018.
5. Cohen KS. *The Way of Qigong: The Art and Science of Chinese Energy Healing.* New York, NY: Random House; 1997.
6. Wudang Internal. Qi Gong. Available at: http://internalstyle.com/energy-art/qi-gong. Accessed April 30, 2018.
7. Wudang Daoist Traditional Kungfu Academy. Qigong: A Brief Introduction to Wudang Qigong. Available at: https://www.wudangwushu.com/qigong. Accessed April 30, 2018.
8. Kuei S, Comee S. *Beginning Qigong: The Ancient Chinese Method of Healing and Strengthening the Body, Mind, and Spirit.* Tokyo, Japan: Tuttle; 1993.
9. Zhao J. *Chinese Soaring Crane Qigong.* Corvallis, OR: Qigong Association of America; 1997.
10. Vera FM, Manzaneque JM, Rodríguez FM, Bendayan R, Fernández N, Alonso A. Acute effects on the counts of innate and adaptive immune response cells after 1 month of Taoist qigong practice. *Int J Behav Med.* 2016;23(2):198-203.
11. Larkey LK, Roe DJ, Weihs KL, et al. Randomized controlled trial of qigong/tai chi easy on cancer-related fatigue in breast cancer survivors. *Ann Behav Med.* 2015;49(2):165-176.
12. Klein PJ, Schneider R, Rhoads C. Qigong in cancer care: A systematic review and construct analysis of effective qigong therapy. *Support Care Cancer.* 2016;24(7):3209-3222.
13. Mayer M. Qigong clinical studies. In: Jonas WB, Crawford CC, eds. *Healing, Intention, and Energy Medicine.* Edinburgh: Churchill Livingstone; 2003:121-137.
14. Lauche R, Cramer H, Häuser W, Dobos G, Langhorst J. A systematic overview of reviews for complementary and alternative therapies in the treatment of the fibromyalgia syndrome. *Evid Based Complement Alternat Med.* 2015;610615.
15. Kelley GA, Kelley KS. Meditative movement therapies and health-related quality-of-life in adults: A systematic review of meta-analyses. *PLoS One.* 2015;10(6):e0129181.
16. Honervogt T. *The Power of Reiki.* London, UK: Gaia; 1998.
17. International Center for Reiki Training. What is Reiki? Available at: http://www.reiki.org/FAQ/WhatIsReiki.html. Accessed April 30, 2018.
18. Muller B, Gunther H. *A Complete Book of Reiki Healing.* Mendocino, CA: LifeRhythm; 1995.

19. Arth Reiki & Healing. Reiki Levels or Degrees. Available at: http://www.healthmantra.com/reiki/reiki_levels.shtml. Accessed April 30, 2018.

20. International Association of Reiki Professionals. Reiki for Pets and Animals. Available at: https://iarp.org/reiki-for-pets-and-animals/. Accessed April 30, 2018.

21. International Association of Reiki Professionals. Reiki for Horses: The Benefits of Equine Reiki. Available at: https://iarp.org/reiki-for-horses-the-benefits-of-equine-reiki/. Accessed April 30, 2018.

22. Swan B. Healing force. *Santa Fe New Mexican*. April 6, 2008. Available at: http://santafescoop.ning.com/profiles/blogs/2014787:BlogPost:4543. Accessed April 30, 2018.

23. Potter P. What are the distinctions between Reiki and Therapeutic Touch? *Clin J Oncol Nurs*. 2003;7(1):89-91.

24. McClintock A. Reiki. In Carlson J, ed. *Complementary Therapies and Wellness*. Upper Saddle River, NJ: Prentice Hall; 2003:214-231.

25. McCormack G. Noncontact therapeutic touch. In Carlson J, ed. *Complimentary Therapies and Wellness*. Upper Saddle River, NJ: Prentice Hall; 2003:186-213.

26. Hallett A. Narratives in therapeutic touch. *Nurs Stand*. 2004;19(1):33-37.

27. Gronowicz G, Secor ER Jr, Flynn JR, Jellison ER, Kuhn LT. Therapeutic touch has significant effects on mouse breast cancer metastasis and immune responses but not primary tumor size. *Evid Based Complement Alternat Med*. 2015;2015:926565.

28. Newshan G, Schuller-Civitella D. Large clinical study shows value of therapeutic touch program. *Holist Nurs Pract*. 2003;17(4):189-192.

29. Rosada RM, Rubik B, Mainguy B, Plummer J, Mehl-Madrona L. Reiki reduces burnout among community mental health clinicians. *J Alternat Complement Med*. 2015;21(8):489-495.

30. Rosenbaum MS, Velde J. The effects of yoga, massage, and Reiki on patient well-being at a cancer resource center. *Clin J Oncol Nurs*. 2016;20(3):E77-E81.

31. Kumar RA, Kurup PA. Changes in isoprenoid pathway with transcendental meditation and Reiki healing practices in seizure disorder. *Neurol India*. 2003;51(2):211-214.

32. Crawford SE, Leaver VW, Mahoney SD. Using Reiki to decrease memory and behavior problems in mild cognitive impairment and mild Alzheimer's disease. *J Altern Complement Med*. 2006;12(9):911-913.

33. Meredith K, Erica L. Reiki improves health of oncology patients: In and out of the hospital. *J Alternat Complement Med*. 2014;20(5):A75.

34. Mackay N, Hansen S, McFarlane O. Autonomic nervous system changes during Reiki treatment: A preliminary study. *J Altern Complement Med*. 2004;10(6):1077-1081.

35. Baldwin AL, Schwartz GE. Personal interaction with a Reiki practitioner decreases noise-induced microvascular damage in an animal model. *J Altern Complement Med*. 2006;12(1):15-22.

36. Rosa L, Rosa E, Sarner L, Barrett S. A close look at therapeutic touch. *JAMA*. 1998;279(13):1005-1010.

37. Novoa MP, Cain DS. The effects of Reiki treatment on mental health professionals at risk for secondary traumatic stress. *Best Pract Mental Health*. 2014;10(1):29-46.

38. Rubik B, Brooks AJ, Schwartz GE. In vitro effect of Reiki treatment on bacterial cultures: Role of experimental context and practitioner well-being. *J Altern Complement Med*. 2006;12(1):7-13.

39. Shiflett SC, Nayak S, Bid C, Miles P, Agostinelli S. Effect of Reiki treatments on functional recovery in patients in poststroke rehabilitation: A pilot study. *J Altern Complement Med*. 2002;8(6):755-763.

40. Anderson E. Introduction to energy therapies. In Carlson J, ed. *Complementary Therapies and Wellness*. Upper Saddle River, NJ: Prentice Hall; 2003:92-99.

41. MagnetTherapyMagnets.com. Measuring magnetic gauss. Available at: http://www.magnetictherapymagnets.com/magnetic-gauss-magnets.html. Accessed May 1, 2018.

42. Ratterman R, Secrest J, Norwood B, Ch'ien AP. Magnet therapy: What's the attraction? *J Am Acad Nurse Pract*. 2002;14(8):347-353.

43. Richmond SJ, Gunadasa S, Bland M, MacPherson H. Copper bracelets and magnetic wrist straps for rheumatoid arthritis–analgesic and anti-inflammatory effects: A randomised double-blind placebo controlled crossover trial. *PLoS One*. 2013;8(9):e71529.

44. National Center for Complementary and Integrative Health. Magnets for Pain. Available at: https://nccih.nih.gov/health/magnet/magnetsforpain.htm. Updated December 7, 2017. Accessed April 30, 2018.

45. National Center for Complementary and Integrative Health. 6 Things To Know When Selecting a Complementary Health Practitioner. Available at: https://nccih.nih.gov/health/tips/selecting. Updated September 24, 2017. Accessed April 30, 2018.

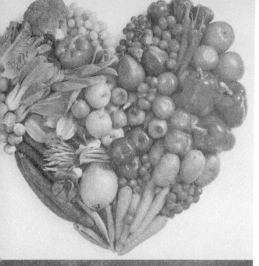

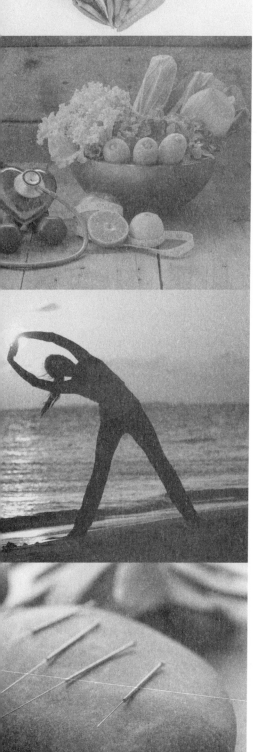

PART 4

Avoidance of Scams and Costly Treatments That Do Not Work

CHAPTER 16

Frauds and Quackery

LEARNING OBJECTIVES

As a result of reading this chapter, students will be able to:

1. Explain what separates conventional medicine from health quackery.
2. Describe the most common forms of consumer health fraud.
3. List guidelines for determining if a health practice is fraudulent.
4. Summarize the quackery of some modern-day scams.
5. Explain the reasons the nutrition market is particularly susceptible to health quackery.

▶ What Is Health Quackery?

Medical or health quackery is not a new problem in the United States. It has always flourished in the areas of disease where no cures had yet been found by legitimate medicine, or where treatment was long and perhaps painful. Quackery, indeed, flourishes because it promises cures, promises which are false, but which a man in pain, unhappy, or afraid would accept without question.[1]

—Congress on Medical Quackery, 1962

Because of the ease of access to health information today, and the skill and design of current advertising, it has become difficult to tell what really has the potential to aid the consumer in addressing personal health issues and what is simply nonsense. Some products have true value in the medical community, others do not. Whether or not there is value is oftentimes, particularly in the medical community, determined based on the kind of evidence found supporting the practice:

- **Scientific medicine**: Reflects established, conventional or mainstream knowledge, based on standard methods of prevention, diagnosis, and treatment, reviewed by medical schools, research centers, professional organizations, professional journals, and governmental offices. This fits the standard for typical Western medicine.

- **Investigational medicine**: Approved testing of medicines or devices on consumers, but not yet fully approved for distribution—under investigation. Treatments are discontinued if they prove to be harmful, outmoded, or not useful.

- **Unproven treatments**: Treatments of unknown value. Not yet proven worthless or proven effective by Western standards.

- **Home or folk remedies**: Some folk remedies can be effective for very specific things, but are not a panacea for all disorders or illnesses, and should not be considered such. It should also be noted some home remedies are not valuable and can be absolutely worthless.

- **Quackery**: False representation of a substance, device, or therapeutic system as being beneficial in treating a medical condition, diagnosing a disease, or maintaining a state of health (e.g., "snake oil" remedies; deliberate misrepresentation of the ability of a substance or device to prevent or treat disease).[2]

You see **quackery** every day, but may not realize what you are looking at. You might be watching television, when an attractive woman appears on the screen and tells you she lost 50 pounds in 3 weeks with this new miracle weight loss drug. Perhaps, you are reading a magazine and somewhere in the final few pages you see an advertisement for a device that can do everything—from relieving arthritis pain, to easing nausea, to curing cancer. If you are a relatively healthy person who is not experiencing any major health issues at the moment, you most likely let those types of claims fade away without much thought. But if you were a consumer who was struggling to overcome the debilitating nature of arthritis or were recently diagnosed with a terminal form of cancer, your reaction may be very different—and that is exactly what the purveyor of quackery is hoping.

Cure-alls, quick fixes, and miracle drugs are promoted and practiced all the time. In the health arena, when these activities have no realistic point of helping you, they are referred to as quackery. Quackery is defined in many different ways, but the central theme of all definitions (like the one described earlier) is that it is the practice of **deceit** or trickery specifically confined to the medical field. In the eyes of the government and the law, it is a form of **fraud**. Most generally, the cure-all is promoted by one of two types of people: (1) the unskilled or ignorant healthcare practitioner searching for financial gain or (2) the person who truly believes their product can help but is promoting something that is useless. In all cases, quackery preys on the unwell or desperate individual who has tried and failed to address their health concern, sees no hope, and is now willing to do anything to find a cure.

▶ What Is a Health Quack?

If "quackery" is the practice of medical fraud or medical deceit, then the person promoting that practice would be referred to as the "quack." Not everyone likes the term and certainly not everyone is comfortable with the term because of its negative connotation, but it is the term used most regularly in the health arena. The *Merriam–Webster* dictionary defines a **quack** as "a pretender of medical skill; an ignorant or dishonest practitioner."[3] The term originated in the 1600s as quacksalver. A physician and alchemist of the time named Paracelsus (**FIGURE 16.1**) was the first physician

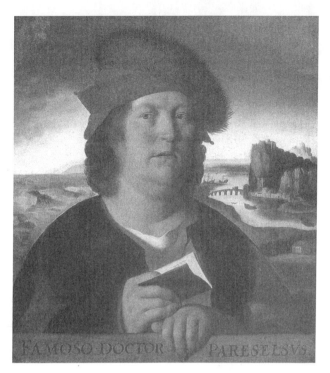

FIGURE 16.1 Paracelsus.
© World History Archive/Alamy Stock Photo.

to be labeled a quack. He had travelled worldwide learning remedies from locals, and he began to integrate those folk remedies into his treatment of patients, in this specific case, those with syphilis. He rubbed a salve containing mercury into a patient's syphilitic rash, healing the sore. Colleague physicians, whose treatment practices Paracelsus had moved away from, called him a quack for using quacksalber.[4]

In the health arena, anyone who offers false hope of recovery or elimination of a healthcare concern through practices, techniques, or use of equipment that has no real chance of resolving the health condition is referred to as a quack. The National Council Against Health Fraud, citing a U.S. House of Representatives, Select Committee on Aging definition, states a quack is "Anyone who promotes health schemes and remedies known to be false, or which are unproven, for a profit."[5] Again, the definition can prove to be challenging. As discussed throughout the book, many remedies based on Eastern philosophies on qi or on energy have no real method of measurement. So, the "proven" criteria refer to the Western, double-blind, research oriented form of proof. And, as discussed, this is simply not possible for many alternative methods. No one would argue that there are methods clearly proven to have no effect, and thus fit the "quackery" label. But many people will argue for methods, ones that have no traditional way of proving or disproving, as legitimate. The remainder of this chapter focuses on methods and modalities known to be without merit.

▶ Why Would Someone Promote a Fraudulent Item?

Financial gain may indeed be a motive for promoting worthless health products. The individuals who do this are deceitful and manipulative, preying on the vulnerabilities of sick people. But not all quacks are outright or even intentionally deceitful. As mentioned earlier, many believe very strongly in their cause (**BOX 16.1**), and have developed their opinions through time and personal experience or through their interpretation of existing research. They may be well educated and many times respected by their peers, and at some point their perspective alters from the mainstream medical community. This is when the great debate begins: Are they crazy or have they gained insight into something others have missed? **Traditional medical practitioners**, who want to see practices tested and researched thoroughly before they are promoted to the public, will dismiss these ideas as quackery. Consumers who are willing to experiment or who have tried all other approaches and failed may very well become immediate believers. Health professionals committed to protecting the latter group, the susceptible and vulnerable, will fight vehemently to protect the consumer.

▶ What Are the Most Common Types of Health Fraud Today?

Clearly, quackery or health fraud is not a new phenomenon. The **Food and Drug Administration (FDA)** estimates that 38 million Americans have used a fraudulent health product within the past year, with 1 out of 10 people who try quack remedies harmed by side effects.[7] The availability of the Internet has created a simple method for **scam** artists and quacks to take advantage of the general public. A review of the May 2009 *Consumer Health Information*[8] from the FDA points to the following as the most common fraudulent health claims:

- **Cancer fraud:** The Hoxsey Cancer Treatment is an herbal procedure that promises to draw cancer out from the skin. The FDA has issued specific warnings against the treatment (**FIGURE 16.2**).

BOX 16.1 Immunizations and Autism

In 1998, British researcher Andrew Wakefield published what was then a landmark paper in *The Lancet*, a highly respected medical journal. In essence, the article drew a link between children who received vaccination (specifically the measles, mumps, rubella vaccine) and an increase in the likelihood of developing **autism**. Since that time, great debate has been held regarding the findings in that study. It was criticized highly for the small number of children actually studied (12) and the associations and conclusions drawn. The work has since been determined to be fraudulent—Wakefield carefully selected the children studied, influenced by a lawyer representing parents involved in a lawsuit against the vaccine maker. The work has been universally debunked by the scientific community, and in 2010 *The Lancet* retracted the article from its publication.[6]

As is the case with many "causes," celebrity support and use of public forums became increasingly visible as performers such as Jenny McCarthy, Jim Carrey, and Holly Robinson Peete called for parents to reconsider vaccinating their children. They claim vaccines are simply promoted for making money (conspiracy theory) and that our children are paying a significant price because of the volume and timing of all the shots. They have been successful, because the number of parents choosing not to vaccinate has continued to grow over the last two decades.

The primary damage here is to the children. Although all the anti-vaccine promotion work is done in good faith, in a perceived effort to help children, it may in fact be hurting them. The reality is that parents are delaying or neglecting important vaccinations for serious illnesses, raising the susceptibility of their children to these diseases. And because a growing number of children are going unvaccinated, all other children are at risk of exposure as well.

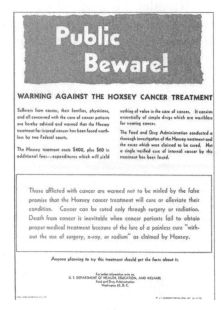

FIGURE 16.2 Announcement issued by the FDA regarding the Hoxsey treatment.

FDA. This week in FDA History – Sept. 21, 1960. Available at http://www.fda.gov/AboutFDA/WhatWeDo/History/ThisWeek/ucm117863.htm. Accessed August 23, 2011.

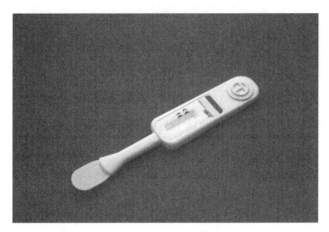

FIGURE 16.3 An at-home HIV test device.

Black salves are marketed as having a similar effect. Neither has been shown to have any benefit and can be corrosive to tissues.

- **HIV/AIDS fraud**: Although treatments exist that can slow the progression of HIV, there is still no cure for the virus. Early initiation of the drug regimen for HIV is important, and experimentation with other products only delays the onset of using medicines demonstrated to have an effect. The FDA has approved only one at-home test device for HIV, called the Home Access HIV-1 Test System or the Home Access Express HIV-1 Test System, which tests for HIV-1 (the viral strain that causes most cases; **FIGURE 16.3**).

- **Arthritis fraud**: There are so many fraudulent arthritis cures marketed today that the U.S. Federal Trade Commission estimates Americans spend nearly $2 billion every year on them. But chronically pained consumers will keep trying to find something to relieve their discomfort. Some of the more common items claimed to cure arthritis are emu oil, colloidal silver, living water, snake venom, bee venom, and gin-soaked raisins. There currently is no proven or consistently demonstrated cure for arthritis.

- **Fraudulent "diagnostic" tests**: Blood, saliva, or urine tests that your physician might normally request are used to assist in the detection of many things such as pregnancy, cholesterol levels, hepatitis, HIV, and blood sugar levels. Unfortunately, there are sources who claim the tests can be used for much more significant purposes. If you are ever curious as to whether a diagnostic test is useful for a particular reason, contact the FDA.

- **Bogus dietary supplements**: There are hundreds of nutritional supplements on the market, and

just about as many wild claims regarding what they are good for. We cannot even begin to list them all. Here is the best rule of thumb: do your homework. Read everything you can, speak to your physician, and get research and facts, not testimonials.

- **Weight loss fraud**: An article in the *Journal of the American Medical Association*[9] indicated that dieting is a constant concern for Americans, with more than 45% of overweight or obese people trying to lose weight, spending $60 billion on weight loss products. That leaves a lot of room for scam artists to promote their products to the general public. The FDA has worked hard to impose **truth in advertising** laws and to ensure that claims made by product developers are accurate. Most of what the consumer hears, however, is overblown and not typical of the true effect of the product. While many products are legitimate weight loss products, many more often contain ingredients not listed on the label, and can be dangerous (**FIGURE 16.4**).

- **Sexual enhancement product fraud**: In 2009,[10] the FDA released its latest warning regarding drugs promoted and sold online for treating **erectile dysfunction** and for enhancing sexual performance. Many of the products are contaminated with drugs that cannot be distributed legally without a prescription and drugs that can cause a significant decrease in blood pressure. One National Institutes of Health (NIH) study found that 77% of the sexual enhancement and erectile dysfunction drugs tested were contaminated and posed a serious risk to users.[11]

- **Diabetes fraud**: The FDA has taken numerous compliance actions against sales of fraudulent

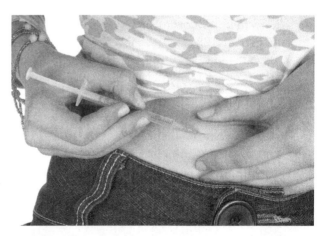

FIGURE 16.4 Questionable practices in weight loss include lipodissolve procedures.
© ajt/Shutterstock

diabetes "treatments" promoted with bogus claims such as "drop your blood sugar 50 points in 30 days," "eliminate insulin resistance," "prevent the development of type 2 diabetes," and "reduce or eliminate the need for diabetes drugs or insulin."

- **Influenza (flu) scams**: Federal agencies have come across contaminated or counterfeit influenza products. Mostly sold through Internet spam, marketers seized on the 2009 scare when the H1N1 virus, or swine flu, hit the headlines. Most of the confiscated products claimed to be generic versions of **Tamiflu**, which is used to prevent influenza. The drugs, however, were mostly vitamin C and other substances, which have not been shown to treat or prevent influenza.

How Do I Avoid Quackery?

The key to success in protecting yourself is to make sure you do your homework on a particular practitioner or treatment modality. The old adage "If it sounds too good to be true, it probably is" holds very true in this case. Ask questions, seek proof, and do not be convinced by testimonials (discussed in Chapter 3). In its *Healthy Aging Guide*,[12] WebMD suggests you be concerned about an alternative therapy if the product or advertisement you are researching:

- promises a quick or painless cure.
- claims its formula is secret or special and only available by mail or from one sponsor.
- claims to have the cure the medical community does not want you to know about.
- uses testimonials or undocumented case histories from satisfied patients.
- claims to be a cure for everything.
- claims to know how to cure a disease no one else understands (like HIV or cancer).
- offers an additional "free" gift or a larger amount of the product as a "special promotion."
- requires advance payment and claims limited availability of the product.

It takes only a moment of consideration to see why a product making these claims is most likely untrue. Why would someone have a cure for cancer and not be using it to provide comfort to the millions suffering from the disease? Why would someone have the cure for AIDS and not help people who were HIV positive? Although the medical community may not be perfect, it is unreasonable to think they are evil and would knowingly withhold a potential cure to a major illness.

What Can I Do If I Feel I Have Been Duped?

The reality of the situation is that consumers are responsible for their own susceptibility to quackery, which means that you are also responsible for protecting yourself (see *caveat emptor* in Chapter 1). It is a matter of due diligence—do your homework! For instance, if you were reviewing cancer treatments, you would easily find that the FDA lists the following "red flags" regarding product fraud and cancer.[13] You should be concerned if a product or device:

- treats all forms of cancer.
- miraculously kills cancer cells and tumors.
- shrinks malignant tumors.
- selectively kills cancer cells.
- more effective than chemotherapy.
- attacks cancer cells, leaving healthy cells intact.
- cures cancer.

Sometimes, it can be challenging to determine if a product or service is legitimate. If you have concerns about a product, device, or service, you can and should file a complaint. If your complaint is about a product that is mislabeled or misrepresented or if you believe it might be harmful to those who use it, contact the FDA or the Federal Trade Commission.

U.S. Food and Drug Administration
Consumer Information
10903 New Hampshire Avenue
Silver Spring, MD 20993
1-888-INFO-FDA

Federal Trade Commission
Bureau of Consumer Protection
600 Pennsylvania Avenue, NW
Washington, DC 20580
1-877-FTC-HELP

One additional place to begin might be your state's attorney or the office of the **attorney general**. That state division will have a mechanism for registering consumer complaints. Search the Internet for your state government website. Depending on the product or device you are concerned about, there are a multitude of organizations that might also be able to assist you. See Chapter 17 for additional details.

▶ What Are Examples of Products Considered Quackery?

The Psychograph

The psychograph was designed based on the pseudoscience of phrenology, the belief that personality and character were determined by the shape of the skull. The skull was measured, and the areas that had bumps (or were bigger) inferred that area of the brain was of greater development, and in turn, a greater part of the personality. The premise was based on the work of Franz Gall, father of phrenology, who divided the brain into 26 areas. The instrument was later patented by Henry Lavery in the 1930s.[14] Throughout the 1800s, this was considered a legitimate science. Have you ever been asked to be a "character reference?" Today, character reference means conveying that someone is trustworthy or a good person. In the early 1800s, however, companies would require you to have a test run by a phrenologist prior to employment to ensure your character was stable! Eventually, the machine became more of a novelty found in theaters and other public places and used for amusement.[15]

Lydia Pinkham's Vegetable Compound

Lydia Pinkham was a midwife, nurse, and schoolteacher in the 1800s.[16] In her later years, Pinkham's family urged her to begin marketing an herbal remedy she had been making in her kitchen to address "female problems," most commonly menstrual cramps. Women of the time did not like to speak with their male doctors about issues related to sex or sexuality, so the idea that they could purchase a remedy at the local store was attractive. The product was made of "black cohosh, life root, unicorn root, pleurisy root, fenugreek seed, and a substantial amount of alcohol,"[16] roughly 20%! As the product gained popularity, the claims for its effectiveness also grew, expanding from treating menstrual cramps to menopause symptoms such as depression and moodiness, to headaches, backaches, and fainting spells.[16] There is little evidence the products contents worked, and by the time the FDA gained enough oversight in the early 1900s, the product was grossing over $3 million per year. Eventually, the FDA required the makers to rein back their claims and reduce the alcohol content, which was approximately the same as today's fortified or dessert wines. You can still purchase the Lydia Pinkham Herbal Supplement over the counter in stores today (**FIGURE 16.5**).

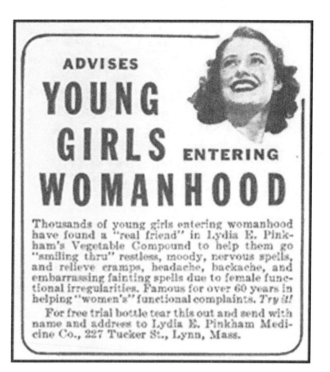

FIGURE 16.5 Advertisement for Lydia Pinkham compound.
Lydia Pinkham

Radithor

Some alternative products have been extraordinarily dangerous. Presently, in the 21st century, we have a very good understanding of the dangers of radiation and radioactive products. That was not the case in the early 20th century. In the 1920s, Radithor was developed by businessman William Bailey.[17] Bailey had passed himself off as a medical doctor, although he never was trained as such. Radithor was a very simple product—radium and distilled water—and Bailey claimed it could cure over 150 different ailments and that it was completely harmless.[17] Bailey's most famous patient was Eben Byers, a successful golfer who suffered an arm injury that was impacting his ability to play golf. Bailey recommended Radithor, and Byers was enamored by the outcomes. He began drinking three doses daily. Within 5 years, Byers was dead. The radium, with a half-life of 1,600 years, did not purge from the body quickly as a vitamin would.

Instead, it stayed in the body, permeating the bones and devouring Byers from the inside out. At the time of his death, Byers had most of his upper and lower jaw removed, nearly all of his teeth had fallen out, and his bones were snapping from their brittle nature.[17] The Federal Trade Commission forced Bailey to pull Radithor from the market, but not before he sold nearly 400,000 bottles (**FIGURE 16.6**).

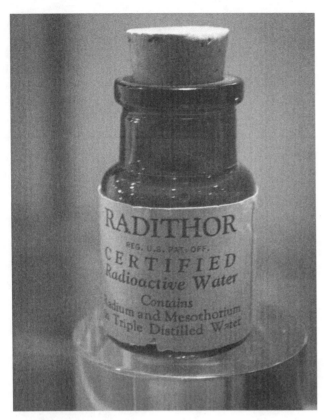

FIGURE 16.6 Radithor bottle, circa 1920.

Spectrochrometry

Spectrochrometry became popular in the 1800s, but gained most of its momentum as a therapeutic approach when Dinshah P. Ghadiali (1873–1966) formed the Spectro-Chrome Therapeutic System in the 1920s.[18] Ghadiali explained that the body is primarily four elements (oxygen, hydrogen, nitrogen, and carbon), and that each of these elements has a primary color wave associated with it. Those color waves respond to their environment. When in balance we are in good health, when out of balance we have illness.[18] Each color, then, had specific ailments it could cure or "attune." Most biographies and histories of Ghadiali do not describe him in positive terms or even suggest he was a scientist. He was arrested for interstate transport of a female for what appears to be prostitution[18] and he served jail time and probation time on two separate occasions for two separate crimes. Ghadiali sold at-home versions of the machine for $150 and professional versions for $750, and by the 1940s had made over $1 million; but by the late 1950s his operations had been shut down as fraudulent. Surprisingly, or maybe not, color spectrum therapy is still popular. You can find more information at the leading organization website, the Dinshah Health Society (**FIGURE 16.7**).

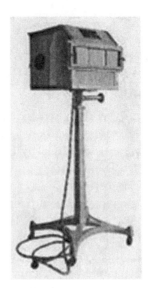

FIGURE 16.7 Spectro-chrome therapy home machine.

Renulife

Renulife was one of several products developed in the early 20th century that claimed to use violet rays for therapeutic purposes.[19] It was a form of electrotherapy, without the major "shocking" that occurred with devices in medical facilities. High frequency violet ray was sent through a vacuum tube and applied directly to the body. In its 1919 manual,[19] Renulife described the benefits as follows:

- Increase blood supply to a given area.
- Increase oxygen in the blood.
- Increase elimination of waste products.
- Increase bodily heat without a corresponding rise in temperature.
- Locally germicidal.
- Mild sparks stimulate or soothe according to length and character of application.
- Strong spirits are caustic.
- Sparks to the spine increase the arterial tension.

The device was claimed to cure over 50 ailments, including abscesses, blackheads, circulatory issues, gout, hemorrhoids, paralysis, toothaches, and wrinkles.[19] Companies producing the devices faced several lawsuits through the 1940s, and by the end of the 1950s, most companies had been ordered by the federal government to stop producing and selling the violet ray (**FIGURE 16.8**).

Sports Bands/Energy Bands

While our previous items have been specific products, this is a categorical item. A quick search on the Internet and you will find a plethora of products called

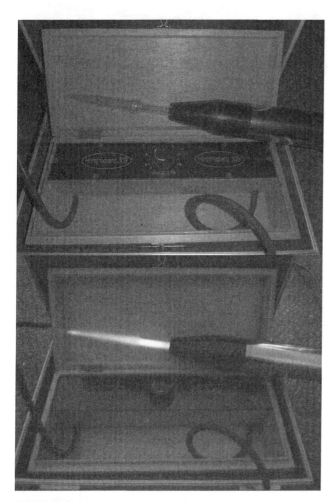

FIGURE 16.8 Renulife violet ray device.

https://en.wikipedia.org/wiki/Violet_ray. License: Wikipedia:Text of Creative Commons Attribution-ShareAlike 3.0 Unported License

"sports energy bands." This product has been growing in popularity, especially as more consumers see professional athletes and popular social figures wearing them. One website tells the consumer that this silicone wristband (which also comes as a pendant or in titanium!) works with your body's natural energy flow to increase strength, balance, and coordination.[20] The site then lists testimonials from dozens of professional athletes supporting the use of the band. The issue here is there is no science presented (and frankly, none exists) that can demonstrate this band has any biological or energy effect on the body. They sell because they are popular.

Diet Products

Another category to be careful of, as the FDA mentions, is diet products. There are hundreds of dietary products on the market that are pure gimmicks. Remember, you should always be cautious when a diet claims to have some unique ingredient unknown to science, or has a system and formula the "experts" do not want you to know about. That is usually a clear sign of fraud. One example is the Blood Type Diet. The diet's creator, a **naturopathic** healer, has posited that one's blood type should dictate one's diet.[21] Again, the diet became popular when promoted by movie stars and athletes who claimed the diet returned their body to its best shape ever. This diet suggests that your blood type is responsible for specific immunity and digestive functions. Because of this, each of the four blood types has a different dietary pattern to follow. However, like all diets and weight loss schemes, if you read far enough into the material, you will see indications that not all people respond positively to the diet designed for their blood type. However, you will find substantial opportunities to spend plenty of money on products designed to help you determine if the diet is best for you.

Many products marketed as dietary supplements are available to consumers. Because dietary supplements are not regulated by the FDA (in fact, all dietary supplement product packaging must contain a disclaimer stating that the FDA has not evaluated the product claims), it is a wide-open market for promotion to the consumer. Consumers should be cautious when choosing supplement products, whether buying them over the counter or online. In 2016 alone, the FDA warned consumers about as many as 20 different dietary supplements.[22] They went on to say that many dietary supplements are tainted with ingredients either not listed on the labels or with drugs that require a prescription. In some cases, the products contained ingredients that had been removed from the consumer market due to dangers posed by their consumption. Some of these products were designed for weight loss, others were marketed as supplements for sexual performance or enhancement, and still others were supplements for bodybuilding. The FDA warns consumers to avoid products that claim to work just like prescription drugs or that claim to contain "legal" alternatives to banned drugs.

▶ Who Are Examples of Recent Quacks?

There are many, many examples of entrepreneurial individuals who used quackery to make fortunes, even though their approaches were at some point determined to be completely bogus. Some contemporary examples include Dr. Wilhelm Reich, Milan Brych, Dr. Hulda R. Clark, and Ruth B. Drown.

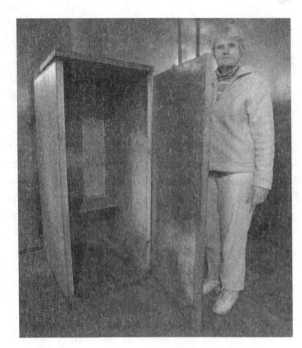

FIGURE 16.9 Orgone energy accumulator.
© Robert F. Bukaty/AP Photos.

Dr. Wilhem Reich was a psychiatrist in the 1950s who promoted a product called the **Orgone energy accumulator**.[23] According to Reich, **Orgone**, was a gas undetected by science, yet it permeated all things in life. Orgone was the central life force, also responsible for the creation of the universe and gravity. Reich told people they could harness this energy and, because it was the most prominent source of energy, they could heal any illness known to man. The Accumulator was essentially a box, sat in by the participant, made of celetex and a steel interior (**FIGURE 16.9**). The individual, according to Reich, would soak up the orgone energy and relieve illness or symptoms related to illness. Even though it is unmeasurable, the notion of a "central life force" is believed by millions, and most likely not a cause for concern with this gadgetry. The Accumulator itself, however, could not be verified to perform as it claimed.

The FDA pursued Reich, and eventually he was arrested for fraud and jailed in 1957, where he died that same year. However, Reich's believers carry on his work still today, promoting products such as discs, pendants, and modules. Each is described as having the power to harness the universal life force, thus balancing the individual and making them healthier.

Milan Brych was a Czechoslovakia-born immigrant in New Zealand in the 1970s, when his claims for curing cancer[24] first surfaced. Brych was injecting patients with a serum (later determined to be some combination of steroids and chemotherapeutic chemicals), and some were showing positive results. However, it was soon determined that Brych was not a doctor, or even trained as one. He was removed from the medical rosters in 1977, and fled from New Zealand authorities to practice in the Cook Islands—a location where the president welcomed him. While practicing, most of his patients died and were buried in a lot behind the treatment center that became known as the Brych Yard. Eventually, the president was removed from office and Brych again fled, this time to the United States where he continued his practice. Brych was arrested in California for practicing medicine without a license and offering a phony cure to cancer sufferers. He was sentenced to 6 years in jail. After 3 years, he was released, and is said to be living in Switzerland under a new name.

Hulda Regehr Clark ran the Century Nutrition clinic[25] in Tijuana, Mexico, until her death in 2009. Dr. Clark, who obtained a PhD in zoology from the University of Minnesota, was the inventor of several devices designed to electrocute pathogens. Her premise was that parasites or pollutants caused all disease. Once parasites were in the system, electrical current could destroy them. Her primary invention[26] was called, appropriately enough, the **Zapper**. The Zapper provided an electrical current designed to kill parasites, and as such, Dr. Clark claimed to be able to cure cancer, HIV,[27] and any other disorder caused by "parasite." She also invented the Syncrometer, which was said to be able to measure the frequency of any disease or organ, much like tuning a radio. If you found the correct frequency, you could adjust the Syncrometer to that wavelength and send the charge directly to where the impulse was needed. This allowed her to cure anything. The mainstream medical community dismissed much of the treatment practice of Dr. Clark. However, her practice remained open until just before her passing in 2009.

In the 1930s, Ruth B. Drown was a promoter of the notion that **radionics**[28] was the solution to health problems. Drown's Therapeutic Machine[29] was said to be able to access etheric life force energy that, when directed though a photographic plate, could produce photographs of tissue found anywhere in the body. The machine required just a dried drop of the patient's blood on a piece of blotter paper. Her techniques, like a few before her, measured the vibration rate of a patient's illness, because it was believed that each organ and each illness produced its own degree of vibration. In 1935, Drown created Radio-Vision.[30] Again, it used radio waves to diagnose and treat a wide variety of illnesses. According to Drown, diagnosis or cure with the device did not even require the patient's presence because radio waves travel over distance. On a side note, a competing radionics developer, Art Tool & Die Company out of Detroit, created

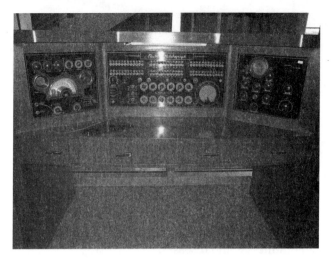

FIGURE 16.10 Electro-metabograph.

Wikipedia. https://commons.wikimedia.org/wiki/File:Electro-metabograph_machine.jpg. License: https://creativecommons.org/licenses/by-sa/3.0/

the electro-metabograph (**FIGURE 16.10**) at roughly the same time period as Drown created her Radio-Vision. Interestingly, it was later determined that while the electro-metabograph was designed for radionics diagnosis and treatment, it did not contain a single piece of radio equipment, so diagnosing or treating illness with radio waves would not have been possible.

By the 1940s, mainstream medical professionals pronounced Drown's work quackery and her inventions useless. Drown's followers of natural healing, however, still believe quite strongly in her philosophies. Natural healing is based in metaphysics, and Drown's followers view auras and orgone energy as legitimate because in metaphysics all existence has a mathematical foundation. In 1950, Drown was asked to come to the University of Chicago to test her diagnostic accuracy. It was a terrible failure, and triggered the beginning of the end for her medical practice. Drown was eventually targeted for fraud by authorities in the state of California, and after a 1963 sting operation[31] set up by the State Department of Public Health, was arrested with all her staff and charged. She died in 1965 awaiting trial.

▶ Is There Quackery in the Nutrition Industry?

Simply stated, people who are overweight make an easy target. According to a report from the Centers for Disease Control and Prevention,[32] 36% of Americans are obese and two in every three Americans are classified as overweight. That is approximately 166 million U.S. adults. Essentially, this creates a tremendous market of consumers looking for a quick solution to their weight issues.

When you have a society obsessed with weight, and 166 million people looking for an easy way to accomplish weight loss, it becomes a simple task for quacks and hucksters to promote the "next greatest weight loss product."

It is evident as well that Americans are buying. In 2016, there were an estimated 75 million Americans on some type of diet.[33] The estimate for spending by Americans on weight loss products was over $60 billion that same year. So, what are people doing? Currently, the low carb diet plans are very popular. This includes diets such as the Atkins Diet, the South Beach Diet, and the Zone. Commercial weight loss companies, such as Weight Watchers and Jenny Craig, are still relatively popular as well. Marketdata, Inc. estimates Americans spent $15 billion last year on meal replacement products alone. Even with all these options, the obesity rates in the United States have not changed significantly in nearly a decade.

When reviewing weight loss options, consumers can protect themselves by assessing a diet in five ways.[34] First, does the diet suggest you make significant calorie reductions? Reducing the calories you consume is a common element of diets, but drastic reductions (diets of 800–1,000 calories or less) are counterproductive. Second, diets that require special pills or powders are usually gimmicks, and will not produce long-term weight loss. In addition, since 2008, the FDA has identified more than 70 weight loss products that have undisclosed components in them, posing serious health risks to the consumer. Third, there is no scientific support for a single food or combinations of foods being the "key" to successful weight loss. If a product makes this claim, you are safe to reject it. Fourth, diets that completely eliminate everything from a single food group have not demonstrated long-term weight loss success. You may see short-term success, but this is more likely due to calorie reductions or reductions in water weight. Once you return to a regular diet, the weight will return. And finally, diets that require you to skip meals will not produce long-term weight loss.

▶ Conclusion

This chapter presented some of the more notable quacks and quackery found in the health arena over the past century. There are many more; we just scratched the surface. Consumers need to remain active in their investigation of treatment options as to not be fooled into utilizing bogus physicians and products when real or serious healthcare issues need to be addressed.

Wrap-Up

Key Terms

Attorney general The principal legal officer who represents a state in legal proceedings and gives legal advice to the government.

Autism A mental condition, present from early childhood, characterized by great difficulty in communicating and forming relationships, and in using language and abstract concepts.

Deceit Concealment or distortion of the truth for the purpose of misleading.

Erectile dysfunction Difficulty in achieving or maintaining an erection; impotence.

Food and Drug Administration (FDA) A division of the U.S. Department of Health and Human Services that protects the public against impure and unsafe foods, drugs, and cosmetics.

Fraud Trickery, unethical practice, or breach of confidence, perpetrated for profit or to gain some unfair or dishonest advantage.

Naturopathic A system or method of treating disease that employs no surgery or synthetic drugs, but uses special diets, herbs, vitamins, massage, and the like to assist the natural healing processes.

Orgone A vital, primal, nonmaterial element believed to permeate the universe.

Orgone energy accumulator A cabinet-like device constructed of layers of wood and other materials claimed by its inventor, Wilhelm Reich, to restore orgone energy to persons sitting in it, thereby aiding in the cure of impotence, cancer, the common cold, and ailments; also called an orgone box.

Quack A person who admits, professionally or publicly, to skill, knowledge, or qualifications he or she does not possess.

Quackery The practice of deceit or trickery specifically confined to the medical field.

Radionics A dowsing technique using a pendulum to detect energy fields emitted by all forms of matter.

Scam A confidence game or other fraudulent scheme, especially for making a quick profit.

Spectrochrometry A pseudoscience that believes the shape and contour of the skull indicates the size of various segments of the brain. The variety in brain sizes is the determinant of character.

Tamiflu An oral antiviral drug that attacks the influenza virus and prevents it spreading inside the body.

Traditional medical practitioner A medical doctor practicing under a Western, pharmaceutical-based philosophy.

Truth in advertising Laws designed to compel advertisers to give accurate, forthright information regarding products, services, and anticipated outcomes.

Zapper A machine created by Hulda Clark that delivers energy to the body in an effort to cure a myriad of illnesses and diseases.

Suggestions for Class Activities

This chapter contains the list of "red flags" for quack product endorsement provided by the FDA. This activity will give you a chance to critically review advertising found on the Internet.

1. Locate the following four items:
   a. A website marketing an herbal supplement
   b. A website marketing a sexual enhancement product
   c. A website page marketing an arthritis drug or technique
   d. A website marketing a nonstandard cancer treatment
2. Using the red flags, determine how likely the product is to be legitimate. Provide a written explanation for each item you believe may be deceptive in nature and why you believe this to be true.
3. For *one* of the websites you identified, create a mock letter to the FDA explaining your concerns and what you believe ought to be done about the issue.

Review Questions

1. Why has quackery always been a part of the medical community?
2. What makes quackery hard to distinguish from more readily accepted forms of treatment?
3. What are the five types of treatments, as defined by the National Council Against Health Fraud?
4. Define "quack." Are quacks always liars and cheats?
5. What are the most common forms of health fraud according to the FDA?

6. What is the most common concern regarding sexual enhancement products?

7. What types of claims should the consumer be careful about when looking into a potential treatment option?

8. Identify some of the claims fraudulent products make to the consumer.

9. What should a consumer do if they feel they would like to file a complaint about a product or service?

10. Describe some of the more recent attempts to deceive the public regarding medical treatment.

11. Why is nutrition a popular area for medical quackery?

References

1. Congress on medical quackery: Conference report. *Publ Health Rep.* 1962;77(5):453-455.

2. Quackery. In: *The Free Dictionary by Farlex.* Free Dictionary Website. Available at: http://medical-dictionary.thefreedictionary.com/quackery. Accessed May 2, 2018.

3. Quack. In: *Merriam-Webster.* Merriam-Webster Website. Available at: http://www.merriam-webster.com/dictionary/quack. Accessed May 2, 2018.

4. Science Museum. Paracelsus (1493-1541). Available at: http://www.sciencemuseum.org.uk/broughttolife/people/paracelsus. Accessed May 2, 2018.

5. National Council Against Health Fraud. Quackery-Related Definitions. Available at: http://www.ncahf.org/pp/definitions.html. Updated March 3, 2001. Accessed May 2, 2018.

6. Eggertson L. Lancet retracts 12-year-old article linking autism to MMR vaccines. *CMAJ.* 2010;182(4):E199-E200.

7. U.S. Food and Drug Administration. Health Fraud Scams. Available at: https://www.fda.gov/ForConsumers/ProtectYourself/HealthFraud/default.htm. Updated April 3, 2018. Accessed May 2, 2018.

8. U.S. Food and Drug Administration. FDA101: Health Fraud Awareness. Available at: https://www.fda.gov/ForConsumers/ConsumerUpdates/ucm235995.htm. Updated November 14, 2017. Accessed May 2, 2018.

9. Snook KR, Hansen AR, Duke CH, Finch KC, Hackney AA, Zhang J. Change in percentages of adults with overweight or obesity trying to lose weight, 1988-2014. *JAMA.* 2017;317(9):971-973.

10. U.S. Food and Drug Administration. 'All Natural' Alternatives for Erectile Dysfunction: A Risky Proposition. Available at: https://www.fda.gov/ForConsumers/ConsumerUpdates/ucm465024.htm. Updated March 18, 2018. Accessed May 2, 2018.

11. Low MY, Zeng Y, Li L, et al. Safety and quality assessment of 175 illegal sexual enhancement products seized in red-light districts in Singapore. *Drug Saf.* 2009;32(12):1141-1146.

12. WebMD. Health Quackery: Spotting Health Scams. Available at: http://www.webmd.com/a-to-z-guides/health-quackery-spotting-health-scams. Accessed May 2, 2018.

13. U.S. Food and Drug Administration Products Claiming to "Cure" Cancer Are a Cruel Deception. Available at: https://www.fda.gov/ForConsumers/ConsumerUpdates/ucm048383.htm. Updated January 8, 2018. Accessed May 2, 2018.

14. Museum of Quackery. History of Phrenology and the Psycograph. Available at: http://www.museumofquackery.com/devices/psychist.htm. Updated June 10, 2015. Accessed May 2, 2018.

15. Paranormal-Encyclopedia. Phrenology. Available at: http://www.paranormal-encyclopedia.com/p/phrenology/. Accessed May 2, 2018.

16. Harvard University Library Open Collections Program, Women Working, 1800–1930. Lydia Estes Pinkham (1819–1883). Available at: http://ocp.hul.harvard.edu/ww/pinkham.html. Accessed September 13, 2017.

17. Cellania M. The strange fate of Eben Byers. *Neatorama.* November 18, 2013. Available at: http://www.neatorama.com/2013/11/18/The-Strange-Fate-of-Eben-Byers/. Accessed May 2, 2018.

18. Museum of Quackery. Dinshah P. Ghadiali and Spectro-Chrome Therapy. Available at: http://www.museumofquackery.com/amquacks/ghadiali.htm. Updated April 13, 2013. Accessed May 2, 2018.

19. Renulife Electric Company. *Renulife Violet Ray (1919 Manual).* Detroit, MI; 1919. Available at: http://www.violetwandstore.com/Articles/renulife_users_directions1919.pdf. Accessed May 2, 2018.

20. Power Balance. Power Balance wristbands and pendants. Available at: http://www.powerbalance.com/default/shop/metal-products/titanium-new.html. Accessed May 2, 2018.

21. Eat Right 4 Your Type®. Blood Type and Your Health. Available at: http://www.dadamo.com/txt/index.pl?1001. Updated March 3, 2015. Accessed May 2, 2018.

22. U.S. Food and Drug Administration. 2016 Warning Letters - Health Fraud. Available at: https://www.fda.gov/ForConsumers/ProtectYourself/HealthFraud/ucm539075.htm. Updated March 7, 2017. Accessed May 2, 2018.

23. The Wilhelm Reich Infant Trust. Biography of Wilhelm Reich. Available at: http://www.wilhelmreichtrust.org/biography.html. Updated October 13, 2017. Accessed May 2, 2018.

24. Kieza G. How a cancer crook hooked Joh Bjelke Petersen. *The Courier Mail.* November 9, 2016. Available at: https://myaccount.news.com.au/sites/couriermail/subscribe.html?sourceCode=CMWEB_WRE170_a_GGL&mode=premium&dest=http://www.couriermail.com.au/news/queensland/state-politics-how-a-cancer-crook-hooked-joh-bjelkepetersen/news-story/37ab35e09138d2014b50e80355bf5d73&memtype=anonymous. Accessed May 2, 2018.

25. Dr. Clark Information Center. Who was Dr. Clark. Available at: http://www.drclark.net/en/about-dr-hulda-clark. Accessed May 2, 2018.

26. Dr. Clark Information Center. Zapper Basics. Available at: http://www.drclark.net/en/the-zapper. Accessed May 2, 2018.

27. Clark HR. *Cure for HIV and AIDS.* Noida, India: B Jain Publishers; 2002.

28. Kook Science Research Associates. Radionics, or Black Box Dowsing. Available at: https://www.kookscience.com/arch/Radionics.html. Accessed May 2, 2018.

29. Adachi K. Dr. Ruth B. Drown, America's Greatest Radionics Innovator: The Untold Story Part 1. Available at: http://www.educate-yourself.org/tjc/ruthdrownuntoldstory.shtml. Published April 7, 2001. Accessed May 2, 2018.

30. Drown RB. *Radio-Vision: Scientific Milestone.* Hollywood, CA: Drown Laboratories. 1960. Available at: https://newearth

.university/wp-content/uploads/sites/13/2017/01/Radio
-Vision-Scientific-Milestone-Ruth-Drown-Laboratories
-1960.pdf. Accessed May 2, 2018.

31. Drown, Ruth B. (1891-1965). In: *Encyclopedia of Occultism and Parapsychology*. Encyclopedia.com Website. Available at: http://www.encyclopedia.com/science/encyclopedias -almanacs-transcripts-and-maps/drown-ruth-b-1891-1965. Accessed May 2, 2018.

32. Ogden CL, Carroll MD, Fryar CD, Flegal KM. Prevalence of obesity among adults and youth: United States, 2011–2014. *NCHS Data Brief*. 2015;219:1-8.

33. Marketdata Enterprises. The U.S. Weight Loss & Diet Control Market, 14th ed. Available at: https://www .marketdataenterprises.com/studies/#WEIGHTLOSS. Published May 2017. Accessed May 2, 2018.

34. TeensHealth. 5 ways to spot a fad diet. Available at: http://kidshealth.org/en/teens/fad-diet-tips.html. Updated October 2013. Accessed May 2, 2018.

CHAPTER 17

Protection and Rights of American Consumers

As a result of reading this chapter, students will be able to:

1. Describe the rights consumers have related to use of the healthcare system.
2. Outline consumers' personal responsibility when making choices related to healthcare system use.
3. Explain the purpose of the Patient Care Partnership.
4. Identify the agencies committed to consumer protection.
5. Compare and contrast the roles various agencies play in consumer protection.
6. Explain how a consumer can determine if a product will be effective.
7. Describe the federal government's role in consumer protection.

▶ Consumer Engagement in Health Decisions

Consumers have increasingly become more involved in decisions related to their health and health care; not everyone is engaged.[1] Based on consumer survey information, the *Deloitte Review* published six categories of healthcare consumers, four actively engaged but in smaller numbers and two inactive types.

Inactive types included the largest segment (34%) "casual and cautious." While they are concerned about the cost of their care, they are not really engaged in healthcare decisions because they do not currently have a need to be. The other inactive group, "content and compliant," make up 22% of the survey, and are inactive in their decisions because they are happy with

their current situation. They like their doctors and hospitals, and they trust that they are being given solid healthcare information. Deloitte refers to this group as the ones who "behave like patients."[1]

Of the four actively engaged consumer groups, the largest segment (17%) is "online and onboard." This group is comprised of online learners happy with their care, but interested in identifying potential alternatives to their care. They will utilize online reference sources to investigate facilities and providers before choosing whom to use. The next largest group, "sick and savvy" (14%) are in the healthcare system more than the other groups. They have illnesses that need to be addressed, are actively engaged with their providers, and work cooperatively to establish a pathway for addressing their issues. The last two groups "out and about" and "shop and save" (9% and 4%, respectively) are actively engaged in establishing options and determining the least expensive path to having their healthcare needs met.[1] The significance in the variety of themes and patterns in consumer behavior requires the providers of health care to establish and market to unique groups in an effort to establish relationships with existing and new clients.

Even with just over half the population not actively engaged in their healthcare decisions, we are still much more active in those decisions than ever before. No longer are we all simply passive receptacles of medical information. Many ask questions, compare costs, demand quality care, research illness, and, yes, review and experiment with alternative care. The result of this shift in health care is the substantial demand from consumers that quality care is a right. With that more active role, however, consumers need to continue to become more responsible for their care.

▶ Consumer Rights and Responsibilities Regarding Health Care

The debate over whether health care itself is a right is more than a 100-year-old debate in the United States. We cover that history more thoroughly in Chapter 18. Here, we look to review the changing role of consumers and providers within the healthcare realm over time. The federal government has passed several laws providing patient protection. Laws protecting your privacy and the privacy of your medical records have been in place for some time. The Health Insurance Portability and Accountability Act of 1996, referred to as the Privacy Law, mandates that your medical records be protected and private. Informed consent laws require that you be notified of the details of your treatment plan and potential risks so you can make a good decision.[2]

Patient rights were most recently addressed nationally with the passage of the Patient Protection and Affordable Care Act (ACA) in 2010. The set of rights included in the passage of ACA was much more specific than historical patient rights documents, and applied primarily to consumer rights related to health insurance. We cover insurance issues more elaborately in Chapter 18. Here, a brief list of rights is included[3]:

- Requires insurance plans to cover people with preexisting health conditions, including pregnancy, without charging more
- Provides free preventive care

- Gives young adults more coverage options
- Ends lifetime and yearly dollar limits on coverage of essential health benefits
- Helps you understand the coverage you are getting
- Holds insurance companies accountable for rate increases
- Makes it illegal for health insurance companies to cancel your health insurance just because you get sick
- Protects your choice of doctors
- Birth control methods and counseling
- Mental health and substance abuse services

A common title or phrase used in documents addressing healthcare rights is Patient Bill of Rights. There have been many different "Bill of Rights" created. For instance, there is one for mental health care and one for hospice care. We cannot cover every specific Bill of Rights in the healthcare arena, but we can focus on two particular documents that helped to establish the groundwork for many of the others: Consumer Rights and Responsibilities (CRR) and the Patient Care Partnership (PCP).

In the early 1990s, healthcare satisfaction was at the front of the political debate during the presidency of Bill Clinton. In early 1997, in response to the limitations placed on consumers by health maintenance organizations, the escalating cost of health care, and increasing consumer dissatisfaction, then-President Bill Clinton created the Advisory Commission on Consumer Protection and Quality in the healthcare industry. The 32-member council was charged with keeping the president informed on the status of the healthcare system, and to recommend actions to improve the quality and value of health care, its consumers, and its employees.

▶ What Was the Result of the Advisory Commission's Work?

The end product of the advisory commission's work was CRR,[4] a document that discusses the rights of consumers related to eight areas of health care: the disclosure of information related to plans, physicians, and facilities; consumer choice of providers and plans; consumer access to emergency services; the participation of the consumer in treatment decisions; respect and nondiscrimination of consumers utilizing the healthcare system; confidentiality of consumer's health information; the right to file complaints and appeals; and the responsibilities of consumers when accessing the healthcare system. Each will be briefly described in the following sections:

- **Information Disclosure**: The commission indicated that information given to consumers should be accurate and easily understood. Also, when necessary, consumers should receive assistance to make informed healthcare decisions. The information provided should include (1) cost, licensure, and emergency services under health plans; (2) certifications, experience, and consumer satisfaction related to healthcare professionals; (3) experience and accreditation of healthcare facilities; and (4) appropriate consumer assistance programs.

- **Choice of Providers and Plans**: Part two of the CRR referred to consumer choice. This included having sufficient providers and emergency services in the network to meet consumer demand, ensuring access to those providers was available, having sufficient women's health services (i.e., gynecology and midwifery), authorizing an appropriate number of specialist visits, and providing a variety of plan options for consumers.

- **Access to Emergency Services**: Part three of the CRR addresses access to emergency services. Specifically, health plans are encouraged to let consumers know the availability of emergency services and other appropriate options, as well as to convey to the consumer that emergency costs, when appropriate, will be covered by the plan.

- **Participation in Treatment Decisions**: The CRR established the right of consumers to play a role in their treatment decisions. Communication and easily understandable information is the key. This section reinforces the consumer's right to choose no treatment, to be told of all risks and potential side effects of treatment options, and to discuss the use of advanced directives.

- **Respect and Nondiscrimination**: The CRR established the consumer right to nondiscrimination. It states, "Consumers who are eligible for coverage under the terms and conditions of a health plan or program or as required by law must not be discriminated against in marketing and enrollment practices based on race, ethnicity, national origin, religion, sex, age, mental or physical disability, sexual orientation, genetic information, or source of payment."

- **Confidentiality of Health Information**: Consumers have a right to the confidentiality of their information and the confidence that information will not be disclosed without their specific consent.

Healthcare practitioners and facilities should make every attempt to use nonpersonal identification numbers (like Social Security numbers) to identify patients under their care.

- **Complaints and Appeals**: When consumers believe they have been treated unfairly, they should have the right to make a complaint and express their concerns. The CRR encourages conflicts to be handled internally whenever possible. The procedure for addressing situations such as incorrect billing, mistreatment by a staff member, or timeliness of services should be clearly explained to the consumer. When consumers act inappropriately, the facility also has the right to terminate services, but should do so in writing, with a complete explanation of the circumstances and resolution done in a timely manner.

  When internal processes do not meet the satisfaction of the consumer, an external appeal may be necessary. This would happen in cases such as refusal of services, denying payment, or reduction in treatment, and should be conducted by individuals trained for that responsibility and not involved in the original decision. Again, completion of the appeal in a timely fashion is recommended.

- **Consumer Responsibilities**: The final component of the CRR reviews consumer responsibilities. Making the healthcare system functional requires all parties, not just providers, to make an effort for success. The following items are included in consumer responsibilities:

  - Take responsibility for maximizing healthy habits such as exercising, responsible alcohol use, managing stress, not smoking, and eating a healthy diet.
  - Become involved in specific healthcare decisions.
  - Work collaboratively with healthcare providers in developing and carrying out agreed-upon treatment plans.
  - Disclose relevant information and clearly communicate wants and needs.
  - Use the health plan's internal complaint and appeal processes to address concerns that may arise.
  - Avoid knowingly spreading disease.
  - Recognize the reality of risks and limits of the science of medical care and the human fallibility of the healthcare professional.
  - Be aware of a healthcare provider's obligation to be reasonably efficient and equitable in providing care to other patients and the community.

- Become knowledgeable about your health plan coverage and health plan options (when available), including all covered benefits, limitations, and exclusions; rules regarding use of network providers; coverage and referral rules; appropriate processes to secure additional information; and the process to appeal coverage decisions.
- Show respect for other patients and health workers.
- Make a good faith effort to meet financial obligations.
- Abide by administrative and operational procedures of health plans, healthcare providers, and government health benefit programs.
- Report wrongdoing and fraud to the appropriate resources or legal authorities.

What Does CRR Mean for the Consumer?

Primarily, CRR spells out what is believed to be the optimal functioning capacity of the U.S. healthcare system. Individual consumers have the right to accurate, professional, and understandable systems and treatments, while at the same time hold the responsibility to be honest, forthcoming, and timely regarding health and personal well-being. When patients, doctors, and hospitals begin the process of trying to accomplish the same goals, the system works for everyone.

▶ What Is the Patient Care Partnership?

The American Hospital Association (AHA) first wrote their Patient Bill of Rights in the 1990s. It was an initial attempt to build a bridge between physicians and patients at a time when consumers believed the system was getting too impersonal. Doctors and hospitals believed that the usage patterns established by consumers were often unnecessary and were creating a financial burden on an increasingly expensive system to run. The AHA document was an attempt to get consumers and the medical system to work together to improve care, and at the same time reduce costs.

In 2003, the AHA released a new version, titled the Patient Care Partnership, or the PCP. The document, like its predecessor, was created to inform consumers of what they should expect during a hospital stay, and what rights and responsibilities the consumer held.

Your Rights Under the PCP

The PCP[5] focuses on areas of care and the consumer's rights associated with them. The consumer should expect high quality hospital care. This includes the right to know the names of your medical staff and their level of expertise, and to receive appropriate care where and when you need it. Consumers should expect a clean and safe environment, and be notified of issues that arise and how they might affect the consumer's care.

The component of the PCP most focused on is the consumer's involvement in their care. The PCP includes the right to discussions regarding your condition and your care (benefits, risks, long-term outcomes, posthospital care, and financial impact). The PCP also includes involvement in the discussion of your personal treatment plan. Usually, this involves the signing of documents signifying you have been consulted about treatment and your agreement or refusal of that treatment. It also includes the consumer identifying who should be responsible for making decisions about health care if the patient cannot make those decisions for themselves. The PCP emphasizes the consumer's role in the provision of complete and accurate information regarding past illness, allergies, medications, and health plan. And finally, being involved in the healthcare decisions means both sides understanding the patient's healthcare goals.

The PCP believes in the consumer's right to the protection of patient privacy, and the healthcare facility's commitment to following state and national laws in that regard. Finally, the PCP discusses ensuring the patient understands posthospitalization guidelines, and can receive assistance in understanding billing and payments when necessary.

What Does the PCP Mean to the Consumer?

Much like the efforts placed behind the creation of the CRR document, the PCP sends the message to consumers that the hospital will do all it can to make your hospital visit the best it can be, but needs the consumer to play an active role in that process. When the hospital and the consumer work together, the quality of care is improved.

▶ Consumer Confidence in Medical Care

In 2005, the Department of Health and Human Services—Centers for Medicare and Medicaid Services (CMS) and Agency for Healthcare Research and

Quality (AHRQ)—approved and mandated the Hospital Consumer Assessment of Healthcare Providers and Services (HCAHPS).[6] It was first implemented in 2007. The intent of the survey was to create a standardized tool to receive consumer feedback about their experience in the healthcare system. This would then allow an "apples to apples" comparison of facilities, so consumers could make choices about where to receive care. CMS requires hospitals to complete the assessment in order to receive full reimbursement for services provided to consumers. Therefore, the data are comprehensive and extensive, pooling 3.1 million surveys from 4,167 hospitals nationwide in 2015.[7] Data covering the Fall 2015–Summer 2016 period indicate consumers are most satisfied with communication with physicians, communication with nurses, and discharge information. Care transition was the greatest concern, followed by quietness of the hospital environment, communication about medicines, and responsiveness of hospital staff with hospitals (nationally) reporting under 70% of their consumers satisfied with these components of the hospital experience.[8] Overall patient satisfaction with hospitals experiences has shown modest yet steady increases since 2010. Level of patient satisfaction was good for smaller facilities, but showed steady decline in satisfaction rates as the facility grew in the number of beds available. Also, emergency department satisfaction among consumers was lower than nonemergency department satisfaction.

There seems to be much agreement about the rights consumers have regarding the use of the healthcare system. Protected privacy, involvement in the decisions regarding treatment and nontreatment options, and communication with doctors and nurses are central to the process of a successful healthcare experience. Continued monitoring through the HCAHPS for long-term comparison of consumer satisfaction will tell the tale as to whether we have been successful in providing a healthcare system that both works and is satisfactory to the consumer.

Am I a "Consumer" of Health Care?

Health care is not usually something we think of in terms of "consumption," but as you have read, we are all consumers of health care. There are the obvious uses in the healthcare system such as seeing your family doctor or a specialist, receiving prescription drugs, or visiting an emergency department; but the consumer market for health care is much larger. If you have ever purchased ibuprofen for a headache, an antihistamine for allergies, a treadmill for a workout, a diet book, nutritional supplements, or self-help books or

videos, you have contributed to the health consumer market. And you are not alone. In 2015, Americans spent about $9,990 each ($3.2 trillion total) on medical health care,[9] plus $44 billion on over-the-counter health-related products,[10] $26 billion on gym memberships and diet plans,[11] and $10 billion on home fitness equipment.[12] Health care is big business in the United States.

Who do you trust? What do you believe? How do you know that a product will be effective? How do you protect yourself? In many cases, laws exist protecting the consumer from fraudulent advertising or product **fraud**. The same is true for products in the health arena, including medical **malpractice**. As the business of health care and the market for health products continue to grow, challenges arise for the consumer. Several organizations are available to assist you if you have an issue. Each has its own area of emphasis, with varying degrees of health-related work, but all are designed to protect the consumer.

▶ What Organizations Are Available to Me If I Have a Consumer Issue?

Consumers have the right to be treated fairly and appropriately whether they are utilizing the healthcare system, purchasing a car, or deciding whether a crib is safe for their newly born child. Fortunately, a wide array of governmental and public agencies has emerged to protect citizens from fraud and danger. Each agency in the following section has been serving consumers for decades and is well established. To obtain more information on a specific agency, see **TABLE 17.1** for agency website addresses.

Public Citizen

In 1971, Ralph Nader's efforts to protect the consumer came to fruition in an organization titled Public Citizen[13] that was dedicated to protecting the consumer. In the health arena, Public Citizen focuses on consumer safety issues and on healthcare issues. Its website states its health and safety division objectives as:

"Public Citizen's health and safety work protects consumers by advocating for safer, more effective drugs, medical devices and other products; equitable healthcare services and more physician accountability; safer cars and trucks; and improvements in worker safety."

The Health Research Group has been a watchdog of the healthcare industry, publicly calling for increased

TABLE 17.1 Websites for Consumer Agencies

Public Citizen	www.citizen.org
U.S. Public Interest Research Group	www.uspirg.org
Consumer Federation of America	www.consumerfed.org
Consumers Union	www.consumersunion.org
Better Business Bureau	www.bbb.org
U.S. Food and Drug Administration	www.fda.gov
Federal Trade Commission, Bureau of Consumer Protection	www.ftc.gov/about-ftc/bureaus-offices/bureau-consumer-protection
Consumer Product Safety Commission	www.cpsc.gov

access to health care for all, promoting safe and affordable drugs and medical devices, and improving work standards. The group also maintains two very popular sites: WorstPills.org, which addresses 18,000 medicines people access, their effectiveness, and potential harm; and Physician Accountability/Doctor Discipline, a site where you can determine what physicians have been disciplined by the state or national boards.

Other efforts of Public Citizen are varied. Four divisions beyond the Health Watch (Congress Watch, Energy Watch, Global Trade Watch, and Litigation Watch) focus on specific aspects of consumer safety.

U.S. Public Interest Research Group

The U.S. Public Interest Research Group (USPIRG) conducts research, provides advocacy, and conducts community organizing to address consumer issues of public concern.[14] The USPIRG is a federation of representatives of Public Interest Research Groups at the state level, and promotes itself as an agency that "stands up to powerful special interests." In fact, the USPIRG's mission promotes **activism** designed to protect health and encourage fair treatment of consumers, free of the influence of lobbying from special interest groups.

Historically, the states' PIRGs have had an influence on several notable changes in consumer safety and public health. Some of these accomplishments include the following:

- Passage of generic drug laws in the 1970s
- Conducting studies that led to the ban on asbestos as an insulation material

- Raising awareness for stronger antiflammable children's sleepwear
- Passage of the nation's first lemon laws (laws protecting consumers when a newly purchased vehicle is defective)
- Superfund laws
- Reforms on toxic pollution control and public notification
- Creation of the Consumer Financial Protection Agency
- Fair credit card fees

One of the more visible efforts of the USPIRG each year is the Toy Safety Report titled *Trouble in Toyland*.[15] Published annually since 1986, the report has resulted in the removal from the market of more than 100 dangerous toys. The group played a significant role in the development of **lobby** reform, prescription drug safety and review reform, and promoted laws designed to protect consumer identity.

Consumer Federation of America

The Consumer Federation of America (CFA) is "an association of nonprofit consumer organizations that was established in 1968 to advance the consumer interest through research, advocacy, and education. Today, nearly 300 of these groups participate in the federation and govern it through their representatives on the organization's board of directors."[16] CFA describes itself as a research, advocacy, education, and service organization that pursues the following:

- CFA investigates consumer issues and publishes findings intended to assist advocates, policymakers, and individual consumers.
- CFA advances policy and policy discussion at all levels of government. They promote policies based on their degree of merit and engage in consumer beneficial debate.
- CFA uses media to disseminate consumer issue information. They provide an online newsletter and conferences related to finance and food as vehicles for information.
- CFA provides assistance to individuals and organizations through the America Saves campaign (since 2000) and, in addition to the above newsletters and conferences, provide a State and Local Resource Center, a Consumer Cooperative Advisory Group, and an annual Awards Dinner that recognizes distinguished public, consumer, and media service.[16]

The CFA's primary contribution in consumer health comes in the areas of financial/identity safety issues, consumer fraud protection, automobile safety, and children's product safety.

Consumers Union

Consumers Union (CU) is the organization responsible for policy and action based on the publication and findings of *Consumer Reports* magazine. CU strives to create a safe marketplace for consumers by providing a thorough analysis of the safety, reliability, and quality of commonly used and purchased items.[17] Unique compared to public magazines and periodicals found on online or at the newsstand, *Consumer Reports* prides itself on not accepting advertising. This allows the organization to be honest, frank, and unbiased in its analyses of consumer products. In the health area, CU is most involved with establishing safe hospital procedures and access to health insurance.

Better Business Bureau

The vision of Better Business Bureau (BBB) is "an ethical marketplace where buyers and sellers trust each other." By design, the BBB strives to enhance the consumer experience by[18]:

- setting standards for marketplace trust.
- encouraging and supporting best practices by engaging with and educating consumers and businesses.
- celebrating marketplace role models.
- calling out and addressing substandard marketplace behavior.

- creating a community of trustworthy businesses and charities.

The BBB builds its relationship with the public in several ways.[19] First, consumers can access BBB Business Profiles. Business Profiles provide an array of information on businesses, including consumer experiences. These reports can assist individuals with making an informed choice on whether to support a business or purchase goods from a business, or the site also allows for consumers to file complaints when necessary. In the health arena, consumers might use the BBB's Scam Tracker, a database of items related to fraud in the marketplace. Second, the BBB provides a dispute resolution service. For example, the BBB Auto Line is a dispute resolution program for consumers who believe their automobile warranty is not being honored. The BBB also provides mediators and arbitrators to resolve consumer conflicts in the areas of telecommunications, and moving and storage. The third method for building a relationship with the public is BBBOnLine, which encourages companies to strive for accuracy and quality on their websites. If companies meet the criteria established by the BBB, they can advertise this on their site, increasing consumer confidence in the company's products. Finally, as mentioned in Chapter 3, the BBB oversees the Children's Food and Beverage Advertising Initiative. Information related to this can be found through the Parents Corner program on the BBB website.[19]

▶ What Governmental Agencies Are Involved in Consumer Protection?

The government has also integrated consumer protection into its structure. As with public agencies, each has a particular area of expertise. In addition, several have the additional responsibility for administering laws applicable to that area of expertise.

The Food and Drug Administration

The FDA is the most significant governmental player in the protection of consumer rights. With origins of the FDA dating back to the 1820s, protecting consumer welfare has long been a priority in U.S. government. The FDA is housed in the federal Department of Health and Human Services and is responsible for regulating a wide range of areas, including the nation's vaccines and blood supply; the safety and labeling of cosmetics; over-the-counter and prescription drug approvals (as well as labeling and manufacturing standards); the labeling and safety of all food products (except for some regulations regarding poultry, eggs, and beef, which the FDA is a secondary agency to the Department of Agriculture); approval, manufacture, performance standards, and malfunction reporting of medical devices; and the standards and assessment of radiation-emitting equipment.[21]

Beginning its work as the Division of Chemistry and later the Bureau of Chemistry, the FDA began to function as a regulatory agency in 1906 with the passage of the Federal Food and Drug Act.[22] Since its original passing, Congress has amended or added to the law more than 40 times. Each amendment added to the FDA's regulatory and oversight responsibility. Examples include the Import Milk Act (1927), Fair Packaging and Labeling Act (1966), Controlled Substances Act (1970), Prescription Drug Marketing Act (1987), Nutrition Labeling and Education Act (1990), Dietary Supplement Health and Education Act (1994), and Pediatric Research Equity Act (2003). A full list of the laws the FDA has regulatory responsibility for are located on the agency's website. For some of the highlights, see **BOX 17.1**.

Bureau of Consumer Protection

The Bureau of Consumer Protection (BCP) is a division of the Federal Trade Commission designed to protect consumers from businesses that choose to **defraud** or deceive through the sale of their products. The BCP will investigate claims from consumers in an attempt to stop unfair practices. The bureau also uses its authority to provide education to the public, establish policy related to fair business practices, and when necessary, file suit against companies that break the law. The BCP, according to its website, provides services through eight divisions. These are summarized as follows.[23]

- **Division of Privacy and Identity Protection**
  - Enforces the laws that prohibit unfair or deceptive acts or practices
  - Enforces the Children's Online Privacy Protection Act (what can online entities collect about children)
  - Enforces the Fair Credit Reporting Act (accuracy of and access to credit bureau information)

BOX 17.1 Influences of the U.S. Food and Drug Administration

The following information shows the major events, milestones, issues, and accomplishments of the U.S. Food and Drug Administration (FDA) during the last 150 years.[20] While not nearly all-inclusive, it shows the broad spectrum of influence the FDA has had on the health and well-being of people in the United States.

1820–1900

First **compendium** of standard drugs for the United States, Drug Importation Act; 1862: Bureau of Chemistry formed, predecessor to the FDA.

1900–1969

Purity of serums, vaccines, and similar products; prohibition of interstate commerce of **adulterated** food/drugs; stops use of poisonous preservatives and cure-all claims for worthless and dangerous patent medicines; prohibits false therapeutic claims in labeling; requires food package contents to be clearly identified on the outside of the package; requires prescriptions for certain narcotics; imposes controls on cosmetics and therapeutic devices; requires new drugs to be shown safe before marketing; regulates **biologicals** and communicable diseases; requires directions and purpose for use on drug labels; imposes safety limits for pesticide residues on vegetables; bans hazardous toys without adequate label warnings.

1970–1990

Categorizes drugs based on abuse and addiction potential compared to their therapeutic value; initiated over-the-counter drug review; ensures safety and effectiveness of medical devices; issues tamper-resistant packing regulations; expedites the availability of less costly generic drugs; approves AIDS test for blood.

1990–Present

Identifies anabolic steroids as controlled substances; requires packaged food nutrition and health labels; accelerates the review of drugs for life-threatening diseases; requires nutrition labeling for supplements; institutes an over-the-counter drug labeling format; requires labeling foods for *trans* fat content; bans OTC materials used to make steroids; bans dietary supplements containing ephedrine.

Source: U.S. Food and Drug Administration. Significant dates in U.S. FDA food and drug law history. Available at: http://www.fda.gov/AboutFDA/WhatWeDo/History/Milestones/ucm128305.htm. Accessed July 15, 2018.

- Enforces the Gramm-Leach-Bliley Act (confidentiality of customer information)
- Operates the Identity Theft Data Clearinghouse

■ **Division of Advertising Practices**
- Enforcing truth-in-advertising laws and deceptive marketing practices
- Monitoring and reporting on advertising food, violent movies, video games, and music to children
- Fairness to Contact Lens Consumers Act
- Federal Cigarette and Smokeless Tobacco Acts
- Dietary supplement guides and restriction of transportation of dietary supplements across borders

■ **Division of Consumer & Business Education**
- Conducts education with public regarding rights
- Works with industry to explain compliance regulations

■ **Division of Enforcement**
- Legal branch that enforces consumer protection laws
- Analyzes and reports on market trends affecting consumers
- Works with FTC on enforcement of court rulings in civil cases

■ **Division of Marketing Practices**
- Works to halt Internet and telecommunications fraud, including **spam**, investment, and work-at-home schemes
- Enforces the Do Not Call component of the Telemarketing Sales Rule, which prohibits unwanted or late-night telemarketing calls
- Enforces the CAN-SPAM Rules, for labeling sexually explicit commercial e-mail
- Requires **franchise** sellers to provide details on business potential to those who might buy into the franchise (Franchise and Business Opportunity Rule)
- Enforces the 900 Number Rule, making charges clear and prohibiting their being marketed to children
- Requires funeral directors to be upfront and complete regarding charges for services
- Enforces the Magnuson-Moss Act, which gives consumers upfront information related to product warranties

■ **Division of Consumer Response & Operations**
- Provides a Consumer Response Center to collect and handle complaints
- Manages the Consumer Sentinel containing millions of FTC consumer fraud complaints

- Administers the core financial, administrative, and consumer **redress** activities of the bureau

■ **Division of Financial Practices**
- Focuses on enforcement in the financial services industry
- Ensures fair and safe lending practices, loan servicing, debt collection, and credit counseling or other debt assistance practices
- Aids consumers in understanding costs and terms related to credit cards and financial services
- Works to stop unfair mortgage lending practices, including discriminatory credit practices as defined in the Equal Credit Opportunity Act
- Works to ensure mortgage payment collection practices are fair and ethical
- Works to halt deceptive telemarketing practices
- Works to ensure that those who work in the debt collection, debt reduction, and credit counseling industries do so ethically

■ **Division of Litigation Technology & Analysis**
- Operates the digital forensics unit, making information available in court
- Analyzes financial information for consumer protection
- Collaborates on the detection and elimination of unfair or deceptive practices
- Identifies consumer protection issues related to new technology

Consumer Product Safety Commission

The U.S. Consumer Product Safety Commission (CPSC) is what is referred to as a federal regulatory agency. The commission has oversight responsibility on a vast array of products around the home and in sports, recreation, and schools. The CPSC investigates claims of products that may cause a fire; pose an electrical, chemical, or mechanical hazard; or cause injury to children. Specifically, based on the CPSC website, the commission is responsible for[24]:

■ developing voluntary standards with standards organizations, manufacturers, and businesses.
■ issuing and enforcing mandatory standards or banning consumer products if no feasible standard would adequately protect the public.
■ obtaining the recall of products and arranging for a repair, replacement, or refund for recalled products.
■ researching potential product hazards.
■ informing and educating consumers directly and through traditional, online, and social media and

🔍 CASE STUDY

Miguel and Maya have just learned that they will be having their first child in 6 months. They are very excited to begin the process of preparing for their new arrival. However, not having had children before, they are unaware of what products are of high quality and what products may present a danger to their new baby.

Question:

1. Where could Miguel and Maya find accurate information on the following products and services:

    a. Cribs
    b. Children's clothing
    c. Infant toys
    d. A reliable minivan
    e. Medications for their child
    f. Child care facilities

by working with foreign, state and local governments, and private organizations.

■ educating manufacturers worldwide about our regulations, supply chain integrity, and development of safe products.

The CPSC provides regular reports and statistical analysis on deaths and injuries related to consumer products, when use results in poisoning, carbon monoxide exposure, electrocution, fire, or sport- and recreation-related injury. All reports are available from the CPSC or on the CPSC website. Consumers can request reports, receive injury statistics, or review specific products' injury history. One can access laws and regulations related to consumer-purchased products. Finally, if a consumer has a grievance with a product's safety, they can file a report with the commission.

The CPSC is not a testing or certification group, nor does it recommend products for consumers to use. Instead, when enough reports have come in regarding a product, the commission may order a recall or replacement for safety reasons. All manufacturers, retailers, and distributors of consumer products are covered under the laws and regulations of the CPSC.

▶ Who Provides Consumer Protection at the State Level?

The agencies discussed so far are either national organizations or federal-level agencies. There are supporting agencies available at the state level as well. Every state in the United States has an attorney general (AG). The AG is the lead legal figure in the state, and is often called the "People's Lawyer."[25] An AG's responsibilities can vary from state to state, but almost all AG's in the

United States have some responsibility for consumer protection. Many states, and some larger cities, also have departments of consumer protection. For some, it is a stand-alone division. For others, it is a responsibility relegated to an agency such as the Department of Health or the Department of Commerce. It may require you to hunt a bit to determine who in particular is responsible for consumer protection in your state, but starting with the AG's office is a good place to start.

▶ What Role Does the Consumer Play?

In 1962, when then-President John F. Kennedy[26] told congress that the American people had the right to safety, information, choice, and voice, he set the parameters clearly for protecting people from consumer misfortune. The primary role the consumer plays comes to life in the "voice" piece. When you believe a company is **misbranding** products, providing false or misleading information, or when you believe a product is unsafe, consumer agencies need to hear your voice. Let businesses know you expect to buy quality products that are safe for you and your family at fair prices.

▶ Conclusion

In most cases, consumers can be confident that they are dealing with ethical, well-intended agencies and health providers. However, in the event that a consumer believes they are being mistreated or have been misled, public and governmental agencies are available to assist with their issue. Consumers have the opportunity to learn the laws related to their situation and access consumer protection agencies to help resolve the situation.

Wrap-Up

Key Terms

Activism A doctrine or practice that emphasizes direct vigorous action, especially in support of or opposition to one side of a controversial issue.

Adulterate To corrupt, debase, or make impure by the addition of a foreign or inferior substance or element.

Biological Any substance, such as a serum or vaccine, derived from animal products or other biological sources and used to treat or prevent disease.

Compendium A brief summary of a larger work or of a field of knowledge.

Consumer A person that uses economic goods.

Defraud To deprive of something by deception or fraud.

Franchise The right or license granted to an individual or group to market a company's goods or services in a particular territory; a business granted such a right or license.

Fraud Intentional perversion of truth in order to induce another to part with something of value or to surrender a legal right.

Globalization Marked especially by free trade, free flow of capital, and the tapping of cheaper foreign labor markets.

Lobby To attempt to influence or sway someone (such as a public official) toward a desired action.

Malpractice An injurious, negligent, or improper medical practice.

Misbranding To brand falsely or in a misleading way; to label in violation of statutory requirements.

Redress To set right; to make up for; to remove the cause of a grievance or complaint.

Spam Unsolicited, usually commercial, e-mail sent to a large number of addresses.

Suggestions for Classroom Activities

1. Find a newspaper or Internet news article related to product fraud or failure. Bring it to class and share. In groups, discuss the appropriate action and agency to address the issue.
2. Investigate the structure within your state's government to determine who has responsibility for consumer protection.

Review Questions

1. What items are covered under information disclosure in the CRR?
2. In what ways can the consumer participate in their own treatment decisions?
3. According to the CRR, what categories should be protected from discrimination?
4. Identify 10 consumer responsibilities related to use of the healthcare system.
5. What is the PCP? What is it designed to accomplish?
6. What seems to be the early trends in survey data related to patient satisfaction in the United States?
7. What consumer protection group was founded by Ralph Nader? What is that agency's role in consumer protection?
8. What do PIRG do? Name three examples of PIRG accomplishments.
9. What organization is responsible for the production of *Consumer Reports*?
10. What organization is responsible for informing the public when a company is deemed untrustworthy?
11. How long has the U.S. FDA been helping to protect U.S. consumers?
12. Identify the different divisions active in the BCP.
13. What agency is responsible for establishing industry standards for product safety?

References

1. Coughlin S, Wordham J, Jonash B. Rising consumerism: Winning the hearts and minds of health care consumers. *Deloitte Review*. 2015;16.
2. Department of Health & Human Services. What are my health care rights and responsibilities? Available at: https://www.hhs.gov/answers/health-care/what-are-my-health-care-rights/index.html. Updated August 11, 2014. Accessed May 2, 2018.
3. Healthcare.gov. Rights & protections. Available at: https://www.healthcare.gov/health-care-law-protections/. Accessed May 2, 2018.
4. President's Advisory Commission on Consumer Protection and Quality in the Health Care Industry. Appendix A: Consumer Bill of Rights and Responsibilities. Washington DC: 1997. Available at: https://archive.ahrq.gov/hcqual/final/append_a.html. Accessed May 2, 2018.
5. American Hospital Association. *Patient Care Partnership: Understanding Expectations, Rights and Responsibilities*. Atlanta, GA: 2003. Available at: https://www.aha.org/system/files/2018-01/aha-patient-care-partnership.pdf. Accessed May 2, 2018.
6. Hospital Consumer Assessment of Healthcare Providers and Systems. CAHPS® Hospital Survey. Available at: http://www

.hcahpsonline.org. Updated April 25, 2018. Accessed May 2, 2018.

7. Hospital Consumer Assessment of Healthcare Providers and Systems. HCAHPS Fact Sheet (CAHPS® Hospital Survey) November 2017. Available at: http://www.hcahpsonline.org /globalassets/hcahps/facts/hcahps_fact_sheet_november _2017a.pdf. Accessed May 2, 2018.

8. Hospital Consumer Assessment of Healthcare Providers and Systems. Summary of HCAHPS survey results: October 2015 to September 2016 Discharges. Available at: http://www .hcahpsonline.org/globalassets/hcahps/summary-analyses /summary-results/july-2017-public-report-october-2015 –september-2016-discharges.pdf. Accessed May 2, 2018.

9. National Center for Health Statistics. Health Expenditures. Available at: https://www.cdc.gov/nchs/fastats/health-expendi tures.htm. Updated May 3, 2017. Accessed May 2, 2018.

10. Brody JE. Over-the-counter medicines' benefits and dangers. *The New York Times*. November 30, 2015. Available at: https://well .blogs.nytimes.com/2015/11/30/over-the-counter-medicines -benefits-and-dangers/?mcubz=3. Accessed May 2, 2018.

11. Fitness for Weight Loss. Diet and weight loss statistics. Available at: http://www.fitnessforweightloss.com/diet-and -weight-loss-statistics/. Accessed May 2, 2018.

12. Zion Market Research. Global fitness equipment market will reach $12.50 billion by 2021. *Globe Newswire*. December 26, 2016. Available at: https://globenewswire. com/news-release/2016/12/26/901669/0/en/Global-Fitness -Equipment-Market-will-reach-12-50-Billion-by-2021 -Zion-Market-Research.html. Accessed May 2, 2017.

13. Public Citizen. About Us. Available at: https://www.citizen .org/about/about-us. Accessed May 2, 2018.

14. United States Public Interest Research Group. Available at: http://www.uspirg.org. Accessed May 2, 2018.

15. United States Public Interest Research Group. Trouble in Toyland 2016. Available at: http://www.uspirg.org/reports /usp/trouble-toyland-2016. Published November 22, 2016. Accessed May 2, 2018.

16. Consumer Federation of America. Available at: http://www .consumerfed.org. Accessed May 2, 2018.

17. Consumers Reports. About Consumers Report. Available at: http://www.consumersunion.org/about/. May 2, 2018.

18. Better Business Bureau®. Mission and Vision. Available at: https://www.bbb.org/en/us/mission-and-vision. Accessed May 2, 2018.

19. Better Business Bureau. Programs. Available at: https:// bbbprograms.org/programs/. Accessed May 2, 2018.

20. U.S. Food and Drug Administration. Milestones in U.S. Food and Drug Law History. Available at: http://www.fda.gov /AboutFDA/WhatWeDo/History/Milestones/ucm128305. htm. Updated February 1, 2018. Accessed May 2, 2018.

21. U.S. Food and Drug Administration. What does FDA regulate? Available at: https://www.fda.gov/AboutFDA/Transparency /Basics/ucm194879.htm. Updated March 28, 2018. Accessed May 2, 2018.

22. U.S. Food and Drug Administration. When and why was FDA formed? Available at: https://www.fda.gov/AboutFDA /Transparency/Basics/ucm214403.htm. Updated March 28, 2018. Accessed May 2, 2018.

23. Federal Trade Commission, Bureau of Consumer Protection. Our Divisions. Available at: https://www.ftc.gov/about-ftc /bureaus-offices/bureau-consumer-protection/our-divisions. Accessed May 2, 2018.

24. U.S. Consumer Product Safety Commission. Contact / FAQ. Available at: https://www.cpsc.gov/About-CPSC/Contact -Information. Accessed May 2, 2018.

25. National Association of Attorney's General. What does an attorney general do? Available at: http://www.naag.org/naag /about_naag/faq/what_does_an_attorney_general_do.php. Accessed on May 2, 2018.

26. Kennedy JF. Special message to Congress on protecting the consumer interest. The American Presidency Project. Available at: http://www.presidency.ucsb.edu/ws/?pid=9108. Published March 15, 1962. Accessed on May 2, 2018.

CHAPTER 18

Health Insurance in the United States

▶ Healthcare Costs in the United States

The healthcare industry in the United States is very complex. In many regards, it is considered one of the best systems in the world. However, due to a myriad of reasons, delivery of healthcare to U.S. citizens is struggling. Ownership of the healthcare system is largely in private hands, although governmental entities at the federal, state, and county, level own many of the health facilities. Coordination of care among doctors and hospitals is improving, but still fairly rare. Specialist care is favored over primary care, and

costs continue to increase at an unsustainable rate. Healthcare spending in the United States rose an estimated 4.3% to $3.3 trillion in 2016.[1] Just to put that in some perspective, if you made $60,000 per year, you would need to work over 53,000 years to pay off a single year of American medical expenditures! Or, if you made $60,000 per year and had a 40-year professional career, it would take you 1,333 professional lifetimes to pay a single year of American healthcare expenditures. The numbers are huge.

As much as 29% of our annual healthcare spending comes from government expenditure. At the current rate of growth, healthcare costs are predicted to keep increasing on average 5.6% per year through 2025.[2]

At that point, it is estimated that output on healthcare will account for 19.9% or almost one-fifth of our gross domestic product (GDP). A quick review of Chapter 4 will remind you where all that money goes.

▶ How Do Americans Pay for Their Healthcare?

With $3.2 trillion dollars going into the healthcare system, the money has to come from somewhere. The primary sources are private health insurance (33%), **Medicare** (20%), **Medicaid** (17%), and consumer out-of-pocket payments (11%). First, we need to summarize the impact passage of the Patient Protection and Affordable Care Act (ACA) in 2010 has had on health insurance coverage.

Patient Protection and Affordable Care Act, 2010

America is still the only developed, high-income nation in the world without a universal health insurance program.[3] A primary objective of ACA was to reduce the number of uninsured Americans, thereby creating greater access to the healthcare system for those in need. This was done in two primary ways: expanding the Medicaid program to make more people eligible, and the creation of tax credits and a health insurance marketplace for adults between 100% and 400% of the federal poverty level (FPL). The law also provides many guarantees and protections[4] related to insurance, such as the following:

- It requires insurance plans to cover people with preexisting health conditions, including pregnancy, without charging more.
- It provides free preventive care.
- It gives young adults more coverage options.
- It ends lifetime and yearly dollar limits on coverage of essential health benefits.
- It helps you understand the coverage you are getting.
- It holds insurance companies accountable for rate increases.
- It makes it illegal for health insurance companies to cancel your health insurance just because you get sick.
- It protects your choice of doctors.
- It protects you from employer retaliation.

The impact on coverage has been immediate and dramatic. When ACA was first passed in 2010, over 18% of the U.S. population (about 44 million people) was uninsured. As of 2016, that has dropped to roughly 9% of the population (28 million people).[5]

The effort is not without controversy. Requiring Americans to purchase health insurance or pay a penalty has been a significant hurdle in the program's survival. It has been expensive for everyone involved—government, providers, and consumers—and conservative politicians have been threatening to repeal or replace the legislation for years. In 2012, challengers to the implementation of the ACA, claiming that requiring coverage was unconstitutional, took the case to the U.S. Supreme Court, but the Court upheld the major provisions in the act as constitutional.[6] The Court did, however, overturn the ruling that states *must* expand their Medicaid programs. As of October 2017, ACA is still in place. The main selling and debate points of this reform include:

- **Overall approach**: The ACA requires most U.S. citizens and legal residents to have health insurance.
- **Cost**: Could be as much as $940 billion over 10 years.
- **Effect on deficit**: The Congressional Budget Office (CBO) estimates it would reduce the deficit by $143 billion over the first 10 years, and further reduce it by $1.2 trillion in the second 10 years.
- **Coverage**: The ACA expands coverage to Americans who are currently uninsured. It provides coverage for those with preexisting health conditions and extends coverage for young adults until age 26. It extends coverage for early retirees who no longer will be eligible for employer insurance but who are not yet eligible for Medicare. It also holds insurance companies accountable for unreasonable rate hikes.
- **Health insurance exchanges**: The uninsured and self-employed are now able to purchase insurance through state-based exchanges with subsidies available to individuals and families with income between 133% and 400% of poverty level. In 2014, separate exchanges were created for small businesses to purchase coverage.
- **Subsidies**: Individuals and families who make between 100% and 400% of the FPL and want to purchase their own health insurance on an exchange are eligible for subsidies. They cannot be eligible for Medicare or Medicaid and cannot be covered by an employer. Eligible buyers receive premium credits, and there is a cap for how much they have to contribute to their premiums (on a sliding scale).
- **Paying for the plan**: The Medicare Payroll Tax was expanded in 2012 to include unearned income. This is a 3.8% tax on investment income for families making more than $250,000 per year ($200,000

for individuals). Beginning in 2018, insurance companies will pay a 40% excise tax on so-called "Cadillac" high-end insurance plans worth over $27,500 for families ($10,200 for individuals). Dental and vision plans are exempt and will not be counted in the total cost of a family's plan. There will be a 10% excise tax on indoor tanning services.

- **Medicaid**: The ACA expands Medicaid to include people at 133% of the FPL, which is $32,319 for a family of four. The act requires states to expand Medicaid to include childless adults starting in 2014. However, as of 2017, 19 states have chosen not to expand their Medicaid programs. The federal government currently pays 100% of the costs for covering expanded programs, and will drop to 90% in 2020.[7] Illegal immigrants are not eligible for Medicaid.

- **Insurance reforms**: Six months after enactment, insurance companies could no longer deny children coverage based on a **preexisting condition**. Starting in 2014, insurance companies could not deny coverage to anyone with pre-existing conditions. Insurance companies must now allow children to stay on their parents' insurance plans until age 26.

- **Abortion**: The bill segregates private insurance premium funds from taxpayer funds. Individuals would have to pay for abortion coverage by making two separate payments. Private funds would have to be kept in a separate account from federal and taxpayer funds. No healthcare plan would be required to offer abortion coverage. States could pass legislation choosing to opt out of offering abortion coverage through the exchange.

- **Individual mandate**: In 2014, everyone must purchase health insurance or face a $695 annual fine. There are some exceptions for low-income people.

- **Employer mandate**: Technically, there is no employer mandate. Employers with more than 50 employees must provide health insurance or pay a fine of $2,000 per worker each year if any worker receives federal subsidies to purchase health insurance. Fines are applied to the entire number of employees minus some allowances. Employers with 25 or less employees with average wages less than $50,000 who offer insurance to their employees will receive a tax credit.

- **Immigration**: Illegal immigrants are not allowed to buy health insurance in the exchanges—even if they pay completely with their own money.

- **Long-term care**: The legislation established a nationwide system for states to run background check programs for employees of long-term care facilities and providers. This proposal builds on a successful pilot program, which operated in seven states and kept thousands of individuals who had disqualifying records out of the long-term care workforce.

▶ What Are My Health Insurance Options?

Private health insurance is insurance that is provided through an employer or insurance you purchase on your own. Health insurance helps individuals and families to afford medical expenses. Health insurance was originally designed to cover extraordinary expenses due to a serious injury or illness, not doctors' visits for colds and minor injuries. It was typically the lifeline for many people (**FIGURE 18.1**).

More than two-thirds of all American adults have private health insurance.[8] Most college students are on the student university health insurance plan or are on their parents' health insurance plan and do not think much about health insurance. Regardless of the type of insurance you have, there are some basic terms you need to be familiar with to successfully navigate the insurance waters[9]:

- **Premium**: This is the amount you pay each month to have health insurance. Costs vary widely.

- **Deductible**: Every plan has an initial amount of money the consumer has to pay before the insurance company pays anything. This can also vary greatly, from as low as $100 to as high as $10,000 for certain plans. Generally, when the deductibles are lower, the premiums for the plan are higher. It is very important to understand the relationship between your premium and your deductible to understand how much money you will expend prior to your insurance beginning to pay.

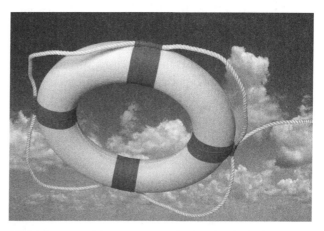

FIGURE 18.1 Health insurance rescues individuals from financial ruin.
© R. Gino Santa Maria/Shutterstock

- **Co-pays and Coinsurance**: This represents either the flat fee (co-pay) or percentage of fees (coinsurance) you will need to pay for each service you obtain. Co-pays and coinsurance do not apply until after the deductible is met.
- **Medical Necessity**: These are procedures that are required for the benefit of a person's physical health. However, note that something like cosmetic surgery is not considered a medical necessity.

Whether you are a student or adult, you should ask yourself certain relevant questions when selecting your insurance plan. For instance: Can I only go to one doctor? If I need a specialist, do I have to get a referral from my doctor? Is there a co-pay for each visit? Do I have to pay for X-rays or other diagnostic tests separately? Should I be concerned about meeting the yearly deductible? These are just some of the questions that would give some clues about the type of health insurance you need and can afford. We will answer several of these questions at the end of the chapter. Next are types of insurance that you should learn about and consider when selecting a plan just for you.

Indemnity Insurance

Indemnity insurance, or fee-for-service insurance, is the most flexible and generally the most expensive type of private insurance. It allows the individual to choose their healthcare providers for all services.[9] An individual can go to any doctor or hospital. An indemnity plan reimburses the person or the healthcare provider for services rendered. For instance, if you go to the doctor for a cough and sore throat, the doctor may order a lab and X-ray to be completed. The doctor then bills and is paid for the lab service, the X-ray service, and their time for the appointment. There is a yearly deductible for the consumer that needs to be met prior to reimbursement. There is also a yearly maximum out-of-pocket expense; after the deductible and out-of-pocket costs are met, the plan begins to pay reimbursable expenses in full. Often, the plan requires preapproval for procedures and hospital stays.

Managed Care Plans

Managed care plans offer health insurance at a greatly reduced cost for the consumer. These plans cover a variety of procedures, but the coverage varies from plan to plan. One insurance provider can have hundreds of variations to the coverage they provide, as they tailor the coverage to the company they are working with. It is extremely important to read the specifics of a managed care plan to be certain of what it covers. The two discussed are **Health maintenance organizations (HMOs)** and **Preferred provider organizations (PPOs)**. The premiums on these types of policies can differ greatly, influenced by age, gender, health status, and geographic location.[10,11]

Health Maintenance Organizations

HMOs are usually provided through an employer and are less expensive than most kinds of insurance. There are restrictions about what physicians are available. These doctors are called "in-network" and have agreed to the insurance company's policies and pay structure. Your primary care doctor will handle all your preventative and nonlife threatening care issues and must make a referral for a consumer to see a specialist.[12] The HMO company must preapprove most tests and procedures. HMOs have an extensive network of physicians and hospitals. Doctors are paid a monthly fee for each patient in their practice rather than by the cost of services from visits and procedures, which is supposed to make the doctors less likely to require extensive medical tests that are unnecessary. The insured chooses a doctor from a list and that doctor becomes the gatekeeper for medical care. All referrals for specialists come from this primary caregiver. The fees are lower than fee-for-service or PPOs. The patient pays a **co-payment** for all doctors' visits that include all services provided during that visit, including lab tests and X-rays. The out-of-pocket expenses can be much lower for the patient with this kind of health insurance. The caveat for this type of insurance is that the patient cannot go out of the network for services, nor can they see a specialist without a referral.[12] Because of the greater control by the provider, premiums, deductibles, and co-pays are lower in an HMO plan.

Preferred Provider Organizations

PPOs are networks of physicians that work with an insurance company. A negotiated rate for services has been prearranged for persons insured under the plan for in-network doctors. Doctors who are not listed as providers are called out-of-network doctors and the co-pay is higher. With PPOs, there is a prenegotiated rate for each kind of service. The insured pays the prenegotiated fees with the plan's doctors. If the insured decides to go outside the plan's providers for services, he or she must pay the difference between the negotiated rate and the outside provider's fee.[12] Because of the greater flexibility in this type of plan, premiums may be comparable or slightly higher to HMOs, but deductibles and co-pays (out-of-pocket costs) are higher than the HMO.[13]

Point of Service Plans

Point of service (POS) plans are similar to both HMO and PPO plans, but you can choose to go with an HMO or a PPO provider each time you receive medical care.[13] With this type of plan, the primary caregivers can refer patients to providers outside the network and the plan will pay most of the bill; but if you choose a specialist outside the plan without the referral, you will have to pay a much higher co-payment.[13]

Health Savings Accounts

Health savings accounts were signed into law by President Bush in 2003. They allow the employee to deduct an amount from their pay each month on a pretax basis that gets deposited into a savings account specifically for health-related expenses.[14] This means the person does not pay taxes on the amount saved or spent on healthcare. Only people with a high-deductible health plans (deductibles over $1,300 for individuals and $2,600 for families per year)[15] can have these types of accounts. These savings accounts can be used for a variety of medical expenses, including over-the-counter drugs, co-pays for doctor visits, co-pays for prescriptions, or any out-of-pocket medical expenses. One benefit of using an HSA is that the money you have placed in the account rolls over from year to year and you do not lose it if it is not spent by year's end.[15]

Flexible Spending Accounts

Flexible spending accounts are similar to the HSA set up by employers that also allow employees to contribute on a pretax basis to reimburse healthcare expenses. These accounts can be used with any type of health insurance, not just high-deductible health plans. The main drawback is that, because the account is employer owned, money placed into the account must be used in the year that the contributions are made. Otherwise, the money is lost. So, this type of account requires careful planning so you do not put more money into the account than you can spend. However, some companies now allow employees until spring of the following year to spend down the account.[16]

High-Deductible Health Plans

High-deductible health plans (HDHPs) are usually called catastrophic insurance because the insurance does not start reimbursing for medical services until the deductible is paid. Out-of-pocket expenses in an HDHP are capped at $6,550 for individuals and $13,100 for families.[15] These plans can be a good choice when a consumer utilizes healthcare infrequently, there is no employer health insurance, and money for premiums is tight. Although the deductible is high, it is still better than being without insurance and paying the entire amount in an emergency or sudden serious illness.

🔍 CASE STUDY

Selecting a Health Insurance Plan

Megan Smith is getting ready to graduate in May. Like many college students, it took her more than 4 years to complete her degree. She has a job offer from a school district in her small hometown to teach for $35,000 per year, or about $2,300 a month after taxes. Her hometown is about 45 minutes from a larger town. Megan has grown up in this town and has gone to the same doctor all her life. When she looked at the insurance options offered through the school district, she had no idea how to choose. One of her choices is an HMO at $50 per month, which includes co-payments of $25 per doctor's visit and $10 for prescriptions. There is a $500 deductible to meet. This insurance includes vision. However, there are no HMO providers in her hometown; she would have to drive 45 minutes to go to a doctor and begin seeing a new primary care physician. She could not go to a specialist without a referral from the new doctor.

The next option is a PPO plan. Her hometown doctor is in the preferred network of providers, so she would not have to travel to see a doctor. The cost for the PPO plan is $200 per month. The plan has a $500 deductible, and then pays 80% of the remaining medical costs for the calendar year, including prescriptions. Vision is not included.

The district also offers vision insurance for $10 a month and dental insurance for $50 a month. They have a free life insurance policy for $10,000, if she dies for any reason after the first 6 months of employment. There is also optional life insurance ($100,000 of coverage for $25 per month), disability insurance ($25 per month), and long-term care insurance ($15 per month). Megan is completely confused about what insurances she will need and chooses the PPO and all of the other insurance choices to make sure she is covered just like her parents are covered. The monthly cost for all of her insurance coverage is $325.

Questions:

1. Did Megan make the right choices?
2. What would happen if she did not have health insurance and later got into a car crash and sustained multiple injuries?

▶ What Are Government Insurance Programs?

One of the main political arguments related to healthcare is whether the federal government should be involved in the process at all. The term "socialized medicine" has been tossed about for decades, with more conservative politicians generally believing the federal government should be out of the way and more liberal politicians painting healthcare as a right to be provided by the government. The reality is that socialized medicine has been in the United States for more than 50 years in multiple forms. Medicare, Medicaid, military insurance programs, and programs for children are all programs that provide healthcare and are managed by the federal government.

Medicare

The Centers for Medicare and Medicaid Services (CMS) is a component of the U.S. Department of Health and Human Services. Medicare accounts for the largest proportion of health spending in the United States, and covers nearly 55 million Americans, including people who are age 65 or older, some disabled people under age 65, and people of all ages with end-stage renal disease (permanent kidney failure treated with dialysis or a transplant).[17] When people retire, if they are on social security and they are age 65, they must go on Medicare, which becomes their primary insurance program. Some people need to apply for Medicare and some are automatically enrolled into the system. If people retire before the age of 65, they must procure their own insurance. Medicare will cover 80% of medical and hospitalization costs, but that leaves people with 20% of their cost that they must cover. Medigap insurance policies called secondary or supplement policies can then be bought to cover that 20%. See **BOX 18.1** for important details about Medicare services.[17]

Medicaid

Medicaid is a medical assistance program that serves more than 69 million people in the United States, and is the largest provider of health coverage.[18] It is a jointly funded program, with costs split by the federal government and the states. The program serves people under the age of 65 who have limited income and

---

BOX 18.1 Medicare Services

Medicare Part A
Part A is hospital insurance. It covers inpatient hospital care, skilled nursing facilities (not custodial or long-term care), and helps cover hospice and home healthcare. Premiums for Part A have usually been covered through payment of payroll taxes while working.

Medicare Part B
Part B is medical insurance. Most people pay a monthly premium for Part B, and it helps cover doctors' services and outpatient care. It covers some services Part A does not cover like physical therapists, occupational therapists, and some home healthcare.

Medicare Supplement Insurance (Medigap)
Medigap is not actually a government program, nor is it a part of Medicare, but it is commonly purchased by those on Medicare to supplement its limitations. If you have Medicare Parts A and B (but are *not* in the Part C Medicare Advantage program) you can purchase an additional insurance policy to fill the "gaps" left by Medicare. These policies are sold by private insurers and have their own premium, deductible, and coverage limitations in addition to what you pay for Part B. There are 10 different options for Medigap, so you must choose the one that best fits your medical situation. It is important to note that Medigap does not cover "everything else" that Medicare misses, as there are no provisions for long-term care, vision care, dental care, hearing aids, eyeglasses, or private duty nursing.

Medicare Part C—Medicare Advantage
The Medicare Advantage program is a managed care program—essentially a blending of Parts A and B, and sometimes Part D. There is no reduction in the benefits you receive compared to traditional Medicare, and in some cases, you may get more. The program will cost you more money up front, in the form of premiums and possible coinsurance, but is designed to reduce costs overall by providing more coordinated services in the long run.

Medicare Part D—Prescription Drug Benefits
Medicare prescription drug coverage is provided by private companies. Consumers will choose a plan and pay a premium. If you decide to enroll in a drug plan after your initial enrollment, you may pay a penalty.

assets, and is focused on children, pregnant women, parents, seniors, and individuals with disabilities. Persons receiving a Supplemental Security Income (SSI) check automatically qualify for Medicaid.

With the passage of ACA, states were given the option to expand Medicaid services to people under 138% of the FPL. As of January 2017, 32 states have chosen to expand Medicaid, while 19 (mostly in the Southern plains and Southeastern United States) have chosen not to expand due to the associated costs. The cost of Medicaid grew an estimated 4.2% in 2016,[19] which puts an increased burden on states even though they receive federal aid. However, the increase in enrollment in Medicaid has slowed dramatically since the initial 2015 eligibility change, with actual spending per consumer in Medicaid flat or lower.[19]

Medicaid will pay for certain goods and services. It is important to note that there are eligibility requirements and limitations on what is covered under Medicaid, and this can vary from state to state. Some examples of services for which regular Medicaid will pay can be seen in **BOX 18.2**.[18]

Children's Health Insurance Program

The **Children's Health Insurance Program (CHIP)** was created in 1997. The program provides federal matching funds to states that provide healthcare services to children age 18 years or younger, whose family income was too high to qualify for Medicaid, but too little to afford health insurance. Almost all states set eligibility for coverage at 200% of the FPL.[20] Like Medicaid, services covered can vary from state to state, but core services provided by all states include the following:

- Routine check-ups
- Immunizations
- Doctor visits
- Prescriptions
- Vision and dental care
- Hospital services
- Lab and X-ray services
- Emergency care

Veterans Health Administration

The Veterans Health Administration (VHA), part of the U.S. Department of Veterans Affairs, provides care for military veterans. The VHA offers many benefits for veterans based upon discharge from active military service other than dishonorable conditions.[21] Services include education, vocational rehabilitation, home loans, and survivor benefits. Those related to healthcare delivery services include healthcare, life insurance, disability compensation, and burial allowances. Disability compensation is a benefit paid to a veteran because of injuries or diseases that happened while he or she was on active duty, or were made worse by active military service. It is also paid to certain veterans disabled from VHA healthcare. The benefits are tax-free.[21]

TRICARE

TRICARE is the U.S. Department of Defense Military Health System healthcare insurance program for active duty service members, retired service members, and their dependents. It is also available for activated National Guard or Reserve members. TRICARE offers 11 healthcare programs, plus pharmacy, dental, and retirement care.[22]

▶ Who Has Health Insurance?

Health insurance coverage in the United States reached an all-time high in 2016, with 91.2% of all Americans having health insurance for part or all of the calendar year. A corresponding 8.8% of Americans remain uninsured, defined by the U.S. Census Bureau (USCB) as having no health insurance for any part of the calendar year.[8] Of those covered, according to the USCB, 55.7% were covered by employer-based insurance plans, 19.7% by Medicaid, 16.7% by Medi-

---

BOX 18.2 Medicaid Services

States design and implement their own individual Medicaid programs. However, some services are considered "mandatory" by the federal government. Those services include:

- Inpatient hospital services
- Outpatient hospital services
- Physician services
- Lab and X-ray services
- Home health services
- Early periodic screening services
- Family planning
- Nurse midwife services
- Transportation to medical care
- Smoking cessation programs

There are dozens of optional services that states can choose to provide, including but not limited to certain dentures, eye care services due to injury or disease, prescription medicines, personal care services, medical equipment, and Medicare premiums, deductibles, and co-payments for certain persons with Medicare.

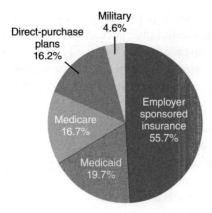

FIGURE 18.2 Health insurance coverage among adults, 2016.

U.S. Census Bureau, Healthcare Coverage in the U.S., 2016.

people covered by employer-sponsored insurance has dropped nearly 10% over the last 20 years. The cost of providing coverage is taking a toll on employers. The average cost of a family insurance plan in 2016 was over $18,000 per year, with the employer covering over 70% of the costs. The percentage of employers offering healthcare may decline even more over time as costs continue to grow and alternatives for coverage potentially expand. The employee's expected contribution to individual plans varies widely, but has generally continued to increase[8] (**FIGURE 18.3**).

care, 16.2% by direct purchase plans, and 4.6% under military coverage plans (**FIGURE 18.2**).

While more than half of those insured are covered by an employer-sponsored plan, the percentage of

Health insurance coverage among children under 18 years of age has remained fairly level since the ACA went into place.[23] Over 93% of youth are covered by some type of health insurance. Employer-sponsored insurance accounts for nearly half of the coverage, while Medicaid covers 38%. Seven percent of children under 18 years of age remain uninsured.

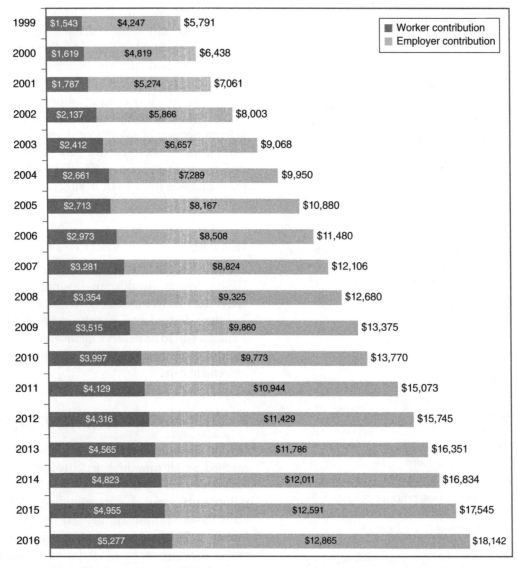

FIGURE 18.3 Annual worker and employer contribution to premiums and total premiums for family coverage, 1999–2016.

Reproduced from Kaiser Family Foundation. HRET Survey of Employer-Sponsored Health Benefits, 1999-2016.

▶ How Does the U.S. Healthcare Delivery System Compare with Other Nations?

In 2000, as the first ranking of its kind, the World Health Organization (WHO) ranked the overall performance of the U.S. healthcare system as 37th out of 191 countries worldwide, and ranked the United States at number one for expenditures per capita.[24] That means that Americans pay more for their healthcare than any other nation in the world. Healthcare has been at the forefront of the national conversation ever since. The greatest reason for the low ranking has to do with access, which has undoubtedly improved since the passage of the ACA and the corresponding drop in the number of people without health insurance. In comparison to our peer nations, however, a 2017 review of the 11 highest income countries by The Commonwealth Fund determined that the United States was last among all nations in healthcare access, equity, and outcomes.[3]

Challenges in the healthcare system may be due to a variety of reasons. We have a healthcare system that has not optimized operations at hospitals and regional networks, and a system that has not developed performance measures regarding quality and scope of medical care. The American Hospital Association states that redesign of the healthcare system should be initiated to improve what they call the "Triple Aim"[25]—improving the patient experience of care, improving the health of populations, and reducing the per capita cost of healthcare. They suggest seven steps to accomplish this[25]:

1. Design the healthcare delivery system with the whole person at the center.
2. Empower people and the care delivery system itself with information, technology, and transparency to promote health.
3. Build care management and coordination systems.
4. Integrate behavioral health and social determinants of health with physical health.
5. Develop collaborative leadership.
6. Integrate care delivery into the community.
7. Create safe and highly reliable healthcare organizations.

The Agency for Healthcare Research and Quality (AHRQ) is a branch of the U.S. Department of Health and Human Services with the mission of reviewing and improving the quality of healthcare in the United States. AHRQ suggests that improving the healthcare system involves incorporating preventative services and self-management support,

empowering all staff to make change within the system, and developing leadership focused on change and improvement.[26] Programmatically, their primary emphases include health literacy, cultural competency, and improving primary care delivery. These efforts are specifically designed to improve acute care while reducing costs.

Another factor that has increased healthcare delivery problems has been changing mortality patterns. By 2050, the group of individuals age 65 or older is projected to increase to 23% of the entire population from the current 15%.[27] The consequence is that people with chronic medical conditions (e.g., diabetes, dementia, arthritis) will be surviving longer and will need medical care for even more years. It will be extremely beneficial, therefore, to improve the U.S. healthcare delivery system. One solution proposed to improve our healthcare system is to allow Medicare to be available for all.

▶ What Can You Do to Become an Informed Health Insurance Consumer?

Many people have high medical bills even if they have health insurance. What can an informed consumer do to prevent themselves from getting stuck with high medical bills?

Understand Your Coverage

HealthCare.gov offers the following advice[29]:

- Ask your health insurance company whether the procedure is covered, not your doctor!
- Review your Summary of Benefits to determine what is covered, your share of the bill, and coverage limitations.
- Know your deductible and whether it has been met for the year.
- Know your co-payments and coinsurances.

Visit In-Network Providers

You will save money by using doctors and hospitals in your health insurance network.

- Get the names of the physicians and facilities you plan to use and ask your health insurer whether they participate before you receive services.
- If you already have a provider you like and want to keep working with, call their office and ask if they accept your coverage.

📄 IN THE NEWS

As the conversation about healthcare reform continues, one economist says it might be quite simple: make Medicare available to all. In a September 2017 editorial,[28] University of Massachusetts-Amherst economist Gerald Friedman suggests that eliminating the "over 65" language in Medicare law, and essentially making it available to anyone who wants it, would allow the government/insurer relationship that currently exists with Medicare to continue. He also suggests it could be much cheaper than moving to a full, single-payer system. Here is how Friedman says the money works out:

- Assuming everyone eligible went into the Medicare program, it would then cover the 28 million uninsured, the 61 million people in Medicaid/CHIP programs, and 171 million with private insurance.
- Savings would come from a reduction in the complexities of medical billing, insurance administration, salaries, marketing costs, and hospitals overcharging private insurers. The savings would total approximately $220 billion dollars based on the current practices.
- Revenues to pay for the additional people would come from each person paying the existing Medicare premiums (about $134 per month), and the elimination of the subsidies currently in place for employer-provided insurance plans, and the ACA subsidy for private insurers. These two total $371 billion.
- The remaining amount needed to pay for the system change would be $246 billion. Friedman states a small increase in the existing Medicare payroll tax, from 2.9% to 5.9% could cover that cost. For the average American worker, this would mean roughly $15 per week.

    Friedman indicates that the plan is affordable for nearly everyone, and it saves the massive leap to a completely single-payer system for the country.

Sources: (1) University of Massachusetts-Amherst. (2) Associated Press. "Medicare for All" could be cheaper than you think. *Washington's Top News*. September 19, 2017. Available at: https://wtop.com/business-finance/2017/09/medicare-for-all-could-be-cheaper-than-you-think/. Accessed May 4, 2018.

- Call your insurance company or state Medicaid and CHIP program. Look at their website or check your member handbook to find providers in your network who take your health coverage.
- Ask your friends or family if they have providers they like and use the tools available to compare healthcare providers in your area.[29]
- Be aware that even though a hospital may participate in your plan, other physicians at the hospital such as anesthesiologists and pathologists may not be part of your plan. Check with your insurer to find out about these costs.
- If you feel that you must use an out-of-network provider, you can request an exception to cover the services at your in-network benefit level.
- Be sure to ask your insurance company before you receive out-of-network services.

Learn About Your Prescription Coverage

Find out which prescriptions your plan covers by visiting the insurance company's website, calling them, reviewing the "Summary of Benefits and Coverage," or reading materials that were mailed to you.[29]

- **Understand your rights:**
    - You have a right to be treated with respect and recognition of your dignity and a right to privacy.
    - You have a right to receive information about your health plan, its services, its practitioners and providers, and your rights and responsibilities.
    - You have a right to participate with practitioners in decision-making regarding your healthcare.
    - You have a right to a candid discussion of appropriate or medically necessary treatment options for your conditions, regardless of cost or benefit coverage.
    - You have a right to voice complaints or appeals about your health plan or the care provided.[30]
- **Understand your responsibilities:**
    - You have a responsibility to provide, to the extent possible, information that the health plan and its practitioners and providers need in order to care for you.
    - You have a responsibility to understand your health problems and participate in developing mutually agreed upon treatment goals to the degree possible.
    - You have a responsibility to follow the plans and instructions for care that you have agreed on with your practitioners.
    - You have a responsibility to pay your co-payments or coinsurance at the time of service.
    - You have a responsibility to be on time for appointments and to notify practitioners/providers when an appointment must be cancelled.[30]

■ **If you do not have insurance:**
- Find out the costs upfront; costs are different for those paying cash than for the insured.
- Ask whether the hospital will negotiate and accept less than the requested amount.
- Get any payment arrangements in writing.
- Ask whether there are programs that can help you afford care.
- Be prepared to show proof of financial need to find out if you qualify.

▶ What Are the Other Forms of Insurance Affecting Health?

Disability Insurance

Disability insurance covers loss of income due to illness or injury that keeps a person from working. Disability insurance comes in long- and short-term varieties. Short-term disability insurance covers the individual after missing only a few days of work, usually 7, 15, or 30 days, and no longer than 26 weeks.[31] Long-term disability insurance covers the individual after several weeks to several months and continues coverage most commonly to the age of 65.[31] Most companies are required to have short-term disability insurance for their employees and can cover up to 60% of their monthly paycheck. According to the Council for Disability Awareness, 24% of women and 21% of men will have a disability incident lasting at least 3 months before they reach 65 years old, and one-third of those will last for more than 5 years.[32]

Social Security can cover unemployment due to disability, but the person has to qualify and not be able to do any form of work. Many people apply for this type of benefit, but few qualify. Another type of loss of income insurance is worker's compensation, if you are injured at work. However, it will only pay a small percentage of your monthly check and is only in force for a limited time frame.[33]

Employer-paid disability will only cover a percentage of the person's paycheck to encourage the person to come back to work, usually 45% to 65%. The money received from employer-based disability insurance is taxable by the federal government. Individually purchased disability insurance is not taxable and can pay up to 100% of the person's paycheck.[31]

Disability premiums are based on how risky your profession is and how much income you are trying to protect. If you have little risk to your job, then your premium should be fairly low.

Dental Insurance

Another choice for insurance from many employers is dental insurance. Each plan will vary in its network of providers. You pay a premium to plans that cover a percentage of specific services up to the plan limit. The network of dentists provides services at a set fee that is well below the regular fee for those services. Most plans usually cover cleanings and exams twice a year without a co-pay, and roughly 50% for dental services up to a maximum of $1,000 per year. Most plans offer a lifetime benefit for orthodontics up to a certain amount, for an additional premium. The premiums for dental insurance can vary widely, so be certain to look at the details of the plan you are offered.

Vision Insurance

Vision insurance helps defray the costs of eye exams, eyewear, and other vision services. Typically, vision insurance covers eye exams with a set co-payment, although many medical plans now cover this part of the process as well. Eyewear is also covered with a co-payment, which varies with the type of insurance. Insurance companies cover a specific dollar amount for frames, lenses, and contact lenses with a co-payment. For instance, one vision insurance company may pay $100 for frames and $100 for lenses with a $25 co-payment. If the person would like $150 frames and $200 lenses, they must pay the $25 co-pay plus the difference between the actual cost of the frames and lenses and the $200 coverage; therefore, the person would pay $175 for the $350 pair of glasses. The same applies to contact lenses. The same insurance company might pay $50 per eye for contact lenses for 6 months. If the contact lenses cost $55 per box per eye and the co-payment is $25, then the person must pay $35 for a 6-month supply of contacts costing $110.

Life Insurance

Life insurance pays money to the **beneficiary** when the policy holder dies. The beneficiary is the person who receives the death benefit. You can name as beneficiary one or more people, a charity, your estate, or a trust fund. If you do not name a beneficiary, the death benefit will go to your estate. There are two levels of beneficiaries—primary and contingent. **Primary beneficiaries** receive the death benefit upon the policy holder's death. The **contingent beneficiaries** receive the death benefit when the policy holder dies and the primary beneficiaries are also deceased or cannot be found. If no contingent beneficiaries are living or cannot be found, the death benefit is paid to the estate. There are basically two types of life insurance—term life and permanent insurance.

Term Life Insurance

Term life insurance comes in two types: level term and decreasing term. **Level term life insurance** pays the same amount at the death of the policy holder at any time during the life of the policy. **Decreasing term life insurance** decreases over the life of the policy. As the amount of years go by, decreasing term life insurance plans diminish in value.[34] Term life insurance does not earn interest and pays the face value of the policy to the beneficiary at the death of the policy holder. The cost of term life insurance is dependent upon the person's age and health status at the beginning of the policy. Premiums usually remain the same throughout the life of the policy and end at a specified age or term. Normally, insurance companies do not sell term life insurance that ends past the person's 80th birthday. Level term policies can be for 5–30 years in 5-year spans. With a 5-year term, it is renewable every 5 years. The premium can change at the end of each fifth year. Policies with 10-, 15-, 20-, 25-, and 30-year terms end at the completion of the term and are not renewable. At the end of the term, a new policy must be purchased with a new premium based on the person's age and health status. For this reason, many people choose 20- or 30-year terms.[34]

Term life insurance can be purchased through an employer, from an insurance agency, from a mortgage lender, or from another lender. Many times, mortgage lenders and motor vehicle dealerships offer term life insurance when a purchase is made, to pay off the loan upon the death of the borrower. If a person thinks that this is necessary, it may be better to buy a whole life policy or term life insurance for a much larger amount to assist the family in paying other expenses at their death, besides just the car or house.

Permanent Insurance

Permanent insurance includes whole life, universal or adjustable life, variable life, and variable universal life.[34] **Whole life insurance** offers a death benefit and a savings account. Part of the premium goes to a life insurance policy and part goes toward a savings account that grows based on the dividends paid by the insurance company. Universal or adjustable life insurance also has a savings account feature called a cash value account, which earns interest at the market rate. If there is enough money in the cash value, either the premiums can be reduced or the cash value can pay the premium until the cash value runs out.

If the financial situation changes for an individual, the cash value can help keep the policy in force; however, if the cash value runs out the policy will be cancelled. **Variable life insurance** uses part of the premium to purchase stocks, bonds, and mutual funds. Variable life can not only increase the earnings of the policy, but can also decrease the value of the cash value and the death benefit depending on the market. Some companies who offer variable life offer a minimum death benefit that cannot change with market fluctuations. **Variable universal life insurance** combines the best features of universal and variable life insurance. The policy has the same risks and benefits of bonds, stocks, and mutual funds, and can adjust the premium with the cash value earnings.[34]

If you have no dependents, enough money saved to pay for your burial, and no indebtedness, you do not need life insurance of any kind. That description fits very few individuals. If you have dependents, you will want to buy enough life insurance to replace the income that you would have earned if you had lived. You may want to purchase life insurance to create an inheritance or give to a charitable organization. Life insurance should be carefully considered to protect those you love from financial burden, while making sure that having life insurance does not become a financial burden.

Long-Term Care Insurance

Long-term care insurance assures coverage when an individual requires supervision and help with activities of daily living (ADL) for more than 90 days. ADL include getting dressed, bathing, taking medication, doing housework, paying bills, and the like. Long-term care insurance also provides coverage for cognitive impairment such as Alzheimer's disease or other brain disorders. It provides financial coverage either in-home, in an assisted living center, or in a skilled nursing facility. Without long-term care insurance, individuals or their families could spend thousands on care, all out of pocket.

Assisted living centers are like apartments that are staffed with people who will help with some ADL. They provide emergency care 24/7; meals are served three times a day and assistance is provided for getting dressed or taking medication. Assisted living is more expensive than an apartment, but not as expensive as a skilled nursing facility.

Skilled nursing facilities offer nursing care and help with ADL. Most people in skilled nursing facilities cannot take care of most ADL, need help with medication and treatments, and are under the supervision of a doctor. They can no longer live independently in either an assisted living center or at home.

In-home care takes place in the person's home, and someone with nursing skills or other skills depending on the need comes to their home and help with the ADL. Sometimes, people only require help with ADL for a short time until they recover from an accident or injury. Sometimes, they require care for the duration of their lives, costing tens of thousands of dollars out of pocket for those without long-term care insurance. For example, expenses associated with long-term care for Alzheimer's disease[35] can include ongoing medical treatment and diagnostic services, medical equipment, prescription medicine, safety monitors, and personal care items. In the United States, the average cost for adult day care services is $1,600 per month, assisted living facilities are $3,700 per month, and nursing home care is $7,200 per month. Each of these may be needed at some point as the disease progresses. Life expectancy after diagnosis with Alzheimer's is 8–10 years, so the costs of care can be very significant.

The premium for long-term care insurance varies depending on the age of the participant—the older the participant the larger the monthly premium. Currently, Medicare pays for long-term hospital care, skilled nursing, some home healthcare, and hospice care, but not long-term care in the home or in assisted living facilities.

The Consolidated Omnibus Budget Reconciliation Act

The **Consolidated Omnibus Budget Reconciliation Act (COBRA)** was passed into law in 1986. COBRA is available for terminated employees, those who lose coverage because of reduced work hours, or children who can no longer be on their parents' policy because of age. It provides those people the opportunity to buy group insurance coverage for themselves and their families for limited periods. COBRA allows the person to continue with health insurance, prescription drug coverage, dental insurance, and vision care. COBRA will not cover life insurance.[36]

COBRA covers employees who work for employers with 20 or more employees in the prior year. The number includes all part-time and full-time employees. If the employee is covered by the employer's health insurance prior to one of the following events, then the person is qualified for COBRA. Qualifying events for employees include voluntary or involuntary termination (other than gross misconduct) or reduction of work hours. Eligible family members

can enroll in COBRA for 18 months after the qualifying event.[36]

Qualifying events for spouses are the same as for employees, plus the employee becoming eligible for Medicare, divorce or legal separation, or death of the employee. Spouses may be insured for 36 months. Children qualify for the events listed for the employee and spouse, plus loss of dependent child status. Children may be covered for 36 months after losing their dependent child status. Qualified persons have a 60-day window to elect to continue coverage through COBRA. The time frame is either the date of qualification or the date the notice to elect COBRA is sent, whichever is later. The premium is paid by the beneficiary of COBRA.[36]

Here is how it might work:

Example 1: Mary has been insured under her mother's health insurance from the university where her mom works. Mary has turned 25 and is no longer allowed to be covered under her mother's insurance. If Mary chooses to pay the premium, she can continue coverage for 36 months.

Example 2: John works but has been under his wife's health insurance plan because it was less expensive. Now, John is getting a divorce and he will not be eligible to enroll in his work insurance for another year. If John chooses, he can be covered for 36 months after the date of his divorce.

Example 3: Allen is married with three children. The company that he works for is downsizing and the company has terminated his employment. He is offered COBRA for 18 months, if he chooses to enroll and pay the premium.

▶ How Do I Choose a Health Insurance Plan?

While most of the chapter was spent discussing group insurance, health insurance can also be purchased as an individual policy. **Individual insurance** is insurance purchased by the individual directly from an insurance company. **Group insurance** is insurance that is available to groups of individuals, such as employers, unions, or professional organizations. Regardless of whether you purchase insurance yourself or receive it through an employer several considerations are necessary to determine if you are choosing the most appropriate plan.

With all of the choices available, you might wonder how you will choose a health insurance plan after you are no longer eligible to participate in your parents'

🔍 CASE STUDY

Roxanne is a divorced mother with a 6-year-old son. Recently, the son needed to have reconstructive surgery on his inner ear to restore his hearing. The chain bones in his inner ear were destroyed during his many ear infections when he was younger. Roxanne is covered by a local HMO through her job at a university. Her provider was happy to refer him to an ear, nose, and throat (ENT) specialist. The visit to the doctor had a co-pay of $25 and the co-pay for the surgery was $100. This is the second surgery her son had to restore his hearing, and the last time the cost was over $5,000 because Roxanne had a PPO rather than an HMO.

Question:

1. In this instance, what could have been a problem with the son's care because of Roxanne's enrollment in an HMO?

health plan. Most people will get a job after graduation and the employer will offer health insurance. Should you choose to participate in your employer's health insurance plan? The answer is yes! Employers pay a portion of the premium of the health insurance plan, which will translate into a lower cost for the employee. Plans are cafeteria style and offer different types of health insurance, including HMOs, PPOs, dental insurance, vision insurance, and life insurance. Larger employers may offer a wider variety of plans. So, how do you choose among the plans?

Many questions need to be answered in order to make an informed choice. You will need to consider how much can you afford now for health insurance, and how much money you have available if you have an accident or contract a serious illness. Most people want to spend as little as possible on a health insurance plan, because the premium is deducted from gross income. However, the premium is deducted before taxes, which means that you pay lower taxes. However, if you have a serious accident or you contract a serious disease, will you be able to pay your medical bills? If you have an automobile accident, the costs can be well over $20,000. If the plan has a $1,000 deductible and then pays 80% of the remaining bill, the total out-of-pocket expenses will be $4,800. Choosing health

insurance should be based on your specific needs and income. See **TABLE 18.1** for an example.

If you do not have a job or you do not have access to group insurance, a high-deductible health plan may be the best route to take. Often called catastrophic insurance, it provides many of the same benefits as a regular plan, but has a very high deductible. You might choose this type of plan if you are young and healthy, you do not access the health system often, you need to have lower premium costs, you do not mind higher out-of-pocket costs, or you are not eligible for Medicaid.[37]

A healthy person without any serious health issues might choose an HMO. If your job offers an HMO, choose a doctor who is in the town where you work, because you will be making most of your doctor's visits during normal working hours. If you have children, it would be better to choose a doctor close to home. The premiums are lower for HMOs than for PPO plans and the co-pays are minimal. One of the most convenient aspects of HMOs is that doctor visits have one co-pay that includes all diagnostic services. HMOs are also one of the most inexpensive plans.

Remember that the caveat with HMO plans is that the main provider works as a gatekeeper for diagnostic services and referrals. The main provider may not want to refer a specialist and may want to handle the disease

TABLE 18.1 Automobile Accident Costing $20,000			
Type of Plan	**Deductible**	**Co-Pay**	**Out-of-Pocket Expenses**
HDHP: $7,500 per person, and pays 80% after deductible	$7,500	$2,500	$10,000
HMO: $50 emergency co-pay		$50	$50
PPO: $1,000 per person deductible, and pays 70% after deductible	$1,000	$5,700	$6,700

⌕ *CASE STUDY*

Since Megan Smith, referred to in the first case study in this chapter, is only 23, she is less likely to have any serious injury or disease. Because of the high deductible on the PPO insurance she will be paying up to $500 out of pocket per year to see her hometown doctor. It may be in her best interest to buy the HMO coverage for anything serious that might happen and pay out of pocket to see her hometown doctor, as she would be paying roughly the same to cover the deductible if she chose the PPO. Also, the HMO covers vision so that she does not have to pay the $10 per month extra. The free life insurance is almost enough to cover funeral costs for Megan, so it is probably enough life insurance for now, until she buys a house or gets married or has children. Disability insurance is probably unnecessary because she does not have a high-risk job and lives near her home, but it is a personal decision. Long-term care insurance may be an important purchase, but it might be good to take a look at the monthly cost and see if putting that into a savings account would earn enough to pay for long-term care without insurance. What do you think?

Questions:

1. Do you agree with the choices in Megan's situation?
2. Considering your personal situation, what choices would you make regarding your coverage?
3. What future events do you suppose will force you to revisit your coverage?

or condition in his or her office. That may or may not be in your best interest. If you have a serious precondition, you may want to choose a PPO. Although the premiums are higher, the plan has more flexibility for specialists. PPOs are also a good choice when there are no HMOs in your area and when you are covering a large family with children going to school outside your area. HMOs cover only emergency care outside the HMO network.

PPOs have an individual and a family deductible that must be met prior to the insurance plan reimbursing you for medical expenses. The family deductible is to help the family if one member has extreme medical costs; however, each person must meet their deductible prior to reimbursement. Most plans have choices for deductible amounts. For instance, there may be a $500 or a $1,000 deductible amount. The higher the deductible, the lower the premiums are. The best way to choose is to determine how often you use medical services. If you rarely go to the doctor, then the higher deductible may be the right choice. If you are a woman, then you may want to consider the lower deductible because of the yearly visits to the gynecologist and tests that are required with each visit. If you are over the age of 40, it also might be wise to choose the lower deductible because of the increased chances of becoming ill and the greater number of tests that are recommended. After the deductible is met, the insured is responsible for the co-pay or coinsurance, usually 20–30% of the medical expenses.

Most health insurance plans cover prescriptions, but payment is different from the type of standardized physician billing. HMOs generally offer prescription benefits with a set co-pay for formulary and generic drugs. Formulary drugs are a list of drugs that have been approved by the insurance company. PPOs have a formulary list as well, and only reimburse up to a certain amount for each drug on their formulary list. Non-formulary drugs are not on the list and need prior approval to be eligible for the prescription plan. Formularies are divided into several tiers and the tiers are established by the price of the drug. Each tier establishes the amount you as the consumer will pay at the pharmacy. Here is an example of a common four-tiered formulary, though they differ from plan to plan[38]:

- **Tier 1, $20 co-pay**: Very low-cost drugs, mostly generics
- **Tier 2, $40 co-pay**: Higher cost generic drugs and low-cost brand name drugs
- **Tier 3, $60 co-pay**: Brand name drugs for which there is no generic
- **Tier 4, $100+ co-pay**: Highest cost drugs or specialty drugs like chemotherapy

▶ Conclusion

The information given in this chapter was intended to raise your awareness about health insurance in the United States. Obtaining employment that offers health insurance benefits will add thousands of dollars to your total employment package. If you are in between jobs, COBRA is a choice. Always keep in mind the fact that if you should get a serious disease or disability and you do not have health insurance, you are at risk of losing everything. Investigate further the marketplace through the ACA to determine if there is aid for you.

Wrap-Up

Key Terms

Beneficiary The person who receives a death benefit.

Children's Health Insurance Program (CHIP) Insurance offered to children whose parents do not qualify for Medicaid, but do not have health insurance.

Consolidated Omnibus Budget Reconciliation Act (COBRA) Terminated employees, those who lose coverage because of reduced work hours, or children who can no longer be on their parents' policy because of age may be able to buy group coverage for themselves and their families for limited periods of time.

Contingent beneficiaries Receive the death benefit when the policy holder dies and the primary beneficiaries are also deceased or cannot be found.

Co-payment The amount of money the insured is responsible for paying for each visit or time of service. These amounts are set by the insurance company.

Decreasing term life insurance Insurance that decreases in value over the life of the policy.

Disability insurance Insurance that covers the loss of income due to illness or injury.

Flexible spending accounts Savings accounts set up by employers that allow employees to contribute on a pretax basis to reimburse healthcare expenses

Group insurance Insurance available to groups of individuals such as employers, unions, or professional organizations.

Health maintenance organization (HMO) Insurance plans usually provided through an employer. Plan has a main provider (doctor) who is a gatekeeper for all services.

Indemnity insurance Allows the individuals to choose their healthcare providers.

Individual insurance Insurance for one individual purchased from an insurance company.

Level term life insurance Life insurance that pays the same amount on the death of the policy holder at any time during the life of the policy.

Medicaid Government insurance for people who meet financial need criteria and for people who are disabled.

Medical necessity A procedure that is required for the benefit of a person's physical health. Cosmetic surgery is not considered a medical necessity, for instance.

Health savings account Allows a person to save pretax dollars to use for medical expenditures that are not covered by insurance.

Medicare Government insurance for everyone who has paid Social Security and is over the age of 65 and some disabled people.

Preexisting condition A medical problem that an insured person already has prior to acquiring health insurance. Some preexisting conditions are not covered by insurance.

Preferred provider organization (PPO) Networks of physicians that work with an insurance company with a negotiated rate for services.

Primary beneficiaries Receive the death benefit upon the policy holder's death.

Variable life insurance Uses part of the premium to purchase stocks, bonds, and mutual funds.

Variable universal life insurance Provides death benefits and cash values that vary when the investment portfolio changes (money market, government bond accounts, equity accounts).

Whole life insurance Offers a death benefit and a savings account.

Suggestions for Class Activities

1. Form groups in the class. Each group should select one of the following to research: Medicare, Medicaid, traditional health insurance, ACA, HMOs, PPOs, and other types of insurance. Each group should write main points about their type of insurance on butcher paper using large markers. Place on a wall and discuss each.

2. Ask people in several age groups to come to the class and form a panel presentation. Before the panel presentation, the members of the panel will be given a list of questions that could be asked. Class members will compose the questions regarding: health insurance, life insurance, views about the ACA, HMOs, PPOs, Medicare, Medicaid, and so forth.

Review Questions

1. What is health insurance?
2. What do you feel should be the rights of U.S. citizens regarding health insurance?
3. What percentage of U.S. citizens are covered by employer-sponsored health insurance?
4. What percentage of U.S. citizens are covered by privately purchased insurance?
5. Why does health insurance cost so much?

6. What are the main provisions of the ACA?
7. What are indemnity plans?
8. What are basic health plans?
9. What are health savings accounts?
10. What are high-deductible health plans?
11. What are managed care options?
12. What are HMOs?
13. What are POS plans?
14. What are PPOs?
15. Who is eligible for government health insurance?
16. What is Medicaid?
17. What is Medicare?
18. Who is eligible for the CHIP?
19. What is military healthcare?
20. What is disability insurance?
21. What is covered under vision insurance?
22. What kinds of life insurance are available?
23. What is long-term care insurance?
24. What is COBRA?

References

1. Centers for Medicare & Medicaid Services. National Health Expenditures 2016 Highlights. Available at: https://www.cms.gov/Research-Statistics-Data-and-Systems/Statistics-Trends-and-Reports/NationalHealthExpendData/downloads/highlights.pdf. Accessed May 4, 2018.
2. Centers for Medicare & Medicaid Services. National Health Expenditure Projections 2016–2025. Available at: https://www.cms.gov/Research-Statistics-Data-and-Systems/Statistics-Trends-and-Reports/NationalHealthExpendData/Downloads/proj2016.pdf. Accessed May 4, 2018.
3. The Commonwealth Fund. Mirror, mirror 2017: International Comparison Reflects Flaws and Opportunities for Better U.S. Healthcare. Available at: http://www.commonwealthfund.org/interactives/2017/july/mirror-mirror/. Accessed May 4, 2018.
4. Healthcare.gov. Affordable Care Act (ACA). Available at: https://www.healthcare.gov/glossary/affordable-care-act/. Accessed May 4, 2018.
5. Henry J Kaiser Family Foundation. Key facts about the Uninsured Population. September 19, 2017. Available at: http://www.kff.org/uninsured/fact-sheet/key-facts-about-the-uninsured-population/. Updated November 29, 2017. Accessed May 4, 2018.
6. eHealth.com. History and timeline of the Affordable Care Act. Available at: https://resources.ehealthinsurance.com/affordable-care-act/history-timeline-affordable-care-act-aca. Updated March 5, 2018. Accessed May 4, 2018.
7. FamiliesUSA. A 50-State Look at Medicaid Expansion. Available at: http://familiesusa.org/product/50-state-look-medicaid-expansion. Updated January 2018. Accessed May 4, 2018.
8. Barnett JC, Berchick ER. *Health Insurance Coverage in the United States: 2016*. United States Census Bureau; 2017:P60-P260. Available at: https://www.census.gov/content/dam/Census/library/publications/2017/demo/p60-260.pdf. Accessed May 4, 2018.
9. WebMD. Understanding Health Insurance—Types of Health Insurance. Available at: http://www.webmd.com/health-insurance/tc/understanding-health-insurance-types-of-health-insurance#1. Accessed May 4, 2018.
10. Botkin M. 10 things that affect your health insurance premium costs. Money Crashers. Available at: http://www.moneycrashers.com/factors-health-insurance-premium-costs/. Accessed May 4, 2018.
11. Torpy JM, Burke AE, Glass RM. JAMA patient page. Health care insurance: The basics. *JAMA*. 2007;297(10):1154.
12. Blue Cross Blue Shield Blue Care Network of Michigan. How to use your HMO benefits. Available at: http://www.bcbsm.com/index/health-insurance-help/faqs/plan-types/hmo/using-your-hmo-benefits.html. Accessed May 4, 2018.
13. Health Coverage Guide. Plan Characteristics and Types. Available at: http://healthcoverageguide.org/reference-guide/coverage-types/plan-characteristics-and-types/. Accessed on May 4, 2018.
14. HealthCare.gov. Health Savings Account (HSA). Available at: https://www.healthcare.gov/glossary/health-savings-account-HSA/. Accessed May 4, 2018.
15. HealthCare.gov. High Deductible Health Plans (HDHP). Available at: https://www.healthcare.gov/glossary/high-deductible-health-plan/. Accessed May 4, 2018.
16. Bera S. HSA vs. FSA: What you need to know for healthcare: *AoL.com*. November 18, 2015. Available at: https://www.aol.com/article/finance/2014/11/18/fsa-vs-hsa/20991918/. Accessed October 3, 2017.
17. Centers for Medicare & Medicaid Services. Medicare Program–General Information. Available at: https://www.cms.gov/Medicare/Medicare-General-Information/MedicareGenInfo/index.html. Accessed May 4, 2018.
18. Medicaid.gov. Medicaid. Available at: https://www.medicaid.gov/medicaid/index.html. Accessed May 4, 2018.
19. Rudowitz R, Valentine A, Smith VK. Medicaid Enrollment and Spending Growth: FY 2016 and 2017. Henry J Kaiser Family Foundation. Available at: https://www.kff.org/report-section/medicaid-enrollment-spending-growth-fy-2016-2017-issue-brief-8931/. Published October 13, 2016. Accessed May 4, 2018.
20. Medicaid.gov. Program History. Available at: https://www.medicaid.gov/about-us/program-history/index.html. Accessed May 4, 2018.
21. U.S. Department of Veterans Affairs. Health Benefits. Available at: https://www.va.gov/HEALTHBENEFITS/apply/veterans.asp. Accessed May 4, 2018.
22. TRICARE. Health Plans. Available at: https://tricare.mil/Plans/HealthPlans. Accessed May 4, 2018.
23. Henry J Kaiser Family Foundation. Health Insurance Coverage of Children 0-18. Available at: https://www.kff.org/other/state-indicator/children-0-18/?currentTimeframe=0&selectedDistributions=employer&selectedRows=%7B%22wrapups%22:%7B%22united-states%22:%7B%7D%7D%7D&sortModel=%7B%22colId%22:%22Location%22,%22sort%22:%22asc%22%7D. Accessed May 4, 2018.
24. Tandon A, Murray CJL, Lauer JA, Evans DB. Measuring Overall Health System Performance for 191 Countries. World Health Organization. Available at: http://www.who.int/healthinfo/paper30.pdf. Accessed May 4, 2018.
25. Committee on Research 2015, Committee on Performance Improvement 2015. *Care and Payment Models to Achieve the Triple Aim*. Chicago, IL: American Hospital Association; 2016.
26. Agency for Healthcare Research and Quality. Health Care/System Redesign. Available at: https://www.ahrq.gov

/professionals/prevention-chronic-care/improve/system/index.html. Updated June 2017. Accessed May 4, 2018.

27. National Institutes of Health. World's older population grows dramatically. Available at: https://www.nih.gov/news-events/news-releases/worlds-older-population-grows-dramatically. Published March 28, 2018. Accessed May 4, 2018.

28. Associated Press. "Medicare for All" could be cheaper than you think. *Washington's Top News*. September 19, 2017. Available at: https://wtop.com/business-finance/2017/09/medicare-for-all-could-be-cheaper-than-you-think/. Accessed May 4, 2018.

29. HealthCare.gov. Get the most out of your 2017 health insurance. Available at: https://www.healthcare.gov/blog/using-2017-coverage-for-health-care/. Published March 23, 2017. Accessed May 4, 2018.

30. CareFirst. Rights and Responsibilities. Available at: https://member.carefirst.com/members/mandates-policies/rights-and-responsibilities.page. Accessed May 4, 2018.

31. National Association of Health Underwriters. What Type of DI Policies Are Available? Available at: https://nahu.org/media/1968/di-policies-available.pdf. Accessed May 4, 2018.

32. Council for Disability Awareness. Chances of Disability. Available at: http://www.disabilitycanhappen.org/chances_disability/disability_stats.asp. Updated March 28, 2018. Accessed May 4, 2018.

33. Social Security. Benefits for People with Disabilities. Available at: https://www.ssa.gov/disability/. Accessed May 4, 2018.

34. Insurance Information Institute. What are the principal types of life insurance? Available at: https://www.iii.org/article/what-are-principal-types-life-insurance. Accessed May 4, 2018.

35. Alzheimer's Association. Planning for Care Costs. Available at: https://www.alz.org/care/alzheimers-dementia-common-costs.asp. Accessed May 4, 2018.

36. U.S. Department of Labor, Employee Benefits Security Administration. An Employee's Guide to Health Benefits Under COBRA. Available at: https://www.dol.gov/sites/default/files/ebsa/about-ebsa/our-activities/resource-center/publications/an-employees-guide-to-health-benefits-under-cobra.pdf. Published September 2016. Accessed May 4, 2018.

37. eHealth. Catastrophic Health Plans. Available at: https://www.ehealthinsurance.com/health-plans/catastrophic-insurance. Accessed May 4, 2018.

38. Glover L. Your drug formulary: How it works and what to know: *NerdWallet*. June 13, 2016. Available at: https://www.nerdwallet.com/blog/health/drug-formularies-and-prescriptions/. Accessed May 4, 2018.

Appendix A

Trusted Websites for Conventional Health Resources and Complementary and Alternative Medicine Practices

▶ What is the Protocol for Evaluating Health Resources on the Internet?

The Health On the Net Foundation (HON) was founded to provide a code of ethics for websites promoting health information. Created in 1995, HON is a nonprofit, nongovernmental organization, accredited to the Economic and Social Council of the United Nations. To cope with the unprecedented volume of healthcare information available on the Net, the HON code of conduct offers a multistakeholder consensus on standards to protect citizens from misleading health information. The HON code is designed for the general public, health professionals, and web publishers. It is used by over 7,300 certified websites in 102 countries. A HON code toolbar is present on their website, which allows for a search to check certification status of websites. More information on HON can be found on their website (www.hon.ch/en).

Consumers can look for the HON designation on a website, in the criterion search in their search engine, or use the descriptions themselves to determine the legitimacy of the information they retrieve.

According to HON, the following eight criteria are used by the HON to award its approval for quality health information found on the Internet:

1. **Authoritative**: Indicate the qualifications of the authors.
2. **Complementarity**: Information should support, not replace, the doctor–patient relationship.
3. **Privacy**: Respect the privacy and confidentiality of personal data submitted to the site by the visitor.
4. **Attribution**: Cite the source(s) of published information, data, and medical and health pages.
5. **Justifiability**: Site must back up claims relating to benefits and performance.
6. **Transparency**: Accessible presentation and accurate e-mail.
7. **Financial disclosure**: Identify funding sources.
8. **Advertising policy**: Clearly distinguish advertising from editorial content.

▶ What Are the Best Websites for Disease and Condition Information?

The Consumer and Patient Health Information Section (CAPHIS) of the Medical Library Association (MLA) compiles the most complete online listing of credible health information websites into what is called the CAPHIS Top 100 List. The criteria used to create the list are quite similar to the HON criteria, and include credibility, sponsorship/authorship, content, audience, currency, disclosure, purpose, links, design, interactivity, and caveats. The website breaks down the list into categories for easy review by the consumer: general health, cancer, breast cancer, diabetes, eye disease, heart disease, HIV/AIDS, and stroke. More detailed information can be found on the website (www.mlanet.org/caphis).

Another valued website is the U.S. National Library of Medicine (NLM), a component agency of the National Institutes of Health (NIH). It is located on the NIH campus in Bethesda, Maryland, and is the world's largest biomedical library. It coordinates a

6,500-member National Network of Libraries of Medicine across the United States. Plenty of information is available in the Health Information section of the NLM website. Links for general health information for patients and families, drugs and supplements, specific populations, genetics, environmental health and toxicology, clinical trials and biomedical literature may be accessed here. For more detailed information, explore the NLM website (www.nlm.nih.gov /hinfo.html). Other examples of Internet resources are MedlinePlus and PubMed (www.nlm.nih.gov/bsd /pmresources.html).

▶ Is There a Simple Way to Identify a Doctor, Specialist, Hospital, or Clinic?

The U.S. NLM division, MedlinePlus, also manages a database of physicians, clinicians, hospitals, clinics, dentists, midwives, specialists, and virtually every type of health care professional you might need. This easy-to-use link-oriented website will redirect you to the appropriate agency or organization that hosts the directory. You can find the listing in the Directory section of the MedlinePlus website. (medlineplus.gov /directories.html).

▶ What Are the Trusted Websites for Complementary and Alternative Medicine Practices?

We have already included the National Center for Complementary and Integrative Health (NCCIH) in many of the chapters in this text. The NCCIH researches, provides funding for research, and trains those interested in CAM. Currently, there are many clinical trials in process and the NCCIH publishes research trial results. For instance, a late study demonstrated that Tai Chi has benefits for those people suffering with fibromyalgia. Continuing education and online lectures are also offered by the NCCIH and their website (nccih.nih.gov) contains information on writing grant applications.

A website at Georgetown University, Dahlgren Memorial Library, contains a *Complementary and Alternative Medicine Resource Guide* (guides.dml .georgetown.edu/c.php?g=288623&p=1924528). The guide is divided into sections with trusted websites in each Nonprofit Organizations, Government, and Academic CAM Centers/Universities. The site contains a link to evaluating websites and contains the CRAAP test, which is defined as follows:

C → Currency

R → Relevance

A → Authority & Authorship

A → Accuracy

P → Purpose

Mayo Clinic too devotes a website (www.mayoclinic .org/tests-procedures/complementary-alternative -medicine/about/pac-20393581) on evaluating complementary and alternative medicine. They promote the following: Look for scientific studies, weed out misinformation by checking dates of articles, checking documentation of sources, and double checking by visiting several health sites and comparing information. The site also offers information and warnings about supplements and what to do when deciding to buy and ingest them. CAM and cancer is becoming very popular. The site offers cautions to people about researching supplements and practices because many could interfere with treatment regimens. It also offers, however, several CAM options that seem to help when combined with standard medical treatment: acupuncture, aromatherapy, biofeedback, massage, meditation, music therapy, and yoga.

We hope that you will use many of these trusted websites when seeking information about health resources and CAM practices. Have a well and happy life.

Dr. Karl and Dr. Linda

Glossary

A

Absolutes Plant extractions that are obtained by using chemical solvents.

Activator A small tool that delivers a light and measured force to correct a misalignment.

Active release technique (ART) Technique designed to treat scar tissue adhesions, which can cause symptoms such as pain, weakness, and restricted range of motion. It is also used to treat overused muscles that may have small tears or are not getting enough oxygen.

Activism A doctrine or practice that emphasizes direct vigorous action, especially in support of or opposition to one side of a controversial issue.

Acupressure The application of pressure or localized massage to specific sites on the body to control symptoms such as pain or nausea.

Acupuncture A traditional Chinese medicine treatment that uses stainless steel needles at specific points in the body to increase the flow of life energy known as qi, or chi. It is a procedure that increases the flow of qi energy to treat illness or provide local pain relief by the insertion of stainless steel needles at specified sites on the body.

Acupuncture point injection Sterile syringes are used to inject vitamins or herbal products into the system via the trigger points.

Adjustment A process of manipulating misaligned vertebrae or other joints in the body (e.g., wrist bones and joints) back into place.

Adulterate To corrupt, debase, or make impure by the addition of a foreign or inferior substance or element.

Advertising The act or practice of calling public attention to a product or service.

Alexander Technique A process in which people can learn to release muscular tension and habitually overtightened muscles that cause our bodies to become distorted, unbalanced, and compressed.

Alkaloids A group of chemicals made by plants and are alkaloid in nature. Examples of alkaloids include cocaine, nicotine, and caffeine.

Allopathic medicine The traditional or conventional system of medicine that uses drugs, surgery, or radiation to prevent or treat diseases.

Allopathic physician A conventional or orthodox physician who is an MD. The medical doctor (MD) or the osteopathic doctor (DO).

Alternative medicine A system of practices not considered to be standard treatments. Examples are chiropractic medicine, Ayurvedic medicine, and traditional Chinese medicine.

Analgesic Any member of a group of drugs used to relieve pain.

Anatripsis The act of rubbing up during massage.

Anointing Involves dipping a finger in oil and touching a person either on the forehead or on another body part as a part of religious ceremony.

Antihistamine Drug used to counteract the physiological effects of histamine production in allergic reactions and colds.

Antitussive Capable of relieving or suppressing coughing.

Aromatherapist A person trained in the use of essential oils.

Aromatherapy Means "treatment using scents"; the use of concentrated plant oils.

Asanas Another name for yoga poses.

Asclepions Sanctuaries of healing. They had their roots in ancient Greece on the island of Kos.

Assessment A process in Therapeutic Touch wherein the practitioner determines where and how the energy of the patient is moving.

Astringent A substance or preparation that constricts tissue. It can lessen discharges such as mucus or blood.

Attorney general The principal legal officer who represents a state in legal proceedings and gives legal advice to the government.

Attunement A Reiki rite of passage where the ability to heal is passed on to a new Reiki practitioner from a Reiki master.

Auricular acupuncture Uses points in the ears that correspond to areas of the body and bodily symptoms.

Autism A mental condition, present from early childhood, characterized by great difficulty in communicating and forming relationships, and in using language and abstract concepts.

Ayurveda A traditional system of medicine of India. The word *Ayurveda* is a Sanskrit word that means science of life or sciences of lifespan.

Ayurvedic medicine A form of holistic alternative medicine that is the traditional system of medicine of India. It may have influenced ancient Chinese medicine and the humoral medicine practiced by Hippocrates in Greece.

B

Bach® Original Flower Remedies Tinctures made from flowers to treat emotions rather than disease.

Bandwagon Advertising technique where mass appeal is used to attract customers.

Basti Medicated enema or colonic irrigation.

Behavioral advertising Tracking a consumer's pattern of Internet use in an effort to display specific types of advertising that might appeal to those use patterns.

Beneficiary The person who receives a death benefit.

Biased research Errors in research during the selection of subjects, the measurements used, or the treatment process (intervention).

Biofeedback A mind–body intervention that helps train people to improve their health by using their own body's electrical signals from the muscles or brain. It is a technique used to train people to control their own involuntary body processes such as heart rate, respirations, and even brain waves. It requires watching a monitor of some sort in order to change the rate using mental control.

Biofield The energy emitted from the human body.

Biological Any substance, such as a serum or vaccine, derived from animal products or other biological sources and used to treat or prevent disease.

Biologically based therapies Use of natural techniques to maintain health and/or treat diseases.

Biomedical physician (or biomedical scientist) These physicians apply research in many fields related to life sciences or body processes (anatomy and physiology, biology, pathology). They research the process of disease causation and attempt to find new treatment modalities.

Biomedicine The application of the principles of the natural sciences, especially biology and physiology, to clinical medicine.

Bioresonance The practice of using an electronic device to measure the body's electromagnetic radiation and electric currents and to detect damaged body cells.

Biotypes Body types or body constitutions that naturopaths use to aid a diagnosis, because they believe each type has certain characteristics that are related to risk of particular diseases.

Blood lactate A chemical associated with stress.

Bonesetters People who set the broken bones of people without conducting surgery.

Botanicals Substances obtained from plants.

Bravewell Collaborative Founded in 2002 by a small group of leading philanthropists dedicated to transforming the culture and delivery of health care and improving the health of the public through integrative medicine.

Buddhism A religion that originated in India by Buddha (Gautama) and later spread to China, Burma, Japan, Tibet, and parts of Southeast Asia. It holds that life is full of suffering caused by desire, and the way to end this suffering is through enlightenment that enables one to halt the endless sequence of births and deaths to which one is otherwise subject to.

Burmese position Sitting on the floor and using a zafu—a small pillow—to raise the hips just a little so the knees can touch the ground. Sitting on the pillow with two knees touching the ground forms a tripod base that gives 360-degree stability.

C

Calibration To adjust instrumentation so that it will be precise.

Cardiac glycosides These chemicals have a marked action on the heart, strengthening the force and speed of systolic contractions.

Carotenoid pigments Pigments found in yellow and red plants such as carrots, sweet potatoes, red and yellow peppers, squash, and tomatoes.

Carrier oils Base or vegetable oils used to dilute essential oils before applying them to skin.

Channeling In Reiki, the role of practitioner. Energy sent to the patient simply flows through the Reiki healer, who is the channel.

Chelation therapy Use of a drug to bind with and remove excess or toxic amounts of metal or minerals from the blood.

Children's Health Insurance Program (CHIP) Insurance offered to children whose parents do not qualify for Medicaid, but do not have health insurance.

Chinese herbal medicine (CHM) The study and use of plants for medicinal purposes.

Chiropractic A discipline and profession that focuses on disorders of the musculoskeletal and nervous systems under the belief that the effects of these disorders negatively impact health.

Chiropractic medicine A method of treatment based on the belief that the nervous system, skeletal system, and muscular system interact, and if that interaction is blocked, disease and/or pain will occur. Chiropractors treat by manipulating the spinal vertebra to release subluxations that cause nerve impingement.

Chiropractic mixers Believe that subluxations can lower resistance to disease or cause a neurological imbalance within the body, thus lowering resistance to disease. They would use adjustments to treat back pain, neck pain, and other musculoskeletal disorders.

Chlorophyll Pigment found in green plants and dark leafy green vegetables such as spinach, parsley, kale, green beans, and leeks.

Cholera An acute, infectious disease characterized by profuse diarrhea, vomiting, and cramps.

Chondritis Inflammation of a cartilage.

Christian Science A healing methodology that does not use medicine. Mary Baker-Eddy founded Christian Science and based it on the healing methods of Phineas Quimby.

Chronic Refers to an illness or medical condition that is characterized by long duration or frequent recurrence.

CO_2 extraction High pressure is placed on the CO_2 turning it into a liquid and a solvent that can extract aromatic molecules. No solvent residue remains because the CO_2 reverts back to gas and evaporates.

Cold-pressed extraction Process involving mechanical pressure to force the oils out of citrus fruit, nuts, and seeds.

Compendium A brief summary of a larger work or of a field of knowledge.

Complementary and alternative medicine (CAM) A group of diverse medical and healthcare systems, practices, and products that are not generally considered to be part of conventional medicine (NCCIH definition).

Computerized axial tomography (CAT) An X-ray procedure aided by a computer so that cross-sectional views are obtained. Many X-ray images are taken at various bodily angles.

Concentration technique Involves concentrating on an external object as a focus point for the mind.

Concrete Waxy mass that remains after solvent extraction. The waxy concrete is then processed to remove the waxy materials.

Consolidated Omnibus Budget Reconciliation Act (COBRA) Terminated employees, those who lose coverage because of reduced work hours, or children who can no longer be on their parents' policy because of age may be able to buy group coverage for themselves and their families for limited periods of time.

Constitution According to Ayurvedic medicine, it is a pattern of energy that comprises or makes up a person.

Consumer A person who buys and uses goods. In this text, it means the person who buys and uses health-related goods.

Contemplation meditative techniques Use introspection, self-study, and reflection. Contemplative meditation is supposed to help people gain a deeper understanding of some aspect of reality.

Contingent beneficiaries Receive the death benefit when the policy holder dies and the primary beneficiaries are also deceased or cannot be found.

Control group This is the population group used as a standard for comparison to the experimental group.

Conventional medicine Mainstream medical practices. Also known as orthodox and traditional medicine.

Co-payment The amount of money the insured is responsible for paying for each visit or time of service. These amounts are set by the insurance company.

Cortisol A chemical associated with stress.

Current Procedural Terminology (CPT) codes Guides for setting physician fees.

D

Deceit Concealment or distortion of the truth for the purpose of misleading.

Decoction The process of boiling a substance in water to extract its essence.

Decongestant Medication or treatment that breaks up congestion, as of the sinuses, by reducing swelling.

Decreasing term life insurance Insurance that decreases in value over the life of the policy.

Defraud To deprive of something by deception or fraud.

Degenerative arthritis Chronic breakdown of cartilage in the joints; the most common form of arthritis, occurring usually after middle age.

Demographic A single vital or social statistic of a human population, such as the number of births or deaths.

Deregulation To remove governmental regulations and control.

Dervish dancers Turkish dancers who dress in a particular style and seem to dance to the rhythm of the cosmos or the universe.

Development assistance for health (DAH) Publicly financed assistance available for underdeveloped countries in the form of financial resources and improved effectiveness of resources.

Diagnosis Identification of a diseased condition.

Diet therapy Prescribed to increase qi energy; it is grounded in the theories of five elements and eight guiding principles.

Direct-to-consumer Advertising sent directly to the consumer, not through a third-party provider.

Disability insurance Insurance that covers the loss of income due to illness or injury.

Distant healing Involves people praying for and healing others at great distances away (sometimes without the ill person knowing it). Also known as intercessory prayer.

Doctor of osteopathic medicine (DO) A conventional or orthodox physician who has similar training as the MD but who has advanced studies in the interconnection of the muscles, bones, and nerves.

Dosha Five elements (ether, air, fire, water, and earth) make up the body's constitution called dosha; there are three doshas: vata, pitta, and kapha.

E

Ectomorph Body type in which the appearance of the body is thin.

Effleurage Massage using contours of the body; uses a smooth stroke.

Electroacupuncture Mild electrical pulses are relayed via acupuncture needles to various trigger points in the skin.

Empirical A word derived from the Greek word for experience or observation.

Empty mind meditation Involves sitting still, often in a full lotus or cross-legged position, and letting the mind go silent on its own.

Endomorph Body type in which the appearance of the body is round and soft. The physique presents the illusion that much of the mass has been concentrated in the abdominal area.

Endorphins Natural pain-killing substances produced in the human body and released by stress or trauma.

Energy therapies Practices that increase natural body energy flow known as Chi energy. Examples are Tai Chi Ch'uan and Qi gong.

Epidemic Refers to an occurrence and rapid rise of an infectious disease in a community or region in a given time period.

Erectile dysfunction Difficulty in achieving or maintaining an erection; impotence.

Essential oils (EOs) Distilled liquid from the leaves, stems, flowers, bark, roots, or other elements of a plant.

Evidence-based research Study evidence or result is integrated with clinical expertise and patient values when making decisions about patient care.

Expectorant Promoting or facilitating the secretion or expulsion of phlegm, mucus or other matter from the respiratory tract.

Experimental Subjects are randomly selected or assigned into a treatment or control group.

Expression A method to extract EOs from the rinds of citrus fruit without using heat. Requires squeezing by hand and collecting oils with a sponge.

External qigong Bodily movement related to the practice of qigong. The practice of transferring the practitioner's qi to another person for healing purposes. This form of qi gong is similar to other bodywork modalities in the West such as Therapeutic Touch.

F

Facet joints These are synovial joints that help support the weight and control movement between individual vertebrae of the spine. Facet joints are at the back on either side of the spinal column, between the discs and the vertebral bodies. The bony prominences of each vertebra form a joint with the vertebrae above and below. The role of the facet joints is to limit excessive movement and provide stability for the spine.

Faith or spiritual energy healing Spiritual energy healing has occurred since earliest times among all cultures, religions, and medicinal practices. Various healing techniques are used (including chants and prayer, touching, or placing the hands close to the body within the energy fields that surround the body). Popular current methods used for energy healing include Reiki therapy, Therapeutic Touch, qi gong healing, and crystal healing.

Fasting To abstain from all food.

Feeling and emotion meditation techniques These may be used independently, but also may be combined with other types of meditation practices.

Five elements In Ayurveda, they are ether (space), air (vayu), fire (agni), water (apa), and earth (prithvi); in TCM, they are water, fire, wood, metal, and earth.

Fixed oils Referred to as vegetable, carrier; or base oils; they contain nutrients such as minerals, antioxidants, and fat-soluble vitamins.

Flavonoids A set of chemicals that include brilliant plant pigments seen in fruits and vegetables.

Flexible spending accounts Savings accounts set up by employers that allow employees to contribute on a pretax basis to reimburse healthcare expenses

Florasols/phytols extraction A process that uses gaseous solvents to extract EOs.

Food and Drug Administration (FDA) A division of the U.S. Department of Health and Human Services that protects the public against impure and unsafe foods, drugs, and cosmetics.

Form A series of predetermined and/or scripted movements designed to increase, unblock, or promote healing through the acquisition of energy (qi).

Franchise The right or license granted to an individual or group to market a company's goods or services in a particular territory; a business granted such a right or license.

Fraud A deceitful, tricky, or willful act committed to gain an unfair or dishonest advantage or to make a profit (make money off someone else). Intentional perversion of truth in order to induce another to part with something of value or to surrender a legal right. Trickery, unethical practice, or breach of confidence, perpetrated for profit or to gain some unfair or dishonest advantage.

Free radicals Unstable oxygen molecules that can cause tissue damage.

Full lotus position A seated position in which each leg is placed on the opposite thigh.

Fumigation Burning of plant oils to create a great deal of smoke.

G

Galvanic stimulation High-voltage pulsed galvanic stimulation using direct current to stimulate deep tissue without producing tissue damage.

Gauss rating The degree of magnetic strength based solely on materials used to construct the magnet.

Ghee A mixture also known as sneha made from cow's milk into an edible oil or medicated butter.

Globalization Marked especially by free trade, free flow of capital, and the tapping of cheaper foreign labor markets.

Gross domestic product (GDP) This is a measure of a country's overall economic output. It is the market value of all final goods and services made within the borders of a country in a year.

Group insurance Insurance available to groups of individuals such as employers, unions, or professional organizations.

Gurdjieff sacred dances A technique wherein the movements are very defined and different parts of the body seem not to be related to each other.

Guru One who is regarded as having great knowledge, wisdom, and authority in a certain area and who uses it to guide others.

H

Half lotus position A seated position in which the left foot is placed onto the right thigh and the right leg is tucked under the left thigh.

Halitosis Offensive odor of the breath.

Health Care Refers to care given to a patient by medical or health professionals.

Health maintenance organization (HMO) A type of health insurance provided at a lower rate and less copay. It requires consumers to go to a doctor in the network or expenses will not be covered. Insurance plans usually provided through an employer. Plan has a main provider (doctor) who is a gatekeeper for all services.

Health savings account Allows a person to save pretax dollars to use for medical expenditures that are not covered by insurance.

Healthcare A system that offers, provides, or delivers health care to individuals.

Healthcare conglomerates Comprised of hospitals, clinics, and research facilities that either include or are affiliated to a medical school.

Herbalist A practitioner of and contributor to the field of herbal medicine.

High-deductible health plan (HDHP) A type of insurance plan that is typically cheaper than the other health plans, but has a much higher deductible (between $1,500 and $5,000). There is no coinsurance, so once the deductible is paid, the remaining expenses are covered 100%.

Histamine Stimulates gastric secretion and causes dilation of capillaries, constriction of bronchial smooth muscle and decreased blood pressure.

Holistic A concept in medical practice upholding that all aspects of people's needs, psychological, physical, mental, emotional, and social, should be taken into account and seen as a whole.

Holistic health Refers to the physical, emotional, spiritual, social, and mental domains of health. All should be seen as making up the whole person.

Homeopathic medicine Medicines prepared by extreme dilution. The fundamental concept of homeopathic is that "like cures like." Substances in the preparations are thought to stimulate the body's own healing response.

Homeopathy The use of extremely diluted substances given to cure disease using the law of similars: *like cures like*.

Hydrosol Floral water or distillate water that remains after distilling an EO.

Hydrotherapy The treatment of physical disability, injury, or illness by immersion of all or part of the body in water to facilitate movement, promote wound healing, and relieve pain. It is usually done under the supervision of a trained therapist. May involve the use of hot, moist soaks or dry heat for pain relief and to promote healing.

Hydrotherapy and heat therapy Use of hot, moist soaks or dry heat for pain relief and to promote healing.

Hypnosis A mind–body technique that focuses on awareness and attention to internal stimuli, much like what is learned while doing meditation. The word "hypnosis" comes from the Greek word *hypnos*, meaning sleep. It was first termed "animal magnetism."

Hypnotherapy Therapy using hypnosis to gain access to the deeper levels of the mind so that a change in thinking and behavior will occur.

Hypothesis A research statement or proposal that the subsequent study will find truthful or not.

I

Immobilization therapies Use of splints, casts, wraps, and traction to immobilize body parts so that the injured part may heal.

Incontinence Inability to control excretion of urine and feces.

Indemnity insurance Allows the individuals to choose their healthcare providers.

Individual insurance Insurance for one individual purchased from an insurance company.

Inference The ability of the researcher to infer what could happen in the future depending on the significance of a predictive type of research study.

Infomercial A product commercial of significant length designed to look like a television show.

Infrastructure The basic, underlying framework or features of a system or organization.

Infused oil Carrier oil that has been mixed with one or more herbs.

Integrative health Coordinated approach to bring alternative medicine and conventional medicine together.

Integrative medicine or integrative health care Combines treatments from conventional medicine and CAM for which there is evidence of safety and effectiveness. Bringing conventional and complementary approaches together in a coordinated way is the healing-oriented medicine that takes account of the whole person (body, mind, and spirit), including all aspects of lifestyle.

Intercessory prayer Involves people praying for and healing others at great distances away (sometimes without the ill person knowing it). Also known as distant healing.

Interferential current (IFC) A kind of TENS therapy in which high-frequency alternate current electrical impulses are introduced into the tissue near the pain center.

Internal qigong A form of qigong emphasizing breathing, meditation, and visualization. Uses certain movements and breath work or visualization to gather and circulate qi in the body.

Iridology The examination of the iris or colored portion of the eye for markings that supposedly reveal changing conditions of every part and organ of the body.

J

Japanese acupuncture Uses fewer and thinner needles with less stimulation than traditional Chinese acupuncture.

K

Kirlian photography Colorful photographs of images surrounding the body and within the body that are made after applying high-frequency electrical currents to a patient's body.

Koan meditation technique Meditations from the Zen School of Buddhism that are designed to break down an ordinary pattern of thinking.

Korean acupuncture Uses points in the hand that correspond to areas of the body and bodily symptoms.

L

Laser acupoint stimulation Uses rays or laser beams rather than acupuncture needles to facilitate the trigger point.

Level term life insurance Life insurance that pays the same amount on the death of the policy holder at any time during the life of the policy.

Lignans Phytoestrogens with weak estrogenic or anti-estrogenic activity.

Lobby To attempt to influence or sway someone (such as a public official) toward a desired action.

M

Macerating (or soaking) Soaking aromatic plants in animal fats or vegetable oils for vacuum distillation.

Magnet therapy The use of magnets on or around the human body to restructure the flow of energy in the human body for purposes of healing and well-being.

Magnetic resonance imaging (MRI) This machine creates a strong magnetic field and combines with radio waves to form a three-dimensional image helpful in viewing the brain and other soft tissue.

Malas Waste products such as urine, feces, or sweat.

Malpractice An injurious, negligent, or improper medical practice.

Mandala Means completion or circle. A word coming from one of the languages of India called Sanskrit.

Mantra A word or phrase repeated during meditation.

Marmas Ayurvedic massage pressure points.

Martial arts Encompass understanding the relationship of the power of breath, the life force (qi energy), the mind, and the concept of oneness.

Massage May come from the Arabic verb *mass*, meaning to touch, or from the Greek word *massein*, meaning to knead. It is manipulating soft tissue and muscles using a variety of physical methods, including applying fixed or moveable pressure, holding, vibrating, rocking, applying friction, kneading and compressing, and/or causing movement to the body.

Medicaid Government insurance for people who meet financial need criteria and for people who are disabled.

Medical acupuncture Acupuncture performed by a Western medical doctor.

Medical necessity A procedure that is required for the benefit of a person's physical health. Cosmetic surgery is not considered a medical necessity, for instance.

Medicare Government insurance for everyone who has paid Social Security and is over the age of 65 and some disabled people.

Meditation A way of being, a way of seeing, and even a way of loving; a state in which the body is consciously relaxed, the mind is allowed to become calm and focused, and deep feelings of well-being are experienced.

Meridians According to traditional Chinese medicine, there are 12 major meridians that link to 12 vital organs, plus six minor meridians that link to other areas of the body.

Mesmerize Term stemming from Dr. Franz Anton Mesmer, who defined the discipline of hypnotism.

Mesomorph Body type in which the appearance of the body is a natural, athletic physique.

Metabolic rate The amount of energy liberated or expended in a given unit of time.

Methamphetamine Used as a stimulant to the nervous system and as an appetite suppressant, and illicitly as a recreational drug.

Mindfulness meditation To become aware of your physical, emotional, and mental activities in the here and now.

Misbranding To brand falsely or in a misleading way; to label in violation of statutory requirements.

Modalities The application of a therapeutic agent, usually a physical therapeutic agent.

Morbidity Refers to illness or disease.

Mortality Refers to deaths.

Mother of tincture The homeopathic mixture first made from plants that is diluted in alcohol and left to sit for 2–4 weeks.

Moxibustion The stimulation of an acupuncture point by burning herbs called moxa, which are placed at or near the point.

Muqame makhssos Muslim massage pressure points.

Muscular dystrophy A genetic disease that is characterized by progressive weakness and degeneration of the skeletal muscles that control movement.

N

Naprapath A person who treats connective tissue disorders

Nasya Nose or sinus irrigation.

National Advertising Review Board (NARB) A group of advertising professionals organized to self-regulate the advertising industry.

Naturopathic A system or method of treating disease that employs no surgery or synthetic drugs, but uses special diets, herbs, vitamins, massage, and the like to assist the natural healing processes.

Naturopathic medicine A holistic, whole body health care system based on the belief that the body has the potential to heal itself and that the physician's role is to support the body's efforts. A system or method of treating disease that employs no surgery or synthetic drugs but uses special diets, herbs, vitamins, massage, and so on to assist the natural healing processes. It is a system of medical practices that relies on more natural healing methods (herbs, massage, exercise). It encompasses a belief in the body's ability to heal itself.

NCCAM National Center for Complementary and Alternative Medicine; former center in the National Institutes of Health. Name has been changed to National Center for Complementary and Integrative Health (NCCIH).

NCCIH National Center for Complementary and Integrative Health. Current name of the NIH center that conducts research to prove the effectiveness of complementary and alternative therapies.

Needs assessment Investigation to determine health needs. May investigate at the community, county, state, or national level.

Neodissociation model A model that suggests hypnosis activates a subsystem of both psychological and physiologic parts.

Neti pot Used to give nose or sinus irrigation, usually using a mild salt solution.

Noetic science The study of the mind and health healing. Noetic means the power of inner knowing, and is a branch of metaphysics.

Nonsteroidal anti-inflammatory drug (NSAID) Used for reducing inflammation and pain.

Nurse practitioner (NP) A registered nurse who has obtained advanced education and clinical training. Most obtain a master's or doctorate degree in nursing practice studies.

Nutritional supplements Also called dietary supplements. Nutritional supplements are preparations that provide additional nutrients and may include such things as green tea, soy preparations, ginseng, red clover, vitamins, and minerals (not an exhaustive list).

O

Objective straights Focus only on the correction of chiropractic vertebral subluxations.

Objectivity in research Findings must not be biased by personal beliefs, perceptions, biases, values, or emotions of the researcher.

Orgone A vital, primal, nonmaterial element believed to permeate the universe.

Orgone energy accumulator A cabinet-like device constructed of layers of wood and other materials claimed by its inventor, Wilhelm Reich, to restore orgone energy to persons sitting in it, thereby aiding in the cure of impotence, cancer, the common cold, and other ailments; also called an orgone box.

Orthomolecular medicine Emphasizes supplementing the diet with mega doses of vitamins, minerals, enzymes, hormones, and amino acids.

Osteoarthritis A type of arthritis of the joints that leads to joint pain, stiffness, and swelling.

Osteopathic A therapeutic system originally based on the premise that manipulation of the muscles and bones to promote structural integrity could restore or preserve health. Current osteopathic physicians use the diagnostic and therapeutic techniques of conventional medicine as well as manipulative measures.

Osteopathy A traditional medical system originally based on the premise that manipulation of the muscles and bones to promote structural integrity could restore or preserve health.

Over-the-counter (OTC) medicine Medicine sold without a prescription.

P

Panchakarma treatment Five types of cleansing therapy (vomiting, purging, colonic cleansing, nose and sinus cleansing, and blood detoxification).

Parasympathetic nervous system Responsible for causing heart rate and breathing to slow down, blood vessels to dilate, and digestive juices to increase.

Pathogen A disease-producing agent such as a virus, bacterium, or other microorganism.

Pathology The science or the study of the origin, nature, and course of diseases.

Pathya vyavastha treatment Use of diet and activity.

Patient Protection and Affordable Care Act (ACA) A health care reform law intended to expand coverage to millions of people and move the country toward a more primary care-based healthcare system.

Peer review Peers review the study usually when it is submitted for publication. It is a means to validate the study design, methodology, and results.

Periodontitis Gum disease that begins when permeability of the mouth tissue permits pathogenic bacterial components to invade deeper periodontal connective tissues and bone leading to tooth loss.

Petrissage The act of kneading using the whole hand, with fingers together and thumbs outstretched so that the rounder contours of the body are squeezed.

Pharmacopoeia A pharmaceutical book that contains a list of drugs, their formulas, methods for making medicinal preparations, requirements and tests for their strength and purity, and other related information.

Physician assistant (PA) A professional who can also provide many healthcare services and works under the guidance of a physician.

Physiology The functions and activities of the body.

Phytoestrogen Estrogen-like chemicals that can act like the hormone estrogen.

Phytotherapy Plant therapy. Using botanical medicine to treat disease conditions.

Placebo A substance having no pharmacological effect but administered as a control in testing experimentally or clinically the efficacy of a biologically active preparation.

Plant coumarins Oral anticoagulants. Coumarin was isolated from the tonka bean (*Dipteryx odorata*), which is in a classification known as coumarou; thus, similar plants were named plant coumarins.

Podiatrist A person qualified to diagnose and treat foot disorders.

Point of service (POS) plan A POS plan is similar to an HMO and PPO. Usually it requires designating a primary care physician who is needed to make referrals to specialists, and the services may include preventative care. The plan may require co-payments and an annual deductible.

Prakriti Dosha balance.

Prana Energy.

Predictive statistics The researcher makes a guess or prediction about the research problem based on the probability that the prediction is accurate. The study tests the prediction using specialized statistical techniques.

Preexisting condition A medical problem that an insured person already has prior to acquiring health insurance. Some preexisting conditions are not covered by insurance.

Preferred provider organization (PPO) A PPO is a type of health insurance that provides a lower rate wherein people can use an in-network provider or pay somewhat more for an out-of-network provider, but the cost may be higher than the HMO. A primary care physician does not need to be selected., and people may see specialists without a referral. It comprises networks of physicians that work with an insurance company with a negotiated rate for services.

Primary beneficiaries Receive the death benefit upon the policy holder's death.

Product claim advertising A form of DTC advertising that reveals the product name and full disclosure of the product uses and side effects.

Prostaglandin Any member of a group of lipid compounds that sensitize the body to pain.

Pseudoephedrine Drug similar in action to ephedrine; used extensively as a decongestant or illicitly to produce methamphetamine.

Pulse taking There are three types of pulses: snake pulse, which denotes vata dosha; frog pulse, which denotes pitta dosha; and swan pulse, which denotes kapha dosha.

Purva-karma treatment Preclensing procedures before shodhanam or shamanam treatment. It involves snehan and swedan treatments.

Putative A type of energy that has yet to be effectively measured by science.

Putrid Having the odor of decaying flesh.

Q

Qi (chi) According to TCM, Qi is a bodily energy that flows through unseen channels in the body called meridians. Illness is believed to occur when Qi is blocked.

Qigong A type of energy therapy that uses gentle movement to access and redistribute energy surrounding and within the human body. Incorporates posture, movement, breathing, meditation, visualization, and conscious intent in order to move qi energy throughout the body. This is purported to improve health and overall life energy.

Quack A person who admits, professionally or publicly, to skill, knowledge, or qualifications he or she does not possess.

Quackery The practice of deceit or trickery specifically confined to the medical field.

Qualitative research Research that seeks to provide understanding of human experience, perceptions, motivations, intentions, and behaviors. It requires observation and personal interaction with subjects rather than the use of a survey instrument.

Quasi-experimental Comparison groups in a study are not randomly selected, and many things may cloud (or confound) the findings.

Quinine A white, bitter, slightly water-soluble alkaloid, having needlelike crystals, obtained from cinchona bark. Used in medicine chiefly in the treatment of resistant forms of malaria.

R

Radiofrequency rhizotomy Application of heated radio frequency waves to the joints' nerves.

Radionics A dowsing technique using a pendulum to detect energy fields emitted by all forms of matter.

Raktamoksha Detoxifying the blood by bloodletting or using certain herbs.

Rancid Having a bad smell or taste. Fats and oils when stale become spoiled or rancid.

Randomized controlled study A study in which the people involved are randomly drawn from a population and then assigned to a treatment protocol by a random draw.

Rebalance A process in Therapeutic Touch to clear or release excess energy from the human energy field into the environmental field.

Redress To set right; to make up for; to remove the cause of a grievance or complaint.

Reflexology A form of massage that involves applying pressure to points on the feet, hands, and ears.

Reform chiropractic Reform chiropractors promote scientific studies and practices and are considered the most biomedical of the groups. Recommend chiropractic care only for musculoskeletal disorders. The group no longer functions.

Reiki An energy therapy characterized by laying hands on an individual at specific locations, and the transfer of energy from the practitioner to the patient.

Reiki degrees Levels of advancement in the art of Reiki.

Reliability The consistency of a measurement, or the degree to which an instrument measures the same way each time it is used under the same condition with the same subjects. It refers to the repeatability of a measurement.

Reminder advertising A form of DTC marketing that only provides the product name without including details about its use or side effects.

Reputable Considered to be respectable or acceptable.

Rescue remedy Five Bach® Original Flower Remedies flowers that make up a formula to treat a crisis.

Research design A design that may be experimental or quasi-experimental.

Research questions Rather than a statement or statements found in hypotheses, research questions are formulated. The study tests each research question for truth or not.

Rheumatoid arthritis A chronic autoimmune disease characterized by inflammation of the joints, frequently accompanied by marked deformities, and ordinarily associated with manifestations of a general or systemic affliction.

Rhythm and song methods of meditation A combination of rhythm, chanting, music, and breath used during meditation to achieve a desired state of calmness.

S

Salicylates and salicins Aspirin-like compounds that have pain-relieving and anti-inflammatory action.

Salvia lavandulaefolia Plant known as Spanish sage. Used for healing purposes.

Sama A ritual practice developed in the mid-9th century that uses music, poetry recital, singing, and dance.

Sanskrit Is one of 22 languages spoken in India and is the liturgical (church language) of Hinduism and Buddhism. The language originated about 1500 BCE.

Saponins Glycosides or chemicals found in plants such as oats, vegetables, and beans that cause plants placed in water to "soap up" or froth to form a lather.

Satvajaya treatment Use of mental hygiene/psychotherapy.

Scam A confidence game or other fraudulent scheme, especially for making a quick profit.

Seer Masters of the healing tradition. A person who knows.

Self-care Personal health maintenance.

Self-correcting If results of a previous research study are later found to be false, the research should be conducted again so that the conclusions or results may be modified.

Serotonin Levels of this chemical influence moods and behavior; low levels are associated with depression, headaches, and insomnia.

Seven tissues (dhatu) Plasma, blood, muscle, lipid, bone, nervous system, and reproductive system.

Shamanam treatment A balancing treatment.

Shamanism An anthropological term referencing a range of beliefs and practices regarding a person (shaman) who is believed to be able to communicate with the spiritual world.

Sherley Amendment The section of the Pure Food and Drugs Act specifically designed to limit the amount of time commercials can be shown during a television program.

Shodhanam treatment A cleansing treatment using five procedures called panchakarma treatment.

Significance levels The levels set before a research study is begun. If the level is not met for a particular hypothesis or research question studied, the research is said to be non-significant and is rejected.

Silent mind meditation Technique involving directly perceiving and feeling the world around us by focusing on how we are thinking.

Snehan treatment Internally it involves ingesting medicated edible oil or butter; externally it is medicated body massage.

Social psychological model A model that suggests that during hypnosis, an altered state of consciousness does not occur; instead, hypnosis is explained by suggestibility, positive attitudes, and expectations

Solvent extraction Process of washing blossoms with a solvent such as hexane to dissolve the nonaromatic waxes, pigments, and volatile aromatic molecules.

Spam Unsolicited, usually commercial, e-mail sent to a large number of addresses.

Spectrochrometry A pseudoscience that believes the shape and contour of the skull indicates the size of various segments of the brain. The variety in brain sizes is the determinant of character.

Spirituality A belief in a higher power; a way to find meaning and hope in one's life; awareness of purpose and meaning in life.

Stagnate To stop developing, growing, progressing, or advancing.

Stark Law Named after the individual who sponsored it. It is supposed to prohibit physicians from referring Medicare and Medicaid patients to a healthcare provider or facility with which they have a financial relationship.

Steam distillation A process that involves heating the plant parts so that plant molecules evaporate, cool down, and then condense into a liquid. Water is drawn off the oil leaving a pure EO.

Subluxation Refers to one or more bones of the spine that have moved out of position and are causing pressure on or irritating spinal nerves.

Subtle energy Generic term used to describe all energy not easily or readily categorized by modern science.

Succession Act of shaking a homeopathic mother of tincture solution during the dilution process.

Sufi dancing Said to be the dance of universal peace and is supposed to bring participants to a mystical experience and cultivate inner peace and harmony. The dance involves whirling by oneself or with partners. Dancers whirl with arms in various positions, such as reaching out and reaching to the heavens.

Sweat lodge Used for a purification ceremony; a place built as a ceremonial sauna lodge.

Swedan treatment Use of dry or wet fomentation or heat therapy to facilitate sweating.

Sympathetic nervous system Responsible for the "fight-or-flight" response produced during times of stress.

T

Tai chi A Chinese exercise system that uses slow, smooth body movements to achieve a state of relaxation of both body and mind.

Tamiflu An oral antiviral drug that attacks the influenza virus and prevents it spreading inside the body.

Tannins Polyphenols obtained from various parts of plants. Found in tree bark, wood, fruit, leaves, and roots.

Tapotement Massage that is given by tapping the body or face. It may be done by cupping, hacking, and pinching.

Temporomandibular disorder (TMD) A condition characterized by pain and tenderness of the jaw when chewing and opening the mouth.

Testimonial An advertising technique in which an individual client is used to share with consumers how a product or service worked for them.

Therapeutic Touch An energy therapy characterized by holding the hands several inches away from the patient, sending energy to the patient via the hands, in an effort to heal.

Tonify Gentle stimulation of an acupuncture point.

Traditional Chinese medicine The traditional medicine of China. Includes practices such as acupuncture, use of Chinese herbs, and energy therapies.

Traditional medical practitioner A medical doctor practicing under a Western, pharmaceutical-based philosophy.

Traditional straights Claim that chiropractic adjustments are a plausible treatment for a wide range of diseases.

Transcendental Meditation® (TM) A technique wherein people repeat a phrase to help themselves relax during medication.

Transcendental A belief in the supernatural; a belief in miracles; a belief in the spiritual.

Transcutaneous electrical nerve stimulation (TENS) Delivery of electrical stimulation through small electrodes placed inside an elastic-type belt. Usually applied to the tissue by the spine before spinal adjustments by chiropractors.

Tri-doshic Having fairly equal characteristics of vata, pitta, and kapha.

Truth in advertising Laws designed to compel advertisers to give accurate, forthright information regarding products, services, and anticipated outcomes.

Tuberculosis An infectious disease that may affect almost any tissue of the body, but especially the lungs. It is caused by the organism *Mycobacterium tuberculosis*, and is characterized by tubercles.

Tuina A type of massage to stimulate or subdue qi energy in the body and bring the patient's body back into balance.

Turmeric A plant that contains curcumin. Used for healing purposes.

U

Ultrasound Use of deep heat by sound waves to treat muscle pain and spasms and to reduce swelling and inflammation.

Universal polarity Concept of all energy being influenced and moved by opposing polar magnetism.

Urinary retention Holding urine in the urinary bladder.

Usual, customary, and reasonable (UCR) Used by the insurance industry to control costs. It began by reimbursing doctors 98% of the fee, and then went to 95%, 90%, 85%, 80%, and even lower.

V

Vacuum distillation A process to remove alcohol and what is left behind to make the floral absolute.

Validity The strength of conclusions, inferences, or propositions. Validity is the extent to which the test predicts the outcome it is supposed to predict.

VALS™ Marketing model used to design advertising to appeal to a particular group of consumers.

Vamana Forced vomiting.

Variable life insurance Uses part of the premium to purchase stocks, bonds, and mutual funds.

Variable universal life insurance Provides death benefits and cash values that vary when the investment portfolio changes (money market, government bond accounts, equity accounts).

Veritable A form of energy that can be measured scientifically.

Veterinary acupuncture Acupuncture used on animals to treat a variety of conditions (e.g., arthritis and hip problems, back pain and disc disease, incontinence and urinary retention).

Vikruiti Dosha imbalance.

Vipassana Is known as insight meditation. Mindfulness is employed during meditation. Requires being watchful of your breath during inhalation and exhalation.

Virechana Forced purging.

Visceral organs Internal organs of the body, specifically those within the chest (as the heart or lungs) or abdomen.

Visualization techniques Used to achieve a meditative state.

Volatile oils Compounds of vegetable origin that evaporate at room temperature and allow us to enjoy the smell.

W

Walking meditation Focuses on awareness of self, the process of walking, and the environment.

WHO AM I Focuses on negating the false self in order to realize one's true nature or enlightenment.

Whole life insurance Offers a death benefit and a savings account.

World Health Organization (WHO) The directing and coordinating authority for health within the United Nations system.

Y

Yin–yang Two energies that control different bodily systems but cannot exist without each other.

Yoga Requires full awareness of posture and movements. Attention is focused on the breath during all movements and helps open up the energy channels. Thought to be a powerful meditation technique.

Z

Zapper A machine created by Hulda Clark that delivers energy to the body in an effort to cure a myriad of illnesses and diseases.

Zazen The breathing technique of Zen meditation, also known as the meditation of the Buddha. This involves awareness and concentration during the breathing process to help build or shape the mind and to free oneself from dualistic thinking (separation of mind and body).

Index

Note: Page numbers followed by *t* indicate material in tables.

V

Vaccinations
    autism and, 266
    chiropractic philosophy and, 205
Vacuum distillation
    defined, 184
    essential oils and, 184
Valerian (*Valeriana officinalis*)
    FDA public health advisory on, 164
    uses for, 175
Validity
    defined, 19
    of health information,
        investigating, 18
Valnet, Jean, 183
VALS Marketing model
    defined, 32
    description of, 27
    motivating factors, types and resource
        level, 27*t*
Vamana, 101, 109
Variable life insurance, defined,
    300, 304
Variable universal life insurance, defined,
    300, 304
Vata (movement), 92
    attributes of, 93
    qualities and manifestations in the
        body, 93
    sign for, 93
Vayu (air), 92
Vedas, 84, 232
Velde, J., 257
Velentzis, L.S., 161
Veritable energy, defined, 250, 261
Vertebrae, spinal manipulation of, 205
Vertebral artery (VBA) stroke, 207
Vervain (*Twelve Helpers*), use for, 196
Veterans Health Administration
    (VHA), 295
Veterinary acupuncture, 121, 134
Vikruti, 93, 100
Vine (*Seven Helpers*), use for, 196
Violence, 51
Vipassana breathing methods, 227
Vipassana meditation, 223
Virechana, 102–103, 109
Visceral organs, defined, 134
Vision insurance, 299
Visual imagery training, 221
Visualization techniques, 73
    defined, 227
    meditation and, 226–227
Vitalism, 88
Vitalists, 204
Vitamins, 2, 159
Volatile oils
    defined, 176
    properties of, 162
Volunteer agencies, health information
        through, 18

Von Peczely, Ignatz, 140
Vyana, 92, 234
Vyayam (exercises), 102

W

Wakefield, Andrew, 266
Walker, David L., 143
Walking meditation, 225
Wallace, Allan, 222
Wallace, Robert, 71
Walnut (*Second Nineteen*), use
    for, 196
Wang Weiyi, 121
Warfarin, alfalfa and, warning, 166
Warm salt water gargle, 54
Warring States Period, 115
Waste in healthcare system, rising
        healthcare costs and, 38
Water
    in Ayurvedic medicine, defined, 92
    in Chinese theory of five elements,
        116
Water fluoridation, chiropractic
        philosophy and, 205
"Water is wet" claim, 23, 24*t*
Watermelon seed oil, 185
Water violet, use for, 196
Watsu, 210
Weasel claim, 23, 24*t*
WebMD, 268
Web sites, health information on, 18
Weight loss fraud, 267
Weight loss product, critique of, 15
Weight Watchers, 273
Weil, Andrew, 68, 72–73
Weiyi, Wang, 121
Wellness
    integrative medicine and, 73
    mind-body interventions and, 222
Wellness programs, development of,
    73–74
Western massage methods, 209
Whirling dervishes, 226
Whistle blower act, 42
White chestnut, use for, 197
White House Commission on
        Complementary and Alternative
        Medicine Policy, 74–75
White willow bark, uses for, 175
WHO. *See* World Health Organization
WHO AM I technique, 228
Whole Food stores, 3
Whole life insurance, defined, 300, 304
Wild oat, use for, 197
Wild rose, use for, 197
Wild yam, uses for, 175
Willow, use for, 197
Women, economy, massage therapy
        and, 213
Wood, in Chinese theory of five elements,
    116

Workforce shortages, hospital costs
        and, 42
World Federation of Acupuncture and
        Moxibustion Society, 124
World Health Organization, 3,
    123, 134
World Parliament of Religions, 232
Wraps, chiropractic medicine and, 206
Writing exercises, 73

X

X-ray studies, chiropractic medicine
        and, 205

Y

Yajurveda, 232
Yarrow (*Achillea millefolium*), uses
    for, 175
*Yellow Emperor's Classic of Internal
    Medicine, The*, 112, 209
Yin–yang
    characteristics, 113
    Chinese diet therapy and, 132
    defined, 134
    five elements and chart for, 117*t*
    herb classification and, 126
    organs, 115
    symbol for, 114
    theory of, 114–115
Ylang-ylang, massage and use of, 212
Ylang ylang oil (*Cananga odorata*),
        source, action, and uses for, 190
Yoga, 8, 71, 88, 221–222, 232–234
    asana poses, 234
    clinical studies on, 234
    function and benefits of, 232–233
    history and description of, 235
    power of the breath and, 234
Yohimbe, uses for, 175

Z

Zafu, 225
Zapper, 272, 274
Zazen, 223, 227
Zeiss, Carl, 85
Zen archery, 225
Zen Buddhist meditation, 223, 227
    breathing (zazen), 223
    guided technique, 248
Zen School of Buddhism, 228
Zhang Zhongjing, 125
Zhong Yi, 112
Zhuang Zi, 250
Zone diet, 273
Zone therapy, 214
Zone Therapy (Fitzgerald), 214